Communication in Nursing

TENTH EDITION

TENTH EDITION

Communication in Nursing

JULIA BALZER RILEY

RN, MN, AHN-BC, REACE, CSL
Faculty, "Caring Science, Mindful Practice
Massive Open Online Course (MOOC)"
through the Watson Caring Science
Institute.
Faculty, Sage-ing® International
President Constant Source Seminars
Ellenton, Florida

ELSEVIER

Elsevier
3251 Riverport Lane
St. Louis, Missouri 63043

COMMUNICATION IN NURSING, TENTH EDITION

ISBN: 978-0-323-87145-7

Previous editions copyrighted 2020, 2017, 2012, 2008, 2004, 2000, 1996, 1992, 1986.

Senior Content Strategist: Yvonne Alexopoulos
Senior Content Development Specialist: Vasowati Shome
Publishing Services Manager: Deepthi Unni
Senior Project Manager: Manchu Mohan
Senior Book Designer: Brian Salisbury

Printed in India.

Last digit is the print number: 9 8 7 6 5 4 3 2 1

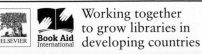

Working together
to grow libraries in
developing countries

www.elsevier.com • www.bookaid.org

As I wrote this tenth edition of Communication in Nursing,
*my husband and I have journeyed with friends
through the ups and downs, the tender mercies,
and missed opportunities of their healthcare experiences.
Especially, we honor Elista and Joe Gerace.*

*I dedicate this book in remembrance of Joseph Robert Gerace
(3/8/50–3/29/22).*

CONTRIBUTORS

Kathleen Sitzman, PhD, RN, CNE, ANEF, FAAN
Professor
Distinguished Watson Caring Science Scholar
Assistant Editor, International Journal for Human Caring
East Carolina University
Greenville, North Carolina

Renee Thompson, DNP, RN, FAAN, CSP
CEO & Founder
Healthy Workforce Institute®
Tampa, Florida

Linda Turchin, RN, MSN, CNE
Professor Emeritus of Nursing
Fairmont State University
School of Nursing
Fairmont, West Virginia

FOREWORD

Effective professional communication is a hallmark of nursing excellence. This textbook has been a staple in nursing education since 1986, and the tenth edition continues to provide comprehensive content that will engage and inspire learners and educators alike.

In this edition, I have joined my long-time colleague, collaborator, and friend, Julia Balzer Riley, to bring mindfully considered *caring* to the forefront of professional communication in nursing and healthcare. We have worked together to add content that highlights the importance of authentic caring for self and others in professional life and beyond. This updated content is meant to help learners simplify and deepen their approach to cultivating caring and understanding between self and others in a variety of situations that include clients, significant others, peers, and leaders in professional settings.

I have been studying, practicing, and teaching Jean Watson's Human Caring Theory since 1981 and have learned through experience that authentic, intentional caring is a powerful force for good in healthcare and in the world. I began to explore caring in online nursing classrooms during my doctoral studies to better understand how instructors could effectively convey and sustain caring online. I have since collaborated with others to complete and publish many studies, book chapters, books, and a Massive Open Online Course (MOOC) related to conveying and sustaining caring for self and others in digital and face-to-face settings. More information on my research and publications can be found at https://www.caringsciencemindfulpractice.com/.

My passion is to teach others simple, mindful, micro-practices to support deep caring for self and others, in face-to-face and digital settings, at work and beyond. In this tenth edition text, research-based content related to conveying and sustaining authentic caring in digital as well as face-to-face situations has been added.

Another addition to this text was inspired by the advent of the new American Association of Colleges of Nursing (AACN) Education Essentials in 2021. Content has been added to reflect AACN *Essentials Core Competencies,* and a mapping table of where these core competencies resonate with content in this text has been provided in Appendix I.

All of the content, both old and new, is meant to inspire readers and help them develop communication habits that reflect their own unique temperaments and personal strengths while grounding them in authentic caring and professionalism.

Kathleen Sitzman, PhD, RN, CNE, ANEF, FAAN
Professor
Distinguished Watson Caring Science Scholar
Assistant Editor, International Journal for Human Caring
East Carolina University
Greenville, North Carolina

ACKNOWLEDGEMENTS

Thank you to Yvonne Alexopoulos, Senior Content Strategist, for shepherding me through two editions of this book; to Ellen Wurm-Cutter, Director, Content Development, and Patricia Geary, Executive Assistant, always just an email away for support and guidance. It takes a dedicated team to bring a revision to life.

I am delighted to have the consultation and contributions of Kathleen Sitzman, PhD, RN, CNE, ANEF, FAAN. Dr. Sitzman's dedication to Caring Science, both in theory and in practice, has added a special touch to this edition. She infuses her research and publication with a remarkable clarity, kindness, and creativity. Her invitation to me to join her faculty team for the "Caring Science, Mindful Practice," a free Massive Open Online Course (MOOC), was the beginning of a treasured connection. Thank you!

I am pleased to have the contribution of Renee Thompson, DNP, RN, CSP, whose dedication to creating a healthy workplace by eradicating bullying and incivility is based on caring and respect for ourselves and each other. After following her work over time and enjoying her coffee conversations on YouTube, I invited her to add her approach to our work. Thank you, Renee, for your personal approach to difficult challenges in nursing.

I am grateful to Susan Hill Crowley, MS, RN, for contributing a detailed clinical scenario. Susan shares my passion for Sage-ing®, one approach to conscious aging. Sage-ing® International has welcomed her writing skills in the revision of our training materials. We have enjoyed exploring creative expression for self-discovery. Thank you!

I am blessed to be on this journey with my supportive, loving, funny husband, Jim Riley, who comes into my office with coffee and an invitation to take a break…and then listens and problem solves with me. Thank you!

INTRODUCTION

As you continue this lifelong journey to have a voice in healthcaring, to use your own gifts to support the health and well-being of those entrusted to your care, communication with patients/clients, families, and the interprofessional healthcare team is essential. This text actively engages you in developing basic and advanced competencies in assertive and responsible communication through skill-building exercises; guided reflective writing (Smith, 2021); mindfulness; and other complementary practices. Finely tuned communication skills serve us as we live our own life stories and bear witness to the stories of others. Nurses provide education that helps clients change lifelong habits. We communicate with people who are stressed, angry, and depressed and who are coping with dementia and psychosis. We are client advocates, part of interdisciplinary teams whose members may have different ideas about priorities for care. We return to school to specialize, write grants for research proposals, and become entrepreneurs, administrators, leaders, case managers, infection control specialists, quality experts, and educators. We blend our understanding of healthcare and technology to offer the skill of nursing informatics. We combine a mission of faith and healthcaring in parish nursing. We move into industry to work in occupational health and into schools and communities to improve the health of large populations and communities. We create new positions in which our voices can affect healthcare quality and inequities and cross international boundaries to share knowledge needed to promote worldwide health. We must be assertive to communicate our own needs to ensure balance in our lives. Without such balance, the high-stress environment may diminish our effectiveness.

The intimate moments of connection can make all the difference in the quality of care and meaning for the client and the nurse. As you refine communication skills and build confidence, with time you can move from novice to expert. Nurses honor, with humility, the differences in clients. As you learn and grow in your ability to trust your intuition, be open to what Martin Buber, a Jewish theologian, called the I–Thou relationship—the sacred moment of connection. You can make a difference in the lives of others even in short spaces of time, in a smile, in rearranging a pillow, in asking, "What's this like for you?" Watch for "Moments of Connection," a place in which seasoned nurses and students share their stories of making a difference in moments during which they were mindful and communicating with warmth and compassion—truly present.

Notice the cover art on this tenth edition—it is a circular design called a mandala. The *mandala,* a Sanskrit word meaning "sacred circle," is a symbol for wholeness. This piece was created with healing intention, a visual prayer for a friend. It emerged as "Healing from Within and Without." The purple became a sacred container for Spirit. The yellow became the light of inner healing. Watercolor flowing offered me comfort and self-soothing. I added words, behaviors of the nurse that support the nurse as cocreator of the healing environment along with the client, family, and friends. Carl Jung, a Swiss psychoanalyst found that patients who created mandalas, art within a circle, gained self-awareness and insight. He suggested that when we make art within a circle, it is as if we are addressing our whole self, our whole world (Marshall, 2003). Mandalas create a symbol of where we are at this moment. Holistic nursing teaches us that each of us is whole in each single moment, not needing to be fixed, but at the right place and time for our personal journey, and that we make meaning from even the illness experience. The nurse uses self as an instrument of healing to support the client's journey. The nurse is called to the healing encounter, drawn by compassion to the vulnerability and/or suffering of another (Enzman Hines, Wardell, Engebretson, Zahourek, & Smith, 2015).

Note: In this text, sometimes we use the word *client* rather than *patient* to emphasize the nature of the service that we render and to honor that people are whole persons—body, mind, and spirit—whose role at this time may be that of "patient," which is one role of many in life.

Other expressive art invitations can support your practice (Riley, 2020). Remember, we embellish our nursing practice with who we are. A nurse who sings might sing to a comatose client or initiate a playful song when colleagues are stressed. A nurse who gardens might bring flowers to work. A nurse who cooks might bring a comfort food so staff can break bread together in a time of crisis. What gifts do you bring?

WHAT'S NEW?

In this edition, you will find three Next-Generation NCLEX® (NGN) Examination style case studies in Chapters 1, 26, and 27. These case studies are in the new format students will encounter on the latest NCLEX® licensure exam.

Dr. Kathleen Sitzman wrote the Foreword for this edition in which she references her mapping of all the chapter objectives in the 30 chapters of this text to the AACN 2021 Essential Domains. (See Appendix I: Chapter Objectives in this Book Mapped to the American Association of Colleges of Nursing [AACN] 2021 Essentials Domains).

This work demonstrates the comprehensive nature of this edition.

This tenth edition emphasizes the need for the nurse to care for self to better care for others. You will find a Holistic Self-Care Assessment for the nurse. You will find simple self-care invitations in each chapter called Self-Care Nudge, with strategies to build resilience (Graham, 2020; Newman, 2016). You will find brief quotations called Simplify and Deepen in each chapter that encourage you to reflect on what's important to help you sharpen your critical thinking to support clinical judgment.

Chapter 5 continues to stress approaching each person as a unique individual and is revised to include cultural humility, gender diversity, and discussion of healthcare disparities.

Dr. Kathleen Sitzman's contributions help you to integrate caring into our digital world (Chapter 23); use Watson's Human Caring Theory; and practice mindfulness in caring for patients and yourself. She presents micropractices to use when you or others are distressed (Chapter 26).

In Chapter 27, the chapter on confronting bullying and incivility in nursing, Dr. Renee Thompson helps us to pause in difficult situations and first ask, "How can I respond to this person in a way that's honest and respectful?"

WHAT'S IMPORTANT?

Honor the sacred nature of your work. Take time each day to connect with your own purpose in your work and set goals for your caring each day. Think of a single word or phrase that reflects your intention and let it support you through the day.

Remember:

Take time for your own spiritual practice.
Honor your own body-mind-spirit connection with self-care.
You cannot give what you do not have.
Take your work seriously but yourself lightly.
To be distracted from the person in front of you is to be otherwise attracted...and at this moment in time, nothing is more important than this person.

Author's note: As you continue your career in nursing, be open to unusual paths to meet new goals, and use your strengths to bring your authentic self to clients. I have been curious about the therapeutic value of art since 1968, when I completed my psychiatric nursing affiliation at St. Elizabeth's Hospital in Washington, D.C. This passion was rekindled as I offered expressive art workshops to nurses. I worked with clients in private homes, hospice houses, nursing homes, and hospital rooms to facilitate art processes. These expressive art invitations provide an opportunity to explore emotions and encourage conversation and reflection about the experience of end of life and illness. They add a bit of whimsy and fun at a difficult time, and clients report that they provide distraction from pain.

Sending love and blessings for this journey of healthcaring for others and for yourself.

Julia Balzer Riley, RN, MN, AHN-BC, REACE, CSL

REFERENCES

Enzman Hines, M. E., Wardell, D. W., Engebretson, J., Zahourek, R., & Smith, M. C. (2015). Holistic nurses' stories of healing another. *Journal of Holistic Nursing, 33*(1), 27–45.

Graham, L. (2020). *Resilience offers three ways to tap into the wisdom of the body.* https://www.mindful.org/resilience-expert-offers-three-ways-to-tap-into-the-wisdom-of-the-body.

Marshall, M. C. (2003). Creative learning: The mandala as teaching exercise. *Journal of Nursing Education, 42*(11), 517.

Newman, K. M. (2016). *5 Science-Backed Strategies to Build Resilience* (mindful.org).

Riley, J. B. (2020). *Art in small spaces: Art at the bedside.* Ellenton, FL: CSP. (This is an expressive arts guidebook for self-discovery and healing, available as an E-book or paperback. For more information email. julia@constantsource.com).

Smith, T. (2021). Guided reflective writing as a teaching strategy to develop nursing student clinical judgment. *Nurs Forum*, 56, 241–248.

FRAMEWORK

Part II: Advanced Competencies for Communication in Nursing

Chapter	Will Help You
16. Requesting Support	Seek the support you need from your colleagues to deliver excellent care to clients
17. Overcoming Evaluation Anxiety	Use a rational approach to feel more confident in nursing situations that make you feel anxious
18. Working with Feedback	Be open to feedback from clients and colleagues about your performance as a helper, and provide feedback to them in an assertive way
19. Using Relaxation Techniques to Become More Mindful	Learn techniques for relieving tension and promoting the relaxation response so that you can remain calm in stressful interpersonal encounters
20. Incorporating Imagery in Professional Practice and Self-Care	Rehearse privately so that you can communicate effectively in real situations
21. Incorporating Positivity into Life and Work	Keep your internal dialogue supportive so that you can communicate with confidence
22. Learning to Work Together in Groups	Understand the dynamics of communication in groups
23. Navigating the Complex World of Digital Communication	Build digital communication skills and access resources to enrich your work and strategies to build and sustain caring
24. Learning Confrontation Skills	Invite your clients and colleagues to examine how their behavior is affecting others
25. Refusing Unreasonable Requests	Say no assertively to unreasonable requests from clients and colleagues
26. Caring Communication with Clients and Colleagues whose Behaviors Are Challenging	Use caring communication strategies and micropractices with distressed clients and colleagues
27. Confronting Bullying and Incivility with Honesty and Respect	Overcome your reluctance to deal with incivility and bullying with assertive approaches
28. Managing Team Conflict Assertively and Responsibly	Use a systematic problem-solving approach to deal effectively with conflict between colleagues
29. Communicating at the End of Life	Reflect on the gifts and challenges of communicating with clients near the end of life and with their families
30. Continuing the Commitment to the Journey	Consider the commitments necessary to grow and embrace change in your professional and personal life

CONTENTS

Communication
in Nursing
TENTH EDITION

Basic Competencies for Communication in Nursing

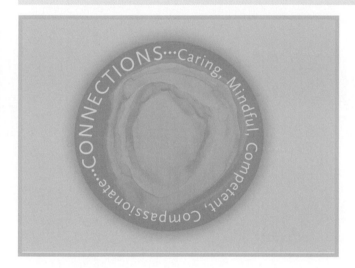

PART 1

Basic Competencies for
Communication in Nursing

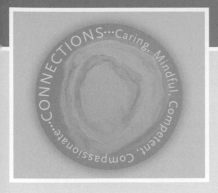

1

Responsible, Assertive, Caring Communication in Nursing

OBJECTIVES

1. Complete a holistic self-care assessment.
2. Identify the functions of interpersonal communication in nursing.
3. Distinguish between assertive, nonassertive, and aggressive communication.
4. Identify a three-step process to build assertiveness skills.
5. Identify assertive rights.
6. Identify irrational beliefs that impede assertive communication.
7. Explain the describe, express, specify, consequences (DESC) script for developing an assertive response.
8. Identify three types of assertions.
9. Identify three essential criteria for presenting an assertive response.
10. Describe the behavior of an assertive nurse.
11. List the advantages of assertive communication.
12. Describe responsible communication in nursing.
13. Discuss the role of caring in nursing.
14. Participate in exercises to build skills in responsible, assertive, caring communication.

From the miracle of birth to the mystery of death, the gift of nursing is the intimate journey we take with the patient and family. *Why* should you study and practice communication? Reflect on your answers to this question as you read this opening chapter. This I believe:

- Communication is a lifelong journey.
- You can make a difference in patients' lives by practicing caring, assertive, responsible communication.
- As you grow in comfort with assertive skills, you will build positive relationships in your professional and personal life.
- You support each other's rights for ethical, competent, caring practice as you have the courage to grow your own assertive communication skills.
- You make a difference even in short moments of connection, and you always have enough time as you learn how to be fully present.
- This text will support your own life journey of meaning making in your work.

Nursing students can use this book as they begin their professional journey. Nurses will find this work useful as they understand clear communication as an essential ingredient for success in a changing healthcare climate.

Practicing clear, assertive communication builds confidence, essential for interprofessional communication to advocate for patient safety (Hanson et al., 2020).

HOW TO USE THIS BOOK

If you have not read this book's introduction and foreword, do so now! It is an important practice when reading a text to learn the intention of the book, to pose questions to yourself as you read, to help fit what you read into your experience, to retain content, and to be an adult learner. This will help grow your own skills for healthcaring. The Active Learning Practice outlined in each chapter's beginning and referenced at the chapter's end will support your deepening understanding of the content.

Purchase a journal, or assemble blank pages, to use for this application, to respond to chapter exercises, and to reflect on clinical or personal experiences for your own problem solving and self-discovery. (See Exercise 3 at the end of this chapter.) Guided reflective writing can help you to build your communication skills and develop clinical judgment (Smith, 2020).

3

Note two features in each chapter to support you: professionally, **Simplify and Deepen;** personally, **Self-Care Nudge.**

PRACTICE SELF-CARE

To be present and caring for others, you must replenish your own energy by caring for yourself. Complete your Holistic Self-Care Assessment, Appendix II, at the end of the book. (See Exercise 1 to process this assessment.) Self-care is the foundation of ethical, responsible practice to help you bring your best self to your work and to your life. To bring love and compassion to others, you practice them on yourself (Kinyon, 2021; Townsend, 2021).

 ACTIVE LEARNING

We know that reading comprehension is improved when the reader is actively asking and answering questions while reading. To build your communication skills, answer the questions in this section in each chapter. Think about how you will write your answers as you read each chapter.

What?
Write one thing you learned from this chapter.

So What?
How will this affect your nursing practice?

Now What?
How will you implement this new knowledge or skill?

Think About It …

Next, you need to understand the meaning of four important concepts introduced in the opening sentence: responsibility, assertiveness, caring, and communication. These concepts are significant because they form the framework of this textbook.

THE MEANING OF INTERPERSONAL COMMUNICATION

Communication involves the reciprocal process in which messages are sent and received between two or more people. This book focuses on the communication exchange among you, the nurse, and your clients and colleagues. Communication can either facilitate the development of a therapeutic relationship or create barriers (Stuart, 2012). A Canadian study of interprofessional communication identified nurses' "embedded-in-care" communication and suggested that it be "recognized, supported and encouraged"

as important in decision making in acute medical units (Strachan et al., 2018). An Australian study identified clear communication from managers as key to intensive care unit nurses' willingness to care for COVID-19 patients in a public health emergency (Lord, Loveday, Moxham, & Fernandez, 2021).

In general, there are two parts of face-to-face communication: the verbal expression of the sender's thoughts and feelings and the nonverbal expression. Verbally, cognitive and affective messages are sent through words, voice inflection, and rate of speech, and, nonverbally, messages are conveyed by eye movements, facial expressions, and body language. Communication by telephone or other electronic media loses the effect of gestures and other nonverbal communication. Powerful nonverbal messages can stand alone, such as a suspicious glance, a warm smile, or eyes widened with fear.

Senders determine what message they want to transmit to the receiver and encode their thoughts and feelings into words and gestures. Senders' messages are transmitted to the receiver through sound, sight, touch, and, occasionally, smell and taste.

Receivers of the messages have to decode the verbal and nonverbal transmission to make sense of the thoughts and feelings communicated by senders. After decoding the senders' words, speech patterns, and facial and body movements, the receivers encode return messages, either verbally through words or nonverbally through gestures.

In an interaction between two people (e.g., a nurse and a client), each person is both a sender and a receiver, and each person alternates between these two roles. When senders are speaking, they also are receiving messages from the person who is listening. Listeners not only are receiving speakers' messages, but they are also simultaneously sending messages. Fig. 1.1 illustrates this reciprocal nature of the communication process.

At any point in an interpersonal communication, verbal and nonverbal messages about thoughts and feelings are sent and received. With little prompting, you know that the complex process of interpersonal communication is influenced by many variables that affect how messages are sent and received. Take a few minutes to think of the variety of factors that can affect the exchange of messages between people. Add your own ideas to those in the following list:

- Environmental factors: formality, warmth, privacy, familiarity, freedom or constraint, physical distance between people, climate, mood, architecture, arrangement of furniture
- Territory and personal space: crowding, seating arrangements, roles, status, position, physical characteristics (size, height)

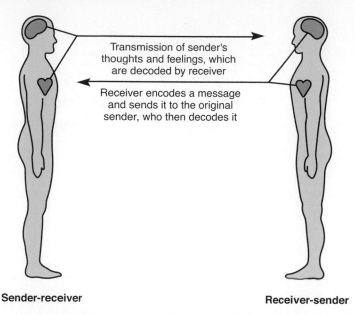

Transmission of sender's thoughts and feelings, which are decoded by receiver

Receiver encodes a message and sends it to the original sender, who then decodes it

Sender-receiver

Receiver-sender

Fig. 1.1 Reciprocal nature of interpersonal communication.

- Physical appearance and dress: body shape, race, body smell, hair, gender, body movements, body adornments, posture, age
- Nonverbal cues: facial expressions, eye movements, vocal cues
- Intrapersonal factors: developmental stage, language mastery, differences in perception, differences in decision-making processes, differences in values, self-concept
- The use of "I" messages to own one's responses, such as, "I don't agree with you," instead of "you" messages, which sound blaming, such as, "You are wrong"

Note that any of the preceding factors have the potential to facilitate communication or to act as a barrier to effective communication, depending on the situation. When these factors are considered, the interpersonal communication process looks something like the diagram shown in Fig. 1.2.

An important function of communication is to transmit messages from one person to another. The real purpose of communication is to create meaning. Senders of messages wish to convey meaning to receivers and vice versa. With this intent, senders choose certain words and gestures in a manner that they believe is congruent with their intended messages. The sender's objective is to transmit a message to receivers that is clear and understandable.

The purpose of communication does not stop there, however. The real purpose of creating understanding in another person is to influence the other person to effect some change. The sender attempts to persuade the receiver to respond to the sender's requests. Requests from clients and colleagues may be for the following:

- Understanding
- Action
- Information
- Comfort

Requests may be stated in obvious or indirect ways. The following examples illustrate both direct and indirect requests.

A client has postoperative pain. His physiologic need is for pain relief. He asks, "When was the last time I had my painkiller?" (He winces and holds his wrist.) His direct request is for information about the time of his last analgesic. His indirect request is for information about when he can have more. He is anticipating action (you giving him the medication) so that he will be comforted.

A nursing assistant says at the beginning of the shift, "I have a terrible headache. I was up for 3 hours last night with my sick daughter. Do you have an aspirin?" Her physiologic need is for rest and pain relief. Her obvious requests are for understanding (for you to empathize with her pain) and action (for you to give her an aspirin). She is possibly hoping that you will comfort her by making allowances for the fact that she is not at her best.

A nurse, newly hired to a unit, needs to feel that he or she belongs to and fits in with the group. When the nurse asks you to show him or her around the unit, the nurse is indirectly asking you to understand that he or she feels alone and unsure. The nurse is directly asking you

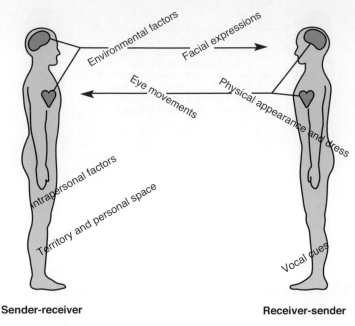

Sender-receiver   **Receiver-sender**

Fig. 1.2 Factors influencing interpersonal communication.

to take action to orient him or her and provide him or her with information about procedures and policy. The nurse is likely hoping that you will make him or her feel welcome (comforted).

In your interpersonal relationships as a nurse, you act as both sender and receiver. You will learn how to deliver assertive and responsible messages and to accurately decode messages from your clients and colleagues. You will be able to confidently interpret both direct and indirect requests and make responsible decisions about how to respond assertively (Box 1.1).

BOX 1.1   Important Functions of Interpersonal Communication in Nursing

- Communication is the vehicle for establishing a therapeutic relationship.
- Communication is the means by which people influence the behavior of others; thus, it is critical to the successful outcome of nursing intervention.
- Communication is the relationship itself because without it, a therapeutic nurse–client relationship is impossible.

From Stuart, G. W. (2012). *Principles and practice of psychiatric nursing* (10th ed.). St. Louis, MO: Mosby.

Self-Care Nudge

Today, as you walk from one patient room to another or from one situation to another, pause and walk mindfully, breathe, and notice your feet on the floor and the sensations of walking.

THE MEANING OF ASSERTIVE COMMUNICATION

MOMENTS OF CONNECTION...
A Nursing Student Reflects

The woman, lying in her hospital bed, was distant in conversation. She had no family members visiting her and no one could get to know her. It was not until I suggested a bath that she began to warm up. She began to talk. Her stories flowed one to another. At the end of her morning washing-up, she said thank you. It was as if she was a different person. As I turned to leave, she grabbed my hand, looked into my eyes, and said, "You made me feel human again." I smiled and said it was my pleasure. I never realized the effect of what, to me, seemed a small part of my day. This was my second semester in nursing school…I felt a real connection.

Assertiveness, a key to successful relationships for the client, the family, the nurse, and other colleagues, reduces interpersonal stress, builds team relationships, improves nursing care, and promotes patient safety (Yoshinaga et al., 2018). Assertiveness is the ability to express your thoughts, ideas, and feelings without undue anxiety and without any expense to others. In other words, it means being clear about what you need and respectful in your language and behavior.

The assertive nurse appears confident and comfortable. Assertive behavior, which is an active behavior, is contrasted with nonassertive or passive behavior, in which individuals disregard their own needs and rights. Aggressive behavior occurs when individuals disregard the needs and rights of others. The assertive nurse is positive, caring, nonjudgmental, clear, and direct without threatening or attacking (Table 1.1).

Assertive communication is a lifelong learning skill that requires time and practice. Be willing to accept the fact that you will make mistakes. Be patient. When a person accustomed to behaving passively tries this new behavior, the results may seem abrupt and abrasive or shy and tenuous. The goal is not to be continually confrontational. When learning this new skill, you must be assertive all the

TABLE 1.1 Assertive and Nonassertive Styles of Communication

Characteristic	Assertive	Nonassertive	Aggressive
Attitude toward self and others	I am OK You are OK	I am not OK You are OK	I am OK You are not OK
Decision making	Makes his or her own decisions	Lets others choose for him or her	Chooses for others
Behavior in problem situations	Engages in direct, fair confrontation	Flees, gives in	Is outright assaultive
Verbal behaviors	Clear, direct statement of wants; objective words; honest statement of feelings	Apologetic words; hedging, rambling; failure to say what is meant	Loaded words; accusations; superior haughty words; labeling of other person
Nonverbal behaviors	Confident, congruent messages	Actions instead of words (not saying what is felt); incongruence between words and behaviors	Air of superiority; flippant, sarcastic style
Voice	Firm, warm, confident	Weak, distant, soft, wavering	Tense, shrill, loud, cold, demanding, authoritarian, coldly silent
Eyes	Warm, in contact, frank	Averted, downcast, teary, pleading	Expressionless, cold, narrowed, staring
Stance	Relaxed	Stooped; excessive leaning for support	Hands on hips; feet apart
Hands	Gestures at appropriate times	Fidgety, clammy	Fists pounding or clenched
Pattern of relating	Puts himself or herself up without putting others down	Puts himself or herself down	Puts himself or herself up by putting others down
Response of others	Mutual respect	Disrespect, guilt, anger, frustration	Hurt, defensiveness, humiliation
Consequences of style	I win, you win; strives for "win–win" or "no-lose" solutions	I lose, you lose; succeeds only by luck or charity of others	I win, you lose; beats out others at any cost

Gerrard, B., Boniface, W., & Love, B. (1980). *Interpersonal skills for health professionals.* Reston, VA: Reston Publishing.
Modified from Piaget, G. (1975). Characterological lifechart of three fellows we all know. In S. Phelps & N. Austin (Eds.), *The assertive woman.* San Luis Obispo, CA: Impact Publishers.

time or you will be seen as nonassertive. When you practice techniques to learn to become more assertive, it is helpful to begin in a supportive environment with people who are accepting of you. Consider sharing your reading material on assertiveness with a roommate, spouse, or friend with whom you can begin practicing your assertive behavior. Start with small issues such as returning a damaged product to a store or offering a compliment.

Assertiveness is a matter of choice. It is important to feel confident that you can speak up for yourself, yet it is not necessary or even wise to speak your mind in every situation. With each person you encounter in any situation, you have the choice of communicating in an assertive or nonassertive style. The words you choose and the way you express them can be assertive, nonassertive, or aggressive. Realistically, you may not always have the energy or desire to assert your rights or express yourself fully. There are times when people cannot respond rationally, such as when they are experiencing high levels of anxiety or panic. A person might fear retaliation from a manager or fear the loss of a job. You must choose the issues for which your assertive behavior is appropriate as well as when, where, and with whom to express your assertiveness. The goal in this text is to help you develop the skills that will enable you to choose to act in the best interests of yourself and your clients. Remember, assertiveness helps you give or receive immediate feedback about a behavior that might have serious consequences if ignored. International nursing literature cites patient safety as a critical issue in healthcare. Clear communication helps prevent errors and adverse events. Speak up for safety (Hanson et al., 2020)!

HOW DO YOU GET STARTED?

As you read and think about assertive communication, begin to analyze situations in your life in which you think you would like to respond assertively. Think about what is happening, what your response to it is, what you want to do or have happen, and what the consequences are of action versus no action. Use this three-step process:

1. Review the list of assertive rights (Box 1.2) to see which right or rights you are giving up by not asserting yourself.
2. Review the irrational beliefs that interfere with acting in your own best interest (Box 1.3).
3. Review the DESC script to formulate an assertive response (Box 1.4).

To build your assertive skills, you will need further study and application. Be patient with yourself and remember that becoming assertive is a lifelong journey (Box 1.5).

BOX 1.2 Assertive Rights

1. You have the right to be treated with respect.
2. You have the right to a reasonable workload.
3. You have the right to an equitable wage.
4. You have the right to determine your own priorities.
5. You have the right to ask for what you want.
6. You have the right to refuse without making excuses or feeling guilty.
7. You have the right to make mistakes and be responsible for them.
8. You have the right to give and receive information as a professional.
9. You have the right to act in the best interest of the patient.
10. You have the right to be human.

From Chenevert, M. (2011). *Mosby's tour guide to nursing school: A student's road survival kit* (6th ed.). St. Louis, MO: Mosby.

BOX 1.3 Irrational Beliefs

Irrational beliefs arise when we are anxious about being assertive and focus on possible negative outcomes. The rational counterparts focus on possible positive outcomes.

Irrational Belief
- If I am assertive, other people will be upset, hurt by it, or angry with me.
- If someone gets angry with me, I will be devastated.
- Assertive people are seen as cold and self-serving.
- It is wrong for me to turn down legitimate requests.

Rational Counterpart
- The other person may not be hurt or angry. This person might prefer being open and honest, too. This person might feel closer to me and help me solve the problem.
- I will not fall apart in the face of anger. The anger is not my responsibility. An angry response is a choice.
- Assertive responses are honest and demonstrate respect for the other person's point of view. Assertion builds healthy relationships.
- It is acceptable for me to turn down even reasonable requests. I can consider my own needs first, and it is not possible to please all people all of the time!

Modified from Ellis, A. (2001). *Overcoming destructive beliefs, feelings, and behaviors: New directions for rational emotive therapy.* Amherst, NY: Prometheus Books.

BOX 1.4   Anatomy of an Assertive Response

A framework for developing assertive responses is known as the DESC script. Although not all steps are used in every situation, it is a useful tool:
Describe the situation
Express what you think and feel
Specify your request
Consequences

Developed by Bower, S. A., & Bower, G. H. (1991). *Asserting yourself*. Reading, MA: Addison-Wesley.

BOX 1.5   Types of Assertions

1. Basic: Simply expresses an idea, belief, or opinion; stands up for your rights or the rights of others, for example, "I want to…," "I don't want you to…," "Would you…?," "I liked it when you…," "I have a different opinion. I think that…," and "I have mixed reactions. I agree with these aspects for these reasons, but I am disturbed by these aspects for these reasons."
   - To buy time to consider: "I can give you an answer tomorrow after I have had time to think about it."
   - To deal with an interruption: "Excuse me, I am almost through. I'd like to finish my thought."
   - To return merchandise: "I am not satisfied with this product, and I would like a refund."
   - To say no: "I cannot loan you any money."
2. Empathic: Conveys sensitivity to the situation while taking an assertive position.
   - "I know the unit is short-staffed, but I have a pressing personal commitment and cannot work a second shift."
   - "I know you cannot tell me the exact time the computer technician will arrive, but I have a full day and would appreciate knowing if it will be in the morning or afternoon."
3. Escalating: Expresses your needs more emphatically when a simple assertion did not accomplish your goals and your rights are still being violated.
   - "I told you that as a nurse I cannot have a social relationship with you. I must insist that you refrain from asking me personal questions."
   - "I asked you not to use my computer without my permission. You have turned it off improperly and some files have been damaged. Please do not use it again."

Developed by Bower, S. A., & Bower, G. H. (1991): *Asserting yourself*. Reading, MA: Addison-Wesley; modified from Lange, J. A., & Jakubowski, P. (1978). *Responsible assertive behavior*. Champaign, IL: Research Press.

BOX 1.6   An Assertive Nurse

- Appears self-confident and composed
- Maintains eye contact
- Uses clear, concise speech
- Speaks firmly and positively
- Speaks genuinely, without sarcasm
- Is nonapologetic
- Takes the initiative to guide situations
- Gives the same message verbally and nonverbally

When you decide to use an assertive response, remember to consider three essential criteria for success:
- Timing
- Content
- Receptivity

Is the person able to hear your concerns at this time, or is this an extremely busy time? Have you gotten the person's attention by calling the person by name (Adubato, 2004)? Are you phrasing your intervention in a way that demonstrates respect for yourself and for others? Is the person receptive now, or is a cooling-off period necessary? Consider this: Sometimes the assertive response is to be quiet and listen for more information (Boxes 1.6 and 1.7).

Remember: Assertive behavior does not guarantee that you will get what you want, but it does increase the probability that you will. If you want to change shifts with another nurse to be able to go to a family gathering, try asking assertively. Which of the following statements is assertive?
A. "Jim, I was wondering if you would mind…it is probably an imposition, but…well, uh, switching this Saturday for next so I could go to a family party?"
B. "Jim, how many times have I traded with you, and you never think of my social life? I insist you trade weekends with me so I can finally have a life, too."

BOX 1.7   Advantages of Assertive Behavior

- It is more likely you will get what you want when you ask for it clearly.
- People respect clear, open, honest communication.
- You stand up for your own rights and feel self-respect.
- You avoid the invitation of aggression when the rights of others are not violated.
- You are more independent.
- You become a decision maker.
- You feel more peaceful and comfortable with yourself.

C. "Jim, my family is having a special party this Saturday that I would really like to attend. I would appreciate it if you could trade with me. I would be glad to return the favor."

Did you select C? If so, you understood that this request honored the nurse's right to make a request and the colleague's right to refuse. The language was clear, nonapologetic, and respectful. Refer back to Box 1.4:

Describe: "My family is having a party."
Express: "I would really like to attend."
Specify: "Trade with me?"
Consequence: "I would return the favor."

Notice that response A is hesitant and apologetic, not straightforward. The wording denies the right of the request. Response B is aggressive and blaming and even a bit whiny.

PUTTING IT INTO PRACTICE

A nursing student babysits regularly, and often at the last minute the children's mom asks the student to stay later than expected. The student would then be late for class. She decided to approach her employer and explain why she could not stay late. "I am finding that when I stay later than planned, I have been arriving late to my class, and this is really stressing me out. It would help me if we could stay with the time I plan to be able to leave." The mom understood and no longer expected her to stay longer.

Nonassertive communication is a failure to stand up for our legitimate rights and possibly for those of others. It means communicating in an uncertain or uncomfortable way. Our nonassertive behavior may be based on thinking that we are inferior to others in some way. When we are passive or do not speak up to share our views, others may interpret our behavior as a sign of lack of interest or knowledge (Sully & Dallas, 2005). Sometimes being nonassertive gets us off the hook for the moment. We may agree to run an errand for someone because it is uncomfortable to say it is not convenient. Consider the phrase "short-term gain, long-term pain" the next time you consider not speaking up for your own needs. When we are nonassertive, we lose because we fail to show respect for ourselves, which lowers our self-esteem. We begin to feel like doormats. Our needs are not met, and we invite others to take advantage of us via aggressive behavior. We may find that our anger and frustration build up, and we may become aggressive ourselves. An outburst of anger resulting from such frustration can serve to reinforce passivity because of embarrassment at a side of ourselves we do not like.

Aggressiveness is that loud, forceful, often confrontational way of trying to get what we want, even at the expense of others. When we act aggressively, our rights are responded to out of proportion to those of others. Although we may temporarily gloat at our achievement, the experience is short-lived when we realize how we may have embarrassed ourselves or, worse, hurt other people in our determination to get what we wanted. Aggressive behavior frequently provokes anger or resentfulness and may lead to retaliation or passive–aggressive behavior. When an aggressive approach is taken, mutual respect is lacking; others are treated as objects standing in our way. Table 1.1 differentiates among assertive, nonassertive, and aggressive styles of communication.

When you are assertive, you feel better about yourself. It may take a while, however, for nurses who have been socialized to put others first to understand that there is a healthy balance between meeting personal needs and responding in a caring way to others. Nurses who have been more aggressive in their style may soon learn that this behavior distances people. It does get easier when you learn you can choose when to speak up and when to remain silent. You can choose lovingly to do something extra for someone, to inconvenience yourself by choice, not because you feel helpless. A good test of whether you have acted assertively is how you feel after the interaction. If you feel good, it is likely you have been assertive. Remember that if you have been passive most of the time, you may still feel guilty for setting your own priorities first, but the resentment that builds if you do not do so will erode the relationship.

On Reflection: As a nursing student in the 1960s, at 18 years old, at St. Elizabeth's Hospital with 8000 psychiatric patients, to make sense of it all, I read. Joyce Travelbee, an early author in psychiatric nursing, wrote that largely, under any given situation, we all do the best we can. Patrick King (2018, p. 58) wrote:

Self-acceptance is accepting that everything that's happened in your life has led you to be who you are and act how you do, and you're doing your best based on your experiences, knowledge, and the situation. The relationship you have with yourself sets the scene for every relationship you will ever have. If you believe that, despite your flaws, you have the right to do what is best for you, you will behave assertively.

Assertive communication skills make interactions more equal. We all have the right to express thoughts, feelings, and beliefs. When you feel irritated with a "demanding" client, consider that today's clients are not passive recipients of care but consumers with the expectation of good customer service. Assertiveness has positive benefits for all: it builds self-confidence to know that you can treat others fairly while taking care of your own needs. This creates a healthy attitude of mutual respect. Speaking out about your thoughts and feelings provides others with clear, direct messages that are easier to receive than passive–aggressive ones. Assertiveness helps build trust between people. Chaharsoughi et al. (2014) reported that more than 60% of deadly hospital events were caused by ineffective communication between healthcare professionals. Trust is built when healthcare professionals have the courage to acknowledge when things go wrong, right the wrong, express regret, and work to find out how to avoid the mistake in the future.

Adubato (2004) reported that nearly 90% of healthcare errors involve communication and suggested that assertiveness is an important strategy to minimize microcommunication.

WIT AND WISDOM

"Don't" versus "Can't"… sometimes a word choice can make a big difference.

When working on healthy eating habits, telling yourself, "I don't eat candy" rather than I "can't" reminds you of your own power. "I don't loan my car." "I don't go to a party on the nights I choose to study." "I don't stay up late when I have a test the next day." "Can't" allows the other to try to persuade you to do so. You have a policy, you are in charge of your own choices.

(King, 2018)

THE MEANING OF RESPONSIBLE COMMUNICATION

Responsible means "liable to be called on to answer" (Definition of 'responsible,' 2018). For nurses, this accountability may be described as being personally responsible for the outcome of their own professional actions, which are based on knowledge.

Sometimes, responsible communication is a simple statement of caring: "The pain medication will make you feel more comfortable." Other times, responsible communication may be the art of listening. If you do not know what to say, you can just sit quietly with a client.

To communicate responsibly when a problem must be solved means to communicate in a logical way based on your nursing knowledge and on the facts presented in the situation. Responsible communication demonstrates accurate problem-solving behavior for the particular situation. The nursing process is a systematic means for nurses to demonstrate accountability and responsibility to clients. The process is organized into five phases: assessment, diagnosis, outcomes/planning, implementation, and evaluation (Bickford et al., 2015):

Assess: Collect information about the client, family, and community to identify the client's needs, problems, concerns, and responses.

Diagnose: Critically analyze and interpret the data collected, and draw conclusions to identify nursing diagnoses that provide a focus for the rest of the process.

Outcomes/Planning: Establish priorities in the problems identified in the nursing diagnosis. Include the client and, at times, the family to create a plan of care that prescribes interventions to attain expected outcomes. Organize your communication strategy such as what the care plan will contain and when, how, and where you will present it.

Implement: Implement the interventions identified in the plan of care. At this point, you respond to your client or colleague. This book encourages you to respond assertively and responsibly.

Evaluate: Conduct an ongoing evaluation of the client's progress toward attainment of outcomes. This is the phase in which you check whether your response was assertive and responsible and whether your objectives (expected outcomes) were achieved.

A problem-solving process becomes a way of examining every client–nurse (or nurse–colleague) interaction, and it becomes a natural part of your day. While you are receiving a message, you are trying to determine its meaning. You decide whether you will meet the sender's request, and then you transmit an assertive and responsible message that conveys your decision. As you send your message, you observe the effects of your words and gestures on the receiver. During the course of your day, you are sending and receiving messages continuously (Box 1.8). Building communication skills supports your contribution to delivery of safe care by the healthcare team in complex and critical care situations (Swinny, 2010).

BOX 1.8 A Nurse Who Communicates Responsibly…

- Is naturally focused on the nursing process and problem-solving process
- Considers the world of the client and the client's family
- Performs the role of client advocate
- Appreciates the sacred role of intimate care of the sick
- Maintains a sense of wonder at the human experience and treats each person as an individual
- Is open to learning to trust intuition as another way of knowing about the client

SIMPLIFY AND DEEPEN

I asked a nurse in an expressive-arts-in-healing workshop to tell us about her collage, a picture she created from magazine images and words. She replied, "This represents my mission in life: to be kind." In psychiatric nursing I was taught that our self is our best therapeutic tool. How do you bring your best self to your work and to your life?

 MOMENTS OF CONNECTION...
Daring to Care

A nurse worked with a client with a brain tumor who was unable to communicate verbally. He sat up in bed, rocking back and forth, crying out in pain. His distress was not alleviated by pain medication. The nurse climbed up into the bed, rocked him, and sang lullabies the way she sang to her son. He relaxed, became quiet, and "nestled" into the nurse's arms. He was able to go to sleep a bit later and died in his sleep that night. The nurse said that never before or since had she been moved to do this and talked about the importance of trusting your intuition. "I guess God must have directed my actions that day. He put me in the right place and time and gave me the courage to step outside the practice...to care in a special way" (Riley, 1999).

THE MEANING OF CARING

Caring is the basis of the nursing profession. Your communication may be technically responsible and assertive, but without caring you still may not be able to facilitate a change in behavior. It is important to examine what caring means.

Caring is not an abstract concept. Both male and female nurses define caring as the essence of nursing (Colby, 2012). There are explicit ways nurses can communicate to show we care. Encompassed by caring is a commitment to the preservation of our shared humanity and respect for the uniqueness and dignity of each individual we encounter. Caring is an essential ingredient in life and must characterize the nurse–client relationship. Nurses at the University of North Carolina Hospitals implemented the Carolina Care model to operationalize Swanson Caring Theory, linking the caring process with patient well-being (Tonges & Ray, 2011). Consider Swanson's five caring processes (Swanson, 1993):

1. Maintaining belief: sustaining faith in the capacity of others to transition and have meaningful lives
2. Knowing: striving to understand events as they have meaning in the life of the other
3. Being with: being emotionally present to the other
4. Doing for: doing for the other what they would do for themselves if possible
5. Enabling: facilitating the capacity of others to care for themselves and family members (Tonges & Ray, 2011)

This model of caring based on the belief in people's capability to manage their own lives combines nursing compassion (knowing and being with) and competence (doing for and enabling) to support patients' healing and well-being (Tonges & Ray, 2011).

Nurses are demonstrating their caring globally in volunteer organizations to bring better healthcare services and quality of life to underserved populations. One nurse says, "Since we live in such difficult times, the best we can do is wage peace one person at a time" (Justin, 2002).

Caring is the moral ideal that guides nurses through the caregiving process, and knowledgeable caring is the highest form of commitment (Watson, 1995). Nurses can have an extensive command of scientific facts and theories and be technically expert without being caring professionals. In addition, nurses can be technically and scientifically correct but still make moral errors. Although there is satisfaction in being technologically competent, that satisfaction is not as lasting as the satisfaction derived from meaningful moments of connection with clients, families, and colleagues. These are moments that focus on the relationship with and support of the client rather than on illness and pathology (Hunter, 2006). Caring communication is holistic, taking into account the entire person and demonstrating respect for clients as people, not just as bodies, requiring nursing interventions. Take a moment to consider that at times a client's family may need to be cared for as a unit, with care delivery organized around its needs instead of the needs of an individual (Guilianeli et al., 2005). How can you ensure that your communication is caring? Although we as nurses may consciously desire to generate the feeling of being cared for in our clients and intend our behavior to convey this desire, we must remember that not all intended caring on our part is perceived as caring by our clients. A nurse may believe caring is being demonstrated by careful drug administration from a computerized cart taken to the bedside (see the following section). Caring is situation specific. Caring includes an ongoing commitment to sharpening knowledge and skills to identify care needs and nursing actions that will bring about positive change while protecting and enhancing human dignity.

 MOMENTS OF CONNECTION...

Putting the Cart before the Patient

Anne, a registered nurse (RN), worked in an older hospital with small patient rooms that were not designed for the mobile nursing workstation. Anne maneuvered the cart carefully, making sure it did not hit the bed. Mr. Rauer, an older adult who had never been hospitalized, seemed intimidated by the cart with its computer screen and scanner, which Anne used to confirm his identity via his armband. "I feel like a piece of meat in the grocery store." Anne realized that she had led with the machine and not herself. She pulled the cart out of the room and reentered, pulling it behind her. "Let's start over! My name is Anne, and I will be your nurse today." They had a good laugh as she quipped, "Never put the horse before the cart!" She demonstrated caring by humanizing the technology, explaining that the cart helped her give him safe care by good documentation and accurate medication administration. She gave good eye contact, listened carefully, and asked him if there was anything else she could do for him (Mikesell, 2013; Winstanley, 2014).

The implications are clear. We must find out what is perceived to be important to our clients in their return to health, validate the effect our caring actions are having on them, and adjust our actions in keeping with their needs. Taking these steps is a necessary component of responsible nursing. Consider these challenges. It is easier to be offended by a client's anger than to gently explore its source. It is easier to tell an abused wife to leave her husband than to listen to her pain. It is easier to instruct an adolescent to make sure her partner uses condoms than to listen to her story of a mother who is an addict, a father who is absent, and her 22-year-old boyfriend who says he will marry her if she gets pregnant (Carpenito, 2000). In a study to understand clients' experience of caring, caring meant that the clients could unburden their heart to express their suffering and discomfort. The experience of not being cared for communicated that clients were of no importance and that they were troublesome. Caring meant that nurses listened to their wishes and showed evidence of thinking of them such as when a nurse saved lunch for a patient after a procedure that required no drinking or eating (Karlsson et al., 2004). The next time you feel pressured and anxious in your caregiving, stop, take a deep breath, and ask yourself how your nonverbal behavior might be interpreted. Consider something as simple as smiling,

which conveys approval, encouragement, and acceptance (Hader, 2006).

Caring communication is as important with colleagues as it is with clients. If caring exists between coworkers, then that sense of well-being will likely be passed on to clients. Conversely, if there is little caring between colleagues, then nurses will be unlikely to feel complete and satisfied enough to demonstrate a sense of caring with their clients. Caring involves being assertive and responsible. If you let others control you because you are nonassertive or if you invade others' rights by being aggressive, you cannot act in a caring way. If you care enough for yourself to be assertive, then you will know how to care for others. Watson (2007) stated that nurses need to love, respect, and care for themselves and treat themselves with dignity before they can respect, love, and care for others and treat them with dignity.

HOW CAN YOU LEARN TO COMMUNICATE ASSERTIVELY AND RESPONSIBLY?

This book is based on the belief that effective and caring nurse communicators are not born; they are made. You can learn to communicate in competent, caring, and confident ways. You can replace ineffective and nontherapeutic communication habits with helpful interventions. You can continually add to your communication repertoire so that you develop confidence in your ability to communicate effectively in a variety of situations. When you lack confidence, remember that being assertive is more about valuing yourself and nursing, and your confidence will increase with success (Sudha, 2005).

Educational psychologists have proposed that learning involves three domains (McCroskey, 1984; Meichenbaum, 1977; Woodruff, 1961). This book attends to the cognitive aspects (understanding and meaning), affective aspects (feelings, values, and attitudes), and psychomotor aspects (physical capability) of your communication learning process.

By observing the guidelines in this text, you will learn basic communication skills (cognitive domain), you will build confidence through a belief in the value and effect of positive communication (affective domain), and you will meet the challenge, putting skills into action in the real world (psychomotor domain).

Cognitive Domain: Basic Communication Competencies

Communication competence is your ability to demonstrate knowledge of the appropriate communicative behavior in any situation. Communication competence is demonstrated by the identification of behaviors that would be appropriate or inappropriate in an observed interpersonal situation.

Affective Domain: Belief in the Value and Impact of Positive Communication

A belief in the value and effect of positive communication motivates the nurse to seek feedback and practice self-care strategies that build confidence.

Psychomotor Domain: Putting It All Together

Communication skill is your ability to perform appropriate communication behaviors in any given situation. To be a skilled nurse communicator, you must be able to successfully implement communication strategies that are assertive and responsible.

Fig. 1.3 illustrates how to become a caring nurse communicator by developing skills in all three domains. The negative consequences of incomplete development in all three aspects are also illustrated.

Assertiveness takes practice. People accustomed to you always saying yes may push back when you choose to act in your best interest. Healthy relationships are balanced: you work to get your needs met and allow others the same rights. Some relationships just are not good for you. Not everyone has your best interest at heart, but even someone who knows you well and cares for you cannot read your mind. Being clear about what

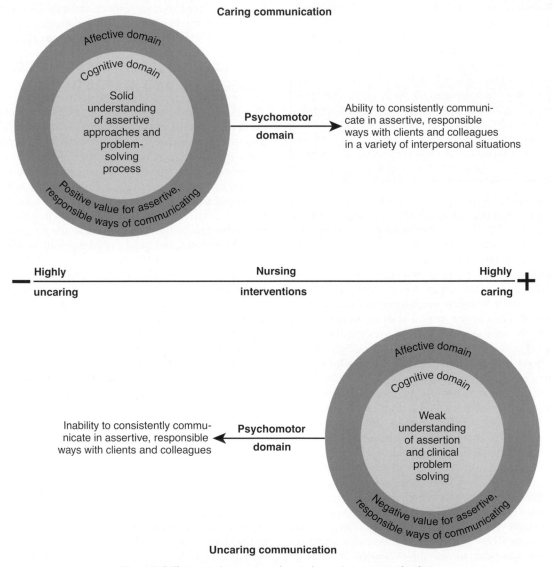

Fig. 1.3 Differences between caring and uncaring communication.

you want makes it more likely that others will work with you.

Consider the word selfless. It is a word we associate with altruism (doing good for others). If you are selfless, you may give so much of yourself away that you have nothing left to give. In your professional and personal life if you do not meet your own needs (body, mind, and spirit), you will have nothing left to give. You may find yourself getting colds and the flu and missing class or work, for which you are penalized. Self-care is an ethical imperative for a nurse. I believe you cannot give what you do not have.

There are no magic words to get your needs met, although this book gives you tools. As you come to value your own needs, set your own priorities, and have compassion for yourself as you would others, you can accept yourself as someone who does the best they can even if they are not perfect. Take a breath and grow into someone with self-respect. Others will come to trust that you say what you mean, respect you, and work with you (King, 2018).

Return to "Active Learning" at the beginning of the chapter and write your responses.

Next-Generation NCLEX® Case Study

Assertive Communication

Scenario: An older adult female client was admitted 4 days ago after a fall that resulted in a fractured right femur. Following surgical stabilization and traction, no family members or friends have visited. Staff members state that she remains distant and seldom engages in conversation when care is being provided. When assessed for pain, the client often states, "It's not bad, don't worry about me"; however, the electronic health record shows that she has been frequently observed grimacing when a change of position is required or skin care is being given. Today, when the nurse states it is time for morning hygiene, the client says, "I like to watch a television show at this time, but you can go ahead with my bath." When the nurse offers to assist the client in identifying her menu preferences, she states, "I'm not a picky eater so anything they bring is fine. I don't want to be a bother because you have many other sicker people to care for than me." The electronic health record shows that the client has consumed less than 50% of all meals, with much of the food left untouched.

Item Type: Cloze

Based on the client's statements and behavior, the nurse identifies that the client's priority need relates to _____1_____. After meeting this need, the client's risk for potential complications, especially related to _____2_____ and _____2_____, can be minimized.

Option 1	Option 2
Lack of assertiveness	Ineffective pain control
Depression	Improper nutrition
Immobility	Diminished sense of self-worth
Aging	Impaired skin integrity

Note: The answer keys for the above NGN case study are given in the back of the book in Appendix III.

PRACTICING RESPONSIBLE, ASSERTIVE, CARING COMMUNICATION

Self-Care Assessment: Exercise 1

In your journal, complete the Holistic Self-Care Assessment, Appendix II, at the end of the book. What surprised you about your scores? Write a reflection about this and begin to include self-care practices in your calendar.

Skill Building: Exercise 2

To build your assertive skills, review Box 1.2 and list any rights you have relinquished. Review Box 1.3. For each relinquished right you listed, identify which irrational beliefs you held that interfered with acting in your own best interest.

Reflective Journaling/Creative Expression/Skill Building: Exercise 3

Begin a "Curious about Communication" journal/log in a spiral or composition notebook. Use this throughout your use of this book. Find images or words in magazines that appeal to you that demonstrate your focus or intention for this journal and glue them on the cover. (A glue stick works well.) This week record events in which you were nonassertive using this format: In what event was I not assertive? Was my behavior nonassertive or aggressive? How would I prefer to have handled this situation?

Skill Building: Exercise 4

Identify a situation in which you want to be assertive. Use the DESC script in Box 1.4 to write your response, or write an assertive response to the following student example, using the DESC script:

"My roommate is super introverted. We had made plans a long time ago to go out. She cancelled at the last minute and said she just didn't want to go. I was so mad. 'Are you bailing on me just so you can stay home alone and do nothing? I don't get it.' Instead, I could have asked her what changed her mind and told her I had really been looking forward to spending time with her. Maybe if I had handled it this way, she would have gone. I ended up apologizing for my reaction and we made up. I was wrong and I acknowledged that."

Skill Building: Exercise 5

Observe other students, faculty, and staff in your clinical area as well as colleagues and family members. Identify one person who could be a role model for assertive communication. Identify one situation in your professional life and one situation in your personal life in which you would have preferred to be assertive. Close your eyes and envision the role model. Ask yourself how this person would have handled the situation and pretend you can see what the person is saying and doing. Write what you imagined, and examine the lessons you learn from this to build your own assertive communication skills.

Quality and Safety Education for Nurses Learning Strategy: Exercise 6

Patient-centered care is a fundamental concept in creating cultures of safety and facilitating continuous improvements in quality. This type of care is threaded through each of the competencies for improving the quality and safety of healthcare identified and described in the Quality and Safety Education for Nurses (QSEN) project (see www.QSEN.org). Communication is the basis for establishing a culture of safety; therefore, many chapters in this book include specific QSEN learning strategies. Mindfully engaging with each client and family as you interact and guide their care can help reduce the potential for error and improve care outcomes. Mindful engagement in a caregiving encounter helps to communicate more effectively with the patient to complete the assessment needed to individualize care and include the patient and family as equal partners. As you plan care for your patient, consider how you can mindfully engage to offer patient-centered care that provides caring communication:

- Clear distractions from your mind and focus on your patient as a unique individual with hopes, values, and health beliefs and as a member of his or her own community.
- What essential information do you need to know to plan effective care for this patient?

- What choices can you offer the patient about their care to demonstrate caring?
- What is the most important thing you can do for this patient at this point in time?
- When is it more important to honor a patient's preferences than strictly adhere to the evidence-based standard of care?

Self-Care: Exercise 7

Visit www.sleepfoundation.org and search Sleep Hygiene. Review suggestions. In your journal, write a brief assessment of how well you sleep. If you identify a need for more sleep, create a simple plan from the suggestions. Write a goal to make one change this week, note your progress, and evaluate it. Discuss sleep issues with others.

REFERENCES

Adubato, S. (2004). Making the communication connection. *Nursing Manage, 35*(9), 33.

Bickford, C. J., Marion, L., & Gazaway, S. (2015). *Nursing: Scope and standards of clinical nursing practice* (3rd ed.). Silver Spring, MD: American Nurses Association.

Carpenito, L. J. (2000). Nurse, always there for you. *Nursing Forum, 35*(2), 3.

Chaharsoughi, N. T., Ahrari, S., & Alikhah, S. (2014). Comparison: The effect of teaching SBAR technique with role play and lecturing on communication skill of nurses. *Journal of Caring Sciences, 3*, 141–147. In N. Lennen & B. Miller (2017), Introducing interprofessional education in nursing curricula. *Teaching and Learning in Nursing, 12*, 59–61.

Colby, N. (2012). Caring from the male perspective: A gender neutral concept. *International Journal of Human Caring, 164*, 36.

Guilianeli, S., Kelly, R., Skelsky, J., et al. (2005). The critical care nurse manager's perspective: The critical care family assistance program. *Chest, 128*(3), 118S.

Hader, R. (2006). If you're happy and you know it…. *Nursing Management, 37*(2), 6.

Hanson, J., Walsh, S., Mason, M., Wadsworth, D., Framp, A., & Watson, K. (2020). 'Speaking up for safety': A graded assertiveness intervention for first year nursing students in preparation for clinical placement: Thematic analysis. *Nurse Education Today, 84*, 104252.

Hunter, L. P. (2006). Women give birth and pizzas are delivered: Language and Western childbirth paradigms. *Journal of Midwifery & Women's Health, 51*(2), 119–124.

Justin, F. (2002). Acting globally. *Adv Nurs, 4*(13), 21.

Karlsson, M., Bergbom, I., von Post, I., et al. (2004). Patient experiences when the nurse cares for and does not care for. *International Journal of Human Caring, 8*(3), 30.

King, P. (2018). *The art of everyday assertiveness*. Lexington, KY: Patrick King Consulting.

Kinyon, K. E. (2021). A stress reduction intervention for first semester nursing students during COVID-19. *Beginnings: American Holistic Nurses Association, 41*(5), 6–9.

Lord, H., Loveday, C., Moxham, L., & Fernandez, R. (2021). Effective communication is key to intensive care nurses' willingness to provide nursing care amidst the COVID-19 pandemic. *Intensive & Critical Care, 62,* 102946.

McCroskey, J. C. (1984). The communication apprehension perspective. In J. A. Daly, & J. C. McCroskey (Eds.), *Avoiding communication: Shyness, reticence and communication apprehension.* Beverly Hills, CA: Sage Publications.

Meichenbaum, D. (1977). *Cognitive-behavior modification: An integrative approach.* New York, NY: Plenum Press.

Definition of 'responsible. (2018). In Merriam-Webster Online Dictionary online. Retrieved from http://www.merriam-webster.com/dictionary/responsible.

Mikesell, L. (2013). Medicinal relationships: Caring conversation. *Medical Education, 47,* 443.

Riley, J. B. (1999). *From the heart to the hands…keys to successful healthcaring connections.* Ellicott City, MD: Integrated Management Publishing Systems.

Smith, T. (2020). Guided reflective writing as a teaching strategy to develop nursing student's clinical judgment. *Nurs Forum, 56,* 241–248.

Strachan, P. H., Kryworuchko, Nouvet, E., et al. (2018). Canadian hospital nurses' roles in communication and decision-making about goals of care: An interpretive description of critical incidents. *Applied Nursing Research, 40,* 26.

Stuart, G. W. (2012). *Principles and practice of psychiatric nursing* (10th Ed.). St. Louis, MO: Mosby.

Sudha, R. (2005). How to be an assertive nurse. *The Nursing Journal of India, 96*(8), 182.

Sully, P., & Dallas, J. (2005). *Essential communication skills for nursing.* Edinburgh, UK: Mosby.

Swanson, K. (1993). Nursing as informed caring for the well-being of others. *Image, 25*(4), 352.

Swinny, B. (2010). Assessing and developing critical-thinking skills in the intensive care unit. *Critical Care Nurse Quarterly, 33*(1), 2.

Tonges, M., & Ray, J. (2011). Translating caring theory into practice. *Journal of Nursing Administration, 41*(9), 374.

Townsend, M. (2021). The moment I became a nurse. *Beginnings: American Holistic Nurses Association, 41*(5), 10–11.

Watson, J. (1995). Postmodernism and knowledge development in nursing. *Nursing Science Quarterly, 8*(2), 60.

Watson, J. (2007). *Nursing: Human science and human care: A theory of nursing.* Sudbury, MA: Jones & Bartlett.

Winstanley, H. D. (2014). How to bring caring to the high-tech bedside. *Nursing, 44*(2), 60.

Woodruff, A. D. (1961). *Basic concepts of teaching.* Scranton, PA: Chandler.

Yoshinaga, N., Nakamura, Y., Tanoue, H., et al. (2018). Is modified brief assertiveness training for nurses effective? A single-group study with long-term follow-up. *J Nurs Manag, 26,* 59.

2

The Client–Nurse Relationship: A Helping Relationship*

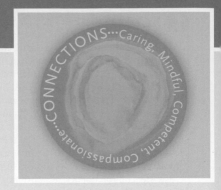

Caring begins with being present, open to compassion, mercy, loving-kindness, and equanimity toward and with self before one can offer compassionate caring to others. It begins with a love of humanity and everything that is living; the immanent, subtle, radiant, shadow-and-light vicissitudes of experience along the way—honoring with reverence the mystery, the unknowns, the impermanence, and changes but actively, joyfully participating in all of it, the pain, the joy, and everything.

Jean Watson (2008)

OBJECTIVES

1. Identify the purpose of the client–nurse relationship.
2. Complete a self-assessment of your communication skills.
3. Identify Peplau's three phases of the nurse–patient relationship.
4. Describe the cognitive, affective, and psychomotor abilities that nurses and clients bring to the therapeutic encounter.
5. Discuss clients' rights as consumers of healthcare service.
6. Identify characteristics of a successful client–nurse relationship.
7. Identify therapeutic communication techniques.
8. Identify nontherapeutic communication techniques.
9. List dos and don'ts in the client–nurse relationship.
10. Identify behavioral dimensions indicative of bonding in the client–nurse relationship.
11. Discuss the FOCUSED model for being present.
12. Identify qualities of a storycatcher.
13. Discuss listening skills.
14. Participate in exercises to build skills in the client–nurse relationship.

For the 20th consecutive year, results of Gallup's annual poll named nursing the most trusted profession (Gaines, 2022). At a time when nurses might have less time with clients, the relationship with the nurse is still our foundation, and we are valued. Consider how nurses' caring communication supports patient safety. A study to examine how nurses recognize and address safety concerns of patients and families identified the creation of space for open safety communication (Groves et al., 2021). In the global health crisis from COVID-19, nurses have creatively faced many challenges in humanizing patient and family care. Using virtual visitations, even supporting family seeing a patient through a window, nurses have balanced the need to see each person as unique with safety needs. Administrators and educators have used reflective practices to support problem solving (Brittany et al., 2021; Guillaumie et al., 2020; Sherwood, 2021). Nurses practice anticipatory compassion when we prevent suffering and when we take steps to help prevent a fall or an infection (Wood, 2018). Have you ever been in the patient role, feeling vulnerable, unsure, and frightened? A friendly word, a smile, or a question about how you are feeling can reassure and calm you, especially in fast-paced care and brief encounters. In the COVID crisis a tender story/photo of an intervention dubbed "the little hands of god/love therapy" depicts gloves filled with warm water to comfort a patient dying in the intensive care unit when no human hands were available (Massey & Lodha, 2021). Encounters we have with our clients can be caring and

---

* With contributions from Margaret E. Erickson, PhD.

Think about how you will write your answers as you read this chapter.

What?
Write one thing you learned from this chapter.

So What?
How will this affect your nursing practice?

Now What?
How will you implement this new knowledge or skill?

Think About It …

helpful or unfeeling and even harmful. In this chapter you will learn how to build effective relationships with your clients.

You will learn about the professional client–nurse relationship so that you can understand how it differs from social, collegial, and kinship relationships. The responsibilities of the nurse in client–nurse relationships have also been outlined so you will be able to articulate your roles and interventions at each stage of the helping relationship. As you read, reflect on the extent to which you foster a helping relationship in your interactions with clients.

SELF-ASSESSMENT TOOL

In the healthcare profession we understand that our clients have a choice of care providers. We need to understand the business of healthcare provision and the importance of being sensitive to good customer service. If you think back to your own experiences as a customer in any industry, you understand that customer service is not common sense; rather, it is a set of skills and attitudes that needs to be central to give good customer service. Your ability to communicate clearly and with compassion and to meet and even exceed your clients' expectations is the essence of customer service. Many complaints are not about clinical issues; they are about perceived rudeness or lack of caring. You also have internal customers, such as colleagues and staff from other departments and disciplines. Complete the following self-assessment not only as a quick check of your skills, but also as a tool to teach the basics of customer service. Just as when you read course or clinical evaluation objectives at the beginning of a class, knowing what is expected of you sets you up to be successful.

Self-Assessment Tool: Communication— The Key to Customer Service

Instructions: Rate yourself from 4 (very skilled) to 1 (not skilled).

1. I feel good about my communication skills.	4	3	2	1
2. I smile at clients, families, and staff.	4	3	2	1
3. I make eye contact.	4	3	2	1
4. I introduce myself and wear my name badge.	4	3	2	1
5. I learn names and use the correct pronunciations.	4	3	2	1
6. If I do not understand, I seek clarification.	4	3	2	1
7. I take a moment to calm myself before interacting with clients.	4	3	2	1
8. I take responsibility for finding answers to questions.	4	3	2	1
9. I answer the telephone promptly and with a smile (that helps!).	4	3	2	1
10. I explain procedures clearly.	4	3	2	1
11. I encourage clients and their families to ask questions.	4	3	2	1
12. I encourage feedback about my work.	4	3	2	1
13. I receive positive feedback about my work.	4	3	2	1
14. I thank a colleague who helps me.	4	3	2	1
15. I offer to help my colleagues.	4	3	2	1
16. I listen, knowing it is OK to be quiet and not have all the answers.	4	3	2	1
17. I respect the client's confidentiality.	4	3	2	1
18. I apologize for delays.	4	3	2	1
19. When I touch a client, I do it gently.	4	3	2	1
20. I dress professionally and pay attention to my grooming.	4	3	2	1
21. I try to do something extra for clients, families, and colleagues.	4	3	2	1
22. I am learning to deal with multiple demands on my time.	4	3	2	1

Continued

Self-Assessment Tool: Communication— The Key to Customer Service—cont'd

Instructions: Rate yourself from 4 (very skilled) to 1 (not skilled).

23. I give compliments to clients, families, and colleagues (yes, doctors, too!).	4	3	2	1
24. I understand that I am still learning and that it is impossible to be perfect.	4	3	2	1
25. I try to be myself, bringing my own special gifts to my nursing practice.	4	3	2	1

Scoring: Add the numbers you have selected. Remember that this is a self-assessment, and feedback from your instructor, peers, and clients adds more data. A score of 77 to 100 = high awareness of necessary skills and 53 to 76 = average awareness of skills. Review your lower scores and select areas for growth. Scores of 25 to 52 = low awareness of necessary skills. Pay more attention to skill development.

WIT AND WISDOM
Hospitality is one form of worship.

Jewish proverb

Self-Care Nudge

Did you know that sleep deprivation compromises nurses' health and patient safety (Ballesion et al., 2020)? Babies respond to a comforting bedtime ritual; adults do, too. Create a sleeping routine to trigger sleep. After a few deep breaths, I say three affirmations to myself: I fall asleep easily; I stay asleep; I awake refreshed. Try it for a few nights.

NATURE OF THE HELPING RELATIONSHIP

A set of preestablished rules and expectations directs the course of client–nurse interactions. There may be some overlap between these interactions and those involving friends and family, but one factor in particular differentiates helping relationships from social relationships. A helping relationship is established for the benefit of the client, whereas kinship and friendship relationships are designed to meet mutual needs. In particular, the client–nurse relationship is established to help the client achieve and maintain optimal health.

Three phases of the nurse–patient relationship, Peplau's interpersonal relations theory introduced in 1952, are still applicable (Hagerty et al., 2017; Way et al., 2021). The phases are the orientation phase in which patients realize they need help and nurses gather essential information, respecting the person as a unique, valued individual; the working phase in which nurses make assessments, using active listening to help clarify their health needs, feelings about their change in health, and work together to problem solve and create a plan of care; and the termination phase, thought of as discharge planning for symptom management and recovery, in which clear boundaries are set to end this relationship to move the patient from dependence to independence and appropriate use of other resources.

A successful helping relationship between nurse and client represents an order of interaction that is different from what occurs in a friendship. This is not because of any superiority in the nurse but because of the mutual trust and the responsibilities for assisting others that characterize true professional relationships.

Nursing care is planned to meet an individual client's unique needs and situation with respect for the goals and preferences of the patient and family. Nurses provide patient education so that clients have the information necessary to make informed decisions about their healthcare, health promotion, disease prevention, and attainment of a peaceful death. Nurses establish a partnership with the client and family and with other healthcare providers. Professional practitioners of nursing bear a responsibility for the nursing care that clients/patients receive as sanctioned by state nurse practice acts (Bickford et al., 2015). Client–nurse relationships are entered for the benefit of the client, but such a relationship is more effective if it is mutually satisfying. Clients are satisfied when their healthcare needs have been met and they sense that they have been treated in a caring manner. Nurses feel a sense of accomplishment when their interventions have had a positive influence on their clients' health status and when their conduct has been competent and caring.

Clients and nurses alike come to the relationship with unique cognitive, affective, and psychomotor abilities that they use in their joint endeavor of enhancing the clients' well-being. Nurses are responsible for encouraging this interchange of ideas, values, and skills. In an effective helping relationship, a definite and guaranteed interchange occurs between clients and nurses in all three dimensions.

Cognitive, Affective, and Psychomotor Abilities in the Therapeutic Encounter

The following sections include some of the cognitive, affective, and psychomotor abilities that clients and nurses bring to their therapeutic encounter. Table 2.1 further illustrates that both clients and nurses start with ideas and expectations that influence the course and outcome of their relationship.

Cognitive

Clients and nurses know something about health and illness in general and about the individual client's health concerns in particular. Clients bring their model or worldview:

TABLE 2.1 Interchange of Knowledge, Attitudes, and Skills between the Client and Nurse in the Helping Relationship

What Clients Bring to the Client–Nurse Relationship	What Nurses Bring to the Client–Nurse Relationship
Cognitive	
Preferred ways of perceiving and judging	Preferred ways of perceiving and judging
Knowledge and beliefs about illness in general and their illness in particular	Knowledge and beliefs about illness in general
Knowledge and beliefs about health promotion and maintenance in general and information about their own healthcare activities	Knowledge about their clinical specialty and knowledge and beliefs about health behaviors that prevent illness and promote, regain, and maintain health
Ability to problem solve	Ability to problem solve
Ability to learn	Knowledge about factors that increase client compliance with the treatment regimen
Affective	
Cultural values	Cultural values
Feelings about seeking help from a nurse	Feelings about being a nurse-helper
Attitudes toward nurses in general	Attitudes about clients in general
Attitudes toward treatment regimen	Biases about nursing treatment regimen
Values about preventing illness	Value placed on being healthy
	Value placed on people's active prevention of illness or enhancement of well-being
Willingness to take positive action about own health status at this time with this particular nurse	Willingness to help clients take positive action to improve their well-being
Psychomotor	
Ability to relate to and communicate with others	Ability to relate to and communicate with others
Ability to perform own healthcare management	Proficiency in administering effective nursing interventions
Ability to learn new methods of self-care	Ability to teach nursing interventions to the client

"the way they perceive life, events, people, and situations… communicate, think, feel, act, and react" (Erickson et al., 1983) to the relationship. Clients have definite knowledge about what has made them ill and has interfered with their growth and fulfillment. They also know "what will make them well, optimize their fulfillment and or promote their growth." This knowledge is called self-care knowledge (Erickson et al., 1983). As nurses we want to help our clients access and use their self-care knowledge to achieve a greater state of health and well-being. Nurses have their own views, which are based on their knowledge and beliefs about what will help their clients. To prevent clients and nurses from operating in isolation or at cross-purposes, they must exchange essential information.

In addition to having different ideas, clients and nurses also have preferred ways of observing their worlds and making decisions about what they see. Each of us has a preferred mental process (the one we have developed most highly, the one we use best) that forms the core of our personalities (Myers, 1998). Clients and nurses have different ways in which they prefer to use their minds, specifically the ways they choose to perceive and to make judgments (Myers, 1998). Perceiving includes becoming aware of things, people, occurrences, and ideas. Judging includes reaching conclusions about what has been observed.

Some clients and nurses, for example, are primarily practical. They are attuned to immediate experiences, literal facts at hand, and concrete realities. Myers used the word *sensing* to describe this preferred way of collecting data in problem solving. Other clients and nurses prefer to think about what could be rather than what is. Their intuitive imaginations fill their minds with ideas and explanations that do not always depend on the senses for verification. Myers called this preferred way of collecting data *intuitive*.

Consider the following situation to understand the differences in these two ways of perceiving and how they affect the client–nurse relationship.

Mr. Zabrick is an 80-year-old resident of a senior citizens' apartment complex where he lives with his retired, 70-year-old widowed sister. In the past 9 months, Mr. Zabrick has had chemotherapy and radiation treatments for lung cancer. His tumor has vanished, and his blood levels are stabilized; yet, to his disappointment, he feels lethargic and anorexic.

Eight days ago, his sister awoke in the night and found Mr. Zabrick in the bathtub in which he had fallen after mistaking it for the toilet. She noticed that her brother is unsteady on his feet and is losing weight.

Clients (or family members) and nurses who prefer concrete details, or sensing, would evaluate Mr. Zabrick's situation by focusing on the visible evidence that might account for his deterioration. They would observe the lack of saliva under the tongue and its brown furry appearance and note his report of an unpleasant taste and odor in the mouth. They would see the small, hard stools and the abdominal distention. They would feel the decreased turgor of his skin and notice the muscle weakness. They would count the amount of fluids and quantity of food consumed by Mr. Zabrick.

Clients or nurses who prefer detailed information would put these pieces together and likely come to the conclusion that Mr. Zabrick is dehydrated. Those who use this way of perceiving prefer information that is measurable, and the thinking process is systematic, with one step taken at a time.

Clients (or family members) and nurses who prefer a more intuitive perceiving process might not gather all these data before jumping to a conclusion about what is happening to Mr. Zabrick. They are likely to look for patterns in the data (as opposed to discrete pieces of information). They would start thinking about possible explanations and then work backward to obtain the facts. They might notice, for example, that Mr. Zabrick has said, "Why bother with trying anymore? If I had a chance to do it again, I'm not sure I'd take the treatments," and wonder if his fatigue and grief are consuming him. They might remember that Mr. Zabrick's daughter-in-law died despite rigorous chemotherapy and that his lifelong friend was diagnosed with brain cancer 3 weeks earlier and wonder if Mr. Zabrick's symptoms reflect his doubt about living with such losses. Another theme on which intuitive individuals might focus is the relationship between the assault on Mr. Zabrick's body from treatments, changes in diet and exercise, and sleep deprivation and the effect of the severe heat and humidity of the previous 7 weeks.

These two perceiving processes, sensing and intuitive, are quite different. It is important for nurses to understand their preferred way of perceiving and try to discover which process their clients prefer. Both ways of seeing the world are valuable; one is not better than the other. Each way simply selects different information on which to focus.

Judging, the process of making decisions about the information collected through perception, is the other mental process in which clients and nurses may differ. Some persons have logical, orderly, and analytical decision-making processes and treat the world objectively (Myers, 1995). Decision makers such as these prefer to fit all experience into logical mental systems. Myers called this preference *thinking* and said that these people make decisions based on critical analysis of facts, valuing fairness. Other clients and nurses prefer to tune into the subjective world of feelings and values. Myers called this preference *feeling* and said that these individuals make decisions by analyzing how they will affect people, valuing harmony.

Each of us prefers one of these decision-making processes over the other (Myers, 1995). Consider the following situation to better understand the two judging processes.

Jossie is a 19-year-old first-year university student who is 8 weeks pregnant and unmarried. She is receiving counseling about her options. She sees three choices and will soon decide whether to have an abortion, continue with the pregnancy and give up her baby for adoption, or carry her baby to term and raise the child herself.

Clients and nurses who prefer a rational, objective way of making decisions would invite Jossie to consider all the facts and then make a logical decision based on them. They would look at the consequences of any decision Jossie might make and judge it using their head rather than their heart. They would be able to remain emotionally uninvolved. They have the ability to see the "long view" and would likely encourage Jossie to consider her future pragmatically and act on the most sensible choice (Myers, 1995).

Clients and nurses who prefer to consider effects on the people in the situation would likely explore how Jossie feels about each of the choices and how each fits her values. Such people would probably emphasize the benefits of any plan Jossie considers rather than criticizing it; they would also likely support Jossie's personal convictions.

This glimpse at two different methods for using our minds alerts us to the misunderstandings that can arise in helping relationships. We cannot assume that clients' minds are guided by the same principles as our own. Clients, their family members, and professional colleagues may reason in the same way that you do, or they may prefer using different ways of perceiving and judging. They may not value the things you value or show interest in the same things you do (Myers, 1998).

We all use different combinations of perceiving and judging, and colleagues and clients with the same preferences are likely to be the easiest to like and understand. They will tend to have similar interests (because they share the same kinds of perceptions) and consider the same matters important (because they share the same kinds of judgment) (Myers, 1998).

On the other hand, it will be harder to understand and predict the behavior of colleagues and clients whose perception and judgment preferences differ from our own. We are likely to take opposite stands on any issue with colleagues and clients who prefer different thinking processes (Myers, 1998). The therapeutic nurse–patient relationship, a mutual learning experience and a corrective emotional experience for the patient, is based on the underlying humanity of nurse and patient, with mutual respect and acceptance of ethnocultural differences (Stuart, 2012).

If you would like to learn more about your preferences for perceiving and making decisions and about other personality preferences, arrange with your school's counseling or guidance department to take the Myers–Briggs Type Indicator (MBTI). Learn more about MBTI online at https://www.mbtionline.com, where you can also complete the assessment for a fee. The aim of the MBTI is to identify, from self-reporting of easily recognized reactions, the basic preferences of people regarding perception and judgment (Myers, 1998). Learning about your own preferences and personality will make you more aware of how your way of thinking influences your behavior in client–nurse helping relationships (see Chapter 3).

Affective

Clients and nurses have positive and negative feelings about helping relationships; each also has biases about the other and each has different priorities for working on particular health concerns. The attitudes of clients and nurses greatly affect whether they work in harmony or discord, their respective knowledge surfaces or is submerged, and they perform the commitment of improving the health of individual clients. In addition, people's "model" or "worldview" (Erickson et al., 1983) includes their definition or perception of what constitutes health. Smith (1981) discovered that people view health from four different models: the clinical model in which there is an absence of disease; the role-performance model in which the person is able to perform his or her role in life; the adaptive model in which health is determined by a person's ability to cope with stress; and the eudemonistic model in which health is perceived as a quality of life, a person's ability to enjoy life, have meaningful relationships, and have a state of well-being. Understanding how a nurse and client define health is very important because it affects the plan of care, the desired goals, and the outcomes. As noted previously, when nurses listen to their client's story, they gain greater insight and knowledge into how a person defines health.

The major source of our value system is our culture. In America today, culture is heterogeneous (with a variety of cultural groups), so nurses and clients are likely to encounter different beliefs and values, particularly because the United States is home to people from all parts of the world. Modern medical and nursing practices become two of the external forces with which immigrants come in contact. This encounter with the American healthcare system is loaded with choices for immigrants to make in deciding how much of their culture's traditional medical practices they wish to maintain. Cultural patterns are one of the important means by which people adapt to recurrent change in their environments (see Chapter 5).

Psychomotor

Clients need to know what skills the nurse has, and the nurse needs to determine clients' abilities to participate in their treatment plan. Consider a scenario in which a client provides detailed information from the Internet. Can you envision a partnering to share information? The nurse can help the client determine which sources are most reliable (see Chapter 23).

CLIENTS' RIGHTS IN THE HELPING RELATIONSHIP

Together nurses and clients share their energy and resources and commit to healing. They also confront issues regarding the meaning of illness to the client and family and work toward self-realization and personal growth. As consumers of our healthcare services, clients have the following rights:

- To expect a systematic and accurate investigation of their health concerns by thorough and well-organized nurses
- To be informed about their health status and have their questions answered so that they clearly understand what nurses mean
- To receive healthcare from nurses who have current knowledge about their diagnosis and are capable of providing safe and efficient care
- To feel confident they will be treated courteously and have nurses show genuine interest in them
- To trust that the confidentiality of personal information will be respected
- To be informed about plans of action to be performed for their benefit
- To refuse or consent to nursing treatments without jeopardizing their relationship with their nurses
- To secure help conveniently, without hassles or roadblocks
- To receive consistent quality of care from all nurses

CHARACTERISTICS OF CLIENT–NURSE HELPING RELATIONSHIPS

Client–nurse relationships are special helping relationships that are characterized by the following features:

- Mindful presence and genuine concern based on an understanding that nurses have an ethical imperative for self-care: be prepared mentally, emotionally, and physically to assist your clients in resolving their health-care problems (ANA Code of Ethics, 2015).

- A purposeful and productive objective: together clients and nurses agree about the nature of the health problem in question. They develop and implement a plan designed to reach agreed-on objectives. Clients and nurses together evaluate the outcomes and decide whether the desired and expected outcomes have been achieved.
- Competence, creativity, practicality, and safe practice in handling health concerns offered.
- Maintenance of the client's present level of health and protection from future health threats because of the increased knowledge gleaned from the helping relationship.
- Easing of clients' worries and fears through nurses' reassurances and easing of pain through soothing comfort measures.
- Consistency in the helping relationship wherever and whenever clients and nurses come together.
- A series of phases, with a beginning (initiation), middle (maintenance), and end (termination) to each encounter.
- Individualized care.
- Safe space and privacy so that clients may disclose intimate details about their life: nurses are responsible for protecting their clients' confidentiality.
- Professional boundaries in the expressions of caring: even though nurses may have strong feelings for their clients, it is expected that they can maintain adequate objectivity and perspective to provide therapeutic assistance. Clients and nurses can develop attachments for each other, which makes the relationship special for each.

Nurses use therapeutic communication techniques (Table 2.2), as contrasted with nontherapeutic communication techniques (Table 2.3), to implement the nursing process.

POINTERS TO GUIDE YOU IN YOUR CLIENT–NURSE HELPING RELATIONSHIPS

This section offers dos and don'ts for conducting yourself in client–nurse helping relationships.

Do

- Be punctual and polite in your manner of relating to clients, and be kind in your approach to clients by putting their needs and concerns first;
- Praise and encourage clients in their efforts to take better care of themselves; and

- Be patient and understanding about clients' reactions to their particular health situations.

Don't

- Patronize clients by using medical jargon or in any way making them feel inadequate or estranged;
- Use labels such as "good," "lazy," or "uncooperative," which prevent you and colleagues from seeing clients as they really are;
- Procrastinate in following through on clients' reasonable requests;
- Make a promise you cannot be sure to keep;
- Judge, criticize, or retaliate against clients for acts of omission or commission that have negatively affected their health;
- Seek to meet your own needs through the client–nurse relationship; and
- Offer information if you are not certain just to avoid looking uninformed.

As a nurse, it is your responsibility to ensure that a thorough assessment is made of your clients' health concerns, that suitable nursing actions are chosen and implemented to help your clients, and that an evaluation of the results is performed. Assuming this leadership does not mean that you take over and do for, or to, your clients. The quality of your nursing care is determined by the completeness of the interchange of knowledge, attitudes, and skills between you and your clients. To be most helpful to all your clients, make sure that you solicit their knowledge, become aware of their feelings and attitudes, and take into account their strengths and limitations in caring for themselves. Use this information to individualize nursing care. Be aware of how your knowledge, attitude, and skills affect your ability to be helpful. Effective nursing requires being assertive and responsible. Chapter 4 will show you how to make problem-solving a mutual process between you and your clients.

BONDING IN THE CLIENT–NURSE RELATIONSHIP

The client and nurse both contribute to the success of the relationship. Bonding is the shared experience between the client and the nurse that occurs when each feels connected to the other. Research has developed instruments to measure the caring behavior of the nurse and others to measure client satisfaction. Tejero (2009) developed an instrument to determine the degree of bonding between the nurse and the client. This instrument was developed using qualitative data from observations and interviews and was corroborated from literature and validated in a bedside setting. The study identified two indicators of bonding, openness, and engagement and delineated behavioral dimensions for each. The bonding

TABLE 2.2 Summary of Therapeutic Communication Techniques

Technique	Definition	Therapeutic Value
Listening	An active process of receiving information and examining one's reactions to the messages received	Nonverbally communicates the nurse's interest in the client
Remaining silent	Periods of no verbal communication among participants	Nonverbally communicates the nurse's acceptance of the client
Establishing guidelines	Statements regarding roles, purposes, and limitations for a particular interaction	Helps the client to know what is expected of him or her
Making open-ended comments	General comments asking the client to determine the direction the interaction should take	Allows the client to decide what material is most relevant and encourages the client to continue
Reducing distance	Diminishing physical space between the nurse and client	Nonverbally communicates that the nurse wants to be involved with the client
Acknowledging	Recognition given to a client for contribution to an interaction	Demonstrates the importance of a client's role within the relationship
Restating	Repetition to the client of what the nurse believes is the main thought or idea expressed	Asks for validation of the nurse's interpretation of the message
Reflecting	Direction back to the client of his or her ideas, feelings, questions, or content	Attempts to show the client the importance of his or her own ideas, feelings, and interpretations
Seeking clarification	Request for additional input to understand the message received	Demonstrates the nurse's desire to understand the client's communication
Seeking consensual validation	Attempts to reach a mutual denotative and connotative meaning of specific words	Demonstrates the nurse's desire to understand the client's communication
Focusing	Questions or statements to help the client develop or expand an idea	Directs conversation toward topics of importance
Summarizing	Statement of the main areas discussed during an interaction	Helps the client to separate relevant from irrelevant material; serves as a review and closing for the interaction
Planning	Mutual decision making regarding the goals, direction, and so forth of future interactions	Reiterates the client's role within the relationship

From Sundeen, S. J., DeSalvo Rankin, E. A., Stuart, G. W., et al. (1998). *Nurse–client interaction: Implementing the nursing process* (p. 113). St. Louis, MO: Mosby.

scores for nurses and patients were higher in relationships of longer duration and in relationships in which there was more frequency of contact. Reflect on these dimensions to provide yourself with clues to the development of bonds with your clients. Box 2.1 lists dimensions that indicate the patient's and nurse's openness or engagement or the lack thereof.

HOW TO LISTEN

Keep your mind from wandering by focusing your attention on what the person is saying, repeat it in your mind,

and reflect on what it might be like to be in the person's situation. The term *mindful listening* means to be fully present and attentive in the moment on purpose, without trying to change anything or judge anything. Mindful listening is not always easy and gets better with practice (Sheridan, 2016). Take a breath and relax. Consciously set aside your own distractions, knowing that if you are distracted, then you are otherwise attracted: Something else is more important than the other person. This distraction can be communicated nonverbally and undermine being seen as an authentic, caring nurse.

TABLE 2.3   Summary of Nontherapeutic Communication Techniques

Technique	Definition	Therapeutic Threat
Failing to listen	Failure to receive the client's intended message	Places the needs of the nurse above those of the client
Failing to probe	Inadequate data collection represented by eliciting vague descriptions, getting inadequate answers, following standard forms too closely, and not exploring the client's interpretation	Generates an inadequate database on which to make decisions; leads to lack of individualization of client care
Parroting	Continual repetition of the client's phrases	Projects the metacommunication that "I am not listening" or "I am not a competent communicator"
Being judgmental	Approving or disapproving statements	Implies that the nurse has the right to a dependency relationship
Reassuring	Attempts to do magic with words	Negates fears, feelings, and other communications of the client
Rejecting	Refusal to discuss topics with the client	The client may feel that not only communication but also the self was rejected
Defending	Attempts to protect someone or something from negative feedback	Negates the client's right to express an opinion
Getting advice	Declaration to the client of what the nurse thinks should be done	Negates the worth of the client as a mutual partner in decision making
Making stereotyped responses	Use of trite, meaningless verbal expressions	Negates the significance of the client's communication
Changing topics	Nurse's direction of the interaction into areas of self-interest rather than areas of concern to the client	Nonverbally communicates that the nurse is in charge of deciding what will be discussed; may cause topics important to the client to be missed
Patronizing	Style of communication that displays a condescending attitude toward the client	Implies that the client–nurse relationship is not based on equality; places the nurse in a superior position

From Sundeen, S. J., DeSalvo Rankin, E. A., Stuart, G. W., et al. (1998). *Nurse–client interaction: Implementing the nursing process* (p. 117). St. Louis: MO: Mosby.

Am I a good listener?
LISTEN:
1. **L**ook at the other person. Make eye contact without staring.
2. Show **I**nterest in what the other person is saying. Lean forward and use open body language such as uncrossed arms.
3. **S**top talking…listen! Mary Kay said, "God gave us two ears and one mouth for a reason."
4. **T**hink about what the other person is saying, NOT what you plan to say next. Stephen (Covey, 2013) in *The 7 Habits of Highly Effective People* says, "Seek first to understand rather than to be understood."
5. Use **E**mpathy skills such as acknowledging, restating, and reflecting (see Table 2.2).

6. **N**ever assume you know what the other person means. Use questions to clarify until the other person agrees that you understand.

You might use these words to keep the person speaking: "I see. I understand. Good point. I can see that you feel strongly about that. I understand how you could see it like that."

A pattern emerged in the data analysis of a study to explore how undergraduate nursing students experience making a difference in practice settings. This pattern was *concernful* practice. Students experienced knowing and connecting with clients to make a difference. The things they learned by staying with clients and listening helped the students negotiate with staff to make changes in the client's care and contributed to one student's first experience with

BOX 2.1 Bonding between Nurse and Patient: Openness and Engagement

Reflect on the following behaviors as indicators of openness and engagement or the lack thereof on the part of the client/patient and the nurse as indicators of bonding. These dimensions were generated from qualitative research observations and interviews with collaboration from literature validated in the bedside setting.

OPEN

The Patient	The Nurse
Looks at the approaching nurse in seeming anticipation of the nurse's arrival	Greets patient, or returns a greeting verbally or nonverbally
Greets the nurse first/initiates greeting	Pauses to visually check on the patient, seemingly trying to validate the assessment or data
Greets the nurse back in a verbal or nonverbal way (e.g., smiles)	Touches the patient for further assessment
Acknowledges the nurse's statements by replying, smiling, nodding, and similar behaviors	Exchanges friendly/light comments or jokes, showing ease with the patient
Manifests at-ease behaviors such as light comments, friendly remarks/jokes	Makes clarifications, asks follow-up questions for further assessment
Volunteers information and elaborates on the patient's physical condition and past and present health status even when not prompted to do so	Enquires about what the patient already knows (e.g., medications, procedures, hospitalization, and so forth) or what the patient would like to know more about
Verbalizes feelings, psychosocial implication of disease in his or her life	Listens attentively to the verbalization of the patient's feelings, health condition, personal/family information
Talks about support persons and other resources	Asks the patient/family about other pertinent information that may not be in the record but is needed for the care of the patient
Talks about other personal concerns	

NOT OPEN

The Patient	The Nurse
Shows avoidance of the nurse as he or she approaches	Ignores patient's questions or comments
Interrupts the nurse in midsentence	Discourages inquiries from the patient by cutting the patient off in midsentence, or makes remarks suggesting that the patient not make more comments or ask questions
Shows cold treatment toward the nurse (e.g., not looking at the nurse, turning his or her back, focusing on something else during the conversation)	Has a stern or aloof facial expression
Demonstrates irritation through facial expression (e.g., pouting, curt replies, high-pitched tone of voice, impatient gestures)	Focuses on tasks, not maintaining eye contact with the patient
Converses in an angry tone	Projects irritable behavior through facial expression, voice tone, and body language
	Shows hurried behavior through terse replies, brisk movements, and fleeting presence
	Converses in an angry tone

ENGAGED

The Patient	The Nurse
Accepts nursing care without reluctance	Implements needed interventions/procedures promptly and competently
"Prepares" for a procedure by voluntarily assuming the needed position	Completes routine tasks with friendly comments or other manifestations of high regard/caring for the patient
Seeks clarification for proper implementation of care	Acknowledges and addresses inquiries of the patient about care
Demonstrates an understanding/agreement with what the nurse tells him or her and readily follows the nurse's instructions	

Continued

BOX 2.1　Bonding between Nurse and Patient: Openness and Engagement—cont'd

Provides data asked for by the nurse	Volunteers needed information without being asked by the patient or family
Asks about other anticipated procedures or interventions	Touches the patient for reassurance when appropriate
Takes time to respond to questions or asks that questions or instructions be repeated	Provides verbal reassurance

NOT ENGAGED

The Patient	The Nurse
Demonstrates verbal or nonverbal cues of reluctance/refusal to comply with what the nurse says	Attends only to the intravenous line and other routine procedures and ignores the patient
	Scorns the patient's questions by laughing with sarcasm or getting irritated
	Sternly demands that the patient comply with instructions, demonstrating irritation

Adapted from Tejero, L. M. (2009). Development and validation of an instrument to measure nurse-patient bonding. *International Journal of Nursing Studies, 47*, 608–615.

feeling a responsibility toward the client and the client's care (Ironside et al., 2005). In hospice care, it has been suggested that quality of care improves when the care is client centered, as evidenced by "caring conversations." The connections between clients and nurses are made by presence, touch, and listening (Olthuis et al., 2006).

Finally, it is important to be aware that humans are always communicating. According to Watzlawick (1967), when two people are within each other's visual field, communication is always occurring whether we are communicating verbally or nonverbally. Communication experts believe that 60% to 75% of our communication is actually done nonverbally. As mentioned previously, how we hold our body, whether our arms are opened or crossed, whether we are leaning into or away from the person, and whether we are giving direct eye contact or staring vacantly all communicate a message. How that communication is received is dependent on the person's perceptions and worldview (Erickson, 2006). As nurses it is extremely important to be aware of what we are communicating nonverbally to our clients and, in turn, what their nonverbal language is telling us. "The bottom line is, we are communicating any time someone else is attending to us directly or indirectly" (Erickson, 2006).

WIT AND WISDOM

Suppose we were able to share meanings freely without a compulsive urge to impose our view or to conform to those of others and without distortion and self-deception. Would this not constitute a real revolution in culture?

David Bohm

True Presence

And what about technology? What does it mean to be a competent nurse? Remember that the dazzling technology that seems to create miraculous recovery is a means to an end, not an end in itself. Nursing care is person focused, not technology focused (Bernardo, 1998). To be truly present is to bear witness to the client's experience, understand the client's perspective, and respect the client's dignity and rights to self-determination. "Intention to nurse is the dynamic that is expressed through being authentically present with the other in the moment"; it is understanding that the person is complete in this moment and does not need to be fixed or made whole again (Locsin, 2002). Presence, "being with" in contrast to "doing to," is a central role for hospice nurses (Krisman-Scott & McCorkle, 2002).

As I have worked with nurses and nursing students to clarify what it means to be truly "present," I developed the FOCUSED model (Box 2.2), which is inspired by the work of Buber (1958). Buber distinguished between two types of relationships, the I–It and the I–Thou. The I–It relationship can be experienced as nurses do the work of patient care. Teaching and caring can become routine and, although excellent in form, may lack substance or a real connection with the patient. The I–It is the world of "experiencing and using…a typical subject–object relationship." The I–Thou relationship can be experienced only with the entire being. The I–Thou is "characterized by mutuality, directness, presentness, intensity" (Friedman, 1966). "The It is the eternal chrysalis, the Thou the eternal butterfly" (Buber, 1958). This moment of connection is the essence of presence. To be present, a nurse must disconnect from personal distractions and *feel* and *observe* for times to be able to *connect* in what may seem to be small gestures but

BOX 2.2 FOCUSED on Moments of Connection…a Model for Being Present

FOCUS on moments. .connections that make a difference
   The I–It and I–Thou relationship (Buber, 1958)…looking for the sacred
   "What is being in the moment but being in touch with God? Who might also be called the Great Now…" (Cameron, 2002)
   I. **F**eel
      Disconnect from personal distractions. Stay in the moment. Anticipate needs of clients, families, staff, and community. Be fully present, one thing at a time.
   II. **O**bserve
      Look for opportunities to connect. Watch for signs of fear, anxiety, grief, and confusion. Pay attention to verbal and nonverbal cues.
   III. **C**onnect
      Take the initiative to approach. Listen, speak, touch, share, recommend resources, offer silent prayer if appropriate, offer a private place, or offer something to drink.
   IV. **U**nderstand
      Seek first to understand before to be understood (Covey, 2013). Share meaning in the illness experience. Use empathy to share your own experience, offer hope. Consider lessons you can learn.
   V. **S**hare
      Share stories of moments of connection. Celebrate the connections, the gifts of intimate moments. Today and each day… making a difference in the future of healthcare. We define our practice by the stories we tell.
   VI. Now…to stayed FOCUSED…renew your commitment to life balance
      A. **E**nergize…find ways to restore your energy
      B. **D**isconnect…take time to be alone, use inner resources
©1997, Julia Balzer Riley, RN, MN, AHN-BC, REACE.

that take on great importance in times of client's, a family's, or a colleague's state of high anxiety. The nurse seeks to *understand* the person rather than focuses on being understood or heard by the other. Sharing these moments of connection is sharing how we define nursing in small increments of time that make all the difference to those with whom we share. For the nurse to continue to have the energy to be focused on others, to engage in an I–Thou relationship, self-care is essential. The nurse does this by finding ways to *energize,* to take time to *disconnect,* and to have time alone for restoration. Chapters 18 to 20 and 30 will give you specifics on self-care. Remember, it is said that you cannot give what you do not have.

Jean Watson's model of human caring calls these moments *caring moments* that necessitate the nurse to act (Simourd, 2013), guided by "intentionality and consciousness of how to be…fully present, open to the other person, open to compassion and connection, beyond the ego-control focus" (Watson, 2008). Rosemary Rizzo Parse's theory of nursing, human becoming, offers the following: "The nurse in true presence with person or family, is not a guide or a beacon but rather an inspiring attentive presence that calls the other to shed light on the meaning moments of his or her life…The person is coauthor of his or her own health…" (Parse, 1992, p. 40).

SIMPLIFY AND DEEPEN

The enemy of the good is the better. What if you could extend compassion to yourself, forgiving yourself from being imperfect, learning from your mistakes or missteps?

MOMENTS OF CONNECTION…

A nurse faculty member, who is also a Parse Scholar, shares a story from a nurse patient who experienced "true presence."

Ele is a 54-year-old active woman with congenital mitral prolapse. She was shocked when she was told by her cardiologist that she needed cardiac surgery. Her cardiac surgeon said she was an excellent candidate for a minimally invasive cardiac surgical technique to insert a ring into her heart through the space between two ribs on her right side. The surgery would diminish the mitral regurgitation, giving her back the stamina she had slowly lost for her regular exercise routine. However, her surgeon also pointed out that potential complications of the surgery could lead to death.

As Ele began her hospitalization for open heart surgery, she was bombarded with the multiple nameless nurses who focused on tasks required for surgery. Ele remembers feeling like "nothing." Yet she recalls the time she spent with Sue, a nurse who demonstrated true presence. Sue introduced herself as she sat down beside Ele's bed and asked what would be most helpful at that time. After Ele's questions were answered, Sue asked, "What is it like for you right now to be awaiting open-heart surgery?" Ele shared that it was a new experience for her and that she was used to being on the other side of the bed as a nurse in a cardiovascular intensive care unit, knowing the possible positive and negative outcomes. They talked about that paradox of confidence in the surgeon, while knowing the risks. Sue asked what were her hopes and dreams. Ele said she saw herself being very active again. Ele shared, too, that she wished to make the surgery look easy so she could alleviate her daughter's anxieties because her daughter may need to undergo the same surgery. Ele expressed her tear-filled emotions in speaking and in silence as Sue waited patiently accepting the silences to fill the air and Ele to speak when she was ready. She described her hopes to stay positive and determined for a successful surgery. Sue left her lingering presence—a calming, much appreciated connection—which made a difference in Ele's recovery.

Catherine Aquino-Russell, RN, BScN, MN, PhD, professor, University of New Brunswick, Moncton Campus, Canada

Nurses and organizations are working internationally to understand and demonstrate caring behaviors. At the University of Montreal, researchers are testing the Caring Nurse Observation Tool (CNOT) to measure verbal and nonverbal caring interactions (Cossette & Forbes, 2012). In the United Kingdom 79 wards in Nottingham University Hospitals are implementing the Caring Around the Clock program, which offers intentional hourly rounding to anticipate fundamental care needs (Hutchings et al., 2013). Snellman and Gedda (2012) in Sweden wrote that six values in nursing are worth striving for including "trust, nearness, sympathy, support, knowledge, and responsibility." They suggested that caring encounters and ethical dialog are prerequisites for demonstrating these values.

Dr. Sullivan, dean of the School of Nursing at the University of Virginia, at the fall 2013 convocation, spoke of the "power of pause" in healthcare, which are brief mindful breaks that build resilience to stress and make it possible for healthcare staff to be fully present and to pay careful attention to patients. At this university medical center, staff take time to pause and reflect after a crisis. Research demonstrated that multitasking reduces productivity and that distractibility causes stress. The University of Virginia's Contemplative Science Center integrates mindfulness practices such as meditation throughout the curriculum to destress, pay more attention, and create meaning and wisdom (Kelly, 2013). Cashman (2012) referred to "the Pause Principle" as stepping back to lead forward. Cashman suggested that leaders pause and reflect before acting to create vision, clarity, and understanding.

WIT AND WISDOM

When things begin accelerating wildly out of control, sometimes patience is the only answer. Press pause.

Douglas Rushkof

In a study of the "technologically induced vulnerability and the inherent uncertainty" of clients undergoing bone marrow transplantation, one participant said, "Care was the nurse just being there" (Cooper & Powell, 1998). When clients did not feel like banter or small talk, they could be "certain of the presence of the nurse" (Cooper & Powell, 1998). This research "depicts a caring presence that appears to transcend the distractions of technology and acknowledged a kinship with patients that derived from an acknowledgment of their shared human experience" (Younger, 1995).

The nurse implements the nursing process based on the client's experience and clarifies the client's and nurse's "responsibilities, expectations, opportunities, and accountabilities" (Bernardo, 1998). "True presence is grounded in nursing science, the essence of nursing as a scholarly discipline" (Lynaugh & Fagin, 1988). Presence, at the very core of nursing practice, is the art of nursing. Moments of "intense presencing, although they may be physiologically driven in our highly technological environment of healthcare today, are 'moments of truth' for both the patient and the nurse, the unique opportunity, with artful caring and expert practice, for nurses to use their hearts and their hands to create a moment in which healing can begin" (Wendler, 2002).

Competence in the advanced technology of critical care nursing has been described as a component of caring, and this view is supported by nurse theorists (Newman, 1999; Orem, 2001; Parse, 1992; Rogers, 1985). The suggestion is made that technological competence is another way of knowing more about the client. The helping relationship uses this information to deliver nursing care that focuses on this person in this moment who is a person with a desire to live fully as a human being with his or her own hopes and dreams and vision of himself or herself. The challenge then is to be competent in many ways and to be able to use technology and follow critical pathways to deliver nursing care to a unique person. Building your skills in communication in the helping relationship helps you and the client find meaning in moments of connection.

BECOMING A STORYCATCHER

Baldwin (2005) said that a storycatcher is a practitioner of the heart of language. Story creates context, context highlights relationships and leads to holistic and connected action, and connected action becomes a force for restoring/restorying the world. Baldwin said that we have lost the space for story and may have lost the understanding of how essential storytelling is to who we are.

Consider these qualities of a storycatcher and see how attention to these might deepen your understanding of clients' experiences as reflected in their stories. Storycatchers are intrigued by human experience; inquisitive about meaning and insight; curious and not judgmental; more in love with questions than answers; able to hold personal boundaries in relationships; present while others experience emotions and have insight; able to hold the sacred space for listening; able to invite forgiveness, release, and grace; and aware of the power of story and use it consciously.

Hearing the client's story is an important assessment tool that allows nurses to access a client's self-care knowledge and gain greater understanding of their worldview (Erickson, Personal communication, 2011). By listening to a person's story, the nurse is able to learn what is important to the client and begin to create a personalized plan of care.

 MOMENTS OF CONNECTION...

In a contribution to this chapter, Margaret Erickson shared the following story. On entering the room, she introduced herself to the older gentleman who had been admitted for angina to rule out myocardial infarction. She asked why he thought he was in the hospital. He replied, "You can check my chart. It is all in there." She replied, "I want to hear your story and why you think you are here." He replied, "My wife and I were married for 61 years. She was my other half and best friend. She died 6 months ago, and I am heartbroken." Based on his story she developed a holistic plan of care that helped him deal with his loss and grief. His angina disappeared.

Return to "Active Learning" at the beginning of the chapter and write your responses.

PRACTICING THE CLIENT–NURSE RELATIONSHIP

Critical Thinking/Discussion/Reflective Journaling: Exercise 1

Identify a time when you knew someone was really listening to you. How could you tell the person was listening mindfully? How does it feel to be listened to? How does it make you feel? Discuss your answers with a classmate or write about it in your journal.

Critical Thinking: Exercise 2

Read the following poetic journal entry written by a nurse after a surgical admission. Identify which of the therapeutic communications techniques in Table 2.2 might not have been used by the nurses assigned to this patient. Do you think these nurses did not "care" for this patient? If you

learned a patient had written such comments, what could the nurses on this unit do, given time constraints, to help this patient feel more cared for?

> *I came to you...patient.*
> *You scurried, in all directions*
> *Returning only to scan a wrist band,*
> *Give a pill, check lung sounds.*
> *I leave you...in-patient.*
> *Transforming from in-patient*
> *To person healing...*
> *Little thanks to you.*
> *The leavings of your time,*
> *Too "well" to deserve*
> *Your full attention*
> *Too "sick" to be totally ignored.*
> *Did you have a*
> *Calling to nursing?*
> *If so, when did you*
> *Stop listening?*
> *Heart of nursing, weakened*
> *Barely beating...I pray*
> *For your resuscitation now*
> *And at every remaining moment of your career.*

Reflective Journaling/Discussion: Exercise 3

Review the content on "Moments of Connection," and in your journal write about a time when you feel you made a difference with a client, family member, or colleague. Share this with a classmate or colleagues in a staff meeting in which others are asked to do the same. I believe we define our nursing practice by the stories we share and combat burnout by remembering who we are and what we do. Continue to collect these in your journal.

Skill Building/Critical Incident: Exercise 4

Identify a time when you think you missed an opportunity to connect with a client, family member, or colleague, perhaps, when you were not fully present. Record this in your journal and write how you could have handled it differently. Continue to collect these in your journal.

Skill Building/Discussion: Exercise 5

Interview someone, perhaps a classmate, who has been hospitalized or had contact with a nurse or nurses in any medical setting. Using open-ended questions, encourage the person to relate the personal story of experiencing the care of a nurse. Look for what this person saw as positive and supportive or negative and nonsupportive. Reflect on this anecdotal evidence and discuss what you learned without breaching confidentiality.

Quality and Safety Education for Nurses Learning Strategy: Exercise 6

Student Nurse Jane is checking her patient's medication to be sure she is applying the five rights of medication administration: right patient, right medication, right dosage, right delivery method, and right time. She enters the patient's room, verifies patient identifiers, calls his name, and offers him two oral medications. The patient looks at the pills and asks: "Why am I getting a blue pill today? I usually get a green pill."

- How should Jane respond?
- In developing the nurse–patient relationship, how can patients and their families be included as part of the care team so that they become safety allies?

SIMPLIFY AND DEEPEN

The enemy of the good is the better. What if you could extend compassion to yourself, forgiving yourself for being imperfect and learning from your mistakes or missteps?

REFERENCES

ANA Code of Ethics. (2015). Code of ethics for nurses with interpretative statements. Retrieved from https://www.nursingworld.org/coe-view-only.

Ballesion, A., Lombardo, C., Lucidi, F., & Violani, C. (2020). *Journal of Sleep Research*. https://doi.org/10.1111/jsr.1309630(1)e13096.

Baldwin, C. (2005). *Storycatcher: Making sense of our lives through the power and practice of story*. Novato, CA: New World Library.

Bernardo, A. (1998). Technology and true presence in nursing. *Holistic Nursing Practice, 12*(4), 40.

Bickford, C. J., Marion, L., & Gazaway, S. (2015). *American Nurses Association*. In *Nursing: Scope and Standards of Clinical Nursing Practice* (3rd ed.). MD: Silver Spring. Nursebooks.org.

Brittany, M., Gomez, C., Furst, C., & Rasmussen-Winkler (2021). Facilitating virtual visitation in critical care units during a pandemic. *Holist Nurs Pract, 35*(2), 60–64. doi:10.1097/HNP.0000000000000432.

Buber, M. (1958). *I and Thou*. New York, NY: Harper & Row.

Cameron, J. (2002). *The artist's way*. Los Angeles, CA: Jeremy P. Tarcher.

Cashman, K. (2012). *The pause principle: Step back to lead forward*. San Francisco, CA: Berrett Koehler Publishers.

Cooper, M. C., & Powell, E. (1998). Technology and care in a bone marrow transplant unit: Creating and assuaging vulnerability. *Holistic Nursing Practice, 12*(4), 57.

Cossette, S., & Forbes, C. (2012). Psychometric evaluation of the caring nurse observation tool: Scale development. *International Journal for Human Caring, 16*(1), 16.

Covey, S. R. (2013). *The 7 habits of highly effective people*. New York, NY: Simon & Schuster.

Erickson, H. (Ed.). (2006). *Modeling and role-modeling: A view from the clients' world*. Cedar Park, TX: Unicorns Unlimited.

Erickson, H., Tomlin, E., & Swain, M. A. (1983). *Modeling and role-modeling: A theory and paradigm for nursing*. Englewood Cliffs, NJ: Prentice Hall.

Erickson, M. (2011). Personal communication.

Friedman, M. S. (1966). *The life of dialogue*. New York, NY: Harper & Row.

Gaines, K. (2022). Retrieved from Nurses Ranked as the Most Trusted Profession for 20 Years in a Row | Nurse.org Accessed 03/22/22 at Nursing Ranked as the Most Trusted Profession for 20th Year in a Row (nurse.org).

Groves, P. S., Bunch, J. L., Sabasosa, K. A., Cannava, K. E., & Williams, J. K. (2021). A grounded theory of creating space for open safety communication between hospitalized patients and nurses. *Nurs Outlook, 69*, 632. doi:10.1016/j.outlook.2021.01.005.

Guillaumie, L., Boiral, O., Desgroseilliers, V., Vonarx, N., & Roy, B. (2020). Empowering nurses to provide humanized care in Canadian hospital care units. *Holistic Nurs Pract, 00*(00), 1–16. doi:10.1097/HNP.0000000000000418.

Hagerty, T. A., Samuels, W., Norcini-Pala, A., & Gigliotti, E. (2017). Peplau's theory of interpersonal relations: An alternate factor structure for patient experience data. *Nurs Sci Q, 30*(2), 160–167. doi:10.1177/0894318417693286.

Hutchings, M., Ward, P., & Bloodworth, K. (2013). 'Caring around the clock': A new approach to intentional rounding. *Nursing Management, 20*(5), 24.

Ironside, P., Diekelmann, N., & Hirschmann, M. (2005). Learning the practices of knowing and connecting: The voices of students. *Journal of Nursing Education, 44*(4), 153.

Kelly, M. (2013). President Sullivan confers intermediate honors, presents Jefferson Awards. Retrieved from http://news.virginia.edu/content/president-sullivan-confers-intermediate-honors-presents-jefferson-awards.

Krisman-Scott, M. A., & McCorkle, R. (2002). The tapestry of hospice. *Holistic Nursing Practice, 16*(2), 32.

Locsin, R. C. (2002). Culture of nursing, preoccupation with prediction, and nursing intention. *Holistic Nursing Practice, 16*(4), 1.

Lynaugh, J., & Fagin, C. (1988). Nursing comes of age. *Image, 20*, 184.

Massey, A, & Lodha, C. P. (2021). A review on little hands of God and love therapy. *International Journal of Research in Engineering, Science, and Management, 4*(7), 342–343.

Myers, I. B. (1995). *Gifts differing*. Palo Alto, CA: Consulting Psychologists Press.

Myers, I. B. (1998). *Introduction to type*. Palo Alto, CA: Consulting Psychologists Press.

Newman, M. (1999). *Health as expanding consciousness*. Bloomington, IN: iUniverse.

Olthuis, G., Dekkers, W., Leget, C., et al. (2006). The caring relationship in hospice care: An analysis based on the ethics of the caring conversation. *Nursing Ethics, 13*(1), 29.

Orem, D. (2001). *Nursing: Concepts of practice*. St. Louis, MO: Mosby.

Parse, R. R. (1992). Human becoming: Parse's theory of nursing. *Nursing Science Quarterly, 5*(1), 35.

Rogers, M. (1985). Science of unitary human beings: A paradigm for nursing. In R. Wood, & J. Kekahbah (Eds.), *Examining the cultural implications of Martha Rogers' science of unitary human beings*. Lecompton, KS: Wood- Kekahbah Associates.

Sheridan, C. (2016). The mindful nurse: Using the power of mindfulness and compassion to help you thrive in your work. Retrieved from http://www.rivertimepress.com.

Sherwood, G. (2021). Quality and safety education for nurses: Making progress in patient safety, learning from COVID-19. *International Journal of Nursing Sciences, 8*, 249–251. doi:10.1016/j.ijnss.2021.05.009.

Simourd, J. (2013). Essay: Caring is part of all nursing. *International Journal of Human Caring, 17*(1), 86.

Smith, J. A. (1981). The idea of health: A philosophical inquiry. *Advances in Nursing Science, 3*(3), 45–50.

Snellman, I., & Gedda, K. M. (2012). The value ground of nursing. *Nursing Ethics, 19*(6), 714.

Stuart, G. W. (2012). *Principles and practice of psychiatric nursing* (10th ed.). St. Louis, MO: Mosby.

Tejero, L. M. (2009). Development and validation of an instrument to measure nurse–patient bonding. *International Journal of Nursing Studies, 47*, 608–615.

Watson, J. (2008). *Nursing: The philosophy and science of caring.* Boulder, CO: University Press of Colorado.

Watzlawick, P. (1967). *Pragmatics of human communication: A study of interactional patterns, pathologies, and paradoxes.* New York, NY: W. W. Norton & Company.

Wendler, M. C. (2002). *The HeART of nursing.* Indianapolis, IN: Sigma Theta Tau International Honor Society of Nursing.

Way, F., Shah, Q., Shaheen, A., & Caroll, K. (2021). Peplau's theory of interpersonal relations: A case study. *Nurs Sci Q, 34*(4), 368–371. doi:10.1177/08943184211031573.

Wood, D. (2018). Compassionate care affects patient outcomes. Retrieved from https://www.travelnursing.com/news/nurse-news/nurses-compassionate-care-affects-patient-outcomes.

Younger, J. B. (1995). The alienation of the sufferer. *Advances in Nursing Science, 17*, 53.

3

Starting with YOU: Understanding Yourself to Build a Foundation for Learning about Communication*

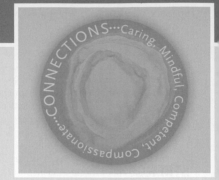

Knowing yourself is the beginning of all wisdom.

Aristotle

OBJECTIVES

1. Recognize the need for self-assessment as a starting point for building communication skills.
2. Learn to identify your own personal strengths.
3. Describe how each person's unique combination of personal strengths can be applied to concepts of communication.
4. Identify four key domains of emotional intelligence, and use tools to identify competency levels.
5. Describe interventions for improving in lower rated areas of emotional intelligence.

6. List five major modes of conflict management, and identify your preferred mode.
7. Identify personal strengths that could be used to learn to use all modes of conflict management as appropriate to the situation.
8. Begin to apply concepts of self-understanding to building responsible, assertive, caring communication skills.

If we are to apply the nursing process to the journey toward caring, assertive, and responsible communication, we must start with a personal assessment to determine your readiness for the journey. What are your natural talents, attributes, and life skills that will assist you in growing your communication skills? How can you know these things about yourself? How will knowing these things help you achieve excellence in your nursing career?

Most of us have tried out some of those Facebook posts that pretend to tell us something profound about ourselves based on whatever information it gleans from our posted data. These are fun and interesting and maybe sometimes frighteningly accurate, but they are not something on which to base your life plan. However, there are some strongly evidence-based, valid, and reliable tools available that can help you make a realistic personal assessment of yourself and build a foundation for applying the vital communication concepts and techniques that are addressed later in this text.

This chapter will assist you in considering areas of talents and strengths that can be used to build your communication skills. It will also challenge you to consider the importance of emotional intelligence (EI) and ways that you can personally grow in this area to enhance your communication with clients and colleagues (Raeissi et al., 2019).

? ACTIVE LEARNING

Think about how you will write your answers as you read each chapter.

What?
Write one thing you learned from this chapter.

So What?
How will this affect your nursing practice?

Now What?
How will you implement this new knowledge or skill?

Think About It …

---

* With contributions from Lyndel Walker, MSN, RN.

Research supports the importance of nurse managers' EI in building team culture and decreasing staff turnover (Majeed et al., 2021). And finally, it will discuss modes of conflict management and how you can apply each of these modes to various situations in your nursing practice. Once you have identified where you are with these foundational building blocks for communication, you will be ready to pack them in your bags as you launch into the journey to caring, assertive, and responsible communication.

STRENGTHS ASSESSMENT

The idea of focusing on personal strengths as opposed to weaknesses was birthed from the Positive Psychology movement that came to prominence around the year 2000. Positive Psychology is now considered a branch of the discipline of psychology that complements the traditional focus on pathology. It focuses on the study of human strengths and virtues and the factors that contribute to a full and meaningful life (Lino, 2016).

Peter Drucker, business professor and guru, made the following observation back in 1967: "one cannot build on weakness. To achieve results, one has to use all the available strengths… These strengths are the true opportunities" (Drucker, 1967, p. 60). Donald Clifton, psychology professor and former chairperson of Gallup, suggested that the two most consistently prevalent assumptions of human nature (that anyone can learn to be competent at almost anything and that a person's areas of greatest potential for growth are in their areas of greatest weakness) are flawed (Hodges & Clifton, 2004). The concept of identifying and focusing on your strengths is based on the idea that when you are using your greatest strengths, you are more engaged, more productive, more successful, healthier, and happier. In other words, by focusing on our strengths, we have less need to worry about fixing our weaknesses and have more opportunity to experience success.

If a baseball player is really good at being a catcher, will the coach force him to focus on his "weak area" and try to turn him into a great pitcher? No, he will encourage him to learn more about catching the ball and how to develop that talent until he is the very best catcher in the league. Too often we focus on our weak areas, thinking that we need to get better in those areas. What if we identify and focus on our strengths and learn to use them to accomplish our goals, whatever they may be? Two comprehensive, evidence-based measures of strengths are now available to help you identify your areas of strength: the Clifton StrengthsFinder, produced through Gallup, which is an analytics and advice organization, and the Values in Action (VIA) Inventory of Strengths, which can be found on the Authentic Happiness website associated with the University of Pennsylvania (Rettew & Lopez, 2008).

According to Clifton et al. (2006), a strength begins with a talent, which is a naturally recurring pattern of thought, feeling, or behavior that can be productively applied. Your own set of talents is what helps to make you the unique person that you are. When you do something well, you are using one or more of your talents, and each of your talents can be applied to multiple areas of performance. Through their research, Gallup identified the 34 most prevalent talent themes and developed the StrengthsFinder assessment tool to measure these. Strengths are defined as the ability to provide consistent, near-perfect performance in a given activity (Clifton et al., 2006). Your natural talents have the potential to become your strengths when refined over time with knowledge and skill (Box 3.1). In the virtual conference, Creating Healthy Work Environments 2021, research was presented to support the integration of knowledge about EI and strengths for leaders and educators (Christman et al., 2021).

The VIA (Peterson & Seligman, 2004) The classification of strengths is based on the belief that strengths are the lived manifestations of virtues and are associated with well-being. It measures 24 character strengths that define what is best about people. These are organized under six over-arching virtues (wisdom and knowledge, courage, humanity, justice, temperance, and transcendence). The VIA list is intended to provide a shared language for describing human strengths. It has been described as the backbone of Positive Psychology. This concept of identifying and focusing on strengths is meant to balance the fact that we already have had shared language for the negative side of psychology in the form of diagnostic terminology (see Box 3.1).

Discovering your strengths has been compared with stumbling across your living room in the dark and then finally making it to the light switch (Rettew & Lopez, 2008). Although you can make it across because of your familiarity with the room and its structures, having the light on makes it much easier. The light of discovery illuminates what you already knew about yourself and gives you terms to describe those things. As demonstrated in the way that those fortune-telling tests on Facebook keep making the rounds, humans have a tendency to be attracted to labels. Labeling things, including ourselves, can give us an improved understanding as well as language to discuss them.

Both of the strengths assessments described previously are available to complete online. The VIA is free of charge for basic information about your results. Expanded information is available for a fee. The Clifton StrengthsFinder

---

BOX 3.1 Strengths Assessments

Gallup StrengthsFinder: https://www.gallupstrengths-center.com/home/en-us

VIA Survey: https://www.viacharacter.org/survey/account/register

has a minimal fee but offers expanded explanations and a number of resources including a book to go along with it so that you can apply the concepts specifically to yourself. Included at the end of this chapter are some suggested application exercises that are less evidence based but will give some meaningful insight into your own strengths. Complete Application Exercises 1A and 1B, then analyze your results as directed and compare them with the lists of strengths from the Clifton StrengthsFinder or the VIA character strengths website. Using this information, you should be able to select a top five list that will closely correspond to what you would find when completing the actual assessments (see Box 3.2).

BOX 3.2   Strengths Lists and Descriptions

List of Clifton StrengthsFinder Theme Descriptions (PDF) is available here: http://news.gallup.com/poll/166991/clifton-strengthsfinder-theme-descriptions-pdf.aspx

Full description of each strength is available here: https://www.strengthsquest.com/193541/themes-full-description.aspx

VIA Character Strengths list is available here with expanded information about each when you click on the symbol: http://www.viacharacter.org/www/Character-Strengths

---

🌹 MOMENTS OF CONNECTION…

A nurse friend of mine shared this story with me. Her grandfather was in the hospital in another state far away from her. He was clearly in his last days, and as he lay there, he called out to a nurse as she passed his doorway. Although she was not assigned to him that day, she came into the room to check on what he needed. "Would you sing for me," he requested. "What would you like me to sing," she asked. The elderly gentleman was a part of a small denomination church that used hymns unique to their faith. Amazingly, as he requested hymn after hymn, she was able to sing each beautifully and drew an audience outside the door beside the very appreciative listener in the bed. What a unique gift she was able to give at this specific time and place for this gentleman. Not only was it a blessing to him, but it was also a comfort to his family, including my friend who was unable to be present with her grandfather. In all probability, no other nurse on that unit that day could have done this.

What are the unique talents/strengths you have that you will be able to use to make a difference in the lives of your

patients? Your unique combination of talents that you grow into strengths will help you to master the communication skills identified in this text and to grow in your profession as a nurse. Who knows when a unique strength of yours will be required to comfort a patient, solve a problem, or even lead a movement? Identifying your talents and learning to build on them will be a good first step to fulfilling all the potential you have within you.

BENEFITS OF DISCOVERING YOUR STRENGTHS

The following are just a few of the benefits that you can experience when you identify your top talents/strengths and begin to use them:

- You will become more aware of your talents and strengths, which will give you labels that you can use and let you discover new ways to apply them.
- It provides validation for some things you felt about yourself but were not entirely sure of. You will gain confidence in doing things you may have felt unsure about in the past.
- You will be able to feel appreciation/thankfulness for your talents and how they have affected your life. Sometimes we are embarrassed about some of the things that make us feel "different." Labeling this "difference" as a "strength" will change your attitude about it.
- You will gain a new excitement for life and the potential that you now see for yourself.
- You will have increased discernment about when to say "no" to activities that do not correspond to your areas of strength. You will feel empowered to say, "that is not a good fit for my talents."
- Knowing your talents/strengths will help you to choose to do the things you have the potential to do best. It will give you more focus for your career and your life.

🌹 MOMENTS OF CONNECTION…

Each year, the students in my interprofessional communications class complete the StrengthsQuest assessment. After discussing the results in small groups, they report their strengths to the class. With each one, I find myself agreeing with the results and being struck by what a great group of strengths this is for a nurse. Each list of five strengths is unique in its combination and ranking, and yet each one sounds perfect for a nurse to have. They will each apply their strengths in different ways as they grow into professional nurses. Keeping in mind their strengths, nurses can find the best environment for using their strengths and for providing their best care to their patients.

MOMENTS OF CONNECTION...

Brandy had been pressured by her instructor to join a professional group based on her high grade point average from school. The group prided itself on its high admission standards and exclusivity. Brandy somehow could not feel comfortable in the group and did not really feel an affinity for its mission. When she did a StrengthsQuest assessment and found that Includer was one of her top five strengths, she felt validated in her feelings and had the freedom to resign from the group and focus her efforts in a direction she felt more called to.

WIT AND WISDOM

Everyone should carefully observe which way his heart draws him, and then choose that way with all his strength.

Jewish proverb

OTHER SELF-ASSESSMENTS

Identifying your natural talents and making plans to develop these into full-fledged strengths is a good start in completing a self-assessment that will get you going on the journey to quality communication skills. Your strengths as measured in the assessments discussed previously are considered to be something you are born with. Although you can further develop these, and there may be times that some will become more prominent than others, they are not likely to change. Next, we are going to discuss a couple of other assessment areas that can be used to further expand your self-understanding. Using these assessments will help you to see where you are strong and highlight areas in which you have room to change and grow.

Self-Care Nudge

What is one self-care practice you can try right now? Stand up and stretch. Walk a few minutes wherever you are. Close your eyes and breathe? Or?

Emotional Intelligence

The term, *emotional intelligence* was first coined by Salovey and Mayer in 1990; however, Daniel Goleman (1995) popularized the concept in his book, *Emotional Intelligence: Why It Can Matter More than IQ*, in 1995. EI is the "something" in each of us that is a bit intangible. It affects how we manage behavior, navigate social complexities, and make personal decisions that achieve positive results (Bleich & Kist,

2013). It is believed that our EI potential can be developed into emotional competence with practice. Goleman et al. (2013) described the four basic domains for EI under two categories. The first category is Personal Competence and within that are the domains of self-awareness and self-management. The second category is Social Competence which contains the domains of social awareness and relationship management (see Box 3.3 for associated competencies for each of these). It has been demonstrated by many research studies that high EI is a more accurate predictor of success in life than a high intelligence quotient (IQ).

It is easy to see how having high EI that involves understanding oneself and others would contribute to quality communication in nursing. Codier and Codier (2017) have identified multiple research studies that demonstrate the importance of EI in nursing. These include areas of workplace functioning, quality patient-centered care, communication in therapeutic relationships, compassionate care, and teamwork and collaboration. Based on these studies, the authors conclude that EI in nurses is requisite for safer patient care. They recommend incorporating EI education skills into nursing education, specifically as they are used in interpersonal communication, interviewing, teamwork, leadership development, and conflict resolution (Codier & Codier, 2017).

Without strong self-reflective skills we cannot grow in EI. Without good self-understanding, work becomes routine and relationships with others will suffer. The emotionally intelligent nurse will have an awareness of individuals, family members, and their community, which is the focus of caregiving. They will have enhanced organization skills having invested in relationships. They will be able to collaborate, show insight into others, and commit to self-growth. The emotionally intelligent nurse is able to connect clinical tasks to critical thinking and action and demonstrates professionalism in all that they do.

There are several ways that you can assess your level of EI. You may want to start by completing Application Exercise 2. There are many free assessments available online as well. See Box 3.4 for a list of a few. If you go online for this testing, you will want to check that the test you do is from a reliable source.

Once you have assessed your level of EI, what can you do with the results? There are many resources available to help you examine ways of raising your EI. You may want to explore some of these resources, which include books and online websites. Listed next are just a few things in each of the four domains that you could do to grow in this vital area. Journaling in each of these areas would be especially helpful in your assessment and growth.

Self-Awareness

- Know your story and how it affects you.
- Make peace with your past and practice forgiveness.

BOX 3.3 Emotional Intelligence Domains and Associated Competencies

Personal Competence: These Capabilities Determine How We Manage Ourselves

Self-Awareness

- Emotional self-awareness: Reading one's own emotions and recognizing their affect; using "gut sense" to guide decisions
- Accurate self-assessment: Knowing one's strengths and limits
- Self-confidence: A sound sense of one's self-worth and capabilities

Self-Management

- Emotional self-control: Keeping disruptive emotions and impulses under control
- Transparency: Displaying honesty, integrity, and trustworthiness
- Adaptability: Flexibility in adapting to changing situations or overcoming obstacles
- Achievement: The drive to improve performance to meet inner standards of excellence
- Initiative: Readiness to act and seize opportunities
- Optimism: Seeing the upside in events

Social Competence

Social Awareness

- Empathy: Sensing others' emotions, understanding their perspective, and taking active interest in their concerns
- Organizational awareness: Reading the currents, decision networks, and politics at the organizational level

Service: Recognizing and Meeting Follower, Client, or Customer Needs

Relationship Management

- Inspirational leadership: Guiding and motivating with a compelling vision
- Influence: Wielding a range of tactics for persuasion
- Developing others: Bolstering others' abilities through feedback and guidance
- Change catalyst: Initiating, managing, and leading in a new direction
- Conflict management: Resolving disagreements
- Building bonds: Cultivating and maintaining a web of relationships
- Teamwork and collaboration: Cooperation and team building

From Goleman, D., Boyatzis, R., & McKee, A. (2013). *Primal leadership: Unleashing the power of emotional intelligence* (p. 39). Boston MA: Harvard Business Review Press.

- Know your beliefs, your emotions, and your behavior patterns.
- Take time to identify your individual feelings and emotions, such as anger, sadness, fear, and joy in various situations.

Self-Management

- Learn new stress management techniques that will help you stay emotionally present in upsetting situations.
- Learn skills for soothing and motivating yourself.
- Maintain healthy eating and exercise habits.

Social Awareness

- Work at understanding nonverbal social signals by focusing on the other person in interactions.
- Develop a positive view of others.
- Work at understanding the basic human emotional needs of your clients and colleagues.
- Understand "games" people play and principles of personal integrity.
- Discomfort when hearing others express certain views tells you something important about yourself. Examine your responses and the reasons for them.

Relationship Management

- Develop skills for reflective listening and developing your capacity for empathy.
- Become aware of ways you use nonverbal communication.
- Learn skills for healthy assertiveness.
- Learn conflict resolution skills; see conflict as an opportunity to grow closer to others.
- Develop skills for support and affirmation of others by becoming an encourager.
- Use humor and play to relieve stress.
  This is adapted from Segal et al. (2018).

WIT AND WISDOM

If your emotional abilities aren't in hand, if you don't have self-awareness, if you are not able to manage your distressing emotions, if you can't have empathy and have effective relationships, then no matter how smart you are, you are not going to get very far.

Daniel Goleman

BOX 3.4 Online Emotional Intelligence Tests

Psychology Today — 146 questions
It is free to take the test and receive a snapshot report. You may purchase the full results for a small fee: https://www.psychologytoday.com/us/test/3203

Mind Tools — 15 questions — free
This one is quick and easy and can give you some baseline information: https://www.mindtools.com/pages/article/ei-quiz.htm

Institute for Health and Human Potential — 17 questions — free
A research company dedicated to helping organizations leverage the science of emotional intelligence: https://www.ihhp.com/free-eq-quiz/

Talent Smart — 28 questions — $$
This is a consulting firm cofounded by emotional intelligence expert Travis Bradberry. Although there is a charge for this test, it includes an unlimited e-learning program with a Goal-Tracking System, emotional intelligence (EQ) lessons, and free retest to track your progress: http://www.talentsmart.com/products/emotional-intelligence-appraisal.php

CONFLICT MANAGEMENT

Conflict can be defined as a disagreement in values or beliefs within oneself or between people that causes harm or has the potential to cause harm. Folger et al. (2012) added that conflict results from the interaction of interdependent people who perceive incompatibility and the potential for interference. Conflict is also a catalyst for change; in fact, some have proposed that conflict is necessary for change. Conflict may widely be considered negative in nature, but it can actually stimulate either detrimental or beneficial effects. Much depends on the manner in which the conflict is handled.

Assessing conflict management skills can provide some additional information about yourself that will help you on your journey to quality communication. Kenneth Thomas (2002) is one of the creators of the Thomas Killman Instrument (TKI), which helps people identify their preferred modes for conflict management. He uses assertiveness and cooperativeness as the most basic dimensions for describing choices for dealing with conflict situations. Assertiveness would be the degree to which you try to satisfy your own concerns, and cooperativeness is the degree to which you try to satisfy the other person's concerns. Assertiveness would be the degree to which you try to satisfy your own concerns while cooperativeness is the degree to which you try to satisfy the other person's concerns. The five modes of conflict handling contain these two concepts in various combination.

The five modes of conflict management identified by Thomas (2002) as well as many others who have done work in this arena are as follows:

Competing: This mode is very assertive but lacking in cooperativeness. The person utilizing this mode is determined to get their own way with no regard for the concerns of the other person. This approach results in a win-lose solution and only one party gets their way.

Collaborating: This mode is a balance between assertiveness and cooperation. Participants using this mode work together to find a solution that satisfies both parties. Collaboration requires extra time and patience to reach the ideal, win-win solution making it less than ideal for situations that need a quick solution.

Compromising: An intermediate answer that only partially satisfies both people's concerns. Each person gives in to some degree and loses some of what they wanted in the process. Although we normally think of compromise as a good thing, this is considered a lose-lose solution since neither party really gets what they wanted.

Avoiding: This mode is both unassertive and uncooperative. The avoidant person does not even air their concerns and the other person gets whatever they wanted. Neither concern is actually addressed, but this is considered a lose-win solution because the other person does get their way.

Accommodating: This mode is very cooperative but lacks assertiveness. The accommodating person chooses to consider the other person's issues without asserting their own wants or needs. This is also considered a lose-win situation. The accommodator has chosen to satisfy the other persons concerns at the expense of their own.

So, which is the best conflict management mode to use? The answer is all of them. Each of these conflict management styles are effective for specific situations. Each of them has benefits and drawbacks to their use. In an emergency situation, the competing mode may be needed for a quick and effective solution. Collaborating may seem like the ideal method because it is a win-win solution, but sometimes there is no time for that and a compromise is necessary for a quicker decision. Avoiding may seem like the most negative mode, but we have all chosen to walk away from a situation that we had a strong opinion about after deciding it really was not worth the effort to get our way. Being in a service-oriented profession, nurses may have a strong tendency toward being accommodating when it comes to conflict situations, but is that always what is best for our patients? We must consider whether it is truly the most assertive, responsible, and caring solution or whether some assertiveness is called for to have the best outcome for our patient.

By completing a conflict management assessment (Box 3.5), you can discover which of the conflict management styles you tend to use most frequently. Once you have determined your most dominant style(s) you will want to take an honest look at some specific situations in your life and determine whether there are better ways to deal with them. Remember this is one of those assessments that is meant to help you grow and change. Which of your strengths identified earlier in this chapter could you use to try some of the conflict management modes that have not been "normal" for you? Note that when we talked about EI, conflict management skills were mentioned as a part of high EI. Consequently, growing in EI and being more aware of your own conflict management tendencies as well

as the other options available to you will help you grow in the area of conflict management as well.

> **WIT AND WISDOM**
> *I am at peace with God. My conflict is with man.*

SUMMING IT UP

How will you apply the things you have learned about yourself through these assessments and as you pursue your journey of caring, responsible communication? As in all areas of personal growth, it is more a journey than a destination. Start by creating a poster or list in a form of your own choosing containing your top five strengths. Post it where you can easily see it throughout this course. Take the time to read more about each of these and add some descriptors, especially as they apply to you. As you learn about the various concepts discussed in the text, think about the ways that you can apply your specific strengths in developing and applying these communication concepts and strategies.

Make notes about the specific ways you plan to grow your EI based on the suggestions here or other resources. Which of your strengths will you use to do this? As you progress through this text, you will find a number of the concepts presented that will contribute to your EI growth. You may want to reassess your EI level when you have completed this course to check for evidence of your personal growth.

Learn to pay attention to the ways that you handle conflict situations. Take the time to journal about situations that you experience and then consider what other mode of conflict management could have been used. In what way would it have changed the outcome? Which of your strengths can help you in learning to handle conflict in different ways? How can you focus your EI development to help in this area?

Actively applying what you have learned in this chapter will help you to make the most of your learning in the remainder of this course. Communication is truly the heart of healthcaring, and starting with the self-assessments described here will give you a strong foundation on which to build those communication skills.

> **SIMPLIFY AND DEEPEN**
> "This above all: To thine own self be true." Polonius in William Shakespeare's *Hamlet*

Return to "Active Learning" at the beginning of the chapter and write your responses.

BOX 3.5 Conflict Management Assessments Available Online

Thomas-Kilmann Conflict Mode Instrument—$$

This research-based tool provides a full assessment with explanations and personalized suggestions for your personal growth in conflict management. There is a charge for completing this one, but results come with a booklet that provides much additional information about conflict management and how to use your results. Visit The Assessment Site – The fastest and easiest way to take the TKI® and more!

The Blake Group—free

This is an organization consulting and solutions group. Their website provides a number of free assessments including ones for communication and emotional intelligence as well as this one for conflict management. This is another simplified version of the TKI: http://www.blake-group.com/sites/default/files/assessments/Conflict_Management_Styles_Assessment.pdf.

United States Institute of Peace—free

This is an independent national institute, founded by Congress and dedicated to the proposition that a world without violent conflict is possible, practical, and essential for U.S. and global security. This assessment is slightly different from the others listed here, but it should still be helpful: https://www.usip.org/public-education/students/conflict-styles-assessment.

PRACTICING COMMUNICATION WITH WHAT YOU HAVE LEARNED ABOUT YOURSELF

Application: Exercises 1A and 1B

Exercise 1A

Consider the following questions in the context of the concept with which it is listed and write out your answers to each.

Passion: To what are you naturally drawn? What do you really care about?

Quick Learning: What kind of activities do you seem to pick up easily?

Process: In what activities do you seem to instinctively know what to do next?

Excellence: During what activities have you had moments of brilliance when you thought, "Wow, did I do that?"

Satisfaction: What activities excite you, either while doing them or immediately after, and you think, "I want to do that again."

Exercise 1B

- Contact six friends and/or family members and ask them simply to tell you what they think of you. Getting them to do this in writing would be especially helpful because it will give you a written record and they may feel freer to be frank.
- Contact six people that you work with and ask them the same thing.
- What were the common themes that emerged from the input you received?
- How can you relate these themes to strengths listed in one of the assessments?

Review the results for the two exercises in the context of one of the lists of strengths referenced in Box 3.2. Can you identify five top strengths that stand out? Are you surprised by any of the results? If possible, go ahead and complete one of the strengths assessments listed in this text. How do these results compare with your own? Which of the list seems more accurate to you?

Application: Exercise 2

1. How aware are you of your own feelings and what has caused them?
2. As a leader, can you be honest with yourself about your own limitations and personal strengths?
3. How well do you manage your distressing emotions? Can you deal easily with upset or stress?
4. How well do you adapt to change?
5. Can you keep focused on your goals and identify steps for achieving them?
6. How well do you understand the feelings of others? Can you see things from their point of view?
7. Can you persuade others to effect change by using your influence with them?
8. Are you a negotiator who can propose effective solutions to arguments between others?
9. Are you a good team player, or do you think you can do better on your own?

And the good news: EI competencies can be upgraded.

REFERENCES

Bleich, M. R., & Kist, S. (2013). Leading, managing, and following. In P. S. Yoder-Wise (Ed.), *Leading and managing in nursing* (6th ed.). St. Louis, MO: Elsevier.

Christman, R. M., Overstreet, R., Racovita, L., Kadatska, P., & Weismeyer, M. (2021). Leadership training creating healthy work environments by enhancing knowledge regrading Clifton Strengths and emotional intelligence. *Creating Healthy Work Environments VIRTUAL 2021.* http://hdl.handle.net/10755/21633.

Clifton, D. O., Anderson, E., & Schreiner, L. A. (2006). *StrengthsQuest: Discover and develop your strengths in academics, career, and beyond.* New York, NY: Gallup Press.

Codier, E., & Codier, D. D. (2017). Could emotional intelligence make patients safer? *American Journal of Nursing, 117*(7), 58.

Drucker, P. F. (1967). *The Effective executive.* New York, NY: HarperCollins.

Folger, J. P., Poole, M. S., & Stutman, R. K. (2012). *Working through conflict: Strategies for relationships, groups, and organizations* (7th ed.). Springer.

Goleman, D. (1995). *Emotional Intelligence: Why it can matter more than IQ.* New York, NY: Bantam Books.

Goleman, D., Boyatzis, R., & McKee, A. (2013). Primal Leadership: Unleashing the power of emotional intelligence. In *Boston MA: Harvard Business Review Press.*

Hodges, T. D., & Clifton, D. O. (2004). Strengths-based development in practice. In A. Linley, & S. Joseph (Eds.), *Handbook of positive psychology in practice.* Hoboken, NJ: Wiley.

Lino, C. (2016). Positive psychology theory in a nutshell, PositivePsychology.com, Positive Psychology Theory in a Nutshell - Positive Psychology Program.

Majeed, N., & Jamshed, S. (2021). Nursing turnover intentions; the role of leader emotional intelligence and team culture. *J Nurs Manag, 29,* 229–239. https://doi.org/10.1111/jonm.13144.

Peterson, C., & Seligman, M. E. P. (2004). *Character strengths and virtues: A handbook and classification.* New York, NY: Oxford University Press.

Raeissi, P., Zandian, H., Mirzarahimy, T., et al. (2019). Relationship between communication skills and emotional intelligence among nurses. *Nurs Manag, 26*(2), 31–35. doi:10.7748/nm.2019.e1820.

Rettew, J. G., & Lopez, S. J. (2008). Discovering your strengths. In S. J. Lopez (Ed.), *1. Positive psychology: Exploring the best in people.* Westport, CT: Praeger Perspectives.

Salovey, P., & Mayer, J. (1990). Emotional intelligence. *Imagination. Cognition and Personality, 9*(3), 185–211.

Segal, J., Smith, M., Robinson, L., & Shubin, J. (2018). Improving emotional intelligence (EQ): Key skills for managing your emotions and improving your relationships. Improving Emotional Intelligence (EQ) - HelpGuide.org, https://www. helpguide.org/articles/mental-health/emotional-intelligence-eq.htm.

Thomas, K. W. (2002). *Introduction to conflict management: Improving performance using the TKI*. Mountain View, CA: CPP.

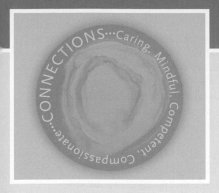

4

Solving Problems Together

For too long both patients and healthcare professionals have thought of healthcare as a car wash, with the patient passively moving through the healthcare system car wash, getting health sprinkled on them, and coming out healthy. This lack of engagement results in dissatisfaction, high costs, and poor quality care. We need to reimagine healthcare as an active collaboration between patient and the healthcare professionals.

Dr. Danny Sands, cofounder and chairman, Society for Participatory Medicine
(2018 https//participatory medicine.org/what-is-participatory-medicine/)

OBJECTIVES

1. Define mutuality in nurse–client relationships.
2. Compare the steps of the nursing process with the Clinical Judgment Measurement Model, (NCJMM), created by the National Council of State Boards of Nursing, (NCJMM).
3. Identify the core competencies of interprofessional collaborative practice.
4. Discuss mutual problem-solving to involve the client in the implementation of the nursing process.
5. Complete exercises to practice a mutual problem-solving approach to the nursing process.
6. Participate in exercises to build skills in solving problems with clients.

MOMENTS OF CONNECTION...

Setting Goals Together

A nurse was called to a client's room to discuss her therapy options for cancer treatment. As they talked, the client began to clearly understand that this disease was going to be what claimed her life. The client cried the most deep, painful, gut-level crying the nurse had ever experienced with an adult. The nurse held her hand and cried with her. They began to talk when the client relaxed. They set goals of her leaving the hospital and experiencing her next Christmas. The nurse said she felt good that she was able to take the time to let the client cry.

ACTIVE LEARNING

Together, think about how you will write your answers as you read each chapter.

What?
Write one thing you learned from this chapter.

So What?
How will this affect your nursing practice?

Now What?
How will you implement this new knowledge or skill?

Think About It ...

MUTUALITY IN NURSE–CLIENT RELATIONSHIPS

An important consideration in mutuality is acknowledging that the people are experts on their own experience (Feo et al., 2021). In a study of depression in family caregivers of Mexican descent, mutuality through culturally appropriate nursing intervention is correlated with less caregiver stress and less depression (Crist et al., 2017). Would you like to learn a way to work with people to make them feel that they are not alone and to help them be more willing to act in their own best interests? At the Dartmouth-Hitchcock Medical Center in New Hampshire, "mutuality" is an emerging concept in professional models of care. They define mutuality as "the convergence of two or more people brought together in a balanced relationship, characterized by understanding and respect for others in order to achieve a shared goal." At this medical center Wiitala, Biernat, and the quality assurance team in psychiatric care reviewing monthly patient satisfaction data found that data collected on the components of mutuality demonstrated a correlation with patient satisfaction. Mutuality, a concept grounded in research, is an essential element in building relationships with the client, although it is not always easy to achieve (Berg, 2005; Chalmers, 2005; Geanellos, 2005; Jack et al., 2005; Porr, 2005; Zoffmann, 2005). Mutuality is characterized by empathy, collaboration, equality, and interdependency (Jeon, 2004). An ongoing sharing of knowledge between healthcare professionals and shared decision making help ensure patient satisfaction (Cerda et al., 2010). A useful mnemonic from motivational interviewing, an intervention designed to promote behavior change, is O.A.R.S., four core interviewing skills. These are *O*pen-ended questioning, *A*ffirming, *R*eflecting, and *S*ummarizing (Barikanit et al., 2021; Dellasega et al., 2012).

SIMPLIFY AND DEEPEN

"When a nurse encounters another, something happens. What occurs is never a neutral event – a pulse taken, words exchanged, a touch, a healing moment. Two persons are never the same."

Barbara Dossey in Helming et al., 2022

INTERPROFESSIONAL COMMUNICATION

In a 4-day hospital stay, a patient can interact with 50 different hospital staff with varying levels of education and occupational training according to the Joint Commission on Accreditation of Healthcare Organizations (2005). Consider how many opportunities there are for inaccurate communication exchange that affects patient safety.

For two decades the goal of practicing in a culture of safety has been an important goal, and yet medical error leading to high morbidity and mortality rates remains a problem, with such errors reported to be the third leading cause of death in the United States. An examination of deficiencies and adverse events indicated that ineffective communication and lack of teamwork can negatively affect clinical outcomes (Griffiths, 2018; Makary & Daniel, 2016).

In 2011, six national associations convened an expert panel of educators in nursing, medicine, pharmacy, public health, dentistry, and osteopathic medicine to determine core competencies for interprofessional collaborative practice. *Interprofessional education (IPE)* is defined by the World Health Organization (WHO) as happening "when two or more professions learn about, from, and with each other to enable effective collaboration and improve health outcomes." (WHO, 2010, p. 13; Yancy et al., 2018.)

As you proceed in nursing, reflect on the following as you fulfill your role in working in mutual problem solving for safe, quality, and competent care from a collaborative practice perspective. The panel identified these four competencies:

1. Ethics for interprofessional practice to work together to maintain a climate of mutual respect with shared values
2. Responsibilities shared using the knowledge of your own role and that of other professions to appropriately assess and deal with the healthcare needs of clients and populations served
3. Communication with other healthcare professionals in a responsible and responsive way to work as a team for health maintenance and treatment of disease
4. Relationship building in teams for shared values in healthcare that is client-centered, safe, timely, efficient, effective, and equitable (adapted from Schmitt et al., 2011, p. 1351)

By 2016, more professional organizations and institutional members joined the Interprofessional Education Collaborative (IPEC). They combined the competencies into a single domain, Interprofessional Collaboration, and expanded it to achieve the "Triple Aim (improve the patient experience of care, improve the health of populations, and reduce the per capita cost of healthcare), with particular reference to population health."

As the complexity of healthcare increases, a variety of models have emerged to support collaboration: tumor boards for cancer treatment may include cardiology, pulmonary care, dermatology, and others; integrated documentation; and simulation of collaboration between healthcare professionals in professional education (Knoop et al., 2017). Nurses know the hospitalized patient on a day-to-day basis and have specific information that can be helpful in individualizing the plan of care. Consider a client who tries to extract a promise from you to hold certain information in confidence from the team. This should be a red flag. You need to tell the client you are obligated to share any information that is important to his or her well-being. Such a request may precede revealing information of thoughts of harm to self or others. If you must reveal information shared in confidence, explain that you cannot withhold potentially harmful information.

Collaborating with other professionals is an important situation in which to use your assertive communication skills. Remember that all team members share the same goals for patient care, and each has an important part on the team. Consider that you and other team members are partners requiring honest communication in mutual respect and trust, especially in regular contact with physicians. Your input is needed to improve safety, quality care, and successful discharge planning. Clear communication among team members can reduce costs such as those from rehospitalization. See Chapter 5 for specific tips about nurse–physician communication.

DEFINING THE DIFFERENCE BETWEEN PROBLEM SOLVING AND MUTUAL PROBLEM SOLVING IN NURSING

Problem Solving: The Nursing Process

In Chapter 1 we identified a classic five-step model of the nursing process called the problem-solving process (ADPIE):
1. Assessment
2. Diagnosis
3. Planning
4. Implementation
5. Evaluation

Building on the nursing process, to prepare nurses to think like clinicians, the National Council of State Boards of Nursing (NCSBN) developed the NCSBN Clinical Judgment Measurement Model (NCJMM), an evidence-based model that identifies six cognitive skills needed. As you collect objective and subjective data, you ask yourself what data is relevant, what is not, and what matters most as you build skills to set priorities in the clinical setting. Review Box 4.1, A Comparison between the Nursing Process and the NCBSN Clinical Judgment Measure Model (NCJMM).

The Mutual Problem-Solving Process in Nursing
Validation

Validation signifies the difference between problem solving for clients and mutual problem solving with clients. Incorporating validation keeps us focused on the rights and

> **BOX 4.1 A Comparison between the Nursing Process and the National Council of State Boards of Nursing Clinical Judgment Measure Model (NCJMM)**
>
> | Nursing Process (ADPIE) | NCJMM |
> | --- | --- |
> | Assessment | Recognize Cues |
> | Diagnosis/Analysis | Analyze Cues |
> | Diagnosis/Analysis | Prioritize Hypotheses |
> | Planning | Generate Solutions |
> | Implementation | Take Action |
> | Evaluation | Evaluate Outcomes |

Ignatavicius and Silvestri, 2021.

obligations of clients to make their own decisions about their health.

The important activity of validation must be incorporated at each step of the problem-solving process in nursing. Validation means consciously seeking out our clients' opinions and feelings at each phase of the nursing process. Validation means unearthing any questions or concerns our clients have about plans for their healthcare and securing their understanding and willingness to proceed to the next step. Incorporating validation into our problem solving stops us from moving too quickly and alienating our clients. It ensures that we obtain complete agreement and commitment from our clients about the plans for the nursing care being considered for their particular health problems. A mutual problem-solving process in nursing looks like this (Iyer et al., 1995):
  I. Assessment
     A. Collecting data regarding the client, client–family system, or community
     B. Identifying needs, problems, concerns, or human responses
 II. Diagnosis
     A. Analyzing data
     B. Validating the interpretation of data with the client
     C. Identifying nursing diagnoses
     D. Validating the nursing diagnoses with the client
III. Planning
     A. Setting priorities for resolution of identified problems with the client
     B. Determining expected and desired outcomes of nursing actions in collaboration with the client
     C. Writing nursing interventions to achieve these outcomes in collaboration with the client
 IV. Implementation
     A. Implementing nursing actions with assistance from the client

B. Encouraging client participation in performing nursing actions to achieve the outcomes

C. Continuing to collect data about the client's condition and interaction with the environment

V. Evaluation

A. Evaluating the outcomes of nursing care in consultation with the client

B. Ongoing evaluation to revise the nursing care plan

Including validation in the nursing process does not necessarily increase time or energy for care. Checking can be done quickly and naturally while interacting with clients. Ensuring that clients understand and agree with each step of the nursing process increases the probability that they will do their part to comply with treatment. Clients who have a clear understanding of their health problems, as well as what they and their nurses can do about them, expend less energy worrying and more energy doing something constructive. Clearly understanding their nursing diagnoses and having a say in how best to respond to them enables clients to maintain a sense of control.

Validation invites the collaboration essential for successful client change. The trust developed from working together is likely to increase the accuracy and validity of the database, enriching the foundation for the rest of the nursing process. The trust growing out of mutuality provides clients with an anchor, giving them the support they need to risk changing health behaviors. Collaboration ensures the benefits of two heads working on a health problem, which is essential because nursing cannot exist in a vacuum. We cannot strive for excellence without including the full participation of clients. "Nursing interactions characterized as task oriented and that disregard the client as an equal participant have been related to acts of resistance" by clients (Hallberg et al., 1995).

Many of today's healthcare customers are speaking up, asking questions, seeking second opinions, demanding alternative healthcare options, and forming their own self-help groups to take action. Their assertiveness and independence reflect the true meaning of the label "client," designating those who claim the rights and privileges of partnership in healthcare.

The client contracts for services with a qualified healthcare provider. This relationship is a negotiated partnership in which the client implicitly agrees to comply with the plan they generate together. The proliferation of advanced nurse practitioners in response to the demands for cost-effective care in a managed care environment demonstrates such a partnership from a holistic perspective. Advanced nurse practitioners identify collaboration with clients and other healthcare professionals as part of their nursing philosophy (Grando, 1998). C. Everett Koop, former US Surgeon General, emphasized that clear communication between clients and physicians could prevent serious medical problems. He reported results from a Louis Harris poll indicating that, of 1000 clients questioned, 25% admitted a hesitancy to talk with their physicians because the physician seemed rushed or distracted or because the client was embarrassed (Koop, 1998). Nurses can build working relationships among nurses, clients, and physicians by assisting with collaborative communication.

Not all healthcare customers think of themselves as active, responsible partners in their care. Some do what healthcare professionals tell them, living out the definition of the label "patient." The passive nature of this role creates an imbalance between the power of the nurse and that of the client. The passivity of this stance creates an inequitable relationship between nurses and others. As nurses, we can help reverse this apathy and listlessness by encouraging our clients to be partners in their own healthcare (Cooper & Powell, 1988). This means appreciating the worth of our clients and calling on their strengths. We can transform our nursing care into a mutual problem-solving process when we invite, even request, the full participation of our partners, the clients.

In the early 20th century, patients were more satisfied with a system of illness care that focused on disease eradication. As the influence of science and technology on healthcare has increased, discontent has emerged, along with resentment of chauvinistic, "all-knowing," healthcare professionals. Clients have begun demanding more influence in their healthcare and requesting more individualized care. Evidence of this movement was seen as early as 1972, with the publication of the Patient's Bill of Rights (presented by the American Hospital Association). This document describes the expectations for respect, knowledge, privacy, and confidentiality and access to any information essential for adequate treatment. Nurses need to focus on the individual's responsibility for healthcare along with his or her rights. It is important to emphasize what clients can do to take care of themselves and to safeguard their right to quality and informed care. The notion of clients as consumers of healthcare that arose in the 1970s has evolved into the idea of clients and their families as customers. In addition to providing informed care, nurses must now give attention to customers' expectations of service. Decreased hospital stays, outpatient surgery, and the movement toward home healthcare make the need for problem solving even more essential because clients and their families and significant others play a more active role. Because clients are frequently discharged from the hospital before they are able to care for themselves, a great deal of client education and care must be done in the home. Clients need to be able to make informed decisions about their choices for insurance. Nurses need to be informed about the differences in the choices of providers and services covered by managed care organizations to assist clients in the selection of and proper procedures for reimbursement.

The standards set forth in *Nursing: Scope and Standards of Clinical Nursing Practice* by the American Nurses Association regarding assessment, diagnosis, outcome identification, planning, implementation, and evaluation provide support for a mutual problem-solving approach with clients. The following statements are taken from two of the standards of nursing practice.

Standard 4: Planning. The registered nurse: Develops an individualized plan in partnership with the person, family, and others considering the person's characteristics including, but not limited to, values, beliefs, spiritual and health practices, preferences, choices, developmental level, coping style, culture and environment, and available technology.

Standard 5: Implementation. The registered nurse: Partners with the person, family, significant others, and caregivers as appropriate to implement the plan in a safe, realistic, and timely manner.

Incorporation of Validation into the Nursing Process

The example given in the following subsections illustrates suggested methods for ensuring maximum client participation in a mutual problem-solving approach.

Validating the interpretation of collected data. From the time clients enter our nursing care, we start asking them questions about their health problems. As we receive information about their situations from the answers they give us, the way they answer our questions, and objective data from laboratory tests and physical assessment, we start to piece together a meaningful picture. That picture is our interpretation of the data. It starts off as fuzzy and develops into a clear explanation of our clients' health problem(s).

Nurses are not the only ones who crave a clear picture of what is going on; clients are usually eager to know as well. Put yourself in the following clinical nursing situation.

Mrs. Cook is 48 years old and has been referred to a home healthcare agency by her family physician to help establish control of her adult-onset diabetes. She has been on oral hypoglycemic agents for the past 2 years. Her most recent blood glucose level was 350 mg/dL.

Mrs. Cook: "Oh, don't worry about me. I'll be fine. You won't need to visit me. I can't be worrying my husband. He wants a healthy wife!"

As you talk, you learn that Mrs. Cook has little knowledge about what special care she must take, how to monitor her nutritional intake, how to pay careful attention to

skin care, and how to check her urine daily for glucose. You learn that sickness is "unacceptable" in her family. She has two sisters who are "perfectly healthy" and a husband she calls a "fitness fanatic."

All her life Mrs. Cook has received verbal and nonverbal messages from her parents and husband that she must be a perfect wife and homemaker and that sickness is not tolerated. When the symptoms of hyperglycemia first occurred, Mrs. Cook tried to ignore them and pretend nothing was wrong. Her neighbor insisted that Mrs. Cook see a doctor when her symptoms of increased thirst and appetite were accompanied by diminished strength and weight loss.

You want to share with Mrs. Cook your assessment that she appears to have little knowledge about how to manage her diabetes to prevent complications. You suspect she has never really learned much about diabetes in an attempt to be "healthy" to live up to her parents' and husband's expectations. It was easier to pretend she was healthy than to admit she had a chronic illness. You sense that she may mistakenly assume that she will not be able to live an active and full life as a diabetic. You validate this interpretation of the information with the following statements:

You: "Mrs. Cook, I know you are eager to feel better, and I have some concerns about your ability to continue to feel healthy without learning more about taking care of yourself and managing your diabetes. From what you've told me, I know it is important to you and your husband that you be healthy. It is my experience that if people exercise proper self-care, diabetes doesn't have to stop them from doing anything they want, but to accomplish this you must accept the fact that you have diabetes. You can do things to be healthy. Tell me what you think about that."

This validation respectfully lets your client know your assessment of her health situation. Your ending allows Mrs. Cook to argue, disagree, or ask questions about your interpretation of her situation.

Identifying actual or potential problems with the client. When Mrs. Cook has either agreed with or amended your assessment, you can then formulate and validate the nursing diagnosis.

Mrs. Cook might say: "What else is there to learn? The nurse practitioner in Dr. Wood's office taught me to give myself insulin. I am fine with that."

Her response presents an opportunity to teach her about potential problems people with diabetes need to avoid. You could respond as follows:

You: "You have mastered taking your insulin; however, there is more to learn. You need to understand the signs of low blood sugar and have a plan for emergencies. Because diabetes affects the circulation, you would benefit from learning about skin care. Taking care to regulate your calories to adjust to your changing levels of energy is also essential to keep you feeling well. Learning how to manage your daily activities can help you stay healthy and active like your family."

This identification of some of the potential problems of diabetes empowers Mrs. Cook to take charge of her own health. You offer hope that she can live normally.

She might respond: "I thought all I had to do was give myself this insulin every day and I'd be OK. I guess there's more to it. My husband wants me to be healthy, and you have to be to keep up with him. He worries about me but doesn't want me to know. He's due home from work early today. Will you talk with him, too? Will you help him understand that I'm OK?"

Validating the nursing diagnoses with the client. *You respond:* "I'd be glad to talk with him. You and I have some work to do, too. The three main areas you need to learn about are adjusting your caloric intake to match your activity level, taking special precautions with your skin care—especially care of your feet, and having a plan to cope with low blood sugar, should that occur. Does that about cover it for you?"

Mrs. Cook: "That sounds like a lot to learn. The thing that surprises me is this talk about skin care. I've always had good skin, and I can't imagine having problems with it."

Setting priorities with the client for the resolution of identified problems. In this case it is appropriate to start with the problem of interest to the client because there is no current crisis.

You: "OK, let's start with skin care."

This validation gives Mrs. Cook some control of the teaching session.

Determining expected and desired outcomes of nursing actions in collaboration with the client. You and your client are concerned about outcomes. It is important for each of you to reveal your goals so that you can work together. To begin the negotiation of the plan, you can clarify expectations:

You: "We both need to have some idea where we are headed in our work together so we know when we have met our goals. I would expect you to be able to have a plan to prevent skin breakdown and low blood sugar and to have a plan to deal with them if they do occur. As for nutrition, it is my hope you will be able to figure out the number of calories you need to have the energy required for your active lifestyle. This sounds like a lot, but I think it's manageable. I'd like to hear what you think."

These suggestions make it clear what you want to accomplish. Now Mrs. Cook needs to indicate her goals.

Mrs. Cook: "It does seem like a lot to learn, but I guess I don't have much choice. I don't want to feel that sick again. I don't think either my husband or I would want to go through that again. What you say makes sense. I'll give it a try."

You: "We can start with these goals. I believe you'll feel more in control of your body, and that will make it easier for you to accept the differences in your body that diabetes causes. Just knowing there are things you can do can take away much of the fear. It will get easier, and these things will become a part of your routine. If you have questions and can't reach me, there is a 24-hour hotline number for the American Diabetes Association."

With this reply you have given Mrs. Cook another good reason for learning about her condition—to be less fearful.

Deciding on nursing strategies to achieve these outcomes in collaboration with the client. You and Mrs. Cook agree on your goals, and you have access to the knowledge, people, and material resources to help this client achieve the expected and desired outcomes.

You: "You indicated you would like to start with learning about skin care. I see you have a DVD player. We have a DVD I can bring that has examples of how to ensure that your skin does not break down. We also have booklets on skin care, and I can answer any questions you have. Which would you prefer?"

Mrs. Cook: "Booklets sound too much like school. I'd like to start with the DVD and then look at the booklets just to make sure I understand."

You have now made a plan with Mrs. Cook's help to start work on the first goal. When she is ready, you can introduce resources for the other goals and supply her with the 24-hour hotline number for the American Diabetes Association. Later on, you can recommend a support group that might be useful as well.

Implementing nursing actions with assistance from the client and encouraging client participation in performing nursing actions to meet the outcomes. In Mrs. Cook's case, your main focus is to encourage her participation in the various forms of learning how to manage the diabetes. One way to show your interest and involvement is to ask open-ended questions about her progress. For example:

"What are your thoughts about the video?"

"What questions do you have about skin care after seeing the video and reading the booklets?"

The answers reveal areas in which additional teaching is needed and provide an opportunity to offer praise and reinforcement.

Evaluating the outcomes of nursing care in consultation with the client. After Mrs. Cook uses the resources, you might adopt a light, humorous approach for evaluation.

You: "Just like being back in school…it's time for a quiz! Are you ready to tell me what you have learned and how you are working on meeting our goals? I know you've been working hard. Tell me what you are doing to prevent skin problems."

Mrs. Cook: "Sure. First, no more tight shoes. They may interfere with the circulation. I threw out my knee-highs. My husband always teases me about those anyway. He says they just aren't sexy. With the rings they leave on my legs, I can see how bad they are for me. The DVD showed me how to cut my toenails straight across. I bought toenail clippers. Oh, yes, I remember to pat dry with the towel instead of rubbing hard. OK, teacher, what grade do I get on skin care?"

You: "I'd say an A, and I just happen to be carrying gold stickers. You are a star. You can use them or share them with your children. I want to add that it's important to stay warm enough in this cold weather and to use body lotion to keep your skin from getting dry and irritated. Rubbing the lotion in will improve your circulation."

Mrs. Cook: "I love those stickers and I feel like I've earned an A. My daughter gave me some fancy lotion for my birthday. I'll use that and thank her for making a good choice."

You can continue to review with Mrs. Cook the other expected outcomes on which you both agreed and discuss her progress. You can encourage her to share what she has learned with her husband and how good she feels about her ability to manage the diabetes. Mr. Cook may need help adjusting to the idea that his wife has a chronic illness. Think of ways to involve the entire family: perhaps a conference during your next home visit. The family context is where the notion of health and illness is learned and fostered. Any support the family can give will likely enhance Mrs. Cook's health and motivate her to continue with preventive care. Joining a support group might also be useful for Mrs. Cook. Seeing that other people lead productive lives, even if their health is not perfect, may alter the idea that Mrs. Cook's diabetes will set her apart as different and unhealthy.

Self-Care Nudge

Take a breath. Close your eyes. Think of three things for which you are grateful.

Benefits of Mutuality that Go beyond the Client–Nurse Dyad

Marck (1990) believed that the benefits of the collaborative client–nurse relationship (which she terms *therapeutic reciprocity*) go beyond any isolated meeting and contribute to growth and development for both clients and nurses. When nurse–client "…communication is reciprocal, the other's humanness is valued and the nursing practice is caring" (Marino, 2017, p. 94).

Matheis-Kraft and colleagues (1990) claimed that clients who take more active roles in their treatments recover faster. This benefits hospitals, which are struggling to contain costs of healthcare. They reported how one American hospital instituted patient-driven healthcare. The goal of the hospital's patient-centered approach is to create a caring, dignified, and empowering environment in which their clients truly direct the course of their care and call on their inner resources to speed the healing process. The staff encourages client awareness of how their own physical, mental, and spiritual resources can promote healing.

In addition to the endorsement by clients and their families, nurses working in an environment with this philosophy report the following spin-offs that have boosted their morale (Matheis-Kraft et al., 1990):

- The opportunity to bring more nurturing and caring into their profession
- The enjoyment of expanded autonomy and authority, which allows them to make a real difference

- The experience of a more equal relationship with physicians who listen to their recommendations and even seek their counsel
- The satisfaction of being client advocates as they were educated to be

Schwertel-Kyle and Pitzer (1990) described their implementation of Orem's self-care model for nursing in a critical nursing care unit as a way of providing optimal care to clients within concise time frames. Originally spurred by the financial constraints of prospective payment systems with set reimbursement rates (which led to shorter hospital stays, more acute illness in those admitted, and decreased caregiving resources), the plan enhanced clients' self-confidence and feelings of accomplishment. Hain and Sandy (2013) described patient–provider agreements with nephrology patients to support compliance with a mutually agreed-on treatment plan for advanced kidney disease. The transformation from passive, dependent patient to active partner is one way for America's nursing clients to start taking responsibility for their healthcare in addition to securing their healthcare rights.

Ways to Make Clinical Problem Solving a Mutual Affair

1. Explore what you believe about the issue of clients having an active part in their healthcare. The extent to which you uphold clients' responsibility for their health mirrors how you involve them in the nursing process. Remember to step back, listen, openly discuss the issue, and focus on collaboration (Grover, 2005).
2. Be aware that an environment in which "questioning, curiosity, risk taking, and skepticism" are tolerated and even encouraged supports critical thinking skills (Seifert, 2010).
3. Watch for "teachable moments," times when events or circumstances may lead to positive behavior change (Lawson & Flocke, 2009). Clients who have had coronary artery bypass surgery may pay more attention to smoking cessation when this risk factor is linked to the possibility of further coronary artery disease and future surgery.
4. Practice revealing your opinions to clients. Increase your confidence in telling clients about your assessment of their particular situations.
5. Avoid giving nursing care without checking with your clients to see where they would like to start. Do not assume you know best because you are the nurse. Clients usually have personal preferences for where to begin working on their healthcare problems. Whereas you might go from easiest to most difficult, your client may want to work on the most complex problem first.
6. Do not negotiate nursing strategy if there is in fact no choice for your client. Occasionally the philosophy of the institution in which you work, technical policies, time, and/or staff shortages dictate the prioritization

and methodology. Most clients resent being given the false impression that they have some choice.
7. Before you do something for your clients, ask yourself, "Could my clients be doing this (turning, transferring, making a telephone call, speaking to a relative, making a bed, changing a dressing) for themselves?" By doing for our clients, we rob them of the opportunity to discover their own power to take care of themselves. Every time we provide clients with the wherewithal (information, equipment, and contacts) to do something for themselves, we save ourselves time and energy, two precious commodities in this time of tight restraint on health dollars, and we empower clients.
8. Remember to evaluate with your clients. If you have been successful in collaborating through all the steps of the nursing process, then continue your good performance through this last phase. The only way to know if your clients are satisfied with the outcomes of your nursing care is to ask for, and listen to, their opinions.
9. Keep in mind that validating is an assertive act. We are not effective when we hesitate to express our points of view or shy away from seeking those of our clients. Validation does not mean commanding or coercing clients. Mutual problem solving is a two-way street; open communication is exchanged between clients and nurses.

🌹 MOMENTS OF CONNECTION...
Partners in Life and Death

> The staff at a neonatal intensive care unit (NICU) were caring for a premature infant who was near death. The parents were concerned that their baby had never experienced anything but the NICU environment in 7 months of life. The nurse and family decided to take the baby outside to feel the sun on his face and to see the flowers. The nurse bagged the baby while the family introduced him to the family dog. There was a brief rain shower that washed the baby's face. It was a beautiful experience to see their final moments with their baby.

It is important to remember that life's problems sometimes require the healing power of time for resolution. Sometimes simply assisting your client to set a goal for the day can start the day on a positive note. Later, review the client's progress to see if the goal needs modification to support success. Multifamily group problem solving to support adolescent diabetics has been helpful, empowering families to share their plans to support improved glycemic control and increasing client satisfaction (Carpenter et al., 2014). Nurses, clients, family members, and colleagues all share in common their own humanity, working to solve problems; this is the beauty and the challenge of the situation!

> **WIT AND WISDOM**
> *We must not talk to them, or at them, but with them.*
>
> **Florence Nightingale [on partnership with clients]**
> **(Atwell, 2010)**

Return to "Active Learning" at the beginning of the chapter and write your responses.

PRACTICING SOLVING PROBLEMS TOGETHER

Critical Thinking/Discussion: Exercise 1

For each of the following client situations, describe what you would say to these clients to encourage them to take a more active part in their healthcare.

1. Mr. Bane is a 33-year-old client newly diagnosed with epilepsy. He has to take medication every 4 hours.
2. Mrs. McNeil is a 63-year-old client with arthritis. She has been urged by her physician to do wrist and finger range-of-motion exercises three times a day.
3. Johnny is a 17-year-old client who has been advised to use specially prepared soap for his facial acne.
4. Beth is a tense young client who has been urged to meditate twice a day to promote relaxation.
5. Mr. Jameson has a high cholesterol level. He has been taught how to reduce the cholesterol in his diet. He selects his own menu daily.

Compare your strategies for approaching each client situation with the suggestions of your colleagues.

Critical Thinking/Discussion: Exercise 2

For each of the following case studies write down how you would discuss the fact that your client has broken your mutual agreement about what actions he or she would take to improve his or her health status. Write out specifically what you would say when you approach the topic with your client.

1. Miss Marson is a 19-year-old client admitted to the hospital for investigation of severe, debilitating headaches. She has agreed not to consume any of her own over-the-counter drugs to alleviate her pain while tests are being done to discover the source of her headaches. On your night rounds you find Miss Marson in the washroom swallowing one extra-strength pain reliever tablet and about to take another.
2. Mrs. Dodds is a 22-year-old client admitted for investigation of severe and rapid weight loss. She has agreed to stick to a bland diet while the reasons for her weight loss are being unearthed. On the evening shift you discover her eating spicy chili her visitor brought her from the local deli.

3. Mr. Jones is a 45-year-old patient who had surgery 5 hours earlier. Preoperatively he agreed to do his deep breathing and coughing after surgery, yet now he is adamant that he has no intention of letting you support his incision so that he can cough. He only wants to sleep peacefully.
4. You are completing a health history on a client who has had chest pain in the past few weeks. She agreed to bring the pertinent information about her family's cardiac health history to you at her appointment today. She comes in without the information, telling you that she was too busy with her friends this week to get the information from her aunt.

After you have done this exercise on your own, compare your responses with those of your colleagues in your class. Be aware of the many ways to assertively inform your clients that they are not completing part of the nursing care plan to which they agreed.

Interprofessional Communication/Online Videos: Exercise 3

Visit https://healthipe.utexas.edu/videos to view one or more videos on each of the four core competencies for collaborative practice. Break into four small groups; each group will watch a different video. Discuss your thoughts about the importance of each competency. Appoint a reporter and reconvene to share your findings.

Interprofessional Communication Observation/Reflection/Discussion: Exercise 4

The next time you are on the nursing unit on which you are doing your clinical course work, identify how many professionals from different disciplines are present. Look for examples of teamwork in solving problems with each other and with the patient and for missed opportunities. Write your reflections in your journal, and share your findings with classmates.

Critical Thinking/Discussion: Exercise 5

The next time you are a client (of a lawyer, nurse, pastor, priest, rabbi, physician, or dentist), make note of how much this professional engages you in mutual problem solving. Notice exactly what the professional does to make you feel included in the planning.

- In what ways does the professional make you feel that your opinions are important?
- In what ways could this professional include you more in the problem-solving process?
- How do your feelings differ in a situation in which you are included and in one in which the professional takes over and does not consult you?

Compare your experiences with those of your classmates. What has this exercise taught you about mutual problem solving?

Creative Expression: Exercise 6

Consider the use of a collage, creating a picture from images and words cut from magazines and glued together onto paper or mat board to help a client envision success and strategies for success for a health challenge such as losing weight. Try it yourself. Create a collage with the intention to see yourself as an expert nurse with a balanced life, or choose another intention for the collage. Take time to reflect on your art and write your thoughts and feelings about it. This will help you to facilitate the client's ability to process and learn from expressive art (Walsh et al., 2004).

Quality and Safety Education for Nurses Learning Strategy: Exercise 7

Solving problems together is a central tenet of teamwork and collaboration, one of the six competencies for the Quality and Safety Education for Nurses (QSEN) framework on which much of nursing education is based. The competencies teamwork and collaboration identify the knowledge, skills, and attitudes (KSAs) required for working together to solve problems and cross-reference with the competency for patient-centered care to define how patients and families are active members of the care team. Including the patient and family in interprofessional care rounds on inpatient units encourages their participation in making decisions about their care. Providing time for patient and family participation provides time to discuss daily care goals for inpatients and overall care goals for outpatients.

- What examples have you observed in clinical settings or from your own personal experience of patient and family inclusion in care decisions?
- What was the impact?
- Was time allotted for patients to ask questions, to teach back, or to rephrase what they heard?
- What examples have you observed when the nurse, the physician, and the pharmacist worked together to discuss a patient's complicated medication regime to determine best times and dosages for administering medications with the patient's lifestyle after discharge?
- Reflect on these observations to identify strategies to work both with your professional colleagues and with patients to coordinate and manage care with all team members to maximize the patient's comfort and recovery.

WIT AND WISDOM

Too often we give children answers to remember rather than problems to solve.

Roger Lewin

REFERENCES

Atwell, A. (2010). Florence Nightingale's relevance to nurses. *Journal of Holistic Nursing, 28*(1), 101.

Barikanit, A., Negarandeh, R., Moin, M., & Fazlollahi, R. (2021). The impact of motivational interview on self-efficacy, beliefs about medicines and medication adherence among adolescents with asthma: A randomized controlled trial. *Journal of Pediatric Nursing, 60*, 116–122. doi:10.1016/j.ijnurstu.2020.103786.

Berg, M. (2005). A midwifery model of care for childbearing women at high risk: Genuine caring in caring for the genuine. *Journal of Perinatal Education, 14*(1), 9.

Carpenter, J. L., Price, J. E. W., Cohen, M. J., Shoe, K. M., Pendley, K. M., & Shroff, J. (2014). Multifamily group problem solving intervention for adherence challenges in pediatric insulin dependent diabetes. *Clinical Practice in Pediatric Psychology, 2*(2), 101.

Cerda, J. C., Prieto Rodriguez, M. A., Perez Corril, O., Lorenzo, S. M., & Danet, A. (2010). Quality of internal communication in health care and the professional–patient relationship. *Health Care Manager, 29*(2), 179.

Chalmers, K. I. (2005). Mothers of children at risk described engaging with home visitors in terms of limiting family vulnerability. *Evidence Based Nursing, 8*(4), 123.

Crist, J. D., Pasvogel, A., Szalacha, L. A., & Finley, B. A. (2017). Depression in family caregivers of Mexican descent. *Research in Gerontological Nursing, 10*(3), 106.

Cooper, M. C., & Powell, E. (1988). Technology and care in a bone marrow transplant unit: Creating and assuaging vulnerability. *Holistic Nursing Practice, 12*(4), 57.

Feo, R., Kumaran, S., Conroy, T., & Heuzenroeder., L (2021). An evaluation of instruments measuring behavioural aspects of the nurse-patient relationship. *Nurs Inq, 29*(2), e12425. doi:10.1111/nin.12425.

Dellasega, C., Anel-Tiangco, R. M., & Gabbay, R. A. (2012). How patients with type 2 diabetes mellitus respond to motivational interviewing. *Diabetes Research and Clinical Practice, 95*, 37–41.

Geanellos, R. (2005). Sustaining well-being and enabling recovery: The therapeutic effect of nurse friendliness on clients and nursing environments. *Contemporary Nurse, 19*(1–2), 242.

Grando, V. (1998). *Articulating nursing for advanced nursing practice.* New York: McGraw-Hill. *Collaboration: A health care imperative.*

Griffiths, B. (2018). Preparing tomorrow's nurses for collaborative quality care through simulation. *Teaching and Learning in Nursing, 13*, 46.

Grover, S. M. (2005). Shaping effective communication skills and therapeutic relationships at work: The foundation of collaboration. *AAOHN Journal, 53*(4), 177.

Hain, D. J., & Sandy, D. (2013). Partners in care: Patient empowerment through shared decision-making. *Nephrology Nursing Journal, 40*(2), 153.

Hallberg, I. R., Holst, G., Nordmark, A., & Edberg, A. K. (1995). Cooperation during morning care between nurses and severely demented institutionalized patients. *Clinical Nursing Research, 4*(1), 78.

Helming, M. A. B., Shields, D. A., Avino, K. M., & Rosa, W. E. (2022). *Dossey & Keegan's holistic nursing: A handbook for practice* (8th ed). Burlington, MA: Jones & Bartlett Learning.

Ignatavicius, D. D., & Silvestri, L. (2021). Getting ready for the Next-Generation NCLEX® (NGN): How to shift from the nursing process to clinical judgment in nursing. *From Nursing Process to Clinical Judgment.* Elsevier Education - Elsevier Education.

Iyer, P. W., Taptich, B. J., & Bernocchi-Losey, D. (1995). *Nursing process and nursing diagnosis.* Philadelphia, PA: Saunders.

Jack, S. M., DiCenso, A., & Lohfeld, L. (2005). A theory of maternal engagement with public health nurses and family visitors. *Journal of Advanced Nursing, 49*(2), 182.

Jeon, Y. (2004). Shaping mutuality: Nurse-family caregiver interactions in caring for older people with depression. *International Journal of Mental Health Nursing, 13*(2), 126.

Joint Commission on Accreditation of Healthcare Organizations. (2005). *The Joint Commission Guide to improving staff communication.* Oakbrook Terrace, IL: Joint Commission Resources.

Knoop, T., Wujcik, D., & Wujcik, K. (2017). Emerging models of interprofessional collaboration in cancer care. *Seminars in Oncology Nursing, 33*(4), 458.

Koop, C. E. (1998). Patient–provider communication and managed care. *Medical Practice Communicator, 5*(4), 1.

Lawson, P. J., & Flocke, S. A. (2009). Teachable moments for health behaviour change: A concept analysis. *Patient Education and Counseling, 76,* 25.

Makary, M. A., & Daniel, M. (2016). Medical error-the third leading cause of death in the US. *British Medical Journal, 353,* i2139.

Marck, P. (1990). Therapeutic reciprocity: A caring phenomenon. *Advances in Nursing Science, 13*(1), 49.

Marino, M. G. (2017). Student paper, therapeutic reciprocity: A concept synthesis. *International Journal for Human Caring, 21*(2), 91.

Matheis-Kraft, C., George, S., Olinger, M. J., & York, L. (1990). Patient-driven healthcare works. *Nurse Manager, 21*(9), 124.

Porr, C. (2005). Shifting from preconceptions to pure wonderment. *Nursing Philosophy, 6*(3), 189.

Schmitt, M., Blue, A., Aschenbrener, C. A., & Viggiano, T. R. (2011). Core competencies for interprofessional collaborative practice: Reforming health care by transforming health professionals education. *Academic Medicine, 86*(11), 1351.

Schwertel-Kyle, B. A., & Pitzer, S. A. (1990). *A self-care approach to today's challenges. Nurse Manager, 21*(3), 37.

Seifert, P. C. (2010). Thinking critically. *AORN Journal, 91*(2), 197.

Walsh, S., Martin, S. C., & Schmidt, L. A. (2004). Testing the efficacy of a creative-arts intervention with family caregivers of patients with cancer. *Journal of Nursing Scholarship, 36*(3), 214.

World Health Organization (WHO). (2010). *Framework for action on interprofessional education and collaborative practice.* Geneva, Switzerland: WHO.

Yancy, N. R., Cahill, S., & McDowell, M. (2018). Transformation in teaching-learning: Emerging possibilities with interprofessional education. *Nursing Science Quarterly, 3*(2), 126.

Zoffmann, V. (2005). Life versus disease in difficult diabetes care: Conflicting perspectives disempower patients and professionals in problem solving. *Quality Health Research, 15*(6), 750.

5

Understanding Each Other: Communication and Culture*

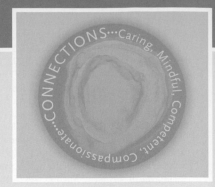

Even as I celebrate differences, I look beyond them to see the divinity that joins us as members of one family, to which we all belong.

Daily Word (2021)

OBJECTIVES

1. Define culture, ethnicity, and ethnocentrism.
2. Define cultural humility.
3. Discuss reasons why nurses need to become informed about the healthcare beliefs and behaviors of diverse cultures.
4. Discuss two common American values that may interfere with nurses' recognition and appreciation of the healthcare beliefs and behaviors of diverse cultures.
5. Describe your own cultural background and its influence on your healthcare beliefs and behaviors.
6. Identify the components of communication suggested for assessment in Purnell's model for cultural competence.
7. Discuss techniques that enhance communication with clients from diverse cultures.
8. Apply communication techniques to improve the care of clients from diverse cultures.
9. Discuss how the variables of age and gender relate to culture and communication.
10. Participate in exercises to build skills in understanding each other.

In an editorial in the *Journal of Hospice & Palliative Nursing,* "The 'Other' Confronting Injustices in 2021 and Beyond" Ferrell and Williams discuss societal and healthcare inequities. They define "other" as a person different than me, which requires "recognizing one's implicit biases…seeking to view another's reality through the lens of the life we are serving (Ferrell & Williams, 2021, p. 1). Nurses have a strong foundation of scholarship and practice—ethical practice, social justice, and transcultural care. Nursing "is based on a commitment to the other, to patient-centered care…sees…through a lens of respect and through action that engenders trust" (Ferrell & Williams, 2021, p. 2).

Some schools of nursing offer a "cultural immersion" trip to another country. Here's a glimpse of a daily event on such a trip. A group of nursing students from the United States was on a 2-week study abroad trip to Ecuador and had to do laundry. Fortunately, there was a local laundromat across the street from the students' hostel in Quito. One morning, two female students went to the laundromat and dropped off their clothes. Afraid of missing the day's field trip, they quickly left, forgetting to leave their names at the laundromat. At the end of the day, they returned to pick up their clothing and found that their clothes were clean and neatly folded with a receipt attached labeled "Dos Gringas" (two foreign girls). The students were speechless. Until this happened, they had never had to consider that they were the "outsiders" in someone else's culture.

Questions:
1. Have you ever had the experience of being an outsider in another culture?
2. Is it possible to get this experience simply by taking a vacation in a foreign country?

---

* With contributions from Lois O. Gonzalez, PhD, APRN, BC, and Kim Curry, PhD, APRN.

3. What types of interactions with the local population do you think would be necessary to more fully experience the various aspects of another culture?

As our society becomes more global and diverse, cultural competence is a major component in the quality and safety of care (Green & Reinckens, 2013; Larson et al., 2010); it is not a static but a dynamic concept that must be evaluated continuously as it relates to patient outcomes (Waite et al., 2014). According to the Quality and Safety Education for Nurses (QSEN) initiative, an understanding of how diverse cultural, ethnic, and social backgrounds function as sources of patient, family, and community values is vital for today's future nurses (QSEN, 2010). QSEN calls patient-centered care, which includes culture and diversity, one of the six pillars of safe and effective nursing care, recognizing this competency as one of the required knowledge, skills, and attitudes (KSAs) needed to promote patient safety (QSEN, 2010). According to their definition, nurses should be able to:

"Provide patient-centered care with sensitivity and respect for the diversity of human experience. Seek learning opportunities with patients who represent all aspects of human diversity. Recognize personally held attitudes about working with patients from different ethnic, cultural, and social backgrounds. Willingly support patient-centered care for individuals and groups whose values differ from own" *(QSEN, 2010).*

? ACTIVE LEARNING

Think about how you will write your answers as you read this chapter.

What?
Write one thing you learned from this chapter.

So What?
How will this affect your nursing practice?

Now What?
How will you implement this new knowledge or skill?

Think About It …

Being culturally aware takes a great deal of commitment and effort on the part of the nurse. Merely talking about culture does not necessarily mean that you have translated knowledge into action. Individuals are not likely to translate cultural knowledge into behavior until they experience direct contact with people from other cultures. This exposure is becoming more and more inevitable in the United States.

Data from the 2020 US census provides evidence that America is more racially and ethnically diverse than in the 2010 census. Most groups had population gains this decade, and the increase in the multiracial population was up to 276%. The White population remained the largest ethnicity. Persons identifying as White alone, not in combination with another group, decreased by 8.6% (Jones et al., 2021). Matveev's conclusions remain timely. This multiracial, ethnically complex population will challenge US healthcare providers who are attempting to offer culturally driven client care. Changing demographic trends indicate that America is making progress in efforts to reduce inequalities and barriers to opportunities. Unfortunately, despite improvements in access to healthcare across US ethnic populations, disparities between the majority population and most ethnic groups still exist. Intercultural knowledge, communication, and competence will become necessities in almost every occupation (Matveev, 2017).

Eliminating racial and ethnic healthcare disparities is urgent, and our efforts must focus on social, cultural, and environmental factors that reach far beyond the traditional medical model. The National Standards for Culturally and Linguistically Appropriate Services (CLAS) were updated in 2012. The principal standard is to "provide effective, equitable, understandable, and respectful quality care and services that are responsive to diverse cultural health beliefs and practices, preferred languages, health literacy, and other communication needs" (US Department of Health and Human Services, 2019). Effective communication between and among cultures is essential because it is the way we interact globally. In the American healthcare setting, nurses indicate an understanding of the importance of communication and demonstrate awareness of the need for cultural awareness, but many have not operationalized into their practice the significance of culture. Because nurses spend more time with clients than do most other healthcare professionals, it is particularly important for nurses to realize that both communication and culture are inextricably connected to healthcare. Nurses need to know about culture, both their own and that of their clients, because it influences both nurses' and clients' healthcare perceptions and behaviors.

The effect of culture and communication-related issues can be life-threatening, particularly in cases in which there are differing perceptions and descriptions of pain. For example, an assessment of the quality of chest pain is a critical piece of data so that an acute myocardial infarction can be distinguished from other conditions causing pain in the chest or epigastric area. Missed diagnoses and delayed treatments occur when responses to pain are culturally dictated, and an individual may delay coming for treatment because of fear, stoicism, or meanings attributed to pain. Such delays can be life-threatening (Sobralske & Katz, 2005).

Negotiating a larger, white-dominated culture can be painful for minorities, particularly when people in the majority are not aware of cultural differences. After living for an extended period of time in a majority culture, a minority person can choose one of two paths. He or she can either become acculturated or live apart in isolation or within the safe boundaries of a familiar cultural neighborhood. The latter prevents participation in and enrichment of the larger culture, thwarting the development of increased multiculturalism in the community.

We are experiencing a nationwide increase in our multicultural society. When nursing experts are asked to predict the skills, education, and perspectives that nurses will need to prosper in the coming era, they suggest that nurses will need to demonstrate transcultural competence to employers and consumers (Reeves & Fogg, 2006). However, some nurses still ask, "What's culture got to do with it?" Everyone is familiar with the meaning of communication, but what is culture?

DEFINITION OF CULTURE, ETHNICITY, AND ETHNOCENTRISM

Madeline Leininger defines *culture* as the learned and shared beliefs, values, and lifeways of a particular group that are generally transmitted intergenerationally and influence one's thinking and actions. For three decades, Leininger has emphasized the need for nurses to become informed about other cultures' healthcare beliefs and practices. Ethnicity also needs to be defined because some confuse its meaning with that of culture. According to Leininger, *ethnicity* refers to the social identity and origins of a social group largely because of language, religion, and national origin; for example, the Amish are an ethnic group. Sociologists and psychologists are more likely to use the term *ethnicity*. The term *culture* is used more frequently by anthropologists and transcultural nurses. Culture is a broader term because it refers to the holistic, patterned lifeways of a group rather than to selected ethnic features or origins (Leininger, 2002).

The term *ethnocentrism* was coined by William Graham Sumner, a social evolutionist and professor of political and social science at Yale University. He defined it as the universal tendency of people to believe that one's own ethnic group is the most important and/or that some or all aspects of its culture are superior to those of other groups (Salter, 2002). Furthermore, ethnocentrism perpetuates the attitude that beliefs differing greatly from one's own are

strange, bizarre, or unenlightened and, therefore, wrong (Purnell, 2012). Within this ideology, individuals will judge other groups in relation to their own particular ethnic group or culture, especially with concern to language, behavior, customs, and religion. These ethnic distinctions and subdivisions serve to define each ethnicity's unique cultural identity.

CULTURAL HUMILITY

The American Nurses Association (ANA) standards guide our practice in all areas of diversity, of differences. "Standard 9: Respectful and Equitable Practice: The registered nurse practices with cultural humility and inclusiveness" (ANA, 2021). We are called to create a culture of caring in which we hold the space for others to be who they are and in which we are open and curious about others, with a moral compass that guides us to compassionate caring. We honor that we each have biases and make assumptions that do not serve us or the client. We reflect on our own discomfort and seek to serve with equity. We honor the other person as whole; we ask when we do not know; we listen with empathy, kindness, and an open heart.

What is cultural humility? It is a lifelong personal commitment to self-reflection and self-critique. It is entering into relationships with the intention to honor the beliefs, customs, and values of another, acknowledging differences and valuing the persons for who they are. We recognize there is so much to learn about the differences between us. We come humble and vulnerable and know we do not have all the answers (Yeager, 2013; Fletcher, 2007).

Self-Care Nudge

When you are in a situation where you don't know what to do, take a breath, and accept that the most confident of colleagues feels uncertain at times, even if they don't show it. Consider: "Life is about not knowing, having to change, taking the moment and making the best of it, without knowing what's going to happen next."

Gilda Radner

REASONS WHY NURSES NEED TO BE CULTURALLY INFORMED

There are several compelling reasons why nurses need to be informed about culture. First, shifting demographics will call for dramatic changes in the US healthcare industry. By 2030, one in five Americans is projected to be 65 and over; by 2044, more than half of all Americans are projected to belong to a minority group (any group other than non-Hispanic White alone). By 2060, nearly one in five of the nation's total population is projected to be foreign born. With the increase in clients of diverse ethnic backgrounds, it is imperative that healthcare professionals understand the importance of culture and its relationship to clients, their families, and the community (Colby & Ortman, 2015).

Second, care is central to the concept of nursing. As technology becomes an increasingly important part of healthcare, the essence of human caring becomes the most valued aspect of nursing. Caring transcends cultural boundaries. Caring is a broad construct that includes general themes such as preserving humanity, authenticity, and promoting health and well-being, which are activities that are valued in all cultures (Cook & Peden, 2017).

Third, although the United States has always been a diverse society, this diversity has not always been recognized by healthcare providers because they have long had the attitude that newcomers should adapt to "us." We as a society are beginning to recognize that this is not desirable, and it will not work in a heterogeneous society.

Fourth, this is an age of economic imperatives. Our healthcare system is evolving toward an integrated system combining hospital and community facilities and physical health and mental health services, Western and traditional medicine, primary and tertiary care, technology and clinical practice, and so on. As providers and systems strive to gain market share, competition for clients increases. The increasing diversity of the overall population forces healthcare plans and organizations to ask whether their employees reflect the communities they serve. If they do, their ability to deliver culturally competent care is enhanced. If they do not, then a chance to improve the care experience for a large portion of their members is being lost, and the organization is missing an opportunity to gain a competitive edge in the marketplace.

The provision of publicly financed healthcare services is now being delegated to the private sector. Issues of concern in the current healthcare environment include the marketing of health services and the cost-effectiveness of healthcare delivery. The potential for improved services lies in state–managed-care contracts that can increase retention and access to care, expand recruitment, and increase the satisfaction of individuals seeking healthcare services. To reach these outcomes, managed care plans must incorporate culturally competent policies, structures, and practices to provide services for people from diverse ethnic, racial, cultural, and linguistic backgrounds.

Finally, the issues of working with older clients and with the chronically ill are of immense importance. Healthcare personnel need to work in community settings and with entire families and in settings in which the outcomes are not (and cannot be) the standard medical outcome of cure.

Clearly, the achievement of nursing outcomes requires working with (versus working on) humans in settings in which the nurse has less control. Consequently, the client and family have more control than does the nurse, and culture has a strong effect on how people act.

In summary, nurses need to know about culture because it influences both nurses' and clients' healthcare perceptions and behaviors. Also, with healthcare moving into the community, if nurses expect to be part of this movement, they must know about the culture of diverse clients and communities. To achieve this outcome, nurses must first recognize and then overcome certain attitudes basic to the American culture.

> **WIT AND WISDOM**
>
> *If civilization is to survive, we must cultivate the science of human relationships—the ability of all peoples, of all kinds, to live together, in the same world at peace.*
>
> **Franklin D. Roosevelt**

BARRIERS THAT INTERFERE WITH TRANSCULTURAL COMMUNICATION

Despite notable progress in the overall health of Americans, there are continuing disparities in health status among African Americans, Hispanics, Native Americans, and Pacific Islanders compared with the US population as a whole. In addition, the healthcare system is becoming more challenged as the population becomes more ethnically diverse. Therefore, the future health of the US population as a whole will be influenced substantially by improvements in the health of racial and ethnic minorities.

Cultural, ethnic, linguistic, and economic differences affect how individuals and groups access and use health, education, and social services. They can also present barriers to effective education and healthcare interventions. This is especially true when health educators or healthcare practitioners stereotype, misinterpret, make faulty assumptions, or, otherwise, mishandle their encounters with individuals and groups viewed as different in terms of their backgrounds and experiences. The demand for culturally competent healthcare in the United States is a direct result of the failure of the healthcare system to provide adequate care to all segments of the population.

Ethnocentrism interferes with the appreciation of diverse cultures and their accompanying beliefs and behaviors. Western healthcare may be seen as delivering top-notch high-technology care, yet it is lacking because often the care is reductionistic rather than holistic. Furthermore, the cost of the care is considered exorbitant relative to the outcome. Recognition of ethnocentrism is necessary to develop an appreciation of diverse cultures. One nurse put it this way:

I always thought of myself as open, flexible, and reasonably unprejudiced; but I am not always! When caring for my friend from Saudi Arabia, I realized that, without knowing, I made value judgments. These judgments reflected my inability to accept that others handle the same data differently; and their perspectives are as important as mine.

Facilitating Effective Communication

We as nurses recognize that we need to know about delivering care to diverse clients, but how do we go about it? First, nurses need to become familiar with their own healthcare beliefs and behaviors because, without self-awareness, nurses cannot recognize that their beliefs and behaviors are not necessarily common to all. Nurses' lack of knowledge about their own culture can distort their perceptions of the beliefs and behaviors of clients from diverse cultures. It is logical that if a nurse does not understand the reasons for a client's behavior, then it is impossible for the nurse to implement appropriate interventions.

Your answers to the following questions are both interesting and important. For example, consider your answer to the question, "What did your family do to stay healthy?" If your family advocated taking a daily vitamin to stay healthy, how do you view a client who drinks a small amount of his own urine daily to promote health? How do you perceive the Cuban mother who tells you her child is very beautiful and healthy because he is fat?

"What did your family believe caused illness?" If you grew up in the United States, your family probably thought that illness was caused by germs and bacteria. Someone from a different culture might believe that her liver cancer is a punishment for a wrongdoing or is a result of witchcraft.

"How were specific illnesses treated?" Americans use medication (over-the-counter or prescribed) to treat illnesses. Some people might prefer meditation rather than medication to treat illness. They believe that illness is a sign that the body is out of balance and that meditation helps restore the body's balance. How do you react when a client refuses morning care or breakfast because it is time to meditate?

"Who was responsible for deciding the appropriate treatment?" Because most Americans place a high value on individualism, the individual adult client usually decides what treatment he or she deems to be most appropriate. How do you perceive a client whose husband decides the preferred treatment for his wife?

"What healthcare practitioners outside of the family were used to treat illness?" Most American families eventually consult a medical doctor if illness persists and if home remedies do not work. How do you perceive a client who prefers that a curandero (folk practitioner), not a physician, treat his liver disease?

It is interesting to compare the healthcare beliefs and behaviors of your family of origin with those of friends or other healthcare professionals. It often becomes apparent that your family's ideas and behaviors are not necessarily common to all. This recognition is an important step in not only identifying but also appreciating the healthcare beliefs and behaviors of diverse cultures.

Because cultures are so diverse, no one can possibly know all the unique aspects of each client's cultural healthcare beliefs and behaviors. To address this need, nurses and other healthcare professionals began to develop conceptual and theoretical frameworks for assessing, planning, and implementing culturally appropriate interventions. One of the most popular transcultural theoretical and conceptual frameworks is Leininger's culture care theory, which was designed for nursing (Leininger, 1988).

Since the development of Leininger's cultural theory in nursing (Leininger, 1988), several transcultural frameworks or models have been proposed for nurses, including cultural assessment frameworks and models (Giger & Davidhizar, 2002; Purnell, 2002). Research suggested that culturally competent care brings positive health outcomes (Lagisetty, 2017; Leininger, 1988). With the movement of healthcare to more community-based settings, nursing researchers have expanded on these models to predict public health outcomes of culturally competent care. Kim-Godwin and colleagues (2001) proposed the Culturally Competent Community Care (CCCC) model built around three constructs of cultural competence, the healthcare system, and health outcomes. Four interdependent dimensions of cultural competence are caring, cultural sensitivity, cultural knowledge, and cultural skills. In the healthcare environment calling for more evidence-based practice, the CCCC model provides specific guidelines for community-based nurses in developing and assessing cultural competence and meeting the healthcare needs of a diverse patient population.

With increasing frequency, a cultural assessment has become a standard of care in the initial client assessment in both acute and primary care settings. Consider reviewing the assessment tool that you use when you admit a client. How is the client's culture addressed in the tool? The model for cultural competence developed by Purnell (2012) provides you with ideas about other cultural components that may need to be addressed. The 12 domains essential for assessing the ethnocultural attributes of an individual, a family, or a group are as follows: overview, inhabited localities and topography; communication; family roles and organization; workforce issues; biocultural ecology; high-risk health behaviors; nutrition; pregnancy and childbearing practices; death rituals; spirituality; healthcare practices; and healthcare practitioners. The domains are interconnected and have implications for health.

When cultural communication similarities and differences are identified, stereotyping should be avoided. All cultural groups share some communication practices, but broad cultural communication differences may also exist. Do not assume that all members of the same cultural group share the same communication characteristics. An individualized assessment is needed to ensure that the client's needs are met.

KEY ASPECTS OF CULTURE TO CONSIDER

Purnell identifies four components of culture for discussion of how culture affects communication in the context of providing healthcare to diverse clients: dominant language and dialects; cultural communication patterns; temporal relationships; and formats for names (Purnell, 2012). We will add both age and gender for a discussion of how culture affects communication in the context of providing healthcare to diverse clients. When cultural communication similarities and differences are identified, stereotyping should be avoided. All cultural groups share some communication practices, but broad cultural communication differences may also exist. Do not assume that all members of the same cultural group share the same communication characteristics. An individualized assessment is needed to ensure that the client's needs are met.

Dominant Language and Dialects

Cultural diversity is the current reality. We have a growing population composed of people from a variety of cultural and ethnic groups. In the 21st century, nurses are confronted with the challenge of providing healthcare services to these clients whose first language is different than theirs. How do you care for clients when communication is significantly impaired because you do not speak the same language? One nurse describes such a situation:

I had a patient from Vietnam who was admitted in for hernia surgery. He had been in this country for 2 weeks, and his hernia needed to be repaired before he could start work. He spoke no English, nor did his family, and an interpreter was not available. The only tools available were body language, and, as hard as that was, we were able to communicate to a small degree. It was very difficult to explain anesthesia. He looked scared;

he kept his eyes closed most of the time in preop. It was as if he was pretending he wasn't there. Surgery moves relatively fast, so there wasn't a lot of time before induction. I'm sure the recovery process was equally as difficult and frightening for this man.

The nurse in the preceding scenario poignantly identifies the difficulties and anxieties inherent in working with hospitalized clients who are not fluent in English. The client's anxiety is much greater than that of the staff. Hospitalization is always a crisis. Add to this crisis the anxiety in not being able to communicate your symptoms, perceptions, needs, and questions. The solution is to provide medical interpreters; they are essential to the delivery of culturally competent care. The National Board for Certification of Medical Interpreters works to ensure a high quality of care to clients who are not fluent in English (www.certified-medicalinterpreters.org/2021). Box 5.1 provides guidelines for communicating with non–English-speaking clients that may be useful until medical interpreters become consistently available.

BOX 5.1 Guidelines for Communicating with Non–English-Speaking Clients

If There Is an Interpreter Available
- Use dialect-specific interpreters when possible.
- Give the client and interpreter time alone together.
- Avoid using children and relatives as interpreters.
- Select same-age and same-gender interpreters.
- Address your questions to the client, not to the interpreter.

If There *Is no* Interpreter Available
- Determine whether there is a third language that both you and the client speak. It is common for clients from diverse cultures to speak several languages.
- Remember that nonverbal communication is more important than verbal communication.
- Be attentive to both your own and the client's nonverbal messages.
- Pantomime simple words and actions.
- Remember: A picture is worth a thousand words. Use paper and pencil and also give them to the client.
- Talk with the administration about the importance of using trained medical interpreters when caring for the non–English-speaking client.
- Until medical interpreters are available, use both formal and informal networking to locate a suitable interpreter. If all else fails, owners of ethnic restaurants and grocery stores may be sources for locating interpreters or translators.

Professional interpreters are better able to communicate medical terms and can be of assistance in reducing the risks of breaches in patient privacy and confidentiality. This risk occurs when medical professionals call on family members or volunteers to serve as go-betweens for the health professional and patient. Patients are often uncomfortable sharing sensitive information through relatives or friends. An interpreter is focused on two-way conversation, interpreting the question from the nurse to the patient, listening to the patient's response, and then relaying the information back to the nurse. A family member who is caught up in a crisis, such as a visit to the emergency department, may relay information about his or her loved one but fail to direct the question from the healthcare provider directly to the patient. A trained interpreter might have avoided this problem (Juckett & Unger, 2014).

Because nurses care for clients from diverse cultures, they can expect that the client's first language is often a language other than English. The use of professionally trained interpreters is ideal, but such interpreters are rarely available. Clients frequently know at least a little English. Nurses often find that they need to just plunge in when communicating with a client who knows little English: "I hope I get over it, but I always feel silly when I try to communicate with someone who speaks only a little English. I feel like a little kid—I try to use a lot of gestures. It is really awkward for me; I get so embarrassed. But then I realize how awkward it is for the client to try to speak English. He's got to feel that he's in a place with a lot of foreigners who are responsible for treating him. That's got to be really scary!" Box 5.2 provides guidelines for communicating with clients who speak some English.

There is more to language than understanding the meaning of words. Tone and volume of voice are also important aspects of communication. A nurse from Thailand says, "Thai people are very quiet because they believe that talking too much is a sign of stupidity and ignorance. If you talk a lot, you probably don't think a lot." A Cuban nurse relates, "Our language (Spanish) is everything to us. We're proud to speak it loudly—we love to socialize anywhere with family and friends." It is important that nurses not misinterpret differences in voice tone and volume because they may be cultural.

It is helpful if language interpreters are also able to function as cultural interpreters who are able to teach healthcare providers about cultural context as an adjunct to language interpretation. If the community has a large percentage of a particular cultural group, additional cultural interpreters may be recruited from the community. Community leaders might be encouraged to become involved in identifying potential volunteers and to become actively involved in their training (Green-Hernandez et al., 2004). Several

---

BOX 5.2   Guidelines for Communicating with Clients Who Are Partially Fluent in English

1. Assess the client's nonverbal and verbal communication.
2. Keep your eyes at approximately the same level as the client's eyes. This probably means you will sit. Assess whether the client is comfortable with eye contact.
3. Speak slowly and never loudly (unless the client has a hearing impairment).
4. Use pictures when possible (remember: a picture is worth a thousand words).
5. Avoid using technical terms.
6. Ask for feedback. Provide the client with paper and pencil.
7. Remember that clients understand more than they can express; they just need time to think in their own language.
8. Remember that stress interferes with the client's ability to think and speak in English.

---

years ago, one of the local health departments in the Tampa Bay area identified a migrant worker from a rural area who was well respected in the community. She was recruited as an interpreter and hired full-time by a satellite clinic of the health department to serve the Spanish-speaking migrant population who did seasonal agricultural work in the area.

Cultural Communication Patterns

Communication patterns are an important part of every culture. Box 5.3 offers general guidelines for improving cross-cultural communications.

The nurse must interact with the client to put into practice the guidelines in Box 5.3. This is very important! This

---

BOX 5.3   Guidelines for Improving Cross-Cultural Communications (LEARN)

- **L**isten with sympathy and understanding to the client's perception of the problem.
- **E**xplain your perceptions of the problem.
- **A**cknowledge and discuss the differences and similarities.
- **R**ecommend treatment.
- **N**egotiate agreement.

From Buchwald, D., Caralis, P., Gany, F., Hardt, E. J., Johnson, T. M., Muecke, M., & Putsch, R. W. (1994). Caring for patients in a multicultural society: five vignettes of cross-cultural care. *Patient Care, 28*, 105.

BOX 5.4 Avoidance of Clients Who Are "Different"

"I've noticed nurses ignoring people who are different. I don't think they do it intentionally, but, out of frustration at not being able to communicate, they stay out of the room. Recently we treated an older Cuban woman who only spoke Spanish. She wouldn't eat the hospital food and took some strange herbs. Her daughter was the only family member who spoke English. When her daughter was at her side, the interaction was easy—when her daughter wasn't, there was no interaction. She would look at us with big, wide-open eyes. It was easier to stay out of there than to go in and feel helpless."

is not the time to follow the old adage, "Don't talk to strangers." All too often, nurses seem to apply this saying to clients from different cultures. It is easy to avoid clients whose healthcare beliefs and behaviors are "different" (Box 5.4).

Knowing that every person is an individual, see how these observations fit your experience. Cultural differences are seen in the willingness of individuals to share thoughts and feelings. Faculty of a college of nursing in California observed that their students who were European Americans were open to discussing feelings about almost any topic. This contrasted with Asian American students, who did not value the display of strong feelings and believed that personal thoughts were to be shared only with close friends and family. These observations were respected by the faculty. Students were no longer required to keep journals as part of course requirements because it was not a culturally appropriate assignment for the many Asian students.

The acceptability of touch varies considerably among cultures. In Arab and Hispanic cultures, male healthcare professionals may not touch or examine certain parts of the female body (Andrews & Boyle, 2011). Visitors to France note that both French men and French women greet each other with a kiss or kisses on the cheek. Young men in India walk down the street with their arms on each other's shoulders.

Proxemics, the study of how different cultures prefer different degrees of closeness in personal space offers helpful information to take into account (Kreuz & Roberts, 2019). In general, the British, Canadians, and middle-class Americans feel uncomfortable when forced to stand close to people they do not know well. The United States is a vast country, and historically Americans are used to a lot of space. Latin Americans, African Americans, Indonesians, Arabs, and the French welcome physical closeness (Luckmann, 2000). In addition, maintaining direct eye contact is an important expectation in American culture. This is not a universal standard, however, as one nurse learned: "Since I am a person who values eye contact, it was interesting to me to find out that this can be cultural. Previously, I assumed a lack of eye contact correlated with a lack of self-esteem."

It is important for nurses to recognize that eye contact is often cultural. For example, some Asians and Native Americans believe that prolonged eye contact is rude and intrusive (Luckmann, 2000). Muslim Arab women may not have eye contact with males, with the exception of their husbands. Hasidic Jewish men have culturally based norms concerning eye contact with women (Andrews & Boyle, 2011).

Variation in greetings is found from one culture to another. The handshake of an East Indian woman consists of a quick touch of the palms. Most East Indians bow the head, put the palms together, and say "Namaste," which means "I bow to you—I respect the God in you, I join my hands in prayer for you because I respect you." In American culture, a firm handshake is expected.

Cultural communication patterns take on particular significance for the nurse making home visits (Narayan & Scafide, 2017. A home visit may be refused if the nurse's communication is viewed as rude or inappropriate. For example, the nurse must keep in mind the social customs that are practiced when visiting a person of a given culture. It is of the utmost importance that the nurse demonstrate respect for the client. The home is the client's turf, and the client has complete control. The following points must be kept in mind: How is respect conveyed in the client's culture? Are shoes removed before entering the home? Should you bow or shake the client's hand? Is a "proper" handshake firm or just a brief, light touch of the palms? The nurse knows the name of the person he or she is visiting, but how does the client prefer to be addressed?

Temporal Relationships

Americans expect punctuality and generally attach a negative meaning to what is viewed as "lateness." We have the expression "time is money." The value placed on punctuality plays out in a strange way with appointments in the healthcare system. Clients are expected to be on time only to find that they must wait at least an hour to be seen by the healthcare professional. Timeliness seems to refer to clients but not to healthcare providers. This double standard of punctuality must change.

The Navajo and other Native American tribes have a present time orientation. Consequently, they often fail to understand the relationship between a person's past activities and present illness (Flowers, 2005; Nelson, 2018).

Numerous other cultures are much more flexible regarding time than are Americans: "I've learned from my

Filipino friend that I don't have to set a specific time when I need to talk to her. I don't have to announce myself before making a visit. I can drop by her house at any time, and it will be accepted in her culture—it's not in mine."

Format for Names

It is important to call a client by the name he or she prefers. Most Americans are comfortable with calling people by their first names. This is perceived by some, however, as a failure to show respect. It is important to ask a person how he or she prefers to be addressed because considerable cultural variation exists.

Age

In the United States the percentage of older adults in the general population is increasing rapidly, and the percentage of ethnic older adults is increasing at an even faster rate. The 65-and-older population is expected to be 87 million in 2050, up from 43.1 million in 2012 (Ortman, 2014). Ageism refers to the devaluing of older individuals, and it exists in the American culture.

Aging is generally viewed differently in Asian cultures. Increasing age is valued and respected because it brings knowledge and experience; the opinions of elders are held in high regard. Evidence of this is seen in India and Thailand in which few nursing homes exist. Elders live with their families and are cared for by them. Furthermore, in Hindi, the national language of India, the word *Buddha* means both "wise" and "old."

Ageism is particularly problematic in American culture because our society is aging. Older adults are avid consumers of healthcare and average nearly twice as many visits to their physicians as does the general population. Older adults and healthcare professionals may experience communication problems because of ageism. Examples of ageism include the healthcare professional's use of patronizing speech or the assumption that the older person does not understand. With older adults, use language and imagery that is inclusive of the wide range of individuals within the category of older adults. Because nurses spend more time with clients than do any other type of healthcare professional, nurses have the perfect opportunity to practice and then role-model care that facilitates communication across generations. Box 5.5 suggests communication strategies that healthcare professionals can use to improve healthcare delivery to older adults.

That the young do patronize the old in American society is commonly accepted. Many nurses have witnessed older clients being addressed with disrespectful words such as "honey," "sweetheart," "gramps," "granny," and other patronizing forms of speech. Older adults often construe improper behavior and communication on the part of caregivers as mistreatment (Mouton et al., 2005). Research conducted by

---

BOX 5.5   Communication Strategies to Improve Healthcare Delivery to Older Adults

Develop an increased awareness of ageist stereotyping in interactions between the healthcare professional and an older client.

View each interaction as a negotiation to reduce miscommunication.

Develop a unique relationship with each client (a relational culture unique to each relationship).

Promote the use of repetition and sensitive interrogation to help older adult clients understand technical jargon, diagnoses, and treatment options.

Use metaphors and examples salient to individual clients' interests to explain medical terms and procedures.

Enhance the relational interaction on an affective level so clients will be satisfied and remain loyal.

Develop a holistic understanding of each client by listening to client narratives and historical life reviews. Consider the use of a tape recorder to collect client information and a database management system to refer to client history before client visits.

Understand clients in relation to their cohort membership and its effects on their expectations of the healthcare professional–client interaction.

From Bethea, L., & Balazs, A. (1997). Improving intergenerational health care communications, *J Health Commun, 2*(2),129.

Chasteen (2002) suggested that patronization and stereotyping is not a one-way street. Many nurses have experienced older adults patronizing youth by using speech patterns such as disapproving and parental tones. This finding suggests the possibility of complex communication problems between healthcare professionals and clients because of the aging of our society. Not only are clients increasingly older, but healthcare professionals are also older and are taking care of young adult clients. Clearly, nurses must be aware of the fact that, in the American culture, age is often a factor that influences verbal and nonverbal communication patterns with clients. If this is true for you, consider how it affects your delivery of healthcare services.

Gender

Some of the most significant communication problems are those that exist between men and women because they transcend all cultures. Worldwide, the majority of males and females are socialized differently, resulting in different approaches to communication, affecting both style and content of communication. According to the US Board of Labor and Statistics, 12.6% of registered nurses are men (2021), up 2.7% from 1970 (Labor Force Statistics from the Current

Population Survey Overview (bls.gov), 2021; Egan, 2021). According to the Association of American Medical Colleges, 36.3% of physicians are female, up 8% from 2007 (Boyle, 2021).

In the United States persistent differences in traditional social assumptions about male and female roles typically credit American women with being more emotionally expressive and to place a higher value on interpersonal relationships. Men, on the other hand, are thought to value power and social status and to be more concerned with gathering and processing information. American society provides us with many examples of the frustrations experienced because of traditional differences in male–female communication styles. Lyrics of popular music often describe situations in which men and women cause each other great grief, television soap operas give day-to-day accounts of the triumphs and tragedies (mostly tragedies) that envelop male–female relationships, and a favorite topic of Broadway plays and movies is the struggle between men and women to communicate.

Current interest in enhancing male–female communication is evidenced by the popularity of books that focus on improving relationships between men and women.

Gender differences and assumptions of traditional gender roles between physicians and nurses can add to organizational power imbalances to create barriers to communication. In the past, the majority of physicians in the United States, unlike many countries in the world, were male. Now, the majority of medical students are female. However, in some practice settings and specialty areas, male physicians continue to outnumber females. Nursing has not been so successful at overcoming its gender gap. About 90% of nurses in the United States are female. Given the persistent gender differences that exist in some organizations, it is important to be informed about the influence that gender may have on communication. Gender issues, combined with organizational characteristics, may contribute to problems with satisfactory communication between nurses and physicians and can even affect the retention of nurses.

The current nursing shortage has drawn attention to the need for more effective ways to recruit and retain nurses. Siedlecki and Hixon (2015) surveyed nurses and physicians in a large magnet hospital. The goal of the survey was to identify how nurses and physicians define respectful behavior, examine perceptions of the relationship between nurses and physicians in clinical settings in which they practice together, and analyze the effect of nurse–physician relationships on nursing care decisions. The investigators found that physicians rated their interprofessional relationships more highly than did nurses. Nurses and physicians perceived their work interactions differently, and neither group perceived their practice environment as optimal. Further,

physician behaviors and attitudes can directly affect nursing patient care behaviors and, consequently, patient outcomes.

Communication between physicians and nurses in hospital settings has been found to be the single most important predictor of mortality rates. Furthermore, one of the characteristics of magnet hospitals (found to have lower mortality rates than nonmagnet hospitals) is good nurse–physician relationships (Shen et al., 2011).

Learning how to deal with gender issues in the current healthcare work environment may be one way of improving the delivery of comprehensive nursing care. The following are five strategies to improve communication between nurses and physicians:

1. *Level the playing field:* Understand the rules of professional communication and apply them. The rules are as follows:
2. *Get to the point:* Simplicity of speech is recommended. "Just the facts" is a valuable communication strategy. Use SBAR (Institute for Healthcare Improvement, 2017) (situation, background, assessment, recommendation) to keep the focus on necessary information. Your time and that of other healthcare providers is valuable. Focus on the goal.
3. *Use powerful prose:* Fear of being viewed as aggressive has stifled many nurses from stating the obvious in client care situations. Terms and phrases such as "I'm not sure" and "maybe" are not nearly as powerful in interactions as are statements such as "I think so" and "I know." A nurse who ends sentences with qualifiers and questions may come across as being unsure of what he or she is communicating.
4. *Exude expertise:* Nurses have information about clients that other members of the healthcare team need. How this information is imparted is important. Speak confidently and present yourself in a manner that makes it clear that you understand your patient's situation and needs. All healthcare providers should acknowledge that differences in values, incentives, and perceptions exist between individuals. Accommodating these different perspectives can improve the likelihood of success. Each member of the healthcare team should be viewed as a full partner in devising solutions to communication differences (Siedlecki & Hixon, 2015).
5. *Expect respect:* In male/female communication, men may interrupt more often than women. A typical female response to being interrupted is to stop speaking. If female healthcare providers believe that what they have to say is important, it may be necessary to change tactics to ensure their voice is heard when communicating with male healthcare providers. We begin all interactions expecting respect.

Given that men and women have been socialized differently, how do we best make use of these differences in nursing? Nurses' future success will be determined by how well they select the behaviors that best fit the situation and that focus on assertive and positive approaches to meeting patients' needs. Male and female healthcare workers can learn from each other.

Consider how you may view the lack of verbal communication, or silence. The meaning of silence is problematic to people who assume others are comfortable with speaking spontaneously, those with a preference for extroversion. The significance may be ambiguous; does silence mean client satisfaction or suppressed dissatisfaction? Silence may also be cultural. For example, silence is highly valued in the Navajo culture. A person who hurries a conversation is thought to be rude. Lengthy periods of silence are used to think so that the spoken word will have significance (Andrews & Boyle, 2011).

Consider, too, gender diversity. In light of the increasing awareness of a gender diverse/gender fluid population, adding two questions in the patient interview/assessment has been found to be respectful: (1) ask the preferred name and (2) the pronoun with which to address the patient (Sanders et al., 2019). Such questions are gender affirming. In Dorsen's exploratory study, "Meaning and Impact of Gender Affirmation," presented at the 2021 International Association for Human Caring Virtual Conference, participants shared that this respectful approach means bringing all of our identities into the light, responses such as . . . I need you to see me, to name this, and to celebrate me (Dorsen, 2021).

SIMPLIFY AND DEEPEN

We may create stereotypes without realizing it. "Once you name something, it stops you seeing the whole of it, or why it matters." Alex Michaelides in *The Silent Patient*.

(Michaelides, 2019, p. 1)

CLOSING THOUGHTS

This chapter has focused on the importance of nurses recognizing and appreciating healthcare beliefs and behaviors of diverse cultures. The QSEN initiative recommends that nurses seek out learning experiences with patients who represent all aspects of human diversity (QSEN, 2010). Consider ways in which you may continue to build your cultural competence. Some schools of nursing have immersion courses in which you travel to another country. Participating students experienced a broader worldview (Larson et al., 2010). A qualitative study of the lived experience of students who were involved in a study abroad program suggested participants gained an increase in awareness of diverse cultures and self-efficacy (Edmonds, 2010). As a nurse you can volunteer for a medical mission nationally or internationally that will immerse you in a different culture and build your transcultural communication skills. A clinical experience in community health can provide service

learning in which you learn about diversity while being actively involved in the community. Such courses, which include structure programs for community assessment and working with defined issues, promote the development of the delivery of culturally sensitive care (Amerson, 2010). Dealing with differences is important, but something can also be said for identifying the commonalities we share as members of the human race. Recognition of commonalities builds bonds. For example, we all value our health and our families, and we all want a better world for our children. Consideration of commonalities emphasizes the sameness of members of the human species. Recognizing and appreciating commonalities and differences provide a holistic or transpersonal way of viewing people.

🌸 MOMENTS OF CONNECTION...
Empathy, Respect, and Genuineness

A nurse was assigned to care for an 83-year-old woman from a coastal mountain fishing village in Thailand. The client was diagnosed with liver cancer. Her two daughters served as interpreters. The client's deep religious beliefs in Buddhism were central to her life. Medications and tests were administered at times that were congruent with her schedule for religious practices (e.g., morning prayer, afternoon meditation, evening devotion). Religious icons were allowed to be placed in close proximity to the client. It was observed that the client was drinking only the tea and juice sent on her dietary tray. Negotiations were made, with the advisement of the attending physician, to have the daughters bring traditional foods cooked at home. The nurse was made to feel welcomed when the dietary changes were made. The daughters brought in a huge basket of fruit for the unit staff. While interacting with the family, the nurse mentioned his interest in Asian cooking and in Buddhism. Soon after, the daughters brought the nurse dumplings and fragrant rice "especially for him." Within a short period of time, the unit was blessed with another huge basket of fruit and what the nurse called "the most fragrant flowers I have ever beheld." He was called into the room and was given special rare fruits that came from the Far East.

The nurse described his final interaction with the client and her family: "This would be the woman's last night at the unit, and she reached out and touched my hand (she had never displayed something like this before). I turned to her family and noticed they were weeping. My throat thickened, and tears filled my own eyes. I bowed to my patient and walked out, knowing what it is like being in the presence of someone so much more aware of life than I will ever be."

Return to "Active Learning" at the beginning of the chapter and write your responses.

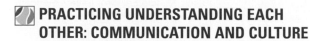

PRACTICING UNDERSTANDING EACH OTHER: COMMUNICATION AND CULTURE

Application: Exercise 1

A group of nursing students from Florida traveled to the mountains of Costa Rica for a language and public health experience. They were required to stay with local families for a language immersion experience. Students knew about home stays, but there was no question that this was the most uncomfortable part of the entire experience. Many host families spoke limited to no English at home, although they had worked with visiting students for years. The families were used to using nonverbal communication and very basic Spanish with students, but students were not used to having to work to communicate their needs. Also, homes in this part of Costa Rica are very small and modest. This reflects the lifestyle of "pura vida": living the simple, pure, and happy life. Showers are small and very basic, with a switch to flip during your shower that supplies limited hot water. Several students found this part of the experience extremely stressful. They were used to taking long, luxurious showers with as much hot water as they wanted. They worried that flipping an electrical switch in the shower could shock them. They found that the switches did not always work properly because there was rust or a wire had broken. Sometimes there was insufficient hot water, but there was always ample cold water. In communicating these problems to the host family, the students quickly learned that a perfectly hot shower every day was not a priority in this part of the world. Students expressed that adapting to this cultural norm was one of the most difficult aspects of the trip.

Questions:
1. What habits and routines in your own lifestyle would be most disrupted by travel to another culture, and how would you adapt to that?
2. What are some ways in which you can prepare for a visit to a foreign country in which another language is spoken?
3. If a nurse accepts a position in an organization in which a substantial portion of patients speak another language, what is the nurse's responsibility for developing skills in that language?

Creative Expression/Reflection: Exercise 2

Think about what you have read about differences in culture. Reflect on what you know about your own culture and communication patterns. What aspects of your own culture might create barriers to communicating with patients from another culture?

Critical Thinking: Exercise 3

Write what you can remember about at least one client from another culture for whom you have cared or observed being cared for and with whom a communication problem existed.

Describe how the application of a few of the communication techniques suggested in this chapter might have improved the outcome.

Skill Building: Exercise 4

Write the first words that come to mind when you contemplate being assigned to care for an "old" client. Reflect on how your expectations may influence the interaction.

Application: Exercise 5

Identify a workplace interaction problem that may have been caused by gender differences in communication. Review the five strategies to improve communication between nurses and physicians and identify possible approaches to the workplace problem you identified.

Critical Thinking and Reflection: Exercise 6

Read the following article: Lim, F. A., Brown. D. V., & Justin Kim, S. M. (2014). Addressing healthcare disparities in lesbian, gay, bisexual, and transgender populations: A review of best practices. *Am J Nurs, 114*(6) 24–34. Respond to this article in an essay in which you describe and discuss the content of the article and the implications for your future nursing practice (Maley, 2019).

Critical Thinking: Exercise 7

The following table depicts the minority population of Canada from the 2011 National Household Survey. Assume that you have been invited to consult with a hospital serving a population with a breakdown in ethnic population similar to Winnipeg. What have you learned in this chapter that might be helpful in training the nursing staff, most of whom are probably members of the dominant White culture, to begin to develop cultural awareness? How might this have affected the provision of healthcare?

Independent Study: Exercise 8

Interview one person from a culture distinctly different from your own, someone who was born in another country and lived there past childhood. Discuss health practices related to that culture, selected traditional therapies used in health promotion, and maintenance and restoration, as well as any other interesting features about the culture and personal responses to the experience. Ask about remedies/

City	Total Population	Visibly Minority Population	Minority (%)	Top Three Visible Minorities
Toronto	5,521,235	2,396,420	47.0	South Asian, Chinese, Black
Montreal	3,752,475	762,325	20.3	Black, Middle Eastern, Latin American
Vancouver	2,280,695	1,030,335	45.2	Chinese, South Asian, Filipino
Ottawa-Gatineau	1,215,735	234,015	19.2	Black, Middle Eastern, Chinese
Calgary	1,199,125	337,420	28.1	South Asian, Chinese, Filipino
Edmonton	1,139,585	254,990	22.4	South Asian, Chinese, Filipino
Winnipeg	714,635	140,770	19.7	Filipino, South Asian, Black
Hamilton	708,175	101,600	14.3	South Asian, Black, Chinese
Canada (overall)	32,852,325	6,264,755	19.1	South Asian, Chinese, Black

From Statistics Canada. (2011). *National Household Survey*. Ottawa, Canada: Statistics Canada.

treatments for a cold, pain, or other ailments. Discuss this person's view of Western medicine. Write a reflective journal entry based on this experience.

Quality and Safety Education for Nurses Learning Strategy: Exercise 9

Communication is a key competency to provide safe, high-quality care.

Like healthcare providers and their patients, healthcare teams also may represent many cultural backgrounds. When English is a second language, people often make assumptions about that person as a member of the team.

How does this dynamic influence interaction among the nurses on the unit or in your clinical learning group? Consider the following situation:

- You have noticed that two students in your clinical group whose country of origin is Saudi Arabia are never included when the group takes a break for coffee, and during the break, others in the group talk about them and wonder why they cover their heads with scarves. You have noticed the two students have become more withdrawn through the course of the semester and do not speak up in clinical conferences unless the instructor asks them questions directly. You would like to change the interactions with the two students because you think it is an example of incivility.
- How can you speak up to help the group recognize the assumptions they are making and how their actions ostracize the two students?
- How can you help the group research and understand why the students wear scarves as part of their values and beliefs?
- Search the literature for the evidence base for the ways civility affects communication and safety culture. How would you organize a clinical conference to focus on incivility and bullying among nurses when they make assumptions and misunderstand cultural backgrounds?

- How can you change your own actions to include the students in group activities?

> **WIT AND WISDOM**
>
> *All communication is more or less cross-cultural. We learn to use language as we grow up, and growing up in different parts of the country, having different ethnic, religious, or class backgrounds, even just being male or female—all result in different ways of talking.*
>
> **Deborah Tannen**

REFERENCES

American Nurses Association. (2021). *Nursing scope and standards of practice* (4th ed). Silver Spring, MD: ANA, p. 93.

Amerson, R. (2010). The impact of service learning on cultural competence. *Nursing Education Perspectives, 31*(1), 18.

Andrews, M., & Boyle, J. (2011). *Transcultural concepts in nursing care*. Philadelphia, PA: J. B. Lippincott.

Boyle, P. (2021). Nation's physician workforce evolves: More women, a bit older, and toward different specialties | AAMC.

Certified Medical Interpreters, National Board for Certification of Medical Interpreters, www.certifiedmedicalinterpreters. org.

Chasteen, A., Schwarz, N., & Park, D. (2002). The activation of aging stereotypes in younger and older adults. *The Journals of Gerontology: Series B, Psychological Sciences and Social Sciences, 57*(6), 540–547.

Colby, S., & Ortman, J. (2015). *Projections of the size and composition of the U.S. population: 2014 to 2060*. Washington, DC: US Department of Commerce.

Cook, L., & Peden, A. (2017). Finding a focus for nursing: The caring concept. *Advances in Nursing Science, 40*(1), 12–23.

Daily Word. (2021). *Belong: Authentic living is my key to belonging*. A Unity Publication June 24, 2021.

Dorsen, C. (2021). Meaning and Impact of Gender Affirmation: An exploratory study presented at the 2021 International Association for Human Caring Virtual Conference.

Edmonds, M. L. (2010). The lived experience of nursing students who study abroad. *Journal of Studies in International Education, 14*(5), 545.

Egan, B. (2021). The Male Nurse: Benefits and Percentages of Men in Nursing (snhu.edu).

Ferrell, B. & Williams, R. (2021). The "other" confronting injustices in 2021 and beyond. *Journal of Hospice & Palliative Nursing, 23*(1), 1–2. doi: 10.1097/NJH.0000000000000720.

Fletcher, K. (2007). Are you practicing cultural humility: The key to success in cultural competency. California Health Advocates blog. Are You Practicing Cultural Humility? – The Key to Success in Cultural Competence - California Health Advocates (cahealthadvocates.org).

Flowers, D. L. (2005). Culturally-competent nursing care for American Indian clients in a critical care setting. *Critical Care Nurse, 25*(1), 45.

Giger, J., & Davidhizar, R. (2002). The Giger and Davidhizar transcultural assessment model. *Journal of Transcultural Nursing, 13*(3), 185–188.

Green, Z. D., & Reinckens, J. (2013). Cultural competency in health care: What can nurses do? *Maryland Nurse News and Journal*.

Green-Hernandez, C., Quinn, A., Denman-Vitale, S., Flakenstern, S. K., & Judge-Ellis, T. (2004). Making nursing culturally competent. *Holistic Nursing Practice, 18*(4), 215.

Institute for Healthcare Improvement. (2017). SBAR: Situation, background, assessment, recommendation. SBAR Tool: Situation-Background-Assessment-Recommendation | IHI - Institute for Healthcare Improvement.

Jones, N., Marks, R., Ramirez, R., & Rios-Vargas, M. (2021). 2020 census illuminates racial and ethnic composition of the country. Improved Race and Ethnicity Measures Reveal U.S. Population Is Much More Multiracial (census.gov).

Juckett, G., & Unger, K. (2014). Appropriate use of medical interpreters. *American Family Physician, 90*(7), 476–480.

Kim-Godwin, Y. S., Clarke, P. N., & Barton, L. (2001). A model for the delivery of culturally competent community care. *Journal of Advanced Nursing, 35*(6), 918.

Kreuz, R. & Roberts, R. (2019). Proxemics 101: Understanding Personal Space Across Cultures. Adapted from Kreuz and Roberts, *Getting through: The pleasures and perils of cross-cultural communication*. The MIT Press, 2018. Proxemics 101: Understanding Personal Space Across Cultures | The MIT Press Reader.

Labor force statistics from the current population survey. (2021). 2020 Annual Averages - Employed persons by detailed occupation, sex, race, and Hispanic or Latino ethnicity Labor Force Statistics from the Current Population Survey Overview (bls.gov).

Lagisetty, P., Priyadarshini, S., Terrell, S., Hamati, M., Landgraf, J., Chopra, V., & Heisler, M. (2017). Culturally targeted strategies for diabetes prevention in minority population. *Diabetes Educator, 43*(1), 54–77.

Larson, K. L., Ott, M., & Miles, J. M. (2010). International cultural immersion: En vivo reflections of cultural competence. *Journal of Cultural Diversity, 17*(2), 44–50.

Leininger, M. (1988). Leininger's theory of nursing: Culture care diversity and universality. *Nursing Science Quarterly, 1*(4), 152.

Leininger, M. (2002). Culture care theory: A major contribution to advance transcultural nursing knowledge and practices. *Journal of Transcultural Nursing, 13*(3), 189.

Lim, F. A., Brown., D. V., & Justin Kim, S. M. (2014). Addressing health care disparities in lesbian, gay, bisexual, and transgender populations: A review of best practices. *Am J Nurs, 114*(6), 24–34.

Luckmann, J. (2000). *Transcultural communication in health care*. Toronto, Canada: Delmar/Thomson Learning.

Matveev, A. (2017). *Intercultural competence in organizations: A guide for leaders, educators and team players*. Cham, Switzerland: Springer.

Maley, B., & Gross, R. (2019). A writing assignment to address gaps in the nursing curriculum regarding health issues of LGBT+ populations. *Nurs Forum, 2019*(54), 198–204. https://doi.org/10.1111/nuf.12315.

Michaelides, A. (2019). *The Silent patient*. New York, NY: Celadon Books.

Mouton, C. P., Larme, A. C., Alford, C. L., Talamantes, M. A., McCorkle, R. J., & Burge, S. K. (2005). Multiethnic perspective on elder mistreatment. *Journal of Elder Abuse and Neglect, 17*(2), 21.

Narayan, M., & Scafide, K. (2017). Systematic review of racial/ethnic outcome disparities in home health care. *Journal of Transcultural Nursing, 28*(6), 598–607.

Nelson, M. (2018). Navajo wellness model: Keeping the cultural teachings alive to improve health. January 2018 Blogs (ihs.gov).

Ortman, J. M. (2014). An Aging Nation: The Older Population in the United States (census.gov).

Purnell, L. (2002). The Purnell model for cultural competence. *Journal of Transcultural Nursing, 13*(3), 193.

Purnell, L. (2012). *Transcultural health care: A culturally competent approach*. Philadelphia, PA: FA Davis.

Quality and Safety Education for Nurses (QSEN). (2010). QSEN Competencies. 2010.

Reeves, J. S., & Fogg, C. (2006). Perceptions of graduating nursing students regarding life experiences that promote culturally competent care. *Journal of Transcultural Nursing, 17*(2), 171.

Salter, F. K. (2002). *Risky transactions: Trust, kinship, and ethnicity*. New York: Berghahn.

Sanders, V., & Pedersen, S. (2019). Guest Editorial: Improving communication with the gender diverse community in diagnostic imaging departments. *Radiography, 24*, S3–S6. https://doi.org/10.1016/j.radi.2018.04.011.

Shen, H. C., Chiu, H. T., Lee, P. H., Hu, Y. C., & Chang, W. Y. (2011). Hospital environment, nurse-physician relationships and quality of care: questionnaire survey. *Journal of Advanced Nursing, 67*(2), 349–358.

Siedlecki, S., & Hixon, E. (2015). Relationships between nurses and physicians matter. *The Online Journal of Issues in Nursing, 20*(3), 6.

Sobralske, M., & Katz, J. (2005). Culturally competent care of patients with acute chest pain. *Journal of the American Academy of Nurse Practitioners, 17*(9), 342.

US Department of Health and Human Services. (2019). National Culturally and Linguistically Appropriate Service Standards. CLAS Standards - Think Cultural Health (hhs.gov).

Yeager, K. A., & Bauer-Wu (2013). Cultural humility: Essential foundation for clinical researchers. *Applied Nursing Research, 26*(4), 251–256. In Distinguishing Cultural Humility from Cultural Competence | Equity and Inclusion (uoregon.edu).

Waite, R., Nardi, D., & Killian, P. (2014). Examination of cultural knowledge and provider sensitivity in nurse managed health centers. *Journal of Cultural Diversity, 21*(2), 74.

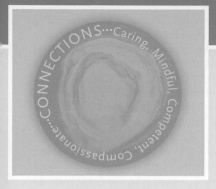

Demonstrating Warmth*

We all need people in our lives who take away the chill of this world with the warmth of their presence.

Author Unknown

OBJECTIVES

1. Discuss the benefits of warmth in communication with clients and colleagues.
2. Identify behaviors that demonstrate warmth.
3. Review a tool to analyze warmth in interpersonal communications.
4. Describe a variety of ways in which warmth is displayed, and articulate the importance of warmth in human interactions.

5. Become aware of opportunities to embellish your life with warmth in day-to-day encounters with clients and colleagues.
6. Participate in exercises to build skills in demonstrating warmth.

❓ ACTIVE LEARNING

Think about how you will write your answers as you read this chapter.

What?
Write one thing you learned from this chapter.

So What?
How will this affect your nursing practice?

Now What?
How will you implement this new knowledge or skill?

Think About It ...

A STUDENT NURSE SHARES

"This chapter stood out to me because I have been told that I am scary to approach because my facial expression is not

---

* With contributions from Margaret E. Erickson, PhD.

welcoming. This chapter says warmth is displayed primarily in a nonverbal manner to convey our inner relaxation and attentiveness to the other person. I can focus on these behaviors to demonstrate warmth, such as making eye contact and facing the client. I am working on these."

DEMONSTRATING WARMTH

How do you demonstrate warmth? As you read, think about someone who demonstrates warmth. Amy Cuddy, a social psychologist and researcher at Harvard Business School, identifies behaviors and cues demonstrating warmth: appropriate self-disclosure, humor, natural smiles, leaning toward the other, communicating on the same physical plane, and being closer physically, remembering that ideal distance varies with culture (Lambert, 2010). Healy (2013), a nurse patient, recounts a long wait before surgery, ponders what it was that distinguished the behavior of one caring nurse, and identifies warmth as the hallmark of compassion, which is also a quality of compassionate listening (Kimble & Bamford-Wade, 2013). "Speak with me in a warm and caring voice" (Lee-Hsiehg, Fang, Kuo, & Turton, 2004). Let your voice inflection say I care about you as we share this moment (Pullen & Mathias, 2010). Warmth is the glue in the bonding between people and the magnetism that draws us to a closer intimacy with others. It is a special ingredient, even a catalyst, in our human relationships. It is comfort, as in the lines of a prayer, "May comfort be yours, warm and soft like a sigh" (Tabron, 2001). The expression of warmth makes us feel welcomed, relaxed, and joyful. Although clients may not be able to judge our intelligence, certifications, or degrees, they can judge our hearts by the care we give and the warmth we demonstrate at their sides (Carver, 1998). A student nurse struggling with injection skills and the potential effect of her lack of confidence on her clients reflected that "a dose of genuine warmth is as essential as skill with a syringe" (O'Connor, 2005).

Warmth has been identified as an essential attribute in psychotherapists. The therapist's warmth, along with empathy and genuineness, contributes to client improvement and leads to more open, full relationships for clients in and out of therapy. Warmth sets the tone for clients, families, and colleagues to share their own stories. Most of you will not be psychotherapists. Your expression of warmth to your clients, however, will make them feel welcomed and not judged. These positive emotions will foster feelings of well-being and likely promote healing. Caring acts that show warmth and genuineness have been associated with increased hope in clients with cancer (Koopmeiners et al., 1997). In a study to identify and validate the dimensions for caregiver reciprocity in intergenerational exchanges, warmth and regard were found to be important factors (Carruth, 1996). Clients who sense your warmth are more likely to engage in dialogue and provide information about their health conditions. This communication helps the nurse to make a nursing diagnosis, determine expected outcomes, work out a nursing care plan, and evaluate the progress of nursing care with the client.

WIT AND WISDOM

The mysteries of human connection, love, and understanding are fully accessible in digital world settings. If we are open to creativity and change, ongoing technological advances coupled with a firm intent to care will continually open new and exciting possibilities for caring across distance, time, and culture.

(Sitzman & Watson, 2017)

A creative way to demonstrate warmth is the "Warm Handoff," defined by the Agency for Healthcare Research and Quality (AHRQ, 2017) as "a strategy to encourage bi (or tri) directional communication with patients, family members, and the care team…moves the conversations between healthcare team members in front of the patient… a safety check!" A nurse took the medication list from the patient, but when medications were discussed in front of the physician with the family present, information surfaced that the evening dose of one medication was often forgotten. This helped the physician readjust the medication with the full picture. The AHRQ offers a comprehensive guide to implement the Warm Handoff process (AHRQ, 2021). Exchanging warmth with colleagues makes the workplace a more pleasant environment. Warmth enhances closeness, which has social and work-related benefits. A study by the American Management Association (Ekeren, 1994) identified eight traits that often lead to failure for executives. The first two were "insensitivity to coworkers" and "aloofness and arrogance." Extending our warmth to our colleagues makes us more approachable. Increased communication among colleagues ensures that important messages about clients or unit policies and procedures are transmitted. Effective leaders demonstrate their considerateness of employees by warmth in their interpersonal relationships, and this helps build rapport (Reece, 2013).

Although we often refer to others as warm, as a human quality warmth is difficult to describe and one of the most difficult interpersonal communication behaviors to learn. Warmth involves not only attitudinal and psychomotor behavior, but also a total way of offering oneself to another person. Showing warmth to others means conveying that you like to be with them and that you accept them as they are. In this sense warmth is a way of showing respect to clients and colleagues.

Warmth is not communicated in isolation. It enhances and is enhanced by other facilitative communication behaviors that you will learn about in later chapters (e.g., respect, genuineness, empathy). By itself, warmth is not sufficient for building an effective helping relationship, developing mutual respect, or solving problems, but warmth enhances these processes.

According to Levine and Adelman (1982), a study conducted in the United States found that 93% of a message is transmitted by tone of voice and facial expression and only 7% by words. We may possibly tune into the nonverbal expression of emotions and attitudes more than the verbal expression. Because expression of warmth is predominantly nonverbal, it is wise to heed these findings.

WAYS TO DISPLAY WARMTH TO YOUR CLIENTS AND COLLEAGUES

Warmth is displayed primarily in a nonverbal manner. Subtle facial and body signs, as well as gestures (small

TABLE 6.1 Facial Signals of Warmth

Facial Feature	How Warmth Is Displayed
Forehead	Muscles are relaxed, and forehead is smooth; there is no furrowing of the brow
Eyes	Comfortable eye contact is maintained; pupils are dilated; gaze is neither fixed nor shifting and darting
Mouth	Lips are loose and relaxed, not tight or pursed; gestures such as biting a lip or forcing a smile are absent; jaw is relaxed and mobile, not clenched; smile is appropriate
Expression	Features of the face move in a relaxed, fluid way; worried, distracted, or fretful looks are absent; the face shows interest and attentiveness

TABLE 6.2 Postural Signals of Warmth

Postural Feature	How Warmth Is Displayed
Body position	Client is faced squarely, with shoulders parallel to the client's shoulders
Head position	Head is kept at the same level as the client's; periodic nodding shows interest and attentiveness
Shoulders	Shoulders are kept level and mobile, not hunched and tense
Arms	Arms are kept loose and able to move smoothly rather than held stiffly
Hands	Gestures are natural, with no clenching or grasping of a clipboard or chart; distracting mannerisms such as tapping a pen or playing with an object are avoided
Chest	Breathing is at an even pace; the chest is kept open, neither slouched nor extended too far forward in feigned attentiveness; a slight forward leaning shows interest
Legs	Whether crossed or uncrossed, legs are kept in a comfortable and natural position; during standing, knees should be flexed and not locked
Feet	Fidgeting, tapping, and kicking are avoided

movements of a hand, brow, or eye), convey our inner relaxation and attentiveness to another person (Table 6.1).

There is a great deal you do with your face to convey warmth. When you are talking to another person, attention is largely focused on the face, so it is important to know how to make facial expressions that maximize your warmth.

During interaction, your face can communicate information regarding your personality, interests, and responsiveness, as well as your emotional state. Your facial expression can open or close a conversation. The context, including the relationship, determines the meaning of facial expressions. Also, the degree of facial expressiveness varies among individuals and cultures. In relationships with clients and colleagues, it is wise to remember that although people from other cultures may not express emotions (e.g., warmth) openly, this does not mean that they do not experience these emotions.

Americans express themselves to varying degrees. People from certain ethnic backgrounds in the United States may use their hands, bodies, and faces more than others. Warmth can be expressed in a variety of ways, but to have a poker face or deadpan expression is usually considered suspicious.

We may interpret insufficient or excessive eye contact as communication barriers. No specific rules govern eye behavior, except that to stare, especially at strangers, is considered rude. Eye contact can have different meanings in different cultures.

Your posture can communicate warmth. Movements or ways of holding yourself that encourage communication and indicate interest and pleasure in being with the other person constitute warmth (Table 6.2). The list in Table 6.2 may sound like your mother telling you to sit up straight at dinner, but the details provide solid guidelines for communicating the warmth you feel, even if you are anxious.

Warmth indicators include a shift of posture toward the other person, a smile, direct eye contact, and motionless hands. In a study by Knapp (1980), gestures such as looking around the room, slumping, drumming fingers, and looking glum detract from warmth. In a dialogue situation, positive warmth cues, coupled with verbal reinforcers such as "mm-hmm," are effective in increasing verbal output from the interviewee (whereas verbal cues alone are insufficient). These findings from an early study have implications for nursing in which so much client information is gathered through interviewing.

Purtilo and Haddad (2002) pointed out that, in addition to whole-body posturing and positioning, gestures involving the extremities, even one finger, can suggest the meaning of a message. Think about how the following gestures would affect your message of warmth: shrugging your shoulders, folding your arms over your chest, rolling your thumb, shuffling your foot, or silently clenching your fist. Even if other parts of your body are focused on conveying warmth, these partial gestures might minimize or erase the message of warmth you are trying to send.

Remember not all gestures have universal meaning. A wink or a hand gesture may not be received in the same mood of warmth in which it is delivered. For example, the American "OK" sign (circle made with thumb and forefinger) is a symbol for money in Japan and is considered obscene in some Latin American countries.

The spatial distance or closeness we create between us and our clients and colleagues can affect the perception of warmth. For Americans, distance in social conversation is about an arm's length to 4 feet. In our exuberance to display warmth, we may invade this unseen but well-defined circumference. Not all clients or colleagues feel comforted by this gesture; some may feel intruded on, and others may feel threatened and act defensively.

Touching is another way to affectionately transmit warmth. From the briefest pat on the shoulder to an embracing hug or extended hand, you can convey warmth to others. Your comfort or lack of comfort with touch is communicated. The gentle, sincere touch of your hand can express warmth, caring, and comfort (Gleeson, 2004; Reynolds, 2002).

Warmth can be conveyed verbally and nonverbally. The volume of the voice is related to warmth. Softer, modulated tones convey warmth more than loud, aggressive tones that are harsh to the ears. A pitch that seems comfortable for the speaker transmits warmth more than an unnatural pitch that seems to be out of the speaker's range. The pacing of words is also important. Pressured, stilted, or stoic speech detracts from the warmth that can be conveyed through rhythmic speech, whose pacing is in keeping with the speaker's natural breathing. The actual words also have the power to extend warmth to others. Loving, soft words are warmer than harsh, thoughtless words: "So, you've never exercised before and now you think you'll become a 'superjock' and take up jogging?" is cold and judgmental compared with "You'd like to improve your fitness level, so you're taking a new lease on life and learning to jog."

As you may have noticed, many of the features of warmth are those of a relaxed person. Not only must you be relaxed, but you can communicate warmth only when you have a genuine interest in the other person and a wish to convey that welcome and pleasure to him or her. A desire to be warm is based on the belief that each person you encounter is worthy of receiving the acceptance and comfort that your warmth generates. The ability to be warm was so valued by a psychiatric facility in Surrey, England, that it was included in an online recruitment ad. When you display high-level warmth, you are completely and intensely attentive to the interaction between yourself and your clients or colleagues, making them feel accepted and important. The opposite, which is cold behavior, conveys disapproval or disinterest.

Self-Care Nudge

Pause, now, and reflect on one positive quality you bring to your life. Take a moment to appreciate that quality, to appreciate yourself.

Stories of Warmth in the Actions of Nurses

A collection of Moments of Connection stories demonstrates the tapestry woven from lessons learned in our professional and personal journeys and illustrates the warmth that is so central to the caring art of nursing.

 MOMENTS OF CONNECTION...

For Our Loved Ones and Yours in Their Final Hours

"My father died suddenly in 1992, alone in a hospital far from family. I can only hope and pray that a kind nurse was with him or, hopefully, held his hand or said a prayer with him as he passed away. I tend to want to hold my patients' hands or pray, or be kind, so their family members can rest assured that a kind person was with their loved one."

 MOMENTS OF CONNECTION...

Pain Management: More Than Analgesia

"I was caring for a pain management patient who was reluctant to take medication. After talking with him, I learned he had lost his only child 3 months before in an automobile accident. He needed to talk. He was frightened and wanted a hand to hold. Despite my busy schedule, I knew this was where I belonged. I left when he was more comfortable. As I walked down the hall, I thanked God for giving me the talent and knowledge to help another person."

MOMENTS OF CONNECTION...
A Pillow, a Washcloth, and Myself

"As an operating room nurse, I had a patient with muscular dystrophy. Her surgery was delayed, and I spent about 30 minutes with her. She was in her twenties, and we laughed and joked. I repositioned her arms and legs for her, since she had many contractures, and gave her pillows and wet washcloths. Our time meant a lot to her, and she asked me if I would see her after surgery. When I did, she was thrilled and asked me to take my hat off so she could see me better. She visited me each time she came to the hospital. Later I learned she and her mother lived alone. She did not have any friends until we met. These comfort measures were just part of my work, but they meant a lot to her."

MOMENTS OF CONNECTION...
Off the Clock

"My story is about my own unplanned C-section. I have been a pain management nurse for 5 years and know many people in the hospital. We all know it can be tough to care for another nurse. A special nurse from the postanesthesia care unit inserted my Foley catheter for my male RN friend who was the circulating RN that day. Then she clocked out after seeing my nervousness and anxiety in the holding area. She comforted me and followed me through surgery. She did everything for me to provide warmth and comfort, including holding my hand during the epidural. I could just picture that 3-inch spinal needle! She took the video for my husband so he could enjoy the first moments of our daughter's life. She provided comfort not only physically but emotionally as well. I will never forget her caring."

MOMENTS OF CONNECTION...
When the Client Is Scared

"I had just begun to work with cancer patients when I met a young woman dying with sarcoma. She required many boluses of medication to relieve her pain, which was worst at night when she was most fearful. I held her hand and patted her shoulder gently to soothe her until the medication took effect."

MOMENTS OF CONNECTION...
Showing Our Sympathy

"Working in the chronic pain setting, we do not have many deaths. When someone does die, as pain clinic coordinator, I call the family to offer condolences. We also send a sympathy card. This time a daughter of a patient was killed in an accident and we chose to send flowers. The patient and family expressed their appreciation for this connection to them at a difficult time."

Factors that make it possible to convey warmth are the physical ability to control the facial, postural, tactile, and verbal indicators of warmth and the ability to overcome any of the cognitive or affective influences mediating against warmth. What are some of the factors working against the expression of warmth? Any thoughts or feelings that distract your attention from other people block the expression of warmth. Being rushed, overcome with strong emotions, shocked, and judgmental about others' behaviors are distractions that divert your attention. When you feel hurried, you are focused on yourself and are unable to enjoy the people around you. Remember to take a deep breath and bring your attention back to the person.

It is only natural to withdraw your warmth when you are angry with another person. When you feel hurt, bitter, irritated, or enraged with a client or colleague, trying to convey warmth would be insincere. At times you may feel insecure about whether you will be accepted or rejected by another person. Then, you might hide behind a crisp facade until you feel safe enough to allow your warmth to surface.

Extension and Withdrawal of Warmth

Any time you wish to become closer to one of your clients or colleagues or to provide the message that you really care, an expression of warmth is appropriate. There are degrees of warmth. An attitude of "I like that client (colleague); I feel warmly toward him with all his strengths and weaknesses" is warmer than "I don't feel dislike for my client (colleague)." The warmth you express should reflect your genuine feelings. Your expression of warmth to a colleague that you would like to date will likely be more open and intense than the warmth you might express to a client in your care.

On the other hand, there may be occasions when you withhold your feelings for fear of being too warm. Perhaps you have romantic thoughts about a client or an unavailable colleague that are inappropriate to express. Sometimes you may have very strong negative feelings toward someone. It is likely that we all have encountered someone who has treated us coldly, with disdain, or even with rudeness or contempt. It would be difficult for most of us to be warm with those who have treated us in this way. When we want to protect ourselves from perceived or actual uncaring or disinterest, we may withdraw our warmth or refrain from offering it.

It is assertive to express your warmth to clients and colleagues when you wish. It is nonassertive to withhold the warmth you feel. In contrast, it is aggressive to exude a warmth beyond the measure of your feelings. When you sincerely convey the warmth you feel, you bring to life the assertive position: "I like myself; I like you." This warmth is nonpossessive and allows others room to be themselves.

The following exercises can make you aware of your warmth and provide you with pointers on how to convey your warmth when you choose.

WIT AND WISDOM

Professionals are those who do their best even when they do not feel like it.

Author Unknown

WIT AND WISDOM

All the statistics in the world can't measure the warmth of a smile.

Chris Hart

SIMPLIFY AND DEEPEN

Kind hearts are the gardens.
Kind thoughts are the roots.
Kind words are the flowers.
Kind deeds are the fruit.

Henry Wadsworth Longfellow

Return to "Active Learning" at the beginning of the chapter and write your responses.

PRACTICING DEMONSTRATING WARMTH

Reflective Journaling/Critical Thinking: Exercise 1

Before you start observing or changing your own behavior, take a few days to observe the warmth displayed by colleagues and friends. In your journal note the following:

- Facial expressions
- Posturing
- Verbal expression
- Touching

What felt good? What warmth behaviors would you like to emulate? Compare your observations with those of your classmates. What did you learn from each other about the communication of warmth?

Critical Thinking/Discussion: Exercise 2

For a few days, focus on your delivery of warmth. What is it you do to show your loved ones that you care? How is this expression different from your display of warmth to coworkers and to clients? How is it the same? Would you like to display more affection for others than you do? Make note of what you could change to be warmer. Find a partner in the class and exchange notes on the self-observations you have made.

Assessment/Skill Building: Exercise 3

Find a full-length mirror and take a good look at yourself. Make a statement about the warmth your image projects. Does the set of your face convey warmth? Why? Why not? Note how you are holding your facial muscles. Do your eyes twinkle, or are they cold? Are your lips softly mobile, or are they tightened? Now change your expression to make it warmer. Note what you do. How does it feel to soften your facial expression? Recall that feeling; you need that memory to call on when you want to convey warmth to another person (when you do not have your mirror handy).

Next, turn away from the mirror and attempt to recapture that same warm facial expression. Then turn to check in the mirror. Have you got it? Or does your head need tilting, your smile broadening, or your eyes crinkling?

If you want to convey warmth, you need to practice these nonverbal gestures so you feel confident that you are sending out the message of warmth you want your clients and colleagues to receive.

Creative Expression: Exercise 4

Identify a situation in which you felt warm toward someone, perhaps one who makes you smile. You might have seen a parent and child playing together or have been playing with your own child. Write a haiku poem describing the scene. This is a three-line, 17-syllable Japanese poem that captures a moment in time from the perception of the poet and usually involves nature.

Use five syllables in the first line, seven in the second line, and five in the third line, for example:

Head on my shoulder
Baby-sleep warmth spreads throughout
New mother delight.

Self-Assessment/Discussion: Exercise 5

This is an assessment of warmth skills. This exercise helps you develop skills in assessing warmth and provides you with feedback on your own warmth skills.

Work in small groups for this exercise. (If you have time, each person can have a turn as interviewer or two

Name of person rated:_____   Name of rater:_____

Interviewer's behavior	1-Minute intervals										
	1	2	3	4	5	6	7	8	9	10	Total
1. Maintains eye contact											
2. Faces interviewee "squarely"											
3. Leans forward slightly											
4. Uses open posture: arms											
5. Uses open posture: legs											
6. Maintains relaxed posture											
7. Nods head to show interest											
8. Smiles											
9. Jokes											
10. Uses warm voice tone											
11. Face shows interest, attentiveness											
12. Speech content shows interest											

Warmth rating scale

Instructions: Place a check mark (✔) in the box beside the rating that
indicates how warm you felt the interviewer's behavior was.

4.0 ☐   Very good response: very warm
3.5 ☐
3.0 ☐   Good response: warm
2.5 ☐
2.0 ☐   Poor response: cool
1.5 ☐
1.0 ☐   Very poor response: cold

Fig. 6.1 Warmth Content Analysis Sheet. (From Gerrard, B., Boniface, W., & Love, B. (1980). *Interpersonal skills for health professionals*. Reston, VA: Reston Publishing.)

students can volunteer for the assessment.) Each person takes a turn interviewing the other about something that person identifies as being of interest to him or her. The interviewer reviews the Warmth Rating Scale (Fig. 6.1) and then focuses on demonstrating warmth in the interview. The rest of the group uses the Warmth Content Analysis Sheet (see Fig. 6.1) to check off the warmth behaviors they see demonstrated by the interviewer.

Instructions for the Warmth Content Analysis Sheet
Note the checklist is for 10 minutes; use it for the number of minutes you are assigned for the activity. Each time you observe the interviewer demonstrate one of the warmth behaviors listed during a 1-minute interval, place a check mark in the appropriate column. For example, if during the first minute the interviewer smiles, has a warm vocal tone, and leans slightly forward, place checks in the

1-minute column beside the appropriate rows. Even if the interviewer engages in a behavior more than once during a 1-minute interval, put only one check mark. During each interval check off only whether a behavior occurs; how often it occurs does not matter. When a minute is up, move to the next minute column and check off any behaviors that occur during that 1-minute interval. During each 1-minute interval you will be making a separate set of ratings. When the interview is over, add up your check marks in each row and write the total in the last column.

After all group members have totaled their scores on the Warmth Content Analysis Sheet, all members use the second scale, the Warmth Rating Scale (see Fig. 6.1), to rate how warm they felt the interviewer's behavior was overall.

Note that these two tools measure different aspects of warmth. The content analysis sheet provides information on specific behaviors that occurred during the interview. The rating scale provides an overall assessment of the quality of warmth provided by the interviewer.

When the ratings are complete, group members give each other feedback on their warmth scores. This feedback includes the overall warmth rating and the specific behaviors used to communicate warmth. As the group members complete their feedback, they should finish by telling the interviewer the one thing the interviewer did best to show warmth.

Self-Assessment/Request for Feedback: Exercise 6

Look for ways to evaluate improvements in your expression of warmth. One of the most important barometers of your warmth is your inner feelings. Are you feeling more relaxed and caring with clients and colleagues? Do you feel like you are expressing more affection and engaging more fully with others? Are your expressions of affection flowing more freely?

For an external evaluation, you can monitor the verbal and nonverbal feedback you obtain from your clients. Do your clients talk more, look at you more, ask questions of you, shift to a relaxing position in the chair, and indicate that they feel cared for by you?

You might wish to receive even more specific feedback about your warmth ability. One way to obtain this feedback is to ask a colleague to watch your interactions with clients and colleagues and to let you know the ways in which your warmth is conveyed and the areas in which you might improve.

Discussion: Exercise 7

Customer service inventories report the value of kindness and warmth in healthcaring relationships. Discuss the value of warmth rather than defensiveness when a client or family member makes a complaint. Consider these phrases to demonstrate warmth. "Tell me about your concerns." "What can we do to make this better for you?"

REFERENCES

Agency for Healthcare Research and Quality (AHRQ). (2017). *Warm handoff: Patient and family engagement in primary care (a slide presentation)*. Warm Handoff | Agency for Healthcare Research and Quality (ahrq.gov).

Agency for Healthcare Research and Quality (AHRQ). (2021). Implementation Quick Start Guide: Warm Handoff (ahrq.gov).

Carruth, A. K. (1996). Development and testing of the Caregiver Reciprocity Scale. *Nursing Research, 45*(2), 92.

Carver, I. (1998). Healthcare with a human touch. *Nursing Spectrum, 8*(18), 7.

Ekeren, G. V. (1994). *Speaker's sourcebook, II: Quotes, stories, and anecdotes for every occasion*. Englewood Cliffs, NJ: Prentice Hall.

Gleeson, M. (2004). The use of touch to enhance nursing care of older persons in long-term mental health care facilities. *Journal of Psychiatric and Mental Health Nursing, 11*(5), 541.

Healy, L. (2013). Warmth is the hallmark of compassion. *Nursing Standard, 27*(25), 28.

Kimble, P., & Bamford-Wade, A. (2013). The journey of discovering compassionate listening. *Journal of Holistic Nursing, 31*(4), 285.

Knapp, M. L. (1980). *Essentials of nonverbal communication*. New York, NY: Holt, Rinehart & Winston.

Koopmeiners, L., Post-White, J., Gutknecht, S., Ceronsky, C., Nickelson, K., Drew, D., et al. (1997). How healthcare professionals contribute to hope in patients with cancer. *Oncology Nursing Forum, 24*(9), 1507.

Lambert, C. (2010). *The psyche on automatic: Amy Cuddy probes snap judgments, warm feelings, and how to become an "alpha dog."* In *Harvard Magazine*. November-December. 1110-48. pdf (harvardmagazine.com).

Lee-Hsieh, J., Fang, Y., Kuo, C., & Turton, M. A. (2004). Patient experiences in the development of a caring code for clinical nursing practice. *International Journal of Human Caring, 8*(3), 21.

Levine, D. R., & Adelman, M. B. (1982). *Beyond language: Intercultural communication for English as a second language*. Englewood Cliffs, NJ: Prentice Hall Regents.

O'Connor, K. (2005). A dose of genuine warmth is as essential as skill with a syringe. *Nursing Standard, 19*(32), 28.

Pullen, R. L., & Mathias, T. (2010). Fostering therapeutic nurse–patient relationships. *Nursing Made Incredibly Easy! 8*(3), 4.

Purtilo, R., & Haddad, A. M. (2002). *Health professionals and patient interaction*. Philadelphia, PA: WB Saunders.

Reece, B. (2013). *Effective human relations: Interpersonal and organizational applications*. Independence, KY: Cengage Learning.

Reynolds, M. (2002). Reflecting on pediatric oncology nursing practice using Benner's Helping Rose as a framework to examine aspects of caring. *European Journal of Oncology Nursing, 6*(1), 30.

Sitzman, K., & Watson, J. (2017). *Watson's caring in the digital world: A guide for caring when interacting, teaching, and learning in cyberspace*. New York, NY: Springer.

Tabron, S. (2001). A prayer. In B. Knight (Ed.). *Blessed are the caregivers: A daily book of comfort and cheer*. Albuquerque, NM: Hartman Publishers.

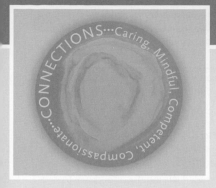

CONNECTIONS···Caring, Mindful, Competent, Compassionate···

Showing Respect*

Imagine what the world would be like if we treated others with inherent and equal dignity and respect, seeing the divine DNA in ourselves and everyone else, too—regardless of ethnicity, religion, gender, sexual orientation, nationality, appearance, or social class.

Richard Rohr (2018)

OBJECTIVES

1. Discuss the benefits of respect in the relationships in healthcare.
2. Identify behaviors that demonstrate respect in relationships.
3. Define workplace bullying.
4. Participate in exercises to build skills in demonstrating respect.

RECOGNIZING THE BENEFITS OF RESPECT

Communication is Standard 9 in the Scope and Standards of Holistic Nursing. The nurse "uses communication styles and methods that demonstrate intention, centering, presence, caring, respect, deep listening, authenticity, and trust" (American Holistic Nurses Association, 2019, p. 93). In a review of literature on respect in philosophy, psychology, sociology, business, theology, and nursing, three themes emerged: respect honors a person's worth when it acknowledges the inherent dignity of worth of each person; respect as a deliberate process contributes to a person's identity and "enhances energy and promotes confidence"; and respect comes when a person earns admiration (Rewakowski, 2018, p. 190). Respect the communication of acceptance of the client's ideas, feelings, and experiences (Haber, Krainovich-Miller, &

McMahon, 1997). When we show respect to our clients and colleagues, we are sending them the message, "I value you. You are important to me." Together, warmth and respect form what is called *unconditional positive regard* (Stuart, 2012). When helpers demonstrate that they care in a nonpossessive way, they transmit unconditional positive regard. This means accepting others for what they are, not on the condition that they behave in a certain way or possess special characteristics. Respect for the client is part of maintaining the person's dignity (Griffin-Heslin, 2005; Milika & Trorey, 2004). Consider the importance of offering respect for the client's family. In a study of respect in older clients in acute care settings, clients and family who felt respected felt free to "ask questions, get help and express their personal wishes" (Koskenniemi, Leino-Kilpi, & Suhonen, 2012), which are important elements to the delivery of individualized care.

---

* With contributions from Margaret E. Erickson, PhD.

77

ACTIVE LEARNING

Beginning competencies for communication in nursing:

Showing Respect
Think about how you will write your answers as you read this chapter.

What?
Write one thing you learned from this chapter.

So What?
How will this affect your nursing practice?

Now What?...
How will you implement this new knowledge or skill?

Think About It ...

 MOMENTS OF CONNECTION...

Respect for the Sacred Relationships in Marriage

"I was the home health nurse for an elderly woman who was dying. Her husband was her primary caregiver. They had been married for more than 50 years and had always slept together. Now, however, the patient was sleeping in a hospital bed. One day the husband seemed more upset than usual. I asked him what was wrong and whether he needed more help. He began to cry and talked about missing her. I suggested he get into her bed with her and snuggle. He was afraid he would hurt her. I convinced him it would probably mean as much to her as it did to him. At the next visit she was comatose. He confided that he had gotten into bed with her the night before and slept all night with her. She had slept through the night without pain medication. He was so grateful I had made the suggestion."

Receiving respect makes people feel important, cared for, and worthwhile. These examples illustrate such reactions. Your coworker tells you, "I love going to my new physician. Besides being a good clinician, she makes me feel so important. She's on time for my appointments, her receptionist remembers my name, and she follows up on all my requests." Your neighbor tells you about her recent experience with the nursing staff on the unit in which her husband is hospitalized: "The nurses are busy, of course, but they seem to have time to say 'hello' and pause for a few minutes to tell me something new about Jack. They never seem too busy for the little touches that make you feel so special. Not like the unit he was on before, where they scowled if you asked for something and gave you the impression that they didn't have time for you."

In contrast, when people do not receive respect, they feel hurt and ignored. For example, a middle-aged woman complains about the health unit coordinator on a busy hospital unit: "She didn't even have the courtesy to raise her head to speak to me when I asked her where Dad's room was. I might as well not have been there." A nurse reports her frustration at the disrespect she encountered: "Boy, I'm glad I don't work there! When I came down to borrow some syringes, the two nurses ignored me and kept on talking! It didn't even register that I was in a hurry and needed the stuff quickly." When people sense that they are not being treated with respect, they feel angry and rejected.

Experience shows that a positive correlation exists among respect, warmth, empathy, and successful treatment outcomes in psychotherapy clients. Indirect evidence supports the notion that respect, in terms of access to the desired physician, provision of convenient clinics, and reduced waiting times for appointments, has a beneficial influence on client compliance with the therapeutic regimen.

SHOWING RESPECT TO YOUR CLIENTS

Respect is communicated principally by the ways nurses orient themselves toward and work with clients. The following ideas about respect reflect the philosophy of holistic nursing. To respect a client is also to have the humility to appreciate that the client is more than a set of symptoms classified as a disease. A person is body, mind, and spirit. These parts of the person are interrelated in such a way that the sum of them is greater than the parts, a whole with inseparable parts. "The whole is in dynamic interaction within itself, between and among other humans and with the universe. When all parts are balanced and in harmony, maximum well-being exists. Well-being can exist in the presence or absence of physical ailment. Although health can be discussed in several ways, such as physical, social, emotional, cognitive, or spiritual health, to be truly healthy, one must experience a sense of well-being. An imbalance and disharmony within the human, human to human, and human to universe interfere with a person's well-being" (Erickson, 2007).

Thus, the effect of treatments, medicines, and nursing interventions is influenced by all parts of the person. A person who is sad may be pessimistic and not open to getting better. A person who has a positive attitude about life, believing that every moment is precious, may not consider a physical symptom or a diagnosis of a disease as the most important thing or the focus of life. This is the person who looks for meaning in illness as a way to reflect on what is most important in a life limited in time, but not in the quality of embracing joy in life even in small moments.

To respect a client, we try to "develop an image and understanding of the client's world, as the client perceives it" (Erickson, Tomlin, & Swain, 1983). "Through this process of 'Modeling' the nurse respectfully gains greater understanding of the client's model or worldview. Based on the client's model of his or her world the nurse is then able to facilitate and nurture the individual in attaining, maintaining, or promoting health through purposeful interventions" (Erickson et al., 1983). To respect a client is to appreciate that a person has an inherent ability to grow and become the most he or she can be, has an inner voice or inner wisdom, and has self-care knowledge. To respect a client is to listen to what the person identifies as a need and to work to incorporate meeting that need into nursing care. To respect a client is to recognize the power of caring in the nurse–client relationship in which a "caring field" (Watson, 2011) is established…when the nurse and client connect on an energetic level…in caring moments…in a relationship that can "create new possibilities for the well-being" (Erickson, 2007) of the nurse and client.

Although respect starts as an attitude, this mental outlook needs to be translated into behavior to demonstrate respect. A behavior that demonstrates respect is acknowledgment.

Acknowledging Clients

Feeling respect for your clients is not enough. They will receive the message that you think they are important and worthwhile only if you deliver the message clearly and directly. The following list provides concrete actions you can take to show respect to your clients:

- Look at your client.
- Offer your undivided attention.
- Maintain eye contact.
- Smile if appropriate.
- Move toward the other person.
- Determine how the other person likes to be addressed.
- Call the client by name and introduce yourself.
- Make contact with a handshake or by gently touching the individual.

Acknowledgment means demonstrating your awareness of your clients as individuals. One nurse wrote about a touching experience with a man sitting in an intensive care unit waiting room across the hall from where she was struggling with paperwork. Seeing his sadness, she walked over to him, sat down, and asked if she could help. Receiving no response, she simply placed her hand on his and sat in silence with him. After a time of silence, he revealed that both his wife and his son had recently died and that now he had been asked to donate his son's organs. The nurse told him she knew this was a difficult time for him and that she was there for him. After more silence, he told her he had made a decision, looked at her sadly, and left.

 MOMENTS OF CONNECTION…
Respect in Quiet Moments

"I work in an outpatient chronic pain center. We needed a piece of equipment that was unavailable, so I went to the intensive care unit to borrow the machine. The nurse told me I could take it from a room in which a patient had just died. I went into the room, which was very quiet, with no sounds of talking family or life-sustaining equipment. I stood in the quiet and honored that person who had died, saying a silent prayer. We face sadness, horror, and death, but in this quiet moment I felt peace, respect, and honor for that person—I felt a connection."

Simple gestures may communicate feelings when words miss the mark (Taylor, 1994). Copp (1993) identified the waiting room as a place of "lost lessons" and comments that students of nursing could learn about the demonstration of caring by being sensitive to the "weary travelers" who have come long distances, the waiting relatives who feel unsure of how to care for the loved one at home, or the waiting friends or relatives who have put their own lives on hold to be there.

Showing respect involves using verbal and nonverbal skills. Looking at our clients or colleagues as they speak shows attention, but it is the quality of our facial expressions that reveals whether we are interested in what our clients or coworkers are saying.

In the United States introductions are accompanied by a firm, brief handshake. This custom may not be the same in all countries from which clients or colleagues come. In some cultures, handshaking is prolonged, and taking our hands away too quickly could be misinterpreted as rejection. Within reason, it is best to allow the client to end the handshake.

In addition, after opening acknowledgments are made, a period of small talk usually follows, during which impersonal and trivial subjects (e.g., the weather) are discussed to break the ice. Some cultures prolong this period of discussion.

Establishing the Nature of the Contact

After you have acknowledged your client, several actions can convey respect at the outset of a new or ongoing client–nurse encounter.

For a first-time contact:

- Make it clear who you are and what your role is in the agency.
- Wear your name pin or identification badge.
- Ask what the other person needs or wants.
- Be clear about how you can be of help.
- Indicate how you will protect your client's confidentiality.

For an ongoing relationship:
- Ensure that the client recalls who you are and your role in the agency.
- Determine the client's needs at this point.
- Indicate that you recall details about the individual.
- Review the issue of confidentiality.
- Refrain from gossiping about other clients.
- If appropriate, suggest a referral so that the client will receive the required assistance.

As nurses we must remember that the most intensely private and personal aspects of clients' lives are revealed in times of crisis and illness, whether in a hospital setting, an outpatient clinic, or the home. At the outset of a client–nurse relationship, we have a duty to tell clients of others with whom we are likely to share the information they give us so that they understand the parameters of confidentiality in the agency. Some private information may need to be shared with other members of the healthcare team in developing a treatment plan. We are obliged to diligently protect the confidences of our clients unless required to reveal them by law or unless our clients give us permission to share these details. Releasing the status of a client's condition to the news media or general public does not create liability exposure, but disclosing more detailed information or a photograph without the client's consent should be avoided. In healthcare facilities in which there is public stigma, such as a psychiatric or drug abuse treatment center, even releasing a client's name would be an automatic invasion of privacy. Clients expect that the information they give will be kept strictly confidential. The need for disclosure should be carefully evaluated before information is shared. Maintaining confidentiality demonstrates respect for the rights of the individual (Erlen, 1998).

MOMENTS OF CONNECTION...

Respect for the Dying Client

"I had a 19-year-old client dying of cancer. His dad had died in Vietnam and his mom could no longer cope. They had no other family, and I would go sit with him, hold his hand, and talk. Finally, the mother said good-bye to him and left. He died 4 hours later. I couldn't leave. I stayed and held him and prayed with him. It was the greatest lesson of my nursing career."

Although the following ethical guidelines for confidentiality were written for psychiatric nurse specialists, these principles are applicable guides in any situation in which nurses are striving to respect clients by protecting their confidentiality (Colorado Society of Clinical Specialists in Psychiatric Nursing, 1990):

- Keep all client records secure.
- Consider carefully the content to be entered into the record:
  - Release information only with written consent and full discussion of the information to be shared, except when release is required by law.
  - Use professional judgment regarding confidentiality when the client is a danger to himself or herself or to others. Do not promise the client that you will keep secrets and acknowledge that you will use your judgment about shared information that might indicate potential harm to the client or someone else.
  - Use professional judgment deliberately when deciding how to maintain the confidentiality of a minor. The rights of the parent or guardian must also be considered.
- Disguise clinical material when used professionally for teaching and writing.
- Maintain confidentiality in consultation and in peer-reviewed situations.
- Maintain the anonymity of research subjects.
- Safeguard the confidentiality of the student in teaching and learning situations.

Establishing a Comfortable Climate

The following list describes the steps necessary to establish a comfortable environment for the client:
- Indicate at the beginning how much time you have so that your client can gauge the length of the discussion and prepare for your leaving.
- Arrange to meet at another time if the allotted period is too brief for the content to be discussed.
- Ensure privacy before engaging in a discussion of confidential matters.
- Ensure that telephones or other people do not interfere with you giving undivided attention to your client.
- Arrange the room so that no barrier, such as a desk, separates you and your client, and avoid standing over a person in a wheelchair.
- Ensure that the environment is comfortable by making space for your client, having a place for a coat and other personal belongings, and adjusting the room temperature and lighting.
- Take care to be on time for appointments and try to avoid inconveniencing a client by switching appointments.
- If you are late or have to change an appointment time, explain the reason to your client so it is clear that the delay was unavoidable.

Promptness for appointments is important to Americans, and we consider it irresponsible to miss scheduled appointments. Time is tangible for Americans as reflected by the phrases "find time," "spend time," "waste time," "save time," and "kill time." Because clients from other cultures may proceed at a pace different from Americans and have different ways of perceiving, regulating, and dividing time, we may have to be creative about considering time customs when making appointments. Clients from cultures with different values about time might have to learn about canceling and rescheduling appointments.

An aspect of mutuality is a sense of equality in the partnership. One nonverbal way to achieve an egalitarian relationship with clients is to arrange the seating so that you are both at the same height.

Authority can be communicated by the height from which one person interacts with another. If one stands while the other sits, the former has subconsciously placed himself or herself in a position of authority…Height is unwittingly used to project a submissive role onto a patient when he or she is confined to a bed, a treatment table, or a wheelchair (Purtilo, Haddad, & Doherty, 2013).

Discussing Sensitive Subjects

Some health issues have an associated stigma or evoke judgment, such as the epidemic problem of obesity in America. Being overweight or obese is grouped as a leading health indicator in Healthy People 2020, which details the nation's health objectives for the first decade of the 21st century (US Department of Health and Human Services, 2010). Although it is easier to avoid addressing such health concerns with a client and family, there are respectful ways to accept this responsibility. A nurse practitioner wrote about her sensitive intervention with an 11-year-old boy weighing 265 pounds. She wanted to preserve his dignity but responsibly address this major health issue. She established rapport, addressed other presenting health issues, then respectfully discussed the challenge of obesity, offering referral to a dietitian for a customized weight-management plan and introducing the child to the activity pyramid (Bollinger, 2001).

Terminating Contact

How nurses end their discussions with clients is just as important as other phases of the interaction. The following are guidelines for terminating the contact:

- If you have to leave early, prepare your client in advance.
- Summarize what you have discussed.
- Follow through with what you said you would do.
- Make notes of any points you want to remember for future contact.
- For ongoing relationships, do the following:
  - Prepare your client for discharge several visits before termination.
  - Allow time and space for the client to talk about the feelings that termination may bring up.

- Express your thoughts and feelings about termination as a way of showing you care.
- If you are going to be away for a limited period of time, make arrangements for client coverage and be sure to check with your client to make sure that these arrangements are suitable.

To maintain cost-effectiveness in American hospitals, the length of stay of patients is decreasing; clients are being discharged earlier. This limits the time for discharge planning, and the transition period from hospital to home is briefer and possibly not as smooth as it once was. Nurses in some hospitals follow a callback system to check on clients at home after discharge for early problem-solving. This kind of follow-up demonstrates respect through a willingness to work with clients by being available and interested in their healthcare problems. Adopting the mutual problem-solving approach is also respectful because it shows good faith in our clients' ability to use their self-care knowledge and self-care resources to facilitate their own healing, health, and well-being (Erickson et al., 1983). Self-care resources refer to the individual's "internal, as well as additional resources…that will help them gain, maintain, and promote an optimum level of holistic health" (Erickson et al., 1983). By facilitating and respectfully recognizing the client's self-care knowledge and resources, the nurse affirms that the client has the means, control, and knowledge necessary to heal and achieve his or her greatest state of well-being (Erickson et al., 1983). Attempts to overcome a language barrier with clients and families is another way of demonstrating respect. Check with the hospital's patient advocate or human resources department to identify employees who could serve as interpreters. LanguageLine Solutions can be purchased for over-the-phone interpretation of 170 languages, 24 hours a day, 7 days a week (call 1-800-752-6096 for information).

SHOWING RESPECT TO YOUR COLLEAGUES

You can apply many of the suggestions given earlier to show respect to your colleagues and to your clients. Being courteous, attentive, and mindful of the unique contribution each colleague makes to the total healthcare team are all ways of conveying respect to colleagues.

Being respectful embodies assertiveness. When we show respect, we are upholding the other person's right to be treated with dignity (Carson & Koenig, 2008) and consideration while not ignoring our own needs to manage our time effectively and perform the role for which we are qualified. Being respectful means acknowledging others' needs to be attended to, understood, and helped within the limits of nurses' abilities and time.

Self-Care Nudge

Reach out. When you are tired and when you feel fed up, too. You don't always know when a few encouraging words can lift someone's spirits. Say thank you to other students after a study session, to a nurse at the end of the shift, or to family and friends for the support they give you (Willard & Kotecha, 2020).

RECOGNIZING DISRESPECTFUL WORKPLACE BEHAVIOR…BULLYING AND INCIVILITY

The American Nurses Association's (ANA) Code of Ethics "…states that nurses are required to 'create an ethical environment and culture of civility and kindness, treating colleagues, co-workers, employees, students, and others with dignity and respect.' The code states that our profession will no longer tolerate violence of any kind…from any source… to create a culture of respect, free of incivility, bullying and workplace violence…" (ANA, 2015).

Bullying, often referred to as incivility (Dellasega, 2021), can be defined as, "anyone who uses his or her perceived strength or power to intimidate another person who, he or she thinks, is weaker in order to gain power over that person" (Ciocco, 2018, p. 9). Examples of such behaviors include being yelled at; the subject of gossip or rumors; sabotaged; ignored when expressing feelings or thoughts; scapegoated; intimidated nonverbally, such as being glared at; and physically threatened (ANA, Tips for Nurses, 2021).

Dellasega (2021) reports a study of 900 nurses in which 39% reported experiencing bullying or harassment at work: 30% from nurses, 25% from patients, 23% from physicians, and 20% from administrators (Cornwall, 2018).

The Joint Commission (http://www.jointcommission. org/), a hospital-accrediting organization, requires a process to create a definition of and policy for addressing disruptive, disrespectful behavior among colleagues. Maimonides Medical Center (Brooklyn, New York) created a code of mutual respect. This code has been implemented in the operating room, in which disrespect can be common. In an operating room, "measures of productivity, efficiency, and safe patient care" are higher when healthcare providers respect one another (Kaplan, Mestel, & Feldman, 2010).

A lack of respect of colleagues has contributed to morale and productivity problems in the American workplace and may contribute to high levels of stress associated with emotional outbursts and violence. Civility is an ethical principle of respect for people. Incivility is "morally destructive patterns of self-absorption, callousness, manipulation, and materialism so ingrained in our routine behavior that we do

not even recognize them" (Peck, 1994). Consider your reaction to the extreme effects of a lack of respect for others in the workplace as you reflect on the importance of respect.

SIMPLIFY AND DEEPEN
Respect yourself and others will respect you.

WE ARE ALL IN THIS TOGETHER

Students, faculty, nurses, and colleagues, we all work to grow in our understanding of how to demonstrate respect and how to intervene when there is disrespect.

Schools of nursing are addressing student incivility. Behaviors that are disrespectful to faculty and other students reflect a lack of value for human dignity and altruism, which are qualities essential for professional nursing. Incivility is rudeness and breaches of common courtesy. Examples of incivility in the classroom are lateness, leaving the class early, inattentiveness, threatening language, or physical violence (Luparell, 2005). Some schools of nursing have instituted disruptive student behavior policies.

At the 2021 virtual conference of The International Association for Human Caring, Chantal Cara presented "Humanizing nursing education by teaching from the heart" from her book, *An Educator's Guide to Humanizing Nursing Education: Grounded in Caring Science* (Cara, Hills, & Watson, 2021). "Teaching from the heart embodies: knowing and living caring; embracing vulnerability; learning and growing together; and being in right relationship." We must understand the effect we can have on people in every single encounter. Being respectful means showing our finely tuned sensitivity to others with the full realization that we can affect their well-being. As nurses, we need to be aware of the power we have to make our clients and colleagues feel cared for and, more important, to use that power consistently and with good intent. Respect for a client is part of nursing excellence. A study was conducted to examine how the coping behaviors of nurses whose own family of origin was dysfunctional helped build competent caring behaviors. It was concluded that the very behaviors that helped these nurses adapt to their own circumstances were valuable behaviors in fine-tuning their sensitivity to clients and their families. One nurse indicated that her own drive to show clients and families respect arose because that was what she longed for as a child (Biering, 1998).

One factor that facilitates nurses' demonstrations of respect is the strong conviction that others have the right to be treated with respect for their feelings of worth. Nurses with less well-integrated values of human dignity might be less consistent in demonstrating their respect. If you find you are inconsistent in conveying respect, examine which of your values conflicts with being respectful in some situations. What is more powerful in influencing your behavior than your desire to be respectful? See Chapter 27 for strategies to deal with aggressive behavior.

WIT AND WISDOM

Never be bullied into silence. Never allow yourself to be made a victim. Accept no one's definition of your life but define yourself.

Harvey S. Firestone

Return to "Active Learning" at the beginning of the chapter and write your responses.

PRACTICING SHOWING RESPECT

Video Demonstration/Reflection/Individual Skill Building or Small Group Discussion: Exercise 1

Take a 5-minute break to watch this excellent video demonstrating concrete ways we can offer compassion and respect to a variety of patients. These concrete examples bring compassion and respect to life. Note how the healthcare team works together. Search YouTube for *Compassion, Dignity, and Respect in Health Care*, a 2014 video from The Health Foundation, or use the link https://www.youtube.com/watch?v=HVF0273iHus. After you watch the video, in your journal write one example of how you can or have demonstrated respect through compassion. If you are working with this video in class, share your response to the video and your example in your small group.

Reflection: Exercise 2

Take a moment to identify a time when you were disrespectful to someone else. Write a brief journal entry about the situation. What happened? In what way were you disrespectful? What were the consequences? How did you feel? Putting yourself in the other person's position, how might that person have felt about the situation? What would you do differently if this happened again? What did you learn from the incident?

Discussion: Exercise 3

Situation: Susan Weeks, a registered nurse, has been working for several days with Mrs. Green, an inpatient. Mrs. Green has elected to refuse chemotherapy for the treatment of cancer, leave the hospital, and be transferred to hospice care. The nurse does not agree with the client's decision, although she believes it to be an informed decision. Discuss how the nurse can demonstrate her respect for Mrs. Green's right to make her own end-of-life decisions.

Discussion: Exercise 4

We speak of the indignities of aging when we speak of the changes in the body as a result of aging and the losses incurred. Consider the respectful use of the word *elder* in some cultures to denote wisdom to honor the years of life experience. Reflect on that connotation of older adults as elders. Discuss why an elder deserves respect and why respect may be especially important. Discuss how you can demonstrate respect to an elder or older adult. Be specific about the behaviors that demonstrate your respect.

Professional Responsibility/Reading and Discussion: Exercise 5

To understand the ethical foundation of our practice, how we are to treat others and how we can expect to be treated, review the ANA's full position statement on incivility, bullying, and workplace violence. For a link to download the document visit Incivility, Bullying, and Workplace Violence | ANA (nursingworld.org) violence. Share your reflection from your reading and examples of these behaviors you have observed or experienced.

Quality and Safety Education for Nurses Learning Strategy: Exercise 6

One of the ways to demonstrate respect to patients and their families is by including them in daily interprofessional care rounds. Establishing eye contact, facing patients, and asking questions about how they are feeling and what they may need to recover helps include patients in their care.

- With your clinical group, role-play a scenario of bedside shift change report with one person acting in the role of the patient.
- Observe ways team members use nonverbal communication to demonstrate respect for the patient.
- Patients often have preferences about the name healthcare providers should use to address patients. How does the team elicit this information and relay it to all team members? Likewise, how do those in the team introduce themselves to the patient to demonstrate respect?
- Note the questions used to elicit key information from patients to be able to establish daily care goals. How does the team work with the patient to reach consensus on the plan of care for the day?
- Many units provide whiteboards in patient rooms to document key information for patients and families. Together with the group, draft a template of the information that should be included to demonstrate respect and inclusion in their care.
- How could you design a quality improvement project to demonstrate the effectiveness of using whiteboards in patient rooms to share critical information?

REFERENCES

American Holistic Nurses Association. (2019). *Holistic Nursing: Scope and standards of practice* (3rd ed.). Silver Spring, MD: ANA & AHNA.

American Nurses Association (ANA). (2015). American Nurses Association position statement on incivility, bullying, and workplace violence. Incivility, Bullying, and Workplace Violence | ANA (nursingworld.org).

American Nurses Association (ANA). (2021). Tips for nurses; Dealing with incivility & bullying. YOU Series: Lessons in Leadership. Cards for distribution, available at Tip Cards: Bullying in the Workplace | ANA Enterprise (nursingworld.org).

Biering, P. (1998). Codependency: A disease or the root of nursing excellence? *Journal of Holistic Nursing, 16*(3), 320.

Cara., C., Hills., M., & Watson, J (2021). *An educator's guide to humanizing nursing education: Grounded in caring science.* New York, NY: Springer Publishing.

Bollinger, E. (2001). Applied concepts of holistic nursing. *Journal of Holistic Nursing, 19*(2), 212.

Carson, V. B., & Koenig, H. G. (Eds.). (2008). *Spiritual dimensions of nursing practice.* West Conshohocken, PA: Templeton Foundation Press.

Ciocco, M. (2018). *Fast facts on combatting bullying, incivility, and workplace violence.* New York, NY: Springer Publishing.

Colorado Society of Clinical Specialists in Psychiatric Nursing. (1990). Ethical guidelines for confidentiality. *Journal of Psychosocial Nursing, 28*(3), 43.

Copp, L. A. (1993). Teaching site: The waiting room. *Journal of Professional Nursing, 9*(1), 1.

Cornwall, L. (2018). RNNetwork 2018 portrait of a modern nurse survey. 2018 Modern Nurse Survey: Nursing shortage leading to nurse burnout (rnnetwork.com).

Dellasega, C. (2021). *Toxic nursing: Managing bullying, bad attitudes, and total turmoil.* Indianapolis, IN: Sigma Theta Tau International.

Erickson, H., Tomlin, E., & Swain, M. A. (1983). *Modeling and role-modeling: A theory and paradigm for nursing.* Englewood Cliffs, NJ: Prentice Hall.

Erickson, H. L. (2007). Philosophy and theory of holism. *Nursing Clinics of North America, 42,* 139.

Erlen, J. A. (1998). The inadvertent breach of confidentiality. *Orthopedic Nursing, 17*(2), 7.

Griffin-Heslin, V. L. (2005). An analysis of the concept of dignity. *Accident and Emergency Nursing, 13*(4), 251.

Haber, J., Krainovich-Miller, B., & McMahon, A. L. (1997). *Comprehensive psychiatric nursing.* St. Louis, MO: Mosby.

Kaplan, K., Mestel, P., & Feldman, D. L. (2010). Creating a culture of mutual respect. *AORN Journal, 91*(4), 495.

Koskenniemi, J., Leino-Kilpi, H., & Suhonen, R. (2012). Respect in the care of older patients in acute hospitals. *Nursing Ethics, 20*(1), 5.

Luparell, S. (2005). Why and how we should address student incivility in nursing programs. *Annual Review of Nursing Education, 3,* 23.

Milika, R. M., & Trorey, G. (2004). Perceptual adjustment levels: Patients' perception of their dignity in the hospital setting. *International Journal of Nursing Studies, 41*(7), 735.

Peck, S. (1994). *A world waiting to be born: Civility rediscovered.* New York, NY: Bantam Books.

Purtilo, R., Haddad, A. M., & Doherty, R. F. (2013). *Health professional and patient interaction* (8th ed.). Philadelphia, PA: WB Saunders.

Rewakowski, C. (2018). Respect: An integrative review. *Nursing Science Quarterly, 3*(2), 190.

Rohr, R. (2018). Daily meditations: From the center for action and contemplation. https://cac.org/daily-meditations/.

Stuart, G. W. (2012). *Principles and practice of psychiatric nursing* (10th ed.). St. Louis, MO: Mosby.

Taylor, C. (1994). Communicating without words: What's left unsaid can make a difference. *Nursing, 24*(6), 30–32.

US Department of Health and Human Services. (2010). Leading Health Indicators. Leading Health Indicators | Healthy People 2020.

Watson, J. (2011). *Human caring science: A theory of nursing* (2nd ed.). Burlington, MA: Jones & Bartlett Learning.

Willard, C., & Kotecha, R. (2020). 8 ways healthcare workers can reduce stress. *Mindful,* November 24, *2020.*

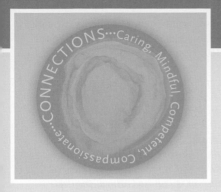

Being Genuine*

My guiding principles in life are to be honest, genuine, thoughtful, and caring.

Prince William

OBJECTIVES

1. Differentiate between genuine and nongenuine behavior.
2. Discuss the importance of being genuine with clients and colleagues.
3. Participate in exercises to build skills in demonstrating genuineness.

BENEFITS OF GENUINENESS IN INTERPERSONAL RELATIONSHIPS

 ACTIVE LEARNING

Think about how you will write your answers as you read this chapter.

What?
Write one thing you learned from this chapter.

So What?
How will this affect your nursing practice?

Now What?
How will you implement this new knowledge or skill?

Think About It ...

A genuine smile from a nurse "conveys acceptance, builds trust," and helps build the relationship with the patient (Thakur & Sharma, 2021, p. 6). From this literature review, the authors conclude that a smile is universal, accepted across cultures. Begin with a genuine smile to indicate

---

* With contributions from Margaret E. Erickson, PhD.

you are approachable, cooperative, and friendly. Middaugh (2017, p. 64) offered suggestions for nurse managers' nonverbal communication. "Genuine smiles begin slowly, light the face, and fade slowly. Because facial expressions trigger corresponding feelings, getting a smile in return is a positive sign. If we say a person is genuine, what does it mean? Why is it important to be "your natural self" in human relationships? We connect with patients by being genuine, attentive, and immersed in the moment with the person…true presence (Robinson, 2014). In a qualitative study of nurse communication behaviors with patients with suicidal ideation, nurses identified building trust through open, genuine communication as ways they showed compassion (Vandewalle et al., 2019). Gilhooley (2017, p. 91), writing on the concept of therapeutic reciprocity, shared that patients identify the nurse's tone of voice, manner of approach, honesty, and being human as barometers of genuineness.

In a study of the lived experiences of women with recurrent ovarian cancer, four themes of sources of comfort were identified: hope of a future, being recognized, genuine presence, and self-preservation. Genuine presence was defined as being "genuine and honest, for better or worse" (Breistig & Huser, 2019, p. 2). A woman diagnosed with cancer shared one thing she thinks nurses need to know, and it is a demonstration of genuine concern. She asked that when you enter a client's room, you stop and see the person first. "Here's what would be so healing that won't take but a moment" (Guilmartin, 2010). "Could you soften your gaze as you look at me? As you approach my bed could you consider whether I need a gentle touch or a positive thought to remind me that I am more than one additional task in a tough day?" Guilmartin (2010) related this story when she discussed the power of a pause. Here a pause is a few moments, perhaps one deep breath, that can reframe how you see your work and its meaning and communicate your genuineness. Carl Rogers (1980), a pioneer in the study of communication, used the two synonyms *realness* and *congruence* for genuineness, which he claims is the basis for the best communication. A fundamental feature of genuineness, in Rogers' view, is the presentation of our true thoughts and feelings, both verbally and nonverbally, to another person. It is not only the words you say or how you say them, but also your facial expression and body posture that signify genuineness. Being genuine means that you send the other person the real picture of you, not a distorted one that differs from how you really think or feel. Genuineness is a spontaneous expression conveying an individual's experience (Haber, Krainovich-Miller, & McMahon, 1997). It is the opposite of self-alienation in which a person suppresses spontaneous reactions to life (Stuart, 2012). You can be open to new possibilities in meeting clients' needs when you are truly present and trust the authenticity of your intention to care for and serve (Bruce & Davies, 2005).

In the classic children's story, *The Velveteen Rabbit* (Bianco, 1996), toys talk about what it means to be real:

> *When a child loves you for a long, long time, not just to play with, but REALLY loves you, then you become Real…by the time you are Real, most of your hair has been loved off, and your eyes drop out and you get loose in the joints and very shabby. But these things don't matter at all, because once you are Real you can't be ugly, except to people who don't understand.*

TO BE REAL IS TO BE YOURSELF

In the helping relationship with clients and in mutually supportive relationships with colleagues in the workplace, being genuine does not mean impulsively dumping your reactions on others. To "hit" clients and colleagues with feelings and then "run" is aggressive. In a therapeutic relationship, genuinely presenting your thoughts and feelings to others can be done assertively and constructively.

As nurses, we make an important judgment call in deciding to genuinely share our inner thoughts and feelings with others. The literature advises nurses to be genuine "when it is appropriate to do so." Appropriateness is linked

to whether our revelations will benefit our clients (or colleagues) and/or our relationships. Read carefully the counsel of Peck (1997) on dedication to the truth:

> *So the expression of opinions, feelings, ideas, and even knowledge must be suppressed from time to time in… the course of human affairs. What rules, then, can one follow if one is dedicated to the truth? First, never speak a falsehood. Second, bear in mind that the act of withholding the truth is always potentially a lie, and that in each instance in which the truth is withheld a significant moral decision is required. Third, the decision to withhold the truth should never be based on personal needs, such as a need for power, a need to be liked, or a need to protect one's map from challenge. Fourth, and conversely, the decision to withhold the truth must always be based entirely upon the needs of the person or people from whom the truth is being withheld. Fifth, the assessment of another's needs is an act of responsibility which is so complex that it can only be executed wisely when one operates with genuine love for the other. Sixth, the primary factor in the assessment of another's needs is the assessment of that person's capacity to utilize the truth for his or her own spiritual growth. Finally, in assessing the capacity of another to utilize the truth for personal spiritual growth, it should be borne in mind that our tendency is generally to underestimate rather than overestimate this capacity.*

We take a risk when we are genuine because sometimes genuineness involves expressing negative thoughts and confronting others with our reactions. When we are genuine, whether expressing negative or positive reactions, the message we give to our clients and colleagues is "You are strong and worthy of my engaging fully with you." When we are genuine, we give careful attention to listening to the other person. We extend ourselves and take the extra step to do the hard work of listening and oppose the "inertia of laziness or the resistance of fear" (Peck, 1997). We enter into a relationship with a client with a fresh perspective, aware that information we have read or heard about a client could influence our ability to be genuine and see him or her as unique. Focusing on making your own observations of the client's behavior will help you avoid stereotyping or stigmatizing a client (Sundeen, DeSalvo Rankin, Stuart, & Cohen, 1998).

To their clients, nurses who are genuine seem to mean exactly what the words they are saying connote, and their accompanying affective behavior matches their words (Arnold & Boggs, 2011). When our verbal message does not correspond to our facial expression, posture, tone of voice, and body language, clients and colleagues decode the disparate information as two distinct and dissimilar messages. It is not hard to imagine that this incongruence of conflicting or mixed messages puts our credibility in question. Furthermore, a meaningful relationship is unlikely to ensue when our clients or colleagues doubt our trustworthiness.

As nurses we have expectations about the behaviors that accompany our assumed roles. Some of the behaviors expected of nurse advocates are providing competent nursing care based on current standards; serving on committees to ensure quality care; and coordinating all services used by clients in an attempt to restore, maintain, or promote health. The roles we assume have cultural, gender, and situational performance expectations. These roles are comforting because they provide guidelines for performance. Being genuine means remembering that roles are filled by individuals with unique personalities, styles, and ideas (Nuwayhid, 1984). Realness means being free from the bonds of the role and not hiding behind the facade of the role. Being a person and a nurse at the same time involves spontaneity; we cannot weigh every word we say or talk in scripts that seem planned or rigid. Congruence includes an openness to sharing without always waiting to be asked and to express directly what is going on inside us without distorting our messages.

Genuineness is a "what you see is what you get" phenomenon. People experiencing your genuineness can trust you because they know you are not sending false signals or hiding something from them. This building of trust is the most important reason for being genuine (Box 8.1). When we believe that we can count on others, we can start to relax in the relationship. We stop worrying about what others might really be thinking and feeling. The energy freed from worrying can be put into the relationship, both deepening it and moving it in the direction for which it was established. Being genuine as a nurse is one major step in gaining credibility with clients and colleagues.

WIT AND WISDOM

Be yourself; everyone else is already taken.

Oscar Wilde

INCONGRUENCE

When a mismatch exists between nurses' experiences of their thoughts and feelings and their awareness, this incongruence is called *denial of awareness* or *defensiveness* (Rogers, 1995). You may notice, for example, that your colleague looks angry. She is stamping her foot, pointing her finger, becoming red in the face, and raising her voice in an accusatory way. When you suggest that she is angry, however, she brushes it off and denies her obvious feelings.

When a mismatch exists between nurses' thoughts and feelings and their communication of this internal experience, it is usually considered falseness or deceit (Rogers, 1995). For example, if you disapprove of the new policy to merge your unit with another unit in the hospital but you hide your anger and tell your boss you think the merger is a good idea because you want to make a good impression on her, this is deceit.

If we pretend that our thoughts and feelings are different from what they really are, then we will say things that we do not believe. If we act on thoughts and feelings that we do not have, we give people the wrong impression about us, leading them astray. In contrast, expressing our genuine thoughts and feelings about issues makes what we stand for absolutely clear to our clients and colleagues. The research findings of Rogers (1957) and Shapiro, Krauss, and Truax (1969) established that genuineness on the part of the therapist has positive therapeutic outcomes.

Even if we can control our verbal communication when we are trying to deceive another about our true thoughts and feelings, our nonverbal cues can give us away (Knapp, 1995). Nonverbal behavior can reveal the information we are hiding or indicate that we are attempting to deceive without indicating specific information about the nature of the deception (Knapp, 1995). We are skilled at manipulating our facial expressions and our postures to coincide with our verbal message, but the way we move our feet, legs, or hands can betray incongruence with our verbal messages,

---

BOX 8.1 Benefits of Nurse Genuineness for Clients and Colleagues

Nurse Genuineness
- Speaks deep from within without apology
- Expresses thoughts, feelings, and experiences in the here and now
- Shows spontaneity
- Conveys openness

Benefits for Clients and Colleagues
- Feel free to express their true thoughts and emotions
- Develop a feeling of trust for the nurse
- Are provided with information they can use in the relationship here and now
- Can unwind in a relaxed atmosphere
- Enjoy a climate of realness

showing that we are not genuine. Some of the foot and leg movements that might alert others to our incongruence are aggressive foot kicks, flirtatious leg displays, autoerotic or soothing leg squeezing, abortive restless flight movements, tense leg positions, frequent shifts of leg posture, and restless or repetitive leg and foot motions. Revealing hand movements might include digging our hands into our cheeks, tearing at our fingernails, or protectively holding our knees while smiling and looking pleasant. Knapp reports studies revealing that one of the reasons we may not expend much effort inhibiting or dissimulating feet and hand behavior is that over the years we have learned to disregard internal feedback, and we do not learn to control areas of our bodies from which we receive little external feedback (Knapp, 1995). Another way we might reveal our incongruence is by neglecting to include the nonverbal action that customarily would accompany the verbal message. Our omission is a signal to clients and colleagues that something is wrong (Box 8.2).

You may ask yourself how anyone could act in any way but genuinely. Occasionally it feels risky to reveal what we think and feel to others. What if they do not agree? What if they think we are ignorant? Sometimes we fear that clients

or colleagues might reject us if they do not like what we say. We worry that others might laugh at us, argue with us, put us down, or gossip about us. We may be threatened by fears that if we are honest, then a colleague might refuse to work with us or a client may request the services of another nurse.

When feeling vulnerable to rejection, we might modify what we think and feel to make ourselves more acceptable to others. We change in an attempt to give others what we think they wish to hear. In so doing, we begin the entanglement of presenting a false impression of ourselves. If others are fooled, they expect the behavior to be repeated, and then we are trapped. We can continue to try to act falsely, or we can confess. If our lack of authenticity is spotted, then others will stop trusting us, question our word, or ask for a second opinion. It is ironic that when we behave insincerely to avoid rejection our worst fears of rejection can come true.

When we are genuine, we have no guarantee that our clients or colleagues will accept us or agree with us, but they will usually be touched by our willingness to present ourselves as we are and our courage to risk rejection. Our honesty is reassuring and refreshing. If others choose to withdraw from a relationship with the genuine us, then they leave us with the satisfaction of knowing we have been honest with ourselves. Being genuine is being assertive; it is an action of standing up for our legitimate rights to express our point of view. When we are authentic, our concept of ourselves as assertive nurses is strengthened.

Self-Care Nudge
Music invites me to move my body and that helps me let go of stress. I write to Zydeco music and fond memories of New Orleans. What song or type of music is calling you now?

DEMONSTRATION OF GENUINENESS

For several days Joyce, a nurse, has been assigned to care for a client who has been flirtatious. He has asked for her telephone number, looked at her seductively, and touched her, as if by accident, as frequently as possible.

Joyce's thoughts: She knows it is her responsibility to behave as a professional. Because the behavior has persisted, she knows she must deal with it. This young man is in a vulnerable position as a patient and needs to have access to a professional who can care for him. A social relationship might alter his ability to make his needs known.

Joyce's feelings: She is attracted to this client but sees his behavior as inappropriate and as a barrier to her providing him with the care he needs. She is worried about embarrassing herself and him by behaving inappropriately.

BOX 8.2   Negative Effects of Nurse Incongruence for Clients and Colleagues

Nurse Incongruence
- Puts up a façade or pretense
- Withholds thoughts or experiences
- Shows a mismatch between verbal and nonverbal messages
- Communicates in a rigid and contrived way that sounds as if it is scripted

Negative Effects on Clients and Colleagues
- Distrust the nurse
- Suspicious of the nurse
- Relate to the nurse in a strained, tense way
- Omit valuable information from the interchange
- Decode the message as two distinct and dissimilar ones
- Feel confusion
- Believe only the nonverbal message
- Question the nurse's credibility
- Have difficulty maintaining a meaningful dialogue in the presence of mixed messages
- Do not believe that they are talking to a real person
- Feel that the nurse is trying to impress them rather than connect with them

The genuine communication is to explain to the client that her relationship with him is professional, not social.

A genuine response could be, "Our relationship here is that of client and nurse. I would ask you to think of it that way so I can provide you with the professional care you deserve."

This statement assertively communicates Joyce's thoughts and feelings in a way that is in keeping with her personal and professional values, making her trustworthy. If she had refrained from expressing her point of view, she would have communicated in a nonassertive and nongenuine way.

A nongenuine nonassertive response would be, "Well, I might go out with you…we'll see."

This message does not clarify the professional nature of the relationship. It might invite more of the flirtatious behavior Joyce wants to avoid.

A nongenuine aggressive response would be, "You guys are all the same. You're a chauvinist…you treat nurses like playthings. Cool it, mister! I have a job to do here."

This approach creates bad feelings and may interfere with Joyce's ability to provide nursing care. Being genuine is an assertive act. In expressing our thoughts and feelings, we need to take care that they are clear, direct, and respectful.

FACTORS INFLUENCING GENUINENESS

Our genuineness springs from three main sources: our self-confidence, our perception of others, and our environmental influences.

When our self-confidence is blossoming, we feel strong enough to risk revealing our true selves. When our self-confidence is withering, it is easier to try to impress others with what we think they want to hear to feel accepted and important. Self-confidence is not something with which we are born; it is something that we must nourish. When we risk being authentic, we feel good about being true to our thoughts and feelings. This good feeling is translated into self-confidence.

When we perceive that others have power and influence over us, we might refrain from being authentically ourselves. If we decide that other people are smarter, more deserving, or more worthy, then we are more likely to show off for these people than relate to them in a way congruent with our thoughts and feelings. Learning to take charge and empowering ourselves to trust our own reactions help us to perceive others as equals with whom we can dare to reveal our true thoughts and feelings.

Environmental variables also influence our ability to be genuine. In front of a large group, many of us might shy away from revealing our true thoughts and feelings. Limited time may prevent us from being genuine. If we know that expression of our thoughts and feelings could cause a reaction in others that would require more than the available time to work out, then we might wait for a better time to express ourselves genuinely.

In one study of patients' perceptions of nurses' knowledge and presence, nurses identified shortened hospital stays, paperwork, and time pressures as barriers to the development of relationships with patients. Both patients and nurses valued the "little things," such as using each other's names or remembering nicknames (Cohen, Hausner, & Johnson, 1994).

To be congruent we need to be aware of our thoughts and feelings (Rogers, 1995). As we get to know ourselves better, expanded self-awareness builds and deepens our self-concept. This greater self-awareness is something we need to relate more genuinely to others (Rogers, 1980).

SIMPLIFY AND DEEPEN

A student spoke of a Buddhist mind-set, that nurses who practice "being-the-work," become *bodhisattvas*, caring nurses who become a blessing to themselves and to others.

A SURPRISING DOORWAY TO HUMAN ENCOUNTERS: TATTOOS—THE SOUL'S WRITING ON THE SKIN?

My son, a minister, recommended a book called *God & Tattoos*. It is the findings of a minister who interviewed more than 300 people with tattoos to answer the question, "Why are people writing on themselves?"

He found when he showed a person respect and patience without judgment, he got genuine stories of "untold pain, the markings of lost or found love, the quest to be loved, maybe by God or the search for a significant other" (Dayhoff, 2016, p. 10). My son suggested that nurses might ask, "Does your tattoo have a story?"

Waiting to get into my classroom, I shared this with several of my early students and the conversation that followed was heartfelt and a confirmation that this is an important question to consider. One student shared her father was in the military and had been deployed many times during her childhood. She felt she did not really know him, but she treasured his letters, always signed, "You are always in my heart." She copied that in his handwriting and had it tattooed near her heart. See Exercise 2 to explore this story-catching experience.

PALLIATIVE CARE: A CALL TO AUTHENTICITY

The approaches used in palliative care nursing, in which the nurse's relationship with client and family has a major effect, are applicable to all nurses and offer intimate opportunities for the nurse to respond genuinely as an authentic caregiver. Palliative care nursing is the active, total care of clients who are not responsive to curative treatments in which control of pain, other symptoms causing distress, and spiritual stress are paramount (Ferrell & Coyle, 2010). Post–World War II babies, known as Baby Boomers, are in their 60s now, and both clients and nurses are turning their thoughts to their own mortality and quality of life. Healing of the body, mind, and spirit (the word *heal* means "to make whole") can occur as the client is dying. It has been said that to "facilitate the process of healing in others, it is necessary to awaken the healer within the self" (Wells-Federman, 1996). The vulnerability of clients and their families becomes a vehicle for the expression of the nurse's authenticity as a real person with genuine empathy and compassion. If we seek to protect our vulnerability, our expression of genuine emotion, we may dehumanize clients. Our own suffering and grief help us to remain compassionate and participate in the healing in which pain and suffering are transformed into wisdom in shared moments (Mulder, 2000).

EVALUATION OF YOUR GENUINENESS

You are the most important judge of your genuineness. If you are behaving in ways that are true to your thoughts and feelings, then you will feel more relaxed and self-assured. The comfort that you feel derives in part from the freedom that comes from living in harmony with yourself. Being genuine protects your right to be integrated. In other words, being genuine is being respectful of yourself.

When you are authentic, it is likely that others will react positively by communicating with you, seeking out your trustworthy companionship, and, in turn, revealing their true feelings and thoughts.

 MOMENTS OF CONNECTION...

Genuine Grief for Real People

"Some of my sweetest experiences have been going to viewings and funerals of patients who have died. The family members share their grief and hug the nurses who cared for their loved ones. They know that we cared with our hearts as well as with our hands and that they don't have to hide their emotions or act 'brave' with us. Although nurses don't go to every funeral of a patient who dies, there are some that give us closure and help us to remember that not all success is measured by patient outcomes. Sometimes success is the ability to connect at a level that is meaningful to the nurse and the patient and family."

Return to "Active Learning" at the beginning of the chapter and write your responses.

 PRACTICING BEING GENUINE

Self-Assessment and Skill Building: Exercise 1

In your day-to-day activities, both professional and personal, notice when you are naturally and easily genuine and when you are untrue to yourself. Also, pay attention to others and ask yourself what behaviors you observe that demonstrate being genuine versus insincere. After several days, note the factors that make it easier for you to be genuine and those that make it more difficult. Record these in your journal. Assessing your genuineness in this way will make clear where you are congruent and where you need to work harder to demonstrate the warmth you feel.

Skill Building/Being a Storycatcher of the Message of Tattoos: Exercise 2

In small groups in class, ask if anyone has a tattoo and does it have a story that he or she would be willing to share. If not, ask if anyone had considered one and what story it would tell. Remember to suspend any judgment you might have about tattoos and use this as an opportunity to be present and genuine. When you have the opportunity and it seems appropriate, pose the question to a client, "Does your tattoo have a story you would share with me?"

REFERENCES

Arnold, E., & Boggs, K. (2011). *Interpersonal relationships: Professional communication skills for nurses* (6th ed.). Philadelphia, PA: WB Saunders.

Bianco, M. W. (1996). *The velveteen rabbit*. New York, NY: Avon/Camelot. (Reprinted from Williams, M. (1922). *The velveteen rabbit, or how toys become real*. London: Heinemann).

Breistig, S., & Huser, B. (2019). Healthcare personnel as a source of comfort in recurrent ovarian cancer. *Norwegian Journal of Clinical Nursing*, pdf-export-78182-en.pdf (sykepleien.no).

Bruce, A., & Davies, B. (2005). Mindfulness in hospice care: Practicing meditation-in-action. *Qualitative Health Research, 15*(10).

Cohen, M. Z., Hausner, J., & Johnson, M. (1994). Knowledge and presence: Accountability as described by nurses and surgical patients. *Journal of Professional Nursing, 10*(3), 177.

Dayhoff, A. (2016). *God & tattoos: Why are people writing on themselves?* Fairfax Station, VA: Evangelize Today Ministry.

Ferrell, B. R., & Coyle, N. (2010). *Oxford textbook of palliative nursing*. New York, NY: Oxford University Press.

Gilhooley, M. (2017). Therapeutic reciprocity: A concept synthesis. *International Journal of Human Caring, 21*(2), 91.

Guilmartin, N. (2010). *The power of pause: How to be more effective in a demanding, 24/7 world*. San Francisco, CA: Jossey-Bass.

Haber, J., Krainovich-Miller, B., & McMahon, A. L. (1997). *Comprehensive psychiatric nursing*. St. Louis, MO: Mosby.

Knapp, M. L. (1995). *Essentials of nonverbal communication*. New York, NY: International Thomson Publishing.

Middaugh, D. (2017). Watch your language. *Nursing Management, 26*(1), 64.

Mulder, J. (2000). Transforming experience into wisdom: Healing amidst suffering. *Journal of Palliative Care, 16*(2), 25.

Nuwayhid, K. A. (1984). Role function: Theory and development. In S. C. Roy (Ed.). *Introduction to nursing: An adaptation model*. (2nd ed.). Englewood Cliffs, NJ: Prentice Hall.

Peck, M. S. (1997). *The road less traveled and beyond: Spiritual growth in an age of anxiety*. New York, NY: Simon & Schuster.

Robinson, S. G. (2014). True presence: Practicing the art of nursing. *Nursing, 44*(4), 44.

Rogers, C. R. (1957). The necessary and sufficient conditions of therapeutic personality change. *Journal of Consulting Psychology, 21*(2), 95.

Rogers, C. R. (1980). *A way of being*. Boston, MA: Houghton Mifflin.

Rogers, C. R. (1995). *On becoming a person: A therapist's view of psychotherapy*. New York, NY: Mariner Books.

Shapiro, J. G., Krauss, H. H., & Truax, C. B. (1969). Therapeutic conditions and disclosure beyond the therapeutic encounter. *Journal of Counseling Psychology, 16*(4), 290.

Stuart, G. W. (2012). *Principles and practice of psychiatric nursing* (10th ed.). St. Louis, MO: Mosby.

Sundeen, S. J., DeSalvo Rankin, E. A., Stuart, G. W., & Cohen, S. A. (1998). *Nurse–client interaction: Implementing the nursing process*. St. Louis, MO: Mosby.

Thakur, K., & Sharma, S. K. (2021). Nurse with smile: Does it make difference in patients' healing? *Ind Psychiatry J, 30*, 6–10.

Vandewalle, J., Beeckman, D., Van Hecke, A., Debyser, B., Deproost, E., & Verhasghe, S. (2019). Contact and communication with patients experiencing suicidal ideation: A qualitative study of nurses' perspectives. *Journal of Advanced Nursing, 75*(11), 2867–2877. Nov 2019. https://doi.org/10.1111/jan.14113.

Wells-Federman, C. (1996). Awakening the nurse healer within. *Holistic Nursing Practice, 10*(2), 13.

Williams, M. (1922). *The velveteen rabbit, or how toys become real*. London: Heinemann.

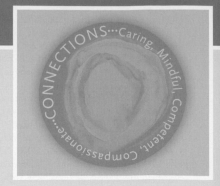

9

Being Empathetic

"Self-absorption in all its forms kills empathy, let alone compassion. When we focus on ourselves, our world contracts as our problems and preoccupations loom large. But when we focus on others, our world expands. Our own problems drift to the periphery of the mind and so seem smaller, and we increase our capacity for connection—or compassionate action."

Daniel Goleman (2007)

OBJECTIVES

1. Define empathy.
2. Identify the preverbal, verbal, and nonverbal aspects of empathy.
3. Discuss the benefits of empathy with clients and colleagues.
4. Identify six steps to empathic communication.
5. Examine steps in breaking bad news.
6. Practice a centering exercise.
7. Participate in exercises to build skills in demonstrating empathy.

WHAT EMPATHY IS

"Health care is an art that must acknowledge the whole of the patient's life (Center for Health Care Progress, 2018). "The Art of Health Care," a 10-minute video on the social determinants of the healthcare of residents of Colorado, evokes thought about what it means to truly understand another person's experience of accessing healthcare (see Art of Health Care: Video - Center for Health Progress).

Do you regularly take the time to ask others their perspective or feelings about a situation? This is good practice for developing skills in empathy (McNamara, 2014), which is an important part of developing trust in the nurse–patient relationship (Dinc & Gastmans, 2013). *Empathy* is the act of communicating to our fellow human beings that we understand something about their world (Dunne, 2005). The empathetic nurse "comprehends the needs of the healthcare users, as the latter feel safe to express the thoughts and problems that concern them" (Moudatsou, Stravropoulou, Philalithis, & Koukouli, 2020, p. 1). The Cleveland Clinic convened its 12th Annual Patient Experience: Empathy and

Innovation Summit in 2021, a digital conference. Two videos showcased in an earlier summit are referenced in Exercise 2 in this chapter. Why host an annual conference on empathy? Empathy research is demonstrating a correlation between empathy and healthcare outcomes (Riess & Reinero, 2014). In a study of 242 Italian primary care physicians caring for a total of 20,961 diabetic patients, patients of physicians scoring highest on an empathy test had significantly fewer acute diabetic complications (Butterfield, 2013).

As a nurse, your practice reflects your understanding of human behavior. How you listen, how you talk, and how you demonstrate empathy and concern are powerful ways to connect with another person (Gallagher, 2009). You are always being observed as a role model, as a communicator…you are "on" all the time (Keefe, 2006). In your education and experience, you grow in self-awareness, build self-confidence, sharpen listening skills, and work on developing nonjudgmental attitudes (Davis, 1990). It is important to note that nurses may become more task oriented than client centered, and patients experience this as a lack of empathy (McCabe, 2004). Taking time to inquire about how the patient is doing, appearing relaxed, and not constantly looking at your watch may demonstrate empathy (McCabe, 2004). You may have the experience of learning and working alongside role models of compassion and empathic communication and negotiating to work with nurses and in settings to foster such ideals. It has been theorized that the ability to experience empathy is the result of a developmental and maturational process (Alligood & May, 2000; Davis, 1990; Olsen, 2001). As a student and novice, you assume the responsibility to work on any problem behaviors such as "prejudice, self-preoccupation, excessive nervous talking, poor listening and poor assertiveness skills, and low self-esteem...that block empathy and interfere with healing" (Davis, 1990). As your own sense of self-identity, personal values, and boundaries develop, it is easier to retain your own identity in interactions with clients and thus to feel at one with others without judgment. You move to the highest level of empathy in which you recognize the other's humanity and personhood regardless of the illness, its circumstance, or stigma. Empathy is more complex than the other interpersonal communication behaviors you have mastered thus far. By the end of this chapter, you will understand what empathy is and be able to explain its importance in interpersonal communication. A number of exercises provide you with the opportunity to practice demonstrating empathy with feedback. Such rehearsal begins the journey to the empathic maturity that benefits clients and colleagues.

 ACTIVE LEARNING

Think about how you will write your answers as you read this chapter.

What?
Write one thing you learned from this chapter.

So What?
How will this affect your nursing practice?

Now What?
How will you implement this new knowledge or skill?

Think About It ...

Think of empathy as occurring in three overlapping stages. The first, self-transposition, occurs when we listen carefully and seek to put ourselves in the client's place. The second, a crossing over, is an emotional shift from thinking to feeling, a deepening of our understanding, and an awareness of the client's experience. This has been called the I–Thou relationship (Buber, 1955), dialogue, or a "shared moment of meaning" (Davis, 1990). The Moments

of Connection in this textbook are examples of interventions that occurred at this level of connection with clients, family, or colleagues. The third stage, getting our "self" back, is when we stand side by side with the other in heartfelt understanding about the experience just shared (Davis, 1990).

American psychologist Carl Rogers contributed immensely to defining the meaning and significance of empathy for helping professionals. He died in 1987, and, in honor of his gifts to us, his direct words are quoted to expand your understanding of the meaning of empathy. This passage is from his book, *A Way of Being* (Rogers, 1980):

An empathic way of being with another person has several facets. It means entering the private perceptual world of the other, and becoming thoroughly at home in it. It involves being sensitive, moment by moment, to the changing felt meanings which flow in this other person, to the fear or rage or tenderness or confusion or whatever that he or she is experiencing. It means temporarily living in the other's life, moving about in it delicately without making judgments; it means sensing meanings of which he or she is scarcely aware, but not trying to uncover totally unconscious feelings, since this would be too threatening. It includes communicating your sensings of the person's world as you look with fresh and unfrightened eyes at elements of which he or she is fearful. It means frequently checking with the person as to the accuracy of your sensings, and being guided by the responses you receive. You are a confident companion to the person in his or her inner world. By pointing to the possible meanings in the flow of another person's experiencing, you help the other to focus on this useful type of referent, to experience the meanings more fully, and to move forward in the experiencing.

A synonym for *empathy* is *communicated understanding*. When we are convinced that others fully understand us without judging us for how we are feeling, questioning why we are reacting that way, or advising us to feel differently, we experience a wonderful sense of acceptance. The process of empathy involves the unconditional acceptance of the individual in need of help; judgments and evaluation of feelings are never offered (Pike, 1990).

This nonjudgmental reception by our fellow human beings is accompanied by feelings of relief and freedom. Once we know we have been understood and accepted, we do not have to struggle to get our point across, nor do we have to justify our reactions to others. When we receive empathic responses, we can relax because we no longer fear being misunderstood or rejected. Acknowledgment of our feelings reassures us that we have a right to be who we are. We may wish to change, and we might change our feelings and reactions in the future, but there is nothing so accepting as having others verbally acknowledge that they understand our feelings.

Another skill associated with empathy is active listening. We can listen passively or actively. Listening passively includes attending nonverbally to our clients or colleagues with eye contact, head nodding, and verbally encouraging phrases such as "uh huh," "mm-hmm," "I see," "yeah," or "I hear you." It is easy to delude ourselves into thinking that when we listen passively we truly communicate that we understand. Passive listening, however, does not include an actual articulation of others' feelings, so it lacks the conviction and reassurance of active listening. The receivers of passive listening have to assume, hope, or pretend that they are being understood. Active listening removes this guesswork. It specifically provides speakers with the knowledge that we know how they are feeling and understand why. Receivers of active listening know that they have been understood.

Natural empathy has been described as a natural and instinctive trait, which is an intrinsic ability to understand the feelings of others. It contrasts with clinical empathy, which is a tool or skill that is consciously and deliberately used to achieve a therapeutic intervention (LaRocco, 2010; Pike, 1990). The goal of empathy is to aid in the establishment of a helping relationship. It is not empathy by itself that is beneficial; it is the intention of the giver and the perception of the receiver. An empathetic nurse helps meet the client's basic need to be understood, which is an important part of establishing a healthy nurse–client relationship (Davis, 2009).

If empathy is truly a curative factor, it must somehow be both communicated to and received by our clients. It is more than a state of mind or attitude. As a concept, empathy is a value-neutral tool that can be used for destructive or manipulative purposes. To be used in a therapeutic or curative way, it must be used to accept, confirm, and validate the total experiences of others. It must be used with the intention of helping.

As nurses in the changing healthcare climate come to accept that the business and caring aspects of patient care must be linked, patients' satisfaction with their caregivers becomes essential. Customer service has become another way to look at delivery of excellent patient care. Patten (1994), in an article about therapeutic hospitality, concluded that "staff interaction skills correlate more highly with patient satisfaction than technical skills." She discussed the ancient practice of hospitality, which has evolved into three levels: public, private, and therapeutic. Therapeutic hospitality involves a high degree of intimacy with a deep personal connection that is the therapeutic use of self. Empathy is an important part of this therapeutic use of self in service recovery when customers' expectations are not met.

HOW TO COMMUNICATE EMPATHICALLY

Empathy includes the ability to reflect, accurately and specifically, in words what our clients or colleagues are experiencing, drawing on the nonverbal behaviors of warmth and genuineness.

Preverbal Aspects of Empathy

In her review article on empathy, Pike (1990) summarized the literature on the mental processes of empathy before the response becomes verbal. Empathy is not total transport into the world of another in which the self is lost in the process. "While there is momentary abandonment, the empathizer never loses sight of her own separateness; she is always aware that the feelings of the other are not her own." Clinical, therapeutic empathy is not subjective. After experiencing the private world of their clients, nurses achieve objectivity by tuning in to their situations. Although they understand what the clients' situations feel like, nurses feel tension and discomfort, which prompts them to action. The empathy is transformed into a verbal connection with the client for the purpose of being helpful (Pike, 1990). This mental shifting requires flexible ego boundaries. Nurses shift from their world into that of their clients, and then back to a processing part of the mind in which they confirm knowledge of their clients' feelings and develop a plan of what to say or do that will be in the clients' best interests.

Verbal Aspects of Empathy

The verbal part of the skill of empathy is reflecting to your clients or colleagues your understanding of their feelings and the reasons for their emotional reactions. The goal is to offer a verbal reflection that is accurate, without exaggerating or minimizing what you are being told. Ideally, the feeling words you use match what the speaker intended; the nuance and strength of the feeling need to be expressed. Your reflection of the rationale for the speaker's feelings specifically needs to be what the speaker intended. The two qualities of verbal empathy that have just been described are accuracy and specificity. It is unrealistic, however, to think that after knowing a client a short time you can always meet these goals. Later you will read about a technique to check the accuracy of your reflection.

Being empathic does not mean repeating verbatim what others have told you. Parroting only irritates speakers and implies that you have not really processed or understood

BOX 9.1 Choosing the "Right" Empathic Word

The following is a list of adjectives describing feelings of being afraid, tense, or worried, which gives you an idea of the range from which you can select the feeling word or phrase.

Afraid	Hesitant	Scared
Agonizing	Ill at ease	Shaken
Alarmed	In a cold sweat	Tense
Anxious	Jittery	Terrified
Apprehensive	Jumpy	Trembling
Cautious	Nervous	Troubled
Concerned	On edge	Uncomfortable
Disturbed	Panicky	Uneasy
Dreading	Petrified	Wary
Fearful	Quaking	Worried
Fidgety	Quivering	
Frightened	Restless	

From Hills, M., & Coffey, M. (1982). On delivering care: An interpersonal skills training manual for nurses. Unpublished manual.

their situation and subsequent reaction. When you respond empathically, you should choose your own words and respond in your own style, yet still be accurate and specific. The following example illustrates how you can accomplish this:

A young patient who has been married for only 6 months has just been told that she has cervical polyps. As she talks, you notice her brow is furrowed, her eyes are glistening, and she hesitantly says, "Can you tell me…what I mean is…I really love my husband…and will these polyps…I mean, I hope I can still make love with my husband.

You pick up several reactions from this young woman. Her stammering and tremulous speech suggest that she is embarrassed about discussing sex. You can most therapeutically deal with her embarrassment by responding in a forthright manner. Her main concern, however, is being able to continue a normal sexual relationship with her husband. You reply empathically as follows:

I can see that you are worried that these polyps you have on your cervix will interfere with your sex life with your husband. Let me explain about cervical polyps. I think I can reassure you.

This response meets the criteria for accuracy and specificity. Your use of the word *worry* accurately reflects the verbal and nonverbal clues you noticed. Reflecting the word *fear* would have been too strong, and using the words *wonder about* or *curious about* (the sexual relationship) would have been too neutral for the level of emotion

she expressed. The feeling words the listener reflects must mirror the nuance the speaker is conveying (Box 9.1). The phrase "that these polyps you have on your cervix will interfere with your sex life with your husband" specifically captures the reason for her worries.

By using your own words and phrasing things in your own style, you avoid parroting and clearly demonstrate that you have understood her worries. Because she felt your understanding before you begin the lesson on polyps, your client is more receptive to the teaching. Hearing a sense of understanding from another person provides a sense of relief and leads us to believe that what the listener says is trustworthy.

Nonverbal Aspects of Empathy

The nonverbal features of empathy are just as important as the verbal aspects. A singer might correctly enunciate each word of a song yet fail to express the mood of the piece. Just as an audience would feel unconnected on hearing an emotionless song, so can disengagement occur when empathy is delivered without being warm and genuine. It is possible to speak an empathic response that is accurate and specific but does not positively affect the other. Only when your empathy is accompanied by warmth and genuineness do the true caring and concern for what your clients and colleagues are experiencing come across. Sympathy is feeling pity for the misfortune of another. Empathy is free of the judgment of sympathy. It is a value-free message showing that you understand the other person's point of view. Empathy is the keynote of an objective, professional relationship respecting boundaries. An example might clarify the necessity for an appropriate level of warmth (Moudatsou et al., 2020).

Your colleague has just told you that she is pregnant and is therefore upset because she will not be able to continue her full-time nursing career. If you were to smother her with a hug or become overly solicitous, your attentive warmth would come across as sympathy. Sympathy focuses on your own feelings rather than the other person's feelings. Being too warm in this situation might suggest that you find her predicament hopeless. Empathy with the appropriate warmth, such as a concerned facial expression and a gentle touch on the shoulder, tells your colleague that you understand. Now she can approach her problem unburdened by your overprotectiveness.

Feeling genuine empathy for others is essential. If you do not care about how your clients or colleagues are feeling, using an empathic response would not be helpful. Even if the verbal part of your empathy is correct, your nonverbal behavior can give away your lack of caring. Usually, our expression of warmth is diminished when we do not genuinely care about the feelings of others. This diminished warmth may speak louder than the words of our empathic response and the message received as one of not caring.

In summary, empathic communication requires a specific and accurate verbal response accompanied by genuine caring and a receivable level of warmth. These attributes of empathy must be spoken in your own style of speaking. In an essay on the lived experience of cancer, a woman writes, "The capacity to recognize and respond to others' distress may be a deep and permeating element of a person's characterological build. For those endowed with the capacity for empathy, its absence is perhaps as unimaginable as color blindness or tone deafness are to those endowed with color perception and perfect pitch" (Charon, 1995).

SIMPLIFY AND DEEPEN

Empathy is simply listening, holding space, withholding judgment, emotionally connecting, and communicating that incredibly healing message of 'you're not alone.'

Brene Brown

 ## MOMENTS OF CONNECTION...

In the Right Place at the Right Time

"When I was a student nurse, I was in my pediatric rotation and had the opportunity to work with a 17-year-old single mom of a child with a cleft palate and lip. The child was 3 months old, and her mom wasn't visiting or holding the child. I asked to speak with her and asked some questions about the baby. I have faint but visible scars from cleft lip surgery, and the mother felt able to talk to me. She told me her parents said the baby was born that way because of the mother's sin of being a single

mother. When I asked what she wanted for her child, she replied, to grow up and be able to sing. I was filled with a warm feeling and told her that her little girl could do anything, that I sing, and then I sang a little song for her. I told her that God doesn't punish. Sometimes you have to search for the blessing. After our talk, the mother began to visit the baby and take part in feeding and caring for the baby. The baby underwent corrective surgery 3 months later."

WHEN TO COMMUNICATE EMPATHICALLY

Rogers (1980) asserted that in some situations empathy has the highest priority of the attitudinal elements and makes for growth-promoting human relationships. When clients or colleagues are hurting, confused, troubled, anxious, alienated, terrified, doubtful of self-worth, or uncertain as to identity, then understanding is called for.

We have as much responsibility for clients' needs to express their feelings on intimate matters as we do for their privacy. We might ask ourselves, "How much should I encourage my clients to tell me? Am I at risk of crossing the line between facilitating communication (with my empathy) and aggressively pursuing their private reactions?" Being empathic can be helpful or invading, and, as nurses, we must strive to use our empathic skills with the intent of being helpful.

It is helpful to be empathic any time people share their thoughts and feelings with you. An empathic reply can be used on its own or with another message or communication strategy. For example, empathy can be used with the following:

- *Statements:* "You feel frustrated because the clinic is not open in the evenings, when it would be more convenient for you to come and have your blood pressure checked. There have been several other requests for extended hours, so I will raise this issue with our office manager." In addition to knowing your plan to follow up on such a complaint, it is reassuring for a client to have you acknowledge the situation and the feelings related to it.
- *Questions:* "Yes, I can see that you are pretty excited about being discharged from the hospital earlier than you had expected. Have you had time to arrange for your babysitter to start earlier and give you a hand with your toddler and your new baby?" Your empathic beginning potentiates the effect of your concern for your client's discharge plans.
- *Alternate points of view:* "You feel pretty adamant that your pack-a-day smoking habit won't harm your health, since your grandfather smoked and lived to be 95. I have

a different way of looking at smoking, since I've recently known several clients who have died of lung cancer. The statistics do indicate a high positive correlation between smoking and lung cancer." Most clients and colleagues hear our side of an argument if we give equal recognition to their point of view.

- *Explanations:* "Being moved to a semiprivate room has really upset you, and you feel that your privacy has been invaded. Switching rooms truly was our last alternative. We need a single room to carry out isolation techniques for an infectious client to protect everyone on the unit." By first acknowledging your client's feelings, you can help pave the way for acceptance of your decision. Examples of invitations for more information are:
- *With a client:* "You're worried about the sharp pains in your kidney area. Have you had any other unusual signs and symptoms lately?"
- *With a colleague:* "From your point of view, our new charting system is cumbersome and pretty frustrating. Do you have any suggestions for streamlining the recording of our nurses' notes?"

Most people engage more fully in our request for additional information when they hear that we understand what they have already told us.

Missing opportunities to convey empathy can create a gulf between speakers and listeners and make speakers feel ignored. When we do not hear others, a new struggle is created for them. They are disappointed at not being understood and, in turn, either withdraw with wounded feelings or fight to convince us of their feelings. When empathy is not offered, our clients and colleagues feel cheated, frustrated, and ignored. Including empathy with other communication strategies lets our clients and colleagues know beyond a doubt that they have been heard and understood.

In any therapeutic relationship it is important that our partners feel cared for. Client–nurse relationships are ones in which we have established ourselves as helpers. That label means that we acknowledge and make public our desire to support others. Empathy is one concrete way to show our caring.

Sometimes when stress levels are high, we get lost in our own concerns and forget that our colleagues have concerns of their own. Simple acts help get us back on track.

HOW EMPATHY BENEFITS CLIENTS AND COLLEAGUES

Clients and colleagues share their thoughts and feelings to be understood, but often it is uncomfortable for them to reveal themselves. As listeners, it is not good enough for us to understand how our clients or colleagues feel without verbally sharing that empathic understanding explicitly and accurately. Communicating our understanding benefits clients and colleagues and our relationships with them.

Empathy increases the feeling of being connected with another person. This positive feeling of belonging helps reduce feelings of loneliness and isolation. Although it has often been said that we are ultimately alone in our journey through life, empathy is a bridge that connects us with others, providing confidence and hope. For colleagues to know they are not alone, responding to each other with empathy provides comfort in times of challenging transitions. The knowledge that you understand your clients and colleagues helps them continue on their way, secure that their feelings have been acknowledged as normal human reactions. The companionship you extend through empathy, however brief the engagement, creates a human bond that adds to your clients' or colleagues' personal strength. Rogers (1980) puts it simply: Empathy dissolves alienation. Consider, too, the family caregivers with whom you come in contact, those giving full-time care in the home or keeping long vigils at the client's bedside in the hospital. These have been called the *hidden patients*. Look for signs of exhaustion caused by a lack of personal time, problems with the behavior of the care recipient, and the demands of their own employment (Ostwald, 1997).

Curry (1994) offered this description of the empathic experience:

> *When I look at patients, I see friends and loved ones on a battlefield of illness and pain. I see my father in the face of a man who can no longer speak because of a brain tumor, but whose eyes still shine when his grandchildren visit. I feel my mother's hands in those of an older woman whose memories have been claimed by Alzheimer's disease. I see my brother in the gaunt young man with AIDS whose family and friends have deserted him.*

Empathy can contribute to feelings of increased self-esteem on the part of those to whom you extend it. The fact that you take the time to listen, hear, process, and reflect what your clients or colleagues say makes them feel important. Caring enough to show that you understand makes others feel significant and worthwhile.

It is impossible to accurately sense the perceptual world of another person unless you value that person and his or her world, unless you, in some sense, care. Hence this message comes through to the recipient: "This other person trusts me, thinks I'm worthwhile. Perhaps I am worth something. Perhaps I could value myself. Perhaps I could care for myself" (Rogers, 1980).

Your empathy demonstrates that you accept how your clients and colleagues feel and helps them to trust that you genuinely accept them as they are.

Your withholding of judgment or advice enhances this trust. When you unconditionally accept others as they present themselves, they can relax and feel free to be who they really are. A consequence of empathic understanding is that others feel valued, cared for, and accepted as the people they are (Rogers, 1980): "True empathy is always free of any evaluative or diagnostic quality. The recipient perceives this with some surprise: 'If I am not being judged, perhaps I am not so evil or abnormal as I have thought. Perhaps I don't have to judge myself so harshly.' Thus, the possibility of self-acceptance is gradually increased." Finely tuned understanding by others gives us all a sense of personhood and identity. Rogers shows us that empathy gives that needed confirmation.

Your empathy can help your clients and colleagues move on to new feelings and change their behavior.

The acceptance your empathy offers frees your clients and colleagues from having to defend or rationalize their feelings; as a result, they are able to experience alternative reactions, freed of any clinging to defensive feelings. When you do not give empathy, then your clients and colleagues believe they have to justify their feelings.

Receiving empathy helps them to be open and move on to different ways of experiencing. It is perfectly natural for people to change their reactions as new information is processed or old data are reexamined in a new light. The acceptance you provide through empathy helps your clients and colleagues remain flexible enough to move to a new awareness.

In our personal and professional lives we are often in relationships with individuals who must make difficult decisions about their lives. More often than not, that person does not need more information, certainly does not need a judgmental presence, and probably does not want the answer or the decision taken from them. What they require from us is real presence that will support them, empower them, and give them the courage to decide (Marsden, 1990).

Presence means more than just showing up. It is the ability to "empathize, listen, reflect, and observe" (Potter & Frisch, 2007). In some instances, your empathic reflection can help your clients or colleagues comprehend more fully how they are reacting. Hearing your reflection of their feelings may increase their self-awareness. Not only is this enlightenment satisfying, but it can widen their perspective of the entire situation. Consider the following example:

You have just empathically reflected to Douglas, a client in the diabetic clinic, that it just does not seem fair that he has diabetes while his roommate's good health allows him the freedom to eat and drink what he wants and to party until all hours of the night.

Douglas: *"Yes, you're right! That's exactly how I'm feeling. I hadn't realized how it gripes me that he isn't restricted like I am. I guess I think about the medical expenses that I have, not to mention the time-consuming treatments I have to put up with. No wonder I'm so short with him when I see him having a good time. In fact, sometimes I'm quite miserable to him…I'd better not let this situation get out of hand."*

Your empathic response increased Douglas' understanding of his behavior and himself. The literature on empathy reports that psychotherapists high in empathy, genuineness, and warmth elicit greater self-exploration in their clients (Shapiro, Krauss, & Truax, 1969).

Now that Douglas is aware of his feelings about his roommate's health and freedom, he can use this self-awareness to help him handle his situation. Douglas could consider all kinds of possibilities. In terms of changing his situation, he could get a roommate with a chronic illness so that he would not have to deal with these feelings, or he could brainstorm ways to minimize the restrictions in his diabetic regimen so that he could live his life more naturally. In terms of changing his feelings, he could stop comparing himself to others and increase his gratefulness for the lifestyle he can lead, or he could be hostile toward his roommate until the roommate can no longer tolerate it and decides either to leave or to fight back.

Being understood makes it possible for clients to listen with greater empathy for their own reactions to what they are experiencing. This greater understanding and prizing of themselves can open new facets of experience, which bring into their awareness a more accurate picture of themselves and a clearer self-concept.

The argument can be made that empathic responses from nurses can enhance healing and well-being in all clients. Illness and hospitalization cause fear, dependency, and upheaval in clients' daily lifestyles and relationships, whether the health problem is surgical, medical, obstetric, or psychiatric. Empathic nurses can tune in to their clients' feelings in a helpful way. Empathy on the part of health professionals can improve the success of the complete clinical problem-solving process and enhance client compliance because of increased client involvement.

Practicing nurses confirm the benefits of empathy in the workplace. Results of a survey of 67 nurses at an ambulatory surgery conference indicated that empathic communication can add joy to the workplace and keep workers enthusiastic about their jobs (Box 9.2).

Copyright © 1995 by Julia W. Balzer Riley.

Nurse leaders who act as giant shock absorbers of uncertainty in an organization can refuel their energy and continue to be empathic by staying in touch with nurses who have direct client contact and listening to their stories of connection (Kerfoot, 2002). Empathy, defined as the ability to understand and interact based on the emotional makeup of others, is one of the key personality traits of emotional intelligence recommended for consideration in hiring employees, along with self-awareness, the ability to recognize one's own emotions and motivation and their effect on others; self-regulation, the ability to control or redirect problematic impulses or moods; motivation, which is a passion for work and pursuit of goals with energy and persistence; and social skills, which are necessary for proficiency in building relationships and networks (Connolly, 2002).

HOW EMPATHY BENEFITS THE NURSE

Consider the warm feeling of compassion you get when you help others feel understood and accepted. Knowing that you have taken the opportunity to make your clients

or colleagues feel better provides immense satisfaction and can augment your feelings of competence.

Nurses want to collect enough information from their clients to assess their concerns accurately and to develop the best nursing care plan for treating their health problems. When clients feel accepted, their trust allows them to open up and provide the information necessary for accurate assessment of their situations. Obtaining sufficient data to make a correct nursing diagnosis is the first and most important step in the systematic problem-solving approach to nursing care. Whether clients' problems are physical, emotional, or a combination of both, empathy can be used to acquire sufficient and comprehensive data.

🌸 MOMENTS OF CONNECTION...
When the Tears Come

"I'm a pediatric nurse, a sensitive one. I have always worried about crying too much. I was with a small child who was dying. I was able to do all the nursing care for her, but all the while, tears ran down my face. After she died, the family came to me and told me how much it meant to them that I cried, because they did not have a sense of caring from other staff. I no longer worry about my sensitivity to my work!"

Empathy can be shown at all stages of the problem-solving process. When you are developing a plan of care, it is essential to determine how your clients feel about the proposed treatment schedule and to empathically reflect your understanding. Acknowledging clients' reactions to treatment regimens and, when possible, adjusting plans accordingly are likely to increase compliant behavior.

As a nurse, you want to know if your nursing care has been effective. Many objective measures of success exist, but one important yardstick is how your clients feel about their treatment outcome. Clients may be sufficiently satisfied and wish to terminate treatment, or they may want to try an alternative plan to achieve their desired outcome. Clients' input has implications for how to proceed in the client–nurse relationship. Showing empathy lets your clients know that you understand and acknowledge their evaluation of progress.

In your working relationships, being empathic with colleagues augments cohesiveness. Showing that you understand your colleagues not only makes working together more enjoyable, it also helps you prevent and work out difficulties in your relationships.

Scenarios Demonstrating Empathy

Clearly, empathy has many positive benefits for our clients and colleagues and has a payoff for ourselves. If we are not conveying empathy at appropriate opportunities in our relationships with clients and colleagues, then it is likely we are relating in ways that are not helpful.

Several activities may result in a failure to express empathy. Be careful not to judge clients or colleagues. If we question the appropriateness of their thoughts and feelings, then we effectively shut off the unbiased and accepting part of our communication. Being truly empathic means being able to put aside our opinions and tune in to how the other person is feeling.

A situation with a client might be:

Your client has come to the physician's office for a colposcopic examination and says to you,

> *"I'm scared to death of this copos…how do you say it? …examination…the whole idea spooks me."*

Empathic response: *"The thought of having a colposcopic examination is really frightening for you. What can I do to relieve some of your fears about it?"*

An example involving a colleague may illustrate this further.

A situation with a colleague might be:

> *You have just started the evening shift on your unit after several days off, and the nurse manager on the day shift remarks,*
> *"Boy! Count yourself lucky to have been off for the past 3 days. It's been like a zoo here! We've had two deaths and five admissions, and we've been short-staffed the whole time. I'm wiped out!"*

Empathic response: *"No wonder you're tired. It sounds like you've had to handle three times the usual workload with the admissions and deaths…and all without enough help. When's your well-deserved time off coming?"*

This empathic reply makes your colleague feel that she has been heard. There is no doubt that you understand what she has been coping with while you were away. All she desired was for you to register how it has been for her. The desire to communicate in a caring way is motivation to use empathy. Being nonjudgmentally empathic requires the desire to show acceptance and the will to focus and concentrate on the concerns of others.

Remember this idea so that as a helping professional you can take care of yourself. It takes courage to be empathic (Pike, 1990): "Entering into a patient's world as if it were his own exposes the nurse to the possibility of pain, despair, anger, fear, and hopelessness. Courage is especially called

for in situations where the nurse is powerless to cure the patient's distress, pain, or suffering."

The greater the maturity and experience of nurses are, the greater is their usable vault of knowledge, attitudes, and learning for enhancing their empathy. All nurses need one important key to open the vault: access to feelings (Pike, 1990).

Empathy is assertive because it takes into account others' thoughts and feelings and protects your right to communicate in a caring way. It is responsible to be empathic because it ensures that your clients feel acknowledged enough to engage in all aspects of the nursing process.

SIX STEPS TO HELP YOU COMMUNICATE MORE EMPATHICALLY

How can we nurture our ability to reliably convey empathy on a consistent basis? The following guidelines are based on a systematic problem-solving approach. If you truly want to be empathic, then these six steps can be helpful:

1. *Clear your head of distracting agendas.* In your busy life you will have many thoughts going through your head, such as personal worries, pressure from expanding work, or perhaps feelings of discomfort related to talking with a client or colleague. To the extent that you can put these aside, do so. If you are able to focus on the person you are with, you will streamline communication. Paying attention to other speakers increases the chances that you will deal with their situations more thoroughly and more effectively. Listening empathically means not having to return time and time again to get complete information, and that means one less item on your long list of things to do. Teach yourself to concentrate (Raudsepp, 1990).

2. *Remind yourself to focus on the speaker.* Remember that your priority is to listen and hear your clients or colleagues so that you can verbally convey your understanding. Remind yourself that your purpose is to tune in to what a speaker is saying. Some people find that a physical gesture, such as removing their glasses or adopting a definite listening stance, reminds them to focus. "Don't interrupt," reminded Raudsepp (1990).

3. *Attend to your clients' and colleagues' verbal and nonverbal messages.* Hear the words that speakers are using to describe how they are feeling and the reasons for their reaction. Look for what your speakers are also saying nonverbally. Take in the entire message that your clients and colleagues are sending you.

4. *Ask yourself, "What does this person want me to hear?"* Attempt to pick out the most important message being delivered. What is the predominant theme? Is anguish the strongest feeling? Is joy the prevailing emotion? Your answer should be what the speaker wants you to

hear, and that very seed is the embryo for your empathic response.

5. *Convey an empathic response.* Verbally reflect the speaker's feelings and the reason for them, ensuring that your response meets the criteria of accuracy and specificity. Pay attention to your nonverbal communication. Convey the amount of warmth you deem appropriate and ensure that the expression is congruent with your intentions to be understanding and accepting.

6. *Check to see if your empathic response was effective.* The purpose of being empathic is to make others feel relieved (that we understand them) and cared for (because of our genuine interest in their situation). Check it out. Do the speakers nod their heads? Do they smile or tell you in other ways that they are delighted you have understood them? Do they visibly relax by letting go of tension or by engaging you in further conversation? These clues let you know that you have been successful.

If your attempt to be empathic has missed the mark, a speaker will let you know in several ways. More assertive clients or colleagues will tell you outright: "No, that's not quite how I'm feeling…It's more like this…." Others may just slowly withdraw from opening up anymore with you. It is acceptable most times to explicitly ask your speaker if your empathy is on target. Try "Is that how you are feeling?" or "Have I understood how it is for you?" or "Let me see if I have this right."

As you spend time fine-tuning your skills as empathetic listeners, the patient's story is revealed. As you learn more about a person's life and coping skills, you can remind him that he is still himself, more than this illness, and has strengths that can be applied in this journey. As you come to know more about the strength of the human spirit in the face of crisis, you can be confident in your support (Ragan & Kanter, 2017).

HOW TO BREAK BAD NEWS

Nurses are often in a position to reinforce and provide clarification when the client and family have received bad news, especially when they work with a dying client. Talking about death may be a difficult task. Although physicians usually break the initial bad news, the nurse can offer support. The actions outlined in Box 9.3 should be taken when breaking bad news.

HOW TO CENTER YOURSELF

The demands of the work of nurses are many and complex. Practice a brief centering technique throughout the day to refocus and bring yourself fully present to the people

---

BOX 9.3 Breaking Bad News

1. Plan what is to be said ahead of time and organize your thoughts. Anticipate questions family members may ask. Knowledge of previous family coping mechanisms is helpful in planning the team response.
2. Establish rapport. If this has not occurred, ask team members who have established rapport with the family to attend.
3. Control the environment as much as possible. Set aside appropriate time; turn off pagers, cell phones, and televisions; take the phone off the hook. Sit down and listen.
4. Find out what the client and family already know.
5. Find out how much given individuals want to know; do not make assumptions about this.
6. Use language the client and family will understand. Be sensitive and respectful of cultural issues.
7. Respond to the reactions of the client and family, using an empathic approach. Continually assess and reassess the client's and family's understanding of the information.
8. When appropriate, explain the treatment plan and prognosis, and summarize.

Modified from American Association of Colleges of Nursing and City of Hope National Medical Center. (2000). *Training program facility guide.* Duarte, CA: End-of-Life Nursing Education Consortium; Matzo, M. L., & Sherman, D. W. (2001). *Palliative care nursing: Quality care to the end of life.* New York, NY: Springer Publishing; Buckman, R. (1992). *How to break bad news: A guide for health professionals.* Baltimore, MD: Johns Hopkins Press.

---

entrusted to your care and those with whom you work (Box 9.4).

 MOMENTS OF CONNECTION…

Keep on Trying…Empathy Is a Lifelong Journey

"This man was such a special person, a quadriplegic for over 30 years who wrote poetry to soothe his spirit and express his deepest feelings. He talked about being able to tell when people who entered his room stopped listening. He said their eyes would just 'glaze over,' and so he would talk 'gobbledygook,' and they never noticed. When I think of empathy, I think of this man. How could we as nurses ever really understand? But knowing him makes me keep trying."

Over time as you see the positive effects of your empathetic response to clients, families, and colleagues, empathy

> **BOX 9.4   Centering Technique to Set the Intention of Being Fully Present with Clients, Family, and Colleagues**
>
> Honor the sacred nature of your work. Take time each day to connect with your own purpose in your work. (This entire process should take less than 30 seconds.)
> 1. Before you interact with a client, family member, or colleague, pause.
> 2. Let go of any distractions or worries just now.
> 3. Close your eyes briefly and take a deep breath.
> 4. Say silently to yourself, "I am here for the greater good of all people involved and will give my full attention to this moment."
> 5. Bring to mind someone or something that evokes love and compassion.
> 6. Hold that feeling of love and compassion, repeating to yourself, "I am present in this moment."

Adapted from Dossey, B. M., & Keegan, L. C. (2008). *Holistic nursing: A handbook for practice* (5th ed.). Sudbury, MA: Jones & Bartlett.

may become a way of being. When describing their work, some nurses say, "It's just the way I am" (Wiseman, 2007).

Self-Care Nudge

When you are upset, try this. Take 5 minutes to write down whatever you are thinking and feeling. You can discard it if you choose or add it to your journal.

Return to "Active Learning" at the beginning of the chapter and write your responses.

PRACTICING BEING EMPATHETIC

Video/Discussion: Exercise 1

Watch the 10-minute video, *The Art of Health Care*, at Art of Health Care: Video - Center for Health Progress. Then download the discussion guide to facilitate your learning about the social determinants of healthcare.

Creative Expression/Discussion/Reflection: Exercise 2

Watch two Cleveland Clinic videos online (less than 10 minutes) on empathy. Search *Empathy: The Human Connection to Patient Care* (4½ minutes) and *Cleveland Clinic's Empathy Series Continues: Patients: Afraid and Vulnerable* (6 minutes). Reflect on how presence and empathy make a difference in interactions with patients. Consider that other students and colleagues each have their own stories, and

you may not know what they are dealing with in their own lives. Write in your journal and/or discuss one behavior you can change to demonstrate your empathy.

Narrative Medicine (Learning through Story)/ Medical Humanities (Learning through the Arts): Exercise 3

Wit is a moving video with Emma Thompson; it is the story of a literature professor's experience with ovarian cancer. Because it is so powerful, arrange to watch it with other students in healthcare. It can be purchased or rented online. This video has been found to be a helpful tool in building empathy skills (Everson et al., 2018). I use it in class. Read about the video online. Reflect on lessons learned in your journal. Share your thoughts with others who have seen the movie.

Reflective Journaling: Exercise 4

Keeping a journal has been found effective in changing beliefs and developing self-reflection, both ways to develop empathy (Webster, 2010; Ketola & Stein, 2013). Continue your own journal keeping by regularly writing a description of and thoughts about your clinical experiences, feelings about the experience, and how and why you are affected by the experience as a person and as a nurse. For this exercise, complete one journal entry following the preceding guidelines.

Skill Building: Exercise 5

This exercise provides you with several hypothetical situations in which clients or colleagues express thoughts and feelings to you. Look at completed responses in Examples 1 and 2. Complete your own empathetic responses to Examples 3 to 5. Remember to meet the criteria of being accurate and specific.

After you have written your initial empathic response, critique it and suggest alternative ways of phrasing your first try to make it more empathic. In your improved response, try to convey complete understanding, and phrase it in your natural way of speaking.

Example 1

A nurse colleague says: "I'm not going to be able to get through that job interview with Mrs. Jones for the position of assistant head nurse. I just know I'll be so uptight that I'll blow it like I did the last time."

First attempt at empathy: "You're feeling pretty nervous about that interview."

Critique: This reply lacks specificity. Including a reference to the fact that it is a job interview would have acknowledged the importance of the event for your colleague. Referring to the reason for her worry about the interview would have made a more complete and accurate empathic response.

Suggested alternative: "You're feeling pretty nervous about your job interview for the assistant head nurse position and worried that it might not go well."

Example 2

A client tells you: "I didn't have to take any pain medication last night for my injured back…and I slept right through the night. It was the first good sleep I've had in four nights."

First attempt at empathy: "That's great! I'm glad you're sleeping better!"

Critique: This statement is more a judgment than a reflection of the client's feelings. The implied feelings are relief (at not having to take the medication) and joy (at sleeping well). These feelings, and the reasons for them, need to be included to make the response empathic.

Suggested alternative: "Boy! What a relief for you to have been comfortable enough to do without your pain medication, and you look overjoyed that you slept so well."

Now it is your turn! For each of the following situations, attempt a written empathic response. Then critique your attempt and suggest how it could be improved.

Example 3

A client says to you: "My husband died a year ago. It's been the longest and saddest year of my life."

Your first attempt at empathy:
Your critique:
Your suggested alternative:

Example 4

A client says to you: "I had a real scare today. My chest x-ray has a spot on it and my doctor has called in a specialist to see what it is. I'm so worried because she told me that cancer can't be ruled out until I've had further tests."

Your first attempt at empathy:
Your critique:
Your suggested alternative:

Example 5

An 18-year-old client says to you: "I never thought I could be HIV-positive. I'm not gay. I don't use drugs. I've only had sex with one person. My life is over."

Your first attempt at empathy:
Your critique:
Your suggested alternative:

After you have completed the preceding examples on your own, get together with the rest of your class and compare your responses. It will be interesting to see how many different ways an empathic response can be phrased and still meet the criteria of accuracy, specificity, naturalness, warmth, and genuineness.

Small Group Work for Skill Building: Exercise 6

This exercise gives you a chance to receive supervised feedback on your ability to be empathic. Work in groups of four. One person takes the role of speaker and one the role of listener; the other two are observers. The speaker chooses a topic about which he or she has strong feelings.

The listener's task is to demonstrate empathic listening to what the speaker has to say during a conversation lasting 4 minutes. The observers use the Empathy Rating Scale (Fig. 9.1) to evaluate the speaker's ability to be empathic. Roles should be rotated so that each person in the group has the chance to be speaker, listener, and observer.

The information on the Empathy Rating Scale that you receive as listener will outline areas in which you are strong and others in which you need to improve your ability to communicate empathically. For example, the Empathy Rating Scale may draw your attention to the fact that you neglect to include the rationale for the speaker's feelings, even though you meet the criteria for accuracy, warmth, naturalness, and genuineness. This exercise can be repeated at intervals after practicing empathy so that over time you can see the pattern of improvement.

Skill Building/Reflection: Exercise 7

Review the centering technique in Box 9.4. For 1 day in the clinical setting, practice this technique immediately before you work with a client. You will find you may shorten the centering further with practice. Write a brief reflection on your response to the use of this centering technique.

Creative Expression: Exercise 8

Consider what clients have to teach us about their experiences. Ask yourself, "If I were a quadriplegic…or…experiencing any disease or disability…how would I feel? What would I think? How would I cope?" The following poem was written by a patient who may have been in residence longer than any other veteran at the Bay Pines Veterans Administration Hospital in Florida. He was a quadriplegic for more than 40 years and the author of more than 100 poems. It was a privilege to meet this poet whose dream was to have his poems published…we are making this

Response No.	Accuracy: matched intensity?	Specificity: rationale included?	Naturalness: own words?	Warmth: verbal? nonverbal?	Genuineness: interest and caring conveyed?
1					
2					
3					
4					
5					
6					
7					

Criteria for Empathy Rating Scale

1. *Accuracy:* Does the intensity of the listener's words match the speaker's intended message?
2. *Specificity:* Does the listener include the rationale for the speaker's feelings?
3. *Naturalness:* Does the listener avoid parroting? Does the listener reflect the speaker's message in a naturally worded style?
4. *Warmth:* Does the listener convey verbal and nonverbal warmth with an empathic response?
5. *Genuineness:* Does the listener convey interest and caring about what the speaker is saying?

Fig. 9.1 Empathy Rating Scale.

dream come true. Howard died in 2006. Howard said he has reframed his life as a teacher of nurses and of the nursing students who cared for him during their clinical rotations…and so he was.

> "Social Malignancy"
> This but one of the little horrors
> We must learn to endure
> And never quite do…
> Quadriplegia is not unlike
> leukemia of the soul
> Always under attack by that social cancer
> Because the severe disability breeds a lack of our credibility.
> Copyright © Howard G. Kirkman. Used with permission.

Creative Expression: Exercise 9

How can you, as a nurse, expand your horizons and your ability to be empathetic? Read poetry. Listen to music. Read literature. View art. These are all expressions of the human experience. In your journal write a poem about a clinical experience that stays on your mind. Perhaps you have a client with whom you have problems connecting or one that touches your heart. You might write a poem that you would share with colleagues. Poetry can help you be more fully present; remind you to listen again to what is being said; increase your ability to tolerate pain, and understand yourself and others; and discover and reflect on clients' feelings to build the skill of empathy (Akhtar, 2000; Connelly, 1999; Goldner, 2005; Raingruber, 2004).

Begin now to consider publishing in your nursing career. Perhaps a reflection or poem from your journal would be a good submission for the Reflections section of *Imprint*, the publication of the National Student Nurses Association (see https://www.nsna.org/get-published-in-imprint.html for more information) (Brown, 2010).

REFERENCES

Akhtar, S. (2000). Mental pain and the cultural ointment of poetry. *International Journal of Psychoanalysis, 81*, 229.

Alligood, M. R., & May, B. A. (2000). A nursing theory of personal system empathy: Interpreting a conceptualization of empathy in King's interacting systems. *Nursing Science Quarterly, 13*(3), 243.

Brown, D. L. (2010). Using art and literature in the clinical setting: An innovative assignment. *Nurse Educator, 3*(2), 53.

Buber, M. (1955). *Between man and man*. Boston: Beacon Press.

Butterfield, S. (2013). New research links empathy to outcomes, American College of Physicians Internist. New research links empathy to outcomes | ACP Internist.

Center for Health Care Progress. (2018). The art of health care. https://centerforhealthprogress.org/blog/publications/art-of-health-care-video/.

Charon, R. (1995). Connections that heal. *Second Opinion, 2*(1), 38.

Connelly, J. (1999). Being in the present moment: Developing the capacity for mindfulness in medicine. *Academic Medicine, 74*, 420.

Connolly, K. H. (2002). *The new IQ. Nursing Management, 33*(7), 17.

Curry, M. C. (1994). What it takes to be a nurse. *Nursing, 24*(5), 33.

Davis, C. M. (1990). What is empathy, and can empathy be taught? *Physical Therapy, 70*(11), 707.

Davis, M. (2009). A perspective on cultivating clinical empathy. *Complementary Therapies in Clinical Practice, 15*(2), 76.

Dinc, L., & Gastmans, C. (2013). Trust in nurse–patient relationships. *Nursing Ethics, 20*, 501.

Dunne, K. (2005). Effective communication in palliative care. *Nursing Standard, 20*(13), 57.

Everson, N., Levett-Jones, T., & Pitt, V. (2018). The impact of educational interventions on the empathetic concern of health professional students: A literature review. *Nursing Education in Practice, 31*, 104.

Gallagher, R. S. (2009). *How to tell anyone anything: Breakthrough techniques for handling difficult conversations at work*. New York, NY: AMACOM.

Goldner, V. (2005). The poem as a transformational third. *Psychoanalysis Dialogues, 15*(1), 105.

Goleman, D. (2007). *Social intelligence: The new science of social relationships*. New York, NY: Bantam.

Keefe, S. (2006). Understanding human behavior. *Advances in Nursing, 7*(5), 29.

Kerfoot, K. (2002). Warming your heart: The energy solution. *Nursing Economics, 2*(20), 74.

Ketola, J., & Stein, J. V. (2013). Psychiatric clinical course strengthens the student–patient relationships of baccalaureate nursing students. *Journal of Psychiatric and Mental Health Nursing, 20*, 23.

LaRocco, S. A. (2010). Assisting nursing students to develop empathy using a writing assignment. *Nurse Educator, 35*(1), 10.

Marsden, C. (1990). Real presence. *Heart & Lung, 19*(6), 540.

McCabe, C. (2004). Nurse–patient communication: An exploration of patients' experiences. *Journal of Clinical Nursing, 13*(2), 41.

McNamara, C. (2014). How to develop skills in empathy. Free Management Library. How to Develop Skills in Empathy (managementhelp.org).

Moreno-Poyato, A. R., & Rodriquez-Nogueira, O. (2021). The association between empathy and the nurse-patient therapeutic relationship in mental health units: A cross-sectional study. *Journal of Psychiatric and Mental Health Nursing, 28*(3), 335–443. https://doi.org/10.1111/jpm.12675.

Moudatsou, M., Stravropoulou, A., Philalithis, A., & Koukouli, S. (2020). The role of empathy in health and social care professionals. *Healthcare (Basel), 8*, 26. doi:10.3390/healthcare8010026.

Olsen, D. P. (2001). Empathetic maturity: Theory of moral point of view in clinical relations. *Advances in Nursing Science, 24*(1), 36.

Ostwald, S. K. (1997). Caregiver exhaustion: Caring for the hidden patients. *Advanced Practice Nursing Quarterly, 3*(2), 29.

Patten, C. S. (1994). Understanding hospitality. *Nursing Management, 25*(3), 80A.

Pike, A. W. (1990). On the nature and place of empathy in clinical nursing practice. *Journal of Professional Nursing, 6*(4), 135.

Potter, P. J., & Frisch, N. (2007). Holistic assessment and care: Presence in the process. *Nursing Clinics of North America, 42*, 213.

Ragan, S. L., & Kanter, E. (2017). Learning the patient's story. *Seminars in Oncology Nursing, 33*(5), 467.

Raingruber, B. (2004). Using poetry to discover and share significant meanings in child and adolescent mental health nursing. *Journal of Child and Adolescent Psychiatric Nursing, 17*(1), 13.

Raudsepp, E. (1990). Seven ways to cure communication breakdowns. *Nursing, 20*(4), 132.

Riess, H., & Reinero, D. (2014). Can empathy be as effective as aspirin? The patient–clinician relationship affects medical outcomes. https://www.gold-foundation.org/can-empathy-be-as-effective-as-aspirin-the-patient-clinician-relationship-affects-medical-outcomes.

Rogers, C. R. (1980). *A way of being*. Boston: Houghton Mifflin.

Shapiro, J. G., Krauss, H. H., & Truax, C. B. (1969). Therapeutic conditions and disclosure beyond the therapeutic encounter. *Journal of Counseling Psychology, 16*(4), 290.

Webster, D. (2010). Promoting empathy through a creative reflective teaching strategy: A mixed-method study. *Journal of Nursing Education, 49*, 87.

Wiseman, T. (2007). Toward a holistic conceptualization of empathy for nursing practice. *Advances in Nursing Science, 30*(3), E61.

10

Honoring Professional Boundaries

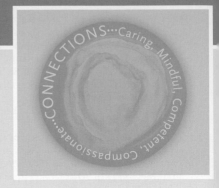

"Boundary crossings can happen to any nurse. The key to avoiding them is continual alertness, self-evaluation, and emphasis on the patient's best interests."

National Council of State Boards of Nursing (NCSBN, 2014a)

OBJECTIVES

1. Discuss professional boundaries in nursing.
2. Define self-disclosure in the helping relationship.
3. Define immediacy in the helping relationship.
4. Identify guidelines for appropriate self-disclosure by the nurse.
5. Discuss helpful self-disclosures.
6. Participate in exercises to build and deepen an understanding of professional boundaries.

As you read this chapter, you will see how essential it is for the nurses to meet their personal needs through self-care and to use clinical judgment in how best to be present for patients.

The nurse–patient relationship is a professional relationship rather than a personal one. Professional boundaries put the patient at the center of the relationship, not the nurse. That is, the main goal is to meet the needs of the patient, not the needs of the nurse. Provision 2 of the American Nurses Association (ANA) Code of Ethics (2015) for nurses states, "The nurse's primary commitment is to the patient, whether an individual, family, group, community or population."

> *"A well-defined therapeutic nurse–patient relationship allows the establishment of clear boundaries that provide a safe space in which the patient can explore feelings and treatment issues…The patient's needs are separate from the nurse's needs. Boundaries are constantly at risk of blurring…Two common circumstances in which boundaries are blurred are (1) when the relationship is allowed to slip into a social context and (2) when the nurse's needs (for attention, affection and emotional support) are met at the expense of the patient's needs" (Halter, 2014, p. 134).*

A nurse's commitment to regular self-care practices, including emotional support, are foundational to the maintenance of professional boundaries. See Exercises 1 and 2 for a brief video and brochure from the National Council of State Boards of Nursing (NCSBN; 2014a, 2014b).

? ACTIVE LEARNING

Think about how you will write your answers as you read this chapter.

Consider what it means to share your experience with clients and families. How has this technique worked for you in the past? Has sharing information ever caused a problem for you? Self-disclosure is a communication skill that takes understanding, experience, and purpose.

What?
Write one thing you learned from this chapter.

So What?
How will this affect your nursing practice?

Now What?
How will you implement this new knowledge or skill?

Think About It …

BEHAVIORS THAT CAN BE INDICATIVE OF BOUNDARY VIOLATION

1. Do you spend a disproportionate amount of time with this patient?
2. Do you think you are the "only" staff member that understands and can care for this patient?
3. Do you find yourself taking this patient's side in discussions with family? Does taking sides serve the patient?
4. Do you keep secrets with the patient?
5. Do you find yourself in social conversation, answering personal questions?
6. Could your behavior be seen as "flirtatious?"
7. Do you spend off duty time with this patient?
8. Do you connect on social media with this patient? Take phone calls? See the patient after discharge?
9. Do you think you are immune to boundary violations (NCSBN, 2014a, 2014b; Coltrane & Pugh, 1978)?

SIMPLIFY AND DEEPEN

"Professional boundaries are the space between the nurse's power and the patient's vulnerability."

A Nurse's Guide to Professional Boundaries, 2014a, p. 4

USING SELF-DISCLOSURE APPROPRIATELY

Self-disclosure, a term attributed to Sidney Jourard, is "the act of making yourself manifest, showing yourself so others can perceive you" (Unhjem, Vatne, & Hem, 2018, p. e798). Jourard believed that self-disclosure evokes reciprocity, and disclosure begets disclosure. It is another interpersonal communication behavior that you can use to show your clients and colleagues that you understand them. Self-disclosure can facilitate movement toward a common goal (Grover, 2005). To bring your unique gifts to the creative process of developing a helping relationship is historically referred to as the "therapeutic use of self" (Halter, 2014). Immediacy is a form of self-disclosure that can facilitate the helping relationship. By the end of this chapter, you will understand what is meant by self-disclosure and appreciate how this skill can be used appropriately in your relationships with clients and colleagues.

SELF-DISCLOSURE IN PERSONAL AND PROFESSIONAL RELATIONSHIPS…MAKING THE DISTINCTION

To self-disclose means to open up the self to others. When we self-disclose, we reveal our thoughts and feelings and make some of our personal experiences known to others. Throughout your life you have used self-disclosure to let others know about you in an effort to develop closer relationships.

Self-disclosures can take a number of forms: complaining; boasting; gossiping; expressing political or religious views; and sharing endearments, secrets, or dreams. In social relationships self-disclosures are traded until the partners establish a mutually agreed-on plateau. Intimate relationships are characterized by more private revelations than those shared between superficial acquaintances. The give and take of self-disclosing can occur with or without formal spoken rules. A specific request for deeper closeness or an observed withdrawal of the usual pattern of sharing influences the relationship and readjusts the established level of intimacy.

"Nursing is inherently characterized by the desire to be connected to others at a very basic level of human significance…in milestone events of birth, death, illness, and growth in the lives of those for whom we care" (Drew, 1997). Nurses are moved to offer self-disclosure in which the need for connectedness "transcends theoretical connections. Sharing…for the sake of connection and to give the interaction life, meaning, and depth" (Drew, 1997). An example of useful information to share with a client with a chronic illness and his or her family members is chronic sorrow. A nurse daughter describes it as "a type of lurking presence that periodically engulfs the life of an individual experiencing chronic illness or disability…it is an intermittent, bearable sadness that is interspersed with periods of joy and satisfaction" (Rosenberg, 1998). To understand this experience as distinguished from the acute grief of traumatic injury or the chronic despair accompanying depression can be helpful in listening to clients' shared experiences of lifestyle changes.

MOMENTS OF CONNECTION…
My Mother Had Cancer, Too

"When my mother was terminally ill in a nursing home, I was torn between sympathy for her and embarrassment. As a nurse daughter, I worried that my mother's complaints would lead the staff to isolate her. I wished she could be a 'good, compliant patient,' even though I understood that her behavior was a reaction to fear. A nurse took me aside, put her hand on my arm, and said, 'My mother died of cancer a year ago. Your mother is a lovely lady and we will take good care of her.' That nurse's sharing of her experience helped me to know that she understood my pain and my mother's pain."

Self-Care Nudge
Give yourself permission to cry.

IMMEDIACY IN THE HELPING RELATIONSHIP

Immediacy is defined as direct, mutual talk about the interpersonal relationship in a helping relationship. Although immediacy may require more attention in a client–therapist relationship, paying attention to how well you are relating to a client in service of his or her health may be necessary. When clients contract for therapy with a counselor, they may have interpersonal relationship problems that also surface in the client–therapist relationship. When the therapist recognizes these issues and brings them to the client's attention for validation, the client's examination of the situation may help in skill building with important relationships outside of therapy. Nurses are engaged in mutual problem solving in the service of the client's health, and relationship issues that prevent the client from participating fully in his or her own healthcare and planning may be appropriate topics to be raised by the nurse.

Egan (2013) identified situations in which immediacy might be helpful. The following are appropriate in the nurse–client relationship:

1. *Tension.* When you are feeling tension in the conversation with a client, try saying, "Let's stop a moment so I can determine whether you are comfortable with what we are discussing. It seems to me there is some tension between us."
2. *Trust.* When it seems the client is not trusting in the relationship, try saying, "It seems to me you are hesitating to answer questions we need to discuss. Are you concerned that what you tell me will not be held in confidence?" It is important to note here that the client needs to understand how information shared will be used. If, for example, the client asks if you will promise not to discuss anything about to be revealed, it is important you let the client know that anything that reveals a danger to the client or to others cannot be kept confidential. This kind of question from a client might precede a client's revealing ideas about suicide, which is information that must be shared for his or her safety. Often a client would be relieved to know you are concerned and that help is available.
3. *Diversity.* When there is diversity of culture, age, or gender between you and the client and you sense that this might be impeding progress in your work with the client, try saying, "You have had more life experience than I have; is this getting in the way of my being able to help you?" Or a female nurse with a male client could say, "It seems to me that it is embarrassing for you to talk with a woman about these issues; is that right? This is information we need to discuss for your health and we will get through it the best we can."
4. *Dependency.* When the client is unable to make decisions and wants advice from the nurse, try saying, "It seems you

want me to give you an answer or direction. I can give you information, but the final decision has to be yours."
5. *Attraction.* When the client is attempting to turn a professional relationship into a social relationship, try saying, "It is important that our relationship remain a professional one so you can get the best possible care." If this issue persists or if you find yourself attracted to a client, seek out support and counsel to meet your obligations to keep the relationship professional.

GUIDELINES FOR SELF-DISCLOSING IN THE HELPING RELATIONSHIP

Self-disclosure by nurses is common but controversial (Unhjem et al., 2018). Client–nurse relationships demand special considerations in the use of self-disclosure. A helping relationship is established for the benefit of the client; in other words, this is a client-centered relationship. It follows that anything you reveal about yourself, such as your thoughts, feelings, and experiences, should be revealed for the benefit of your clients. The focus of the relationship is the client. To continue to maintain healthy boundaries, a characteristic of a professional relationship, you must consider the why, what, when, and how of self-disclosing with your clients (Stuart, 2012).

Why Nurses Should Use Self-Disclosure with Clients

Whereas in a social relationship you might self-disclose to allow others to understand you better, the opposite is true in the professional client–nurse relationship. Self-disclosure is a skill that you can use to show clients how much you understand them because of your similar thoughts, feelings, or experiences and to increase their comfort with the interaction.

When inquiring about breast self-examination practices, for example, a nurse might remark, "Sometimes, as busy as I am, I have difficulty remembering if I examined my breasts that month. Do you have trouble remembering?" The client then feels free to agree. This allows the nurse to introduce information about self-examination reminder systems. The intent of a self-disclosure is to be empathic or to show that you really understand your clients because you have walked a similar path. An effective self-disclosure can transmit all the benefits of empathic responses outlined in the previous chapter.

Because self-disclosure is a sharing of your personal self with your clients, it can deepen the bond between you. Although still within the boundaries of a professional helping relationship, your self-disclosure lets your clients know that you are a normal human being and intend to lead the client into an exploration of deeper feelings (Blaszko

Helming, Shields, Avino, & Rosa, 2022). Such therapeutic self-disclosure may promote comfort, honesty, openness, and risk taking by the client but never burdens clients with your problems (Keltner, Schwecke, & Bostrom, 1999). Corbett and Williams (2014) conducted a qualitative study regarding communication between home care nurses and older adult clients in a rural community in Wales. They found that sharing nonclinical information supported a sense of community, provided "social connectivity," and improved the older adults' well-being. They caution that nurses may still need support to distinguish between appropriate and inappropriate disclosure while still having close relationships with patients. Remember to seek support from your manager or other seasoned colleagues when you are unsure about relationship boundaries.

🌿 MOMENTS OF CONNECTION...

Making Meaning Out of Suffering...A Nursing Student's Journey in Use of Self

"A few days ago, in my preceptorship at a cancer center, I had a 19-year-old patient, newly diagnosed with osteosarcoma on her first day as an inpatient. She was to begin chemotherapy that night after a port placement. As a cancer survivor myself, I am very careful to share my story only when I believe it will truly be helpful. This young girl was so afraid, curious, and anxious about what lay ahead. Most of the clients here are older and, as I walked into her room, I immediately felt myself revisiting my own emotions at 16, newly diagnosed with cancer, with a full head of hair, waiting to have my port placed and begin chemotherapy. Not wanting to cross boundaries, I talked with my preceptor about sharing my own experience with my client and her family. She agreed it would be beneficial. I told her I had cancer 5 years earlier and that I was now doing well. I told her I would be there all day and that if she wanted to talk or ask me questions, I would be happy to do that. She asked what it was like when your hair falls out and how it comes back. As I shared my experience, I knew we stood on common ground, something I know is valuable when you have cancer. Her mom told me I had given them hope by sharing my story. I am so thankful to have had this special opportunity."

What Nurses Should Reveal to Clients in Self-Disclosures

As nurses we have to use our judgment about what we reveal to clients. There are two questions to answer before self-disclosing: "Is what I am planning to reveal likely to demonstrate to my clients that I understand them?" and "Do I feel comfortable (safe from repercussions and embarrassment; legally and morally secure) about revealing this information to my clients?"

When you self-disclose, it is important to set up a client-wins/nurse-wins situation. If your client wins, your self-disclosure makes the client feel understood. If you win, you feel good that you have been skillful in making your client feel better. If your client loses, it is because your self-disclosure is irrelevant; thus the client is distracted from the major issue of concern and is left feeling misunderstood. If you lose, it is because your self-disclosure leaves you feeling uncomfortably exposed or embarrassed.

When Nurses Should Use Self-Disclosure with Clients

The purpose of a therapeutic self-disclosure is to let your clients know that they have been understood. When you wish to increase your level of understanding and strengthen that trust and you feel comfortable revealing the content of your self-disclosure, then self-disclosure is the right choice.

Mary Bateson (1994), a noted anthropologist, wrote a book of stories reflecting her experience in many cultures. "Our species thinks in metaphor and learns through stories." Human beings can join and communicate and learn despite profound differences. As we meet people we have never met before in situations we've never faced and as we try to apply communication skills to real people in real crises, we must "improvise responsibly and with love." This "quality of improvisation characterizes more and more lives today, lived in uncertainty, full of the inklings of alternatives." Consider this as you struggle to choose communication techniques: to say just the right thing, to disclose just the right incident and amount of detail, and to be helpful without being self-absorbed. "Rarely is it possible to study all the instructions to a game before beginning to play, or to memorize the manual before turning on the computer... We can carry on the process of learning in everything we do...Ambiguity is the warp of life, not something to be eliminated... [We learn] to savor the vertigo of doing without answers or...making do... [as we face difficult situations]. We are called to join in a dance whose steps must be learned along the way, so it is important to attend and respond. Even in uncertainty, we are responsible for our steps."

I remember my first communication course in a diploma nursing school, taught from a simplistic text. It all seemed so obvious when I was 17 years old. Not until years later did I realize that clear communication takes work, and the skills to achieve it are anything but obvious. Take the skills and tools you read about here and practice as much as you can with a serious intent to learn. Communication is a part of your journey and may cause great pain and joy in your personal and professional life as you learn from experience.

BOX 10.1 Recommendations for the Sharing of Self in Geriatric Practice

- Understand that the connection is dynamic. The client likes and trusts the nurse who shares. The perception of the nurse as a real person aids in establishing the helping relationship. One nurse shared an interest in pottery with the wife of a resident. This topic provided a nonthreatening common ground that established the foundation for the nurse to help the wife cope and grieve.
- Remember that nurses control how much information they want to share. Nurses who use this technique learn how to let the client get to know them without the burden of high levels of intimacy.
- Recognize that the nurse's sharing of self may help decrease the client's level of anxiety and decrease the stress of illness and treatment.
- Although an intuitive sharing of self can be useful, consider the value of self-disclosure as a preplanned intervention chosen with a therapeutic goal in mind.
- Remember that reminiscence is enhanced in elders when they are encouraged to share about specific events. Speak of personal holiday traditions and question clients about theirs.

Modified from Nowak, K. B., & Wandel, J. C. (1998). The sharing of self in geriatric clinical practice: case report and analysis. *Geriatric Nursing, 19*(1), 34.

How to Self-Disclose in the Helping Relationship

To successfully implement a helpful self-disclosure, you need to follow all the guidelines for conveying empathy outlined in the previous chapter. Here is a concise list of those steps:

1. Clear your head of distracting agendas.
2. Remind yourself to focus on the speaker.
3. Attend to your clients' (and colleagues') verbal and nonverbal messages.
4. Ask yourself, "What does this person want me to hear?"
5. Convey empathy, beginning with an empathic response followed by a self-disclosure. It is usually better to self-disclose after you have made an empathic response. Using an empathic response first keeps the focus on others before shifting it to you. Your self-disclosure enhances and augments your empathic reflection. Beginning with an empathic response and following up with a self-disclosure deepens other people's convictions that they have been understood.
6. Check to see if your empathic response and self-disclosure were effective.

In short, use the four following steps for implementing self-disclosure:

1. Listen
2. Reply empathically
3. Self-disclose
4. Check it out

You may find that you begin to see life as a collection of experiences, your own stories and those of others. Listen with the understanding that the experiences of clients, family, or staff members may serve you in the future. These moments can enrich your practice of nursing and your life.

Geriatric clinical practice offers rich opportunities for connections made through self-disclosure (Box 10.1).

EXAMPLES OF HELPFUL SELF-DISCLOSURES

Here you will read a situation with a client and one with a colleague. The helpful response to each includes the four steps for an effective self-disclosure: listen, reply empathically, self-disclose, and check it out.

Situation 1: With a Client

A client, Mrs. Kern, has just relayed the following information to you:

"I was so scared this weekend when I had Jack at home on a pass from the hospital. He started coughing and got all red in the face…and then he bent over with this violent chest pain. I thought he was going to die. Luckily his nitroglycerin was right on the windowsill. As soon as I gave it to him, he calmed down. His pain left within minutes, thank goodness!"

Helpful Response

"I'm thinking you were scared that your husband might have a fatal heart attack when he doubled up with chest pain. It was probably even more frightening because you were home alone. What a relief for you when the nitroglycerin worked. My husband had severe angina, too, and I felt so helpless and desperate when all I could do was wait and see if the medicine worked. Did you feel this way this weekend?"

Situation 2: With a Colleague

Another nursing student, Joan, says the following to you:

"I'm just thrilled! I've had the most wonderful day on the neuro unit where I am doing my practicum. I'd been paying close attention to this young client's pupillary response and blood pressure. I kept checking his vital signs, and I was sure I could detect a rising trend in his blood pressure and some sluggishness in

this pupillary reflex. I decided to point out my observations to the neurosurgeon on rounds. He checked out my concerns and promptly arranged for my client to go to surgery. In the OR they removed a life-threatening hematoma. I felt so pleased that my careful attention helped save his life. Days like this make all the hard work and study worthwhile."

Helpful Response

"No wonder you are ecstatic! Thanks to your vigilance, his life was saved. It was a life and death situation, and your observation and courage to report them made a difference. I had that proud feeling of knowing I made a difference. I discovered a patient having a myocardial infarction. I called a Code and started CPR…and he lived! Isn't it a relief to know you can remember what to do from what we studied and apply it in the real world?"

PROFESSIONAL BOUNDARIES AND PROFESSIONAL INTIMACY

In 2020, Antonytheva, Oudshoorn, & Garnett conducted a concept analysis of professional intimacy in nursing. Here, intimacy refers to the closeness a nurse experiences with a patient relating to physical activities, such as taking a bath, and psychological and spiritual interventions (Antonytheva et al., 2020). The nurse partners with the patient and family on the healing journey. In holistic nursing, we say the nurse co-creates the healing environment with the patient. The nurse's presence becomes part of that environment. We think of the intimacy with the patient and family in oncology and end-of-life care at other times along life's continuum where the nurse may choose to attend a patient's funeral. There is the tension between how much closeness is healthy and supportive and what is a blurred boundary.

You can use the assessment questions at the beginning of the chapter to help you judge and hold the nurse's behavior up to the imperative to put the patient's needs before those of the nurse. Attention to professional boundaries is important in all situations, and yet personal judgment and individual situations will always be necessary. See Exercise 4 in which a clinical situation is presented in which an open discussion with other students/colleagues will examine the variables in what constitutes a healthy extension of self and what is a boundary violation. Remember, too, that some nurses' approach to being professional can cause them to be detached from the patient. As you grow in experience, in questioning yourself what you do to put the patient first, you will become more comfortable with exploring boundaries in the care as you are witness to the joys and suffering of those you serve.

 MOMENTS OF CONNECTION…

Out of Our Struggle, We Offer Others Our Comfort

"Although I have always known my career was in the Lord's hands, it wasn't until the past 10 years that I realized that my own struggles could help me offer comfort to patients in our chronic pain clinic. My spouse had a kidney transplant and bilateral hip replacements. My mother had fibromyalgia and posttraumatic stress and had become depressed and inactive. I recently had a herniated disc and needed two epidural steroid injections. My husband is doing fantastically despite his physical trials. My mother is goal-setting and moving off the couch. I am able to calm anxious patients through my experience of epidurals and surgery. I have made a great recovery both spiritually and physically. Through adversity, comfort and connections can heal."

Return to "Active Learning" at the beginning of the chapter and write your responses.

PRACTICING SELF-DISCLOSURE

Online Video for Skill Building/Discussion: Exercise 1

Watch the 9-minute 2014 video *Professional Boundaries in Nursing* from the NCSBN (2014b) at Professional Boundaries in Nursing | NCSBN. Identify five behaviors of the nurse that may indicate a shift from therapeutic to nontherapeutic relationships. Share lessons learned and applications.

Online Brochure/Skill Building/Discussion: Exercise 2

Appropriate self-disclosure is a part of maintaining professional boundaries. Read *A Nurse's Guide to Professional Boundaries* (NCSBN, 2014a) (a PDF download at ProfessionalBoundaries_Complete.pdf [ncsbn.org]), reflect on what you have learned about professional boundaries, and discuss your questions and experiences with other students or colleagues.

Skill Building/Discussion: Exercise 3

During the next few days, note when people self-disclose to you. Are these self-disclosures relevant, brief, and personal? Are they conveyed to make you feel understood? Note your reactions to these self-disclosures from colleagues, salespeople, teachers, or friends. Consider what characteristics of their self-disclosures led you to feel cared for and what features jarred you and made you question the genuine interest of the self-disclosure.

Ask yourself, too, to whom do you self-disclose your own concerns? Knowing nurses are vulnerable to burnout and that sharing with a trusted person can support you, consider those people you trust with your own challenges and frustrations (Adair, 2017).

After you have done this exercise individually, get together with your classmates and compare your findings about the communication behavior of self-disclosure.

Clinical Judgment: Exercise 4

A student shared an example of what she saw as "caring" by a nurse colleague. As you read her description of the nurse's actions, prepare to fully discuss if the actions of the nurse were caring or were in any way a possible question of professional boundaries:

A. What other information do you need to decide?

B. Do you see any details that make you question if there were boundary issues?

C. What examples can you share from your own life or practice that further develop the discussion of what professional boundaries are?

"I was a new graduate on an oncology unit. I loved my work, but it was very emotional. In orientation, I worked with a nurse with many years of experience who was passionate about this work. You watch patients slowly decline over time. In this case a woman with four children was admitted, the oldest having just graduated high school. At her yearly physical, blood work and scans showed she had stage 4 colon cancer. Her world changed immediately. The oldest child, her only son, arrived at the hospital, at change of shift, upset because he did not understand what was happening to his mother. The nurse stayed with the family for 5 hours after her shift had ended and explained what was occurring physically to the patient and what would happen in the future. She provided much comfort for the family. She was present in the physical and trusting forms. She instilled faith that there could be some treatments that might not cure the cancer but might extend life and make the woman as comfortable as possible. The nurse was truly dedicated to provide kindness to her patients. I was so lucky to be taught by her!"

Creative Expression: Exercise 5

One of the purposes of self-disclosure in the nurse–client relationship is to demonstrate empathy. As you reflect on your own experiences you can distill the lessons learned, which might be useful in self-disclosure in the clinical setting. Select a chronic illness or disease process or other life experience with which you or someone close to you has personal experience. Write a poem to express what you know about the effects. For example:

Arthritis is stiff mornings and achy days
Arthritis is aging before its time
Arthritis is abandoned wedding rings
Single parenting is all the decisions
Single parenting is being the heavy
Single parenting means pizza for Thanksgiving and a movie on Christmas day…

REFERENCES

Adair, C. (2017). Who are you talking to? The important connection between disclosure and well-being: A relational perspective on Healthy Nurse. *The New Mexico Nurse,* Oct, Nov, Dec, 4.

ANA Code of Ethics. (2015). b. Code of Ethics for Nurses | ANA Enterprise (nursingworld.org).

Antonytheva, S., Oudshoorn, A., & Garnett, A. (2020). Professional intimacy in nursing practice: A concept analysis. *Nursing Forum,* 56(1), 151–159. https://doi.org/10.1111/nuf.12506.

Bateson, M. C. (1994). *Peripheral visions: Learning along the way.* New York, NY: HarperCollins.

Blaszko Helming, M. A., Shields, D. A., Avino, K. M., & Rosa, W. E. (2022). *Dossey & Keegan's Holistic Nursing: A handbook for practice* (8th ed.). Burlington, MA: Jones & Bartlett Learning.

Coltrane, F., & Pugh, C. (1978). Danger signals in staff/patient relationships in the therapeutic milieu. *Journal of Psychiatric and Mental Health Services,* 16(6), 34–36.

Corbett, S., & Williams, F. (2014). Striking a professional balance: Interactions between nurses and their older rural patients. *British Journal of Community Nursing,* 19(4), 162.

Drew, N. (1997). Expanding self-awareness through exploration of meaningful experience. *Journal of Holistic Nursing,* 15(4), 406.

Egan, G. (2013). *The skilled helper: A problem-management and opportunity-development approach to helping* (10th ed.). Independence, KY: Cengage Learning.

Grover, S. M. (2005). Shaping effective communication skills and therapeutic relationships at work: The foundation of collaboration. *AAOHN Journal,* 53(4), 177.

Halter, M. J. (2014). *Varcarolis' foundations of psychiatric mental health nursing* (7th ed.). St Louis, MO: Elsevier.

Keltner, N. L., Schwecke, L. H., & Bostrom, C. E. (1999). *Psychiatric nursing.* St. Louis, MO: Mosby.

National Council of State Boards of Nursing (NCSBN). (2014a). Professional boundaries in nursing (brochure). ProfessionalBoundaries_Complete.pdf (ncsbn.org).

National Council of State Boards of Nursing (NCSBN). (2014b). Professional boundaries in nursing (video). Professional Boundaries in Nursing | NCSBN.

Rosenberg, C. J. (1998). Faculty–student mentoring. A father's chronic sorrow: A daughter's perspective. *Journal of Holistic Nursing, 16*(3), 399.

Stuart, G. W. (2012). *Principles and practice of psychiatric nursing* (10th ed.). St. Louis, MO: Mosby.

Unhjem, J. V., Vatne, S., & Hem, M. H. (2018). Transforming nurse-patient relationships—A qualitative study of nurse self-disclosure in mental health care. *Journal of Clinical Nursing, 27*, e798.

11

Being Specific

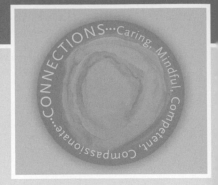

"For it may safely be said, not that the habit of ready and correct observation will by itself make us useful nurses, but that without it we shall be useless with all our devotion."

Florence Nightingale

OBJECTIVES

1. Define specificity.
2. Identify the usefulness of specificity and its effect on communication behavior.
3. Explore an online resource for the use of the SBAR tool.

4. Identify strategies to communicate with specificity.
5. Discuss tips for handoff in nursing change of shift report.
6. Contrast the placebo effect and the nocebo effect.
7. Participate in exercises to build skills in specificity.

RECOGNIZING WHEN SPECIFICITY IS USEFUL

Have you ever been given unclear, nonspecific driving directions and ended up being lost? Details, mileage, landmarks, and a phone number for questions all help. Being specific means being detailed, clear, and concrete. Vagueness can be frustrating, and lack of clarity creates distance between people who are trying to communicate. Miscommunication may cost up to $1.7 billion and 2000 lives, and that is just the beginning. A study published by Controlled Risk Insurance Company (CRICO) Strategies "looked at 30% of malpractice cases in the United States between 2009 and 2013 and found that the most common forms of miscommunication include information around a patient's condition, inadequate amount of informed concern, poor documentation, and unsympathetic response to patient's complaints" (Kern, 2016). The Institute for Healthcare Improvement (IHI, 2017) provides a downloadable brochure on the *The SBAR tool (situation, background, assessment, recommendation)* at SBAR Tool: Situation-Background-Assessment-Recommendation | IHI - Institute for Healthcare Improvement (see Exercises 3 and 4). This frequently used tool provides a framework for specific communication between healthcare professionals.

A lack of specificity contributes to miscommunication. In addition to clarifying our own speech, the technique of specificity assists clients (or colleagues) in moving from broad, elusive areas of discussion to narrower, more pinpointed areas of concern. Assessment of a patient's need for information and level of understanding helps the nurse choose the right amount of detail to include and the appropriate language level to use (Black, 2014).

❓ ACTIVE LEARNING

Think about how you will write your answers as you read this chapter.

What?
Write one thing you learned from this chapter.

So What?
How will this affect your nursing practice?

Now What?
How will you implement this new knowledge or skill?

Think About It …

Using concrete communication is useful in interpersonal situations. Being specific is important when we are doing the following:

- Explaining our thoughts and feelings
- Reflecting others' thoughts and feelings
- Asking questions
- Giving information or feedback
- Evaluating

This list covers situations that nurses repeatedly encounter with clients and colleagues. Being specific or concrete benefits communication in three ways (Arnold & Boggs, 2019; Stuart, 2012):

1. Communicating is more satisfying when we are "on the same wavelength" as those with whom we are communicating.
2. Communicators become clearer about their own thoughts and understand better the thoughts of others.
3. The foundation for problem solving is complete and accurate, which enhances success in communications with clients and colleagues.

BEING SPECIFIC WHEN EXPLAINING YOUR THOUGHTS AND FEELINGS

If you are communicating an emotion, choose words that say exactly what you want to convey. When angry, for example, you might be very angry or irritated. If you tell clients that you are angry with them for being late for their clinic appointments when you are really only mildly irritated, you may create a gulf between you by overstating your case.

When sad, you might feel "blue," depressed, hopeless, or discouraged. If you tell your coworkers that you are merely out of sorts when you are really in despair because your child support check has not arrived and your taxes are due, minimizing your feelings risks diminishing the intimacy and trust between you.

When we are not specific in describing our thoughts and feelings, we invite misunderstanding. Because the purpose of communicating is to build understanding, being indirect or unclear is unproductive.

Saying specifically what makes you feel a certain way clarifies your feelings. For example, you are happy that your client has initiated a reduced-calorie diet and has begun to walk two miles a day. You convey your pleasure by saying the following:

"Mr. Weller, I'm pleased that you are working to improve your health with diet and exercise. I know it can be a challenge, but you will find that you have more energy when you take time for yourself."

Being specific by adding a rationale for your feelings enhances the sincerity of your message. Your explanation has built-in rewards for Mr. Weller. Such a response would make a lot more sense to him than the following:

"That's great, Mr. Weller. Glad to see you are doing well."

Here is another example from the workplace. You are grateful that your colleague on the night shift has highlighted all abnormal laboratory results and displayed them clearly for your review when you arrive for the day shift. You tell her:

"I'm thrilled with this chart you prepared, Jo, and grateful for the time it'll save us on the day shift. Your highlighting will streamline our alerting the physicians and indicate at a glance which patients need temperatures taken or repeat laboratory work. Thank you."

This specific articulation about why you feel grateful adds depth and conviction to your feelings.

Some clients, families, and colleagues prefer logical, rational thinking processes; they are proficient at appreciating and being specific about facts. They may not readily consider feelings or be comfortable dealing with them. Because their strength lies in logical, objective thinking, they may lack the vocabulary to be specific when discussing feelings. Those who prefer thinking over feeling tend to decide things impersonally, are more analytical, and respond more easily to others' thoughts. Nurses, clients, families, and colleagues who prefer to make decisions on the basis of personal feelings and human values are more attuned to others' feelings and likely have more vocabulary and the comfort to talk about feelings. They tend to be more concerned about the human feelings and values in communication than with factual, objective information (Myers & Myers, 1995).

You can learn more about specificity in relation to expressing your thoughts and feelings in Chapter 13.

> **WIT AND WISDOM**
> Be specific and precise about what you want. Some people hold an entire conversation without saying what they want while others can be too blunt. Say what you want and say it in a way that is appropriate for the conversation.
> **Sherrod et al., 2009**

BEING SPECIFIC WHEN REFLECTING OTHERS' THOUGHTS AND FEELINGS

Listening is not a silent pastime. It is active and vocal. Through your warmth and respect, you can show that you are attending to what your clients or colleagues are saying. By being specific, you can convince them that you have heard and understood them.

When you reflect others' thoughts and feelings, you give them a chance to hear what they are really saying. When we respond with clear, concise, detailed statements about others' concerns, it helps the people with problems to clarify them.

For example, one of your clients has given you a lengthy description of her son's epilepsy:

Mrs. Cant: *"I'm so frightened he'll forget to take his medication that I often call the school nurse to check that he's taken it. And when he's late getting home from school, I worry to death that he's lying on a sidewalk somewhere having a seizure. When he plays soccer I'm right there on the sidelines—not so much cheering as praying that all that running won't fire off a seizure. My Lord, will it always be like this?"*

Here is an example of a specific reflection:

Specific response: *"You're wondering if your son will be able to live a normal life, and whether you'll ever be free from worrying about his health and safety."*

You can pinpoint the essence of other people's meanings by being specific when they become engrossed in relating their thoughts and feelings. This tactic helps them grasp more fully both the sense and the significance of what they are saying.

Contrast the clarity of this response with these nonspecific alternatives:

Nonspecific response 1: "You must be very tense, fretting about your son."
   Nonspecific response 2: "It sounds like you spend a lot of time worrying."

Neither of these statements captures the exact meaning that Mrs. Cant was trying to convey. Replying accurately and specifically demonstrates that you fully understand your listener.

BEING SPECIFIC WHEN ASKING QUESTIONS

As an interviewer, at times you might wish purposefully not to be specific so that the interviewee takes the lead. This open-ended strategy generally is used at the beginning of an interview ("How may I be of help to you?" or "What is the pain like?") or at a point in an interview at which you want more information ("Could you tell me more about your family?" or "Could you describe your exercise habits?").

As clinicians, we often want specific information from our clients. To get exactly what we want, we must specifically ask for it. You may wish to know more about a client's family health history, for example. If you ask, "Tell me more about your family's health," you might get everything from "It's fine!" to "Well, let me see, in 1901 my great-grandfather was ill on his sailing venture." A brief response provides you with no information, and a lengthy response requires sifting through to glean the essential details.

Occasionally clients' historical recountings may be jumbled or confused, either because they are unsure of dates and details or because their emotional reactions to their changed health status are interfering with their clarity. When this occurs, it is helpful to stop undirected digressions, backtrack, and reestablish specific points. This process helps clients' thinking to become clearer and more focused.

You likely will need to know specific aspects of your clients' family history such as history of cancer, history of cardiovascular diseases, and so on. Getting to the point and asking for specific information simplifies what you want and increases your chances of getting it from your clients. Using the skill of specificity, you can prevent frustration or fruitlessness in the communication encounter. As nurses, if we fail to achieve clarity, our clients may be left feeling confused and may even doubt our ability to contribute to the interaction. Phrases such as "I'm not sure I understand that," or "Would you go over that again?" let our clients know we are interested and that we need help in understanding what they want us to know (Sundeen, Rankin, & Stuart, 1998).

BEING SPECIFIC WHEN GIVING INFORMATION OR FEEDBACK

As nurses, we are often involved in teaching clients about their treatments, tests, medications, and health behaviors. To provide clients with material that is new to them and to avoid the disrespect of boring them, it is important to focus on the aspects that they particularly want to know. A good general screening question for clients is, "What would you like to know about your treatment (test, medication, diet)?" Posed in an inviting way, this question makes your clients delineate the most important areas for them. Jumping right in with a complete and chronologic explanation wastes time, might be irrelevant, and may even focus on material that is too frightening to them.

The same approach can be used with clients or colleagues who want feedback from you. Clarifying the nature of their request at the outset ensures that your feedback is focused on the area that is important to them.

Imagine, for example, a situation in which a newly hired nurse with 6 months of postgraduate experience asks you for feedback on her performance as a team leader during the past five shifts. At this point you could enthusiastically jump in with praise and advice, but you pause before bombarding her. Instead, you respond to her request for feedback with, "I'd love to comment on your team leadership abilities. What specific areas would you like me to focus on?" This approach allows her to clarify that her abilities to delegate and to handle unforeseen crises are what she wants you to address. Requesting specificity allows you to focus your feedback so that it is helpful to the other person.

 MOMENTS OF CONNECTION...

Never Assume, Clarify!

"I was working with a 16-year-old young man with Hodgkin's disease who had just been told by his doctor that he would be infertile. After the doctor left the room, the look on the man's face told me he was devastated. I asked if he knew what the word 'infertile' meant, and he replied, 'I won't be able to have sex.' I was able to clarify what the term meant and put his mind somewhat at ease. He did well, had a complete remission, and went off to college. We need to be specific in the use of language."

 MOMENTS OF CONNECTION...

To Reduce Anxiety, Provide

Information
"One of my patients had been having extreme pain from postherpetic neuralgia and was not able to sit or lie still at all for about 6 weeks. She was exhausted and scared. I went to see her 4 days in a row to explain how epidurals are done and how they can help to control pain. She said she finally understood, believed it would help, and agreed to have the medication. About 5 minutes after the medication was injected, she fell asleep. When she awoke, she said she had never slept so deeply, hugged me, and thanked me for making a difference in the quality of her life. She received two injections and needed no more."

BEING SPECIFIC WHEN EVALUATING

After you have implemented any nursing action, it is important to evaluate its success. Whether you have led a training session or performed a treatment, it is important to find out if you have accomplished your goals. Your evaluation questions can be phrased specifically. Instead of

asking a vague question such as "How was that?" or "Have you got the hang of it now?," you can phrase your questions to reflect the objectives that necessitated your nursing action.

For example, you could ask your colleague who wants feedback on her team leadership, "Has my feedback on your abilities to delegate and to handle crises been helpful to you?" To the client who wants to know what would be facing him in the week after surgery, you could say, "Did I cover all the points you wanted to know about the recovery phase after your open-heart surgery?" You could ask the first-time father who feels awkward and nervous about bathing his baby, "Has my demonstration on how to bathe your son improved your confidence?" These specifically focused questions assist nurses in evaluating whether they have been helpful. Asking these follow-up questions completes the nursing process.

SIMPLIFY AND DEEPEN
A goal is a dream with a deadline.
Napoleon Hill

PROVIDING SPECIFIC DOCUMENTATION

The use of specificity to collect information from clients needs to be complemented by systematic recording of the data. Clear documentation increases the likelihood that clients will receive the best care. Today, when the courts are holding nurses liable for their own actions, as many as one of four malpractice suits is decided from nursing documentation in clients' charts. Obviously, good care and avoidance of a malpractice suit are two solid reasons for completing the nursing record in a clear and logical manner (Mosby, 2007). Your nursing records should follow the care plans and indicate that the care you provided responded to specific client needs and was appropriate for specific nursing and medical diagnoses. When nursing documentation is written with specific problems and outcomes in mind, the nurses' notes provide a concise, chronologic, factual, and easy-to-audit record of clients' progress (Mosby, 2007). Careful documentation affects the ability of a healthcare agency to be reimbursed for services. Greater precision and detail are being demanded to offer legal protection (Krantz, 1998). There is an old adage, "If it isn't documented, it wasn't done." Although this may not be literally true, an agency's documentation procedures must be followed to ensure a complete representation of the care given and assessments completed. Review the documentation procedures of the organization in which you work to make sure you are being as specific as is required.

Philpott (1985) outlines 22 reasonable and prudent nursing recording policies, practices, and systems. A few of Philpott's key points pertinent to the skill of specificity follow:

- The complexity of the health problems and the level of risk posed by clients themselves, by their condition, or by the use of medical, nursing, or other therapies dictate the detail and frequency of documentation.
- The higher the risk to which a particular client is exposed, the more comprehensive, in depth, and frequent the nursing recordings should be.
- Effective nursing recording is factual, honest, and based on accurate data taken directly from visual, verbal, and/or olfactory cues and palpation.
- Effective recording shuns bias, avoiding tendencies to prejudge or label patients.
- Effective documentation is quantitative, avoiding vague generalizations. For example, with a client who is experiencing a sleeping problem, recordings such as "usual night" or "fair night" offer no useful understanding, waste charting space and nursing time, and may mask a serious problem. Specific documentation such as "slept from 0200 hours to 0300 and states she slept soundly and feels refreshed" provides a clear, accurate, and concise picture of the client's situation; it also enhances credibility for the nurse writer.

SPECIFICITY IN THE HANDOFF

A patient handoff is any time when the responsibility of care is transferred from one member of the healthcare team to another. Miscommunication in the handoff is reported to represent 80% of serious errors in care in part because of communication at the time of handoff (The Joint Commission Center for Transforming Healthcare, 2010).

Work to master handoff skills early in your career. "They will help you set the priorities of the day, learn to summarize your patients' plan of care, and guide communication across disciplines" (Anderson, 2018, p. 56). The research of Rosanne Beuthin, a Canadian nurse, stresses the narrative practice of the handoff: that sharing patients' stories "face-to-face keeps patients safe, keeps us safe, and helps us to cultivate the soul of our nursing practice" (Beuthin, 2015).

In Chapter 6 you read about "the warm handoff," which involved staff, patients, and family in transferring a patient to another facility. A daily occurrence for nurses in a hospital setting is the handoff at change of shift. A study of "best" handoffs revealed four facets: information giving; information seeking; information verifying; and relational communication, conveying trust, warmth, and concern (Streeter & Harrington, 2017; Box 11.1).

BOX 11.1 Handoff Tips for Nursing Change of Shift Report

Best Handoffs

Provide pertinent, accurate, patient information;

Encourage questions and answers;

Encourage checking information for clarity, accuracy;

Create trusting, respectful relationships with a shared goal of quality patient care; and

Occur at the bedside.

Outgoing Nurses

Organize relevant patient information (using unit-based checklists/forms, as required);

Encourage incoming nurses to ask questions, clarify, verify; and

Facilitate positive patient relationship for incoming nurse.

Incoming Nurses

Listen carefully, pay attention;

Take notes;

Ask pertinent questions, clarify, verify;

Offer useful information; and

Are respectful, appreciative, supportive.

Streeter, A. R., & Harrington, N. G. (2017). Nurse handoff communication. *Seminars in Oncology Nursing, 33*(5), 536–543.

Self-Care Nudge

Try the three-good-things (3GT) strategy right now, a promising brief intervention to improve healthcare workers' well-being (Sexton & Adair, 2019). Write three good things that happened to you today. Make this a nightly practice. It's self-soothing to focus on something positive before you go to sleep.

Understanding the Power of the Placebo Effect and the Nocebo Effect

Consider the power of the choice of language in supporting or undermining your client's healing. You may have heard of the *placebo effect,* which is language or expectations of a clinician that positively affect the course of the client's illness by suggestibility. The *nocebo effect* produces negative responses. Both can "influence symptom development, adverse event rate, and treatment efficacy…it is crucial to be aware of these effects to develop strategies for prevention to optimize treatment outcomes" (Kleine-Borgmann & Bingel, 2018, p. 271). Both are "clinical outcomes…not attributable to the actual pharmacologic or physiotherapeutic intervention and are susceptible to attention, expectation, suggestion, and conditioning" (Lang et al., 2005; Schenk, 2008). The nocebo effect can occur when a nurse or other healthcare provider sends a negative message through choice of language, words, or tone of voice.

Patients, especially in situations perceived as life-threatening, are more vulnerable to misunderstandings coming from the following:

Literal interpretations: "We're putting you to sleep now, it'll soon be all over" (before anesthesia).

Emphasizing the negative: "You are a high-risk patient."

Trivializing the patient's concerns: "You don't need to worry" (to a patient after an open-heart coronary artery bypass procedure (Hauser, Hansen, & Enck, 2012).

Examples of language choices include some of the following:

Rather than: "Here's your pill for pain" (suggesting that pain is expected), say "This medicine will help you be more comfortable" (suggesting the medication will increase comfort).

Rather than: "Try not to miss a dose of this medication" (suggesting the client is likely to miss a dose), say "It is important to take this medicine regularly and at the times it is prescribed" (suggesting that the client will comply).

Rather than speculating or carelessly thinking aloud: "Sometimes people have terrible scars from plastic surgery," say "Your surgeon has prescribed a cream you can use to promote healing" (Schenk, 2008).

More extreme examples of careless or just-thinking-out-loud language are actually inflammatory or alarming. A cardiac surgeon, after performing a quadruple coronary bypass, speculated at the client's bedside, "There was one vessel we just couldn't get…we try to do no harm, you know,…but it probably won't make a difference." This was no doubt a conscientious physician who was reviewing the procedure in his mind but was giving the client more information than was needed. Later, this same patient had an initial visit with a new primary physician who commented about the surgery, "Well, bypass surgery is a good thing unless the grafts fail and you bleed out." Perhaps, the physician's comment came from a painful memory of the death of another client, but this client would have been better served to have reinforcement of positive eating habits and regular exercise.

Healthcare providers may be seen as experts by the client who trusts that what they say is to be taken literally. A client, normally anxious in a situation in which personal health is threatened, may be hypervigilant, paying attention to nuances of nonverbal behavior from the healthcare provider. Remember to remain matter of fact when you first see an incision or wound or when the client's symptoms alarm you. A calm approach and appropriate intervention are supportive of the client.

Return to "Active Learning" at the beginning of the chapter and write your responses.

PRACTICING BEING SPECIFIC

Skill Building/Expressive Photography: Exercise 1

Being observant is a skill that can be built into a habit. Consider the famous fictional detective, Sherlock Holmes, who solved cases quickly with his skills of observation and deduction. Konnikova (2013) suggested taking one interesting photo a day. She mentions the 365 project (see https://365project.org). Christine Valters Paintner (2018) called this a photo pilgrimage, a contemplative walk with a camera, with the goal not to take pictures but to "receive the gift of images." We know that mindfulness, slowing down and paying attention, helps us be more present, which can support being observant, which is an essential skill in the practice of nursing. This week take one interesting photo a day, with your smartphone if you use one and share them with classmates. Discuss the experience and how it affected your ability to pay attention and observe.

Skill Building/Specificity in your Personal Life: Exercise 2

"Just the facts, ma'am, just the facts." This is a quote from detective Joe Friday on an old television show called *Dragnet*. A psychiatric nurse consultant was called into a critical care unit to facilitate communication between a nurse manager and a physician. The nurse manager frequently needed to discuss unit issues that needed a response. The physician was busy and wanted brief, specific communication about unit problems. The nurse manager always gave extra details, which led to the physician limiting access to the manager, compromising communication. The consultant suggested the manager use a 3- × 5-in. index card to list a few specific points to be made. Preparing this card helped streamline the issues. Think of a situation in your life where you need to bring up several issues, for example, with a roommate or spouse in which you need to be brief. Using an index card, list a few important points to practice specificity in communication in your personal/work/student life.

Skill Building/Specificity in Your Professional Life, SBAR: Exercise 3

The SBAR tool is a framework for communication between members of the healthcare team about a patient's condition. This tool is used in Exercise 4. Download and review the brochure at SBAR Tool: Situation-Background-

Assessment-Recommendation | IHI - Institute for Healthcare Improvement.

This format is useful when a nurse needs to call a physician at night.

Quality and Safety Education for Nurses Learning Strategy: Exercise 4

When communicating with team members, it is important to be concise, clear, and to the point yet convey critical information accurately and timely. Standardized communication strategies are one way to ensure that you are effectively conveying information. The SBAR technique is widely used to improve safe, team-based communication. Practice SBAR by recalling a recent patient. Record how you would place a call to a physician to request assistance or intervention.

- *Situation:* Describe the situation; what is going on ("I am calling about Mr. Smith, a 45-year-old…").
- *Background:* Describe the clinical background to provide a relevant context ("His blood pressure has been dropping, from 140/90 to…").
- *Assessment:* State the problem of what you think may be going on, your conclusion ("I think he may be…").
- *Recommendation:* State the recommendation or the assistance needed ("I need a physician to check…") (see site for SBAR tool in Exercise 3).

REFERENCES

Anderson, A. (2018). Getting and giving report. *American Journal of Nursing, 118*(6), 56.

Arnold, E., & Boggs, K. U. (2019). *Interpersonal relationships: Professional communication for nurses* (8th ed.). St. Louis, MO: Elsevier.

Beuthin, R. E. (2015). Cultivating a narrative sensibility in nursing practice. *Journal of Holistic Nursing, 33*(1), 98.

Black, B. P. (2014). *Professional nursing: Concepts & challenges.* St. Louis, MO: Elsevier.

Hauser, W., Hansen, E., & Enck, P. (2012). Nocebo phenomena in medicine: Their relevance in everyday clinical practice. *Deutsches Ärzteblatt International, 26*, 109.

Institute for Healthcare Improvement (IHI). (2017). *The SBAR tool (Situation, Background, Assessment, Recommendation), SBAR Tool.* Situation-Background-Assessment-Recommendation | IHI - Institute for Healthcare Improvement.

The Joint Commission Center for Transforming Healthcare. (2010). Facts about hand-off communications. Hand-off Communications | Center for Transforming Healthcare.

Kern, C. (2016). Healthcare miscommunication costs 2000 lives and $1.7 billion. Healthcare Miscommunication Costs 2000 Lives and 17 Billion (healthitoutcomes.com).

Kleine-Borgmann, J., & Bingel, U. (2018). Nocebo effects: Neurobiological mechanisms and strategies for prevention and optimizing treatment. *International Review of Neurobiology, 138*, 271.

Konnikova, M. (2013). *Mastermind: How to think like Sherlock Holmes.* New York, NY: Viking.

Krantz, J. (1998). Taming the new E&M guidelines. *Physicians Management, 38*(3), 41.

Lang, E. V., Hatsiopoulou, O., Koch, T., Berbaum, K., Lutgendorf, S., Kettenmann, E., et al. (2005). Can words hurt? Patient–provider interactions during invasive procedures. *Pain, 114*(1–2), 303.

Mosby. (2007). *Mosby's surefire documentation: How, what, and when nurses need to document.* St. Louis: MO: Mosby.

Myers, I. B., & Myers, P. (1995). *Gifts differing.* Palo Alto, CA: Consulting Psychologists Press.

Paintner, C. V. (2018). *Eyes of the heart: Photography as a Christian contemplative practice.* Notre Dame, IN: Ave Maria Press. Quote in email newsletter from subscription from www.abbeyofthehearts.com, 2018.

Philpott, M. (1985). *Legal liability and the nursing process.* Philadelphia, PA: WB Saunders.

Schenk, P. W. (2008). "Just breathe normally": Word choices that trigger nocebo responses in patients. *American Journal of Nursing, 108*(3), 52.

Sexton, J. B., & Adair, K. (2019). Forty-five good things: A prospective pilot study of the Three Good Things well-being intervention in the USA for healthcare worker emotional exhaustion, depression, work-life balance and happiness. *British Medical Journal Open, 9*, e022695. doi:10.1136/bmjopen-2018-022695.

Sherrod, D., Sherrod, B., & Sherrod, T. (2009). Expand your communication style. *Nursing, 39*(3), 18.

Streeter, A. R., & Harrington, N. G. (2017). Nurse handoff communication. *Seminars in Oncology Nursing, 33*(5), 536–543.

Stuart, G. W. (2012). *Principles and practice of psychiatric nursing* (10th ed.). St. Louis, MO: Mosby.

Sundeen, S. J., Rankin, E. A. D., & Stuart, G. W. (1998). *Nurse–client interaction: Implementing the nursing process* (6th ed.). St. Louis, MO: Mosby.

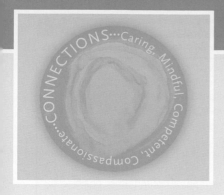

12

Asking Questions

Many of life's treasures remain hidden from us simply because we never search for them. Often we do not ask the proper questions that might lead us to the answer to all our challenges.

English proverb (Andrews, 2011)

OBJECTIVES

1. Discuss the importance of the skill of asking effective questions.
2. Discuss the importance of patients feeling safe to ask questions.
3. Define closed, open, and indirect questions.
4. Identify six points to keep in mind when asking questions.
5. Identify common errors in asking questions and strategies to avoid them.
6. Identify behaviors that support patients asking questions.
7. Participate in exercises to assess and build skills in asking questions.

? ACTIVE LEARNING

Think about how you will write your answers as you read this chapter.

What?
Write one thing you learned from this chapter.

So What?
How will this affect your nursing practice?

Now What?
How will you implement this new knowledge or skill?

Think About It ...

IMPORTANCE OF ASKING QUESTIONS EFFECTIVELY IN NURSING

Questions are important to everyone. Note that a commencement speech given by James Ryan for Harvard's School of Education went viral and became a book with an important question as its title, "Wait, what?", which is a question we might pose when we think we are listening but realize we are not. Another hc lists as one of five most important questions is also important for nursing, "How can I help?" (Ryan, 2017). Stanier, in a book on coaching, identifies seven questions to simplify supporting change (Stanier, 2016). Consider, "What is the real challenge here for you?"

A favorite question I use in mentoring is, What's on your mind?"

The word *question* is derived from the Latin *quaerere* (meaning "to seek"), and this is the very power of good questions. When you take the time to ask questions, you demonstrate interest and respect (Gallagher, 2009). Asking thought-provoking questions can empower clients to think critically about their health and self-care (Nickitas, 2012). Encouraging clients to ask questions supports shared decision making and may improve client satisfaction (Judson, Desky, & Press, 2013).

Wilkenfeld and Campbell (2021) affirm that the nurse's caring relationship with patients supports their comfort with asking important questions, such as when

BOX 12.1   Asking Questions—Closed, Open, and Indirect

Closed questions evoke a simple yes or no answer and may provide little information:
Are you feeling ok? Do you have pain? Have I answered your questions?

Open questions invite details:
Tell me about how you are feeling. What brings you to the emergency room today? How might you use the information we have talked about?

Indirect questions may be more inviting and comfortable:
I would like to know how you are feeling. Can you tell me about what brings you here today? I am wondering if I have answered all your questions.

The more effective you are in asking questions, the more time you save yourself and others, the more pertinent and useful the information you collect, and the more effective your interviewing experience. Effective questioning ensures that you collect the data you need to provide quality nursing care. As you become accustomed to asking questions about nursing practice, you build a foundation for contributing to the profession by posing the questions that stimulate research to support evidence-based practice.

From Knoll, S., & Leifso, G. (2009). Asking questions—Improving practice. *Canadian Operating Nursing Journal, 27*(3), 6.

 MOMENTS OF CONNECTION...

Questions to Help Move beyond the Obvious

"I was working with a 31-year-old woman with myelitis who was in tremendous pain. As I was doing the morning assessment and we were discussing her pain, she began to cry. Upon further exploration, the client revealed that it was not the pain that was her worst concern. With support, she began to tell me about her grandfather, who was dying, and her grandmother, whose cancer was no longer in remission. She was afraid she would never see her grandfather again to be able to tell him what he had meant to her. She touched me deeply because I had had a similar experience. To help her regain some control of her situation, I helped her place a call to her grandfather, and she was able to find closure."

they don't understand an informed con sent form for a procedure. Asking questions effectively is fundamental to nursing assessment and to building the helping relationship (Box 12.1).

For example, if you ask a client if he has chest pain, which is a closed question, you will receive less data than if you ask an open question, "Would you describe your pain to me?"

To open a conversation, you might choose an indirect question such as "I'd like to know what brought you here today." Consider that as you make initial contact with clients, they are performing their own assessments to see if you measure up to their expectations (Sundeen, Rankin, & Stuart, 1998). Illness often makes clients feel vulnerable; they are forced to depend on an unfamiliar person to support them through a frightening life experience. The client needs to trust that the information you seek will be used appropriately and with discernment for promotion of health, dignity, and privacy (Carter, 2009; Matiti & Trorey, 2008). Pay careful attention to building your skills at asking questions, and remember to listen for what is said and what is left unspoken.

From the time your clients enter your care until the completion of your helping relationship, you will be asking them questions. You will ask them about the nature of their concerns so that you can agree on a nursing diagnosis. Finding out what they hope to achieve with the help of your nursing services requires effective questioning. You will discover their preferences for a treatment plan and frequently check with them about its effectiveness. Determining their readiness to take care of their own health concerns after discharge demands that your questioning skills be clear and focused. Remember, too, that helping clients learn how to ask questions of healthcare team members is an essential part of being an active part of their own team.

A study on how clients' communication styles affect physicians' communication concluded that physicians engaged in significantly more client-centered communication when interacting with clients who actively participated in their care by asking questions and providing information (Cegala & Post, 2009).

In your role as a nurse, the main reason for asking questions is to secure data that are essential to providing quality care. Six questions need to be answered to ensure that you obtain the facts you need.

WIT AND WISDOM

R.E.A.L. conversation: Recognize judgments. Express thoughts neutrally. Ask questions. Listen for verbal and nonverbal messages.

John Stoker, 2013

SIX POINTS TO KEEP IN MIND WHEN ASKING QUESTIONS: WHY, WHAT, HOW, WHO, WHEN, AND WHERE OF ASKING QUESTIONS

If obtaining the information you want is important, then it is worthwhile to spend the time planning the strategy that is most likely to secure these facts.

Why to Ask Questions

Before you make any inquiries, you should be sure about why you need the information. Irrelevant questions send the message that you are unfocused (Gallagher, 2009). Questions rooted in personal curiosity may offend your clients. Before you speak, silently answer this question: "How will the information I am seeking direct me in helping my clients?" If you can justify the question, then ask it. If there is any doubt as to whether your clients will understand your reasons for asking, then explain those reasons in advance. Consider the following example.

In your investigations of your client's fall off a ladder, you want to learn about his safety habits in general to determine whether he is in danger of future home accidents. Before asking what might seem to be unrelated, you can clarify your objective by saying something like this:

"I'd like to ask you some questions about your safety precautions with the ladder and about your home safety measures in general. About 80% of accidents occur in the home. My questions might trigger some ideas that could make your home a safer place in which to work and live. Are you agreeable to exploring this area with me?"

Here is another example.

Within the past year, your 79-year-old client has been brought to the emergency department three times after fainting. The cause of the fainting has not been discovered, and your observations about her thinness and lack of energy make you wonder whether inadequate nutrition might be an issue. The following statement can clarify the purpose of your questions:

"We still don't know what is causing your fainting, Mrs. Jones, and we want to investigate every likely source. One possible cause could be a lack of the nutrients essential to keep you going. I'd like to ask you some questions about your diet to determine whether you are getting all you need from the foods you eat. Is that OK with you?"

Both of these examples illustrate how you can prepare your clients for your line of questioning. When clients understand your purpose, they are more likely to be open and reveal information rather than being guarded because they are uneasy about your intentions.

What and How to Ask Questions

What you ask and how you ask it are the next considerations in your strategy. When you have determined why you require the information, then you must plan what to ask to ensure that you are clear in your intentions and know how to phrase your question in a way that invites your client to respond. What you say must be phrased clearly and in a logical progression. Questions should show respect for your clients' privacy and personal information. Any judgments you have about the responses should remain unspoken.

For example, imagine that you require some information about a client's overall activity level and day-to-day schedule to help him fit in his colostomy care. Having explained your purpose and secured his permission, you choose to proceed in a systematic order starting with the following:

"Let's begin with your mornings. Could you outline what you do, hour by hour, on a typical weekday morning, from the time you get up until lunchtime?"

This question outlines for your client exactly what you want to know. He can focus on the mornings, and it is apparent that you will proceed to other times in his weekly schedule.

Consider another example.

You are completing a health history on a client who has just arrived in an outpatient surgical center. He will be receiving an anesthetic, and you need information about his past health status, past illnesses, and family health history. Your facility uses a concise preoperative assessment tool to efficiently obtain this extensive material from clients. Having secured your client's permission, after explaining the purpose of your line of questioning, you proceed with the following:

"As you know, this is a lot of material to cover. To streamline things, I'm going to use this checklist our unit has developed to ensure that we cover everything. Please ask me if there's anything I say that isn't clear to you. Beginning with your childhood, did you ever have diphtheria?…or whooping cough?…or rheumatic fever?"

Explaining your format helps clients accept what might otherwise seem like a barrage of unrelated questions.

Any material that clients provide is of a personal nature, and some areas are more sensitive than others. For some clients, talking about sexual activity or birth control practices may be difficult. For others, talking about personal hygiene or alcohol consumption may be embarrassing. Some clients do not feel comfortable revealing their self-care practices. Others hesitate to reveal family issues or job-related information. You cannot know in advance which topics might be difficult for your clients, so you must keep in mind that any information clients reveal about themselves, their significant others, or their healthcare practices might be sensitive for them.

To help clients feel more comfortable in revealing this information, at the beginning of an interview or as early as possible, reassure them about the confidentiality of your relationship. If you wait until later, you may lose opportunities for uncovering important information.

Confidentiality has a wide range of meanings, and you must be honest and clear with all your clients so that they clearly understand the parameters. Does confidentiality mean that you will not repeat what your clients have said? Does it mean that you will verbally pass the information along to a trustworthy colleague but not put it in writing? Does it mean that you will convey information to team colleagues at client-care conferences? Or does it mean that confidential information will be written on a chart for other team members to read? Exactly what your clients reveal will likely be determined by what you intend to do with the information they contemplate telling you. Sundeen and colleagues (1998) reminded us that clients may feel betrayed if they have been under the impression that client–nurse relationships are confidential and then discover that you have revealed what they consider personal information to another health team member or have written it on their charts.

Another way you can increase your clients' comfort is to treat all areas you discuss respectfully and professionally. Making the effort to ensure that your clients have privacy and the time to respond unhurriedly facilitates their replying openly and fully. Being equally relaxed and straightforward, whether you are discussing sexual matters, family health history, bowel habits, or exercise patterns, contributes to putting your clients at ease. If you show discomfort with any topic by losing eye contact or lowering your voice, for example, your clients get the message that this topic is a sensitive one for you, and they may feel even more embarrassed. To improve your ability to be at ease when asking questions in a variety of areas, you may find rehearsal with colleagues helpful.

Who to Ask Questions

Whom to ask is another important consideration. If your clients are able to speak for themselves, then they are the ones to approach. Occasions may arise, however, when you need information that your clients might not be able to provide. There are times when the observations of significant others can shed light on a client's situation, and this perspective is also valuable to have. For example, if your client has been on a mood-elevating medication, you may wish to have his wife's observations of any changes in addition to your client's sense of the effectiveness of the drug, or on one of your home health visits to a client with multiple sclerosis, you may wish to obtain family members' perspectives on the client's ability to manage at home. Whenever you consult family members or friends, it is courteous and respectful if you do so with the knowledge of and, when possible, in the presence of your client. In some agencies it is the policy to secure written consent from clients before questioning significant others and previous or concurrent healthcare providers. To respect client confidentiality and protect the legality of your actions, it is important that you make yourself aware of such policies.

There are times when clients cannot answer questions. For example, unconscious, aphasic, or psychotic clients are not able to provide information that might be important in their recovery. In these instances, you must do some detective work to discover the essential people from whom to obtain this information.

When and Where to Ask Questions

The physical setup of many hospitals and clinics makes it difficult to secure a completely private place to interview your client. You should make every effort, however, to arrange for a time and place in which you will not be interrupted by telephone calls, noise, other clients, agency activity, or visitors. Arranging such a time and place may require patience because both you and your client have days filled with scheduled and unscheduled activities. It does not usually pay to rush an interview or talk about sensitive issues in an open area. Clients have every right to privacy and a sense of unhurried attention from you.

Keeping in mind these six aspects of asking questions will improve your effectiveness by making you a systematic and sensitive interviewer.

SIMPLIFY AND DEEPEN

Wisdom is a love affair with questions. Knowledge is a love affair with answers.

Julio Olalla (Plews-Ogan, Owens, & May, 2012)

COMMON ERRORS IN ASKING QUESTIONS AND WHAT TO DO ABOUT THEM

Long-Winded Build-Up

In efforts to explain the purpose of our line of questioning to our clients and colleagues, we sometimes go overboard. With a rambling, detailed introduction, we may confuse or bore the other person. The KISS principle is best: Keep It Short and Simple!

Long-winded approach: *"Mr. Haddon, I'd like to ask you some questions about your allergies so that we can eventually work out a lifestyle plan that will allow you to avoid or minimize the stressful reactions you suffer from the various things that irritate you. As you know, repeated allergic reactions can be stressful for the body when it has to constantly fight to return bodily functions to normal. When you are in an allergic reactive state, your body is in the alarm phase and is working overtime trying to return things to normal. When you feel miserable because of the allergies, you also feel tense and anxious and maybe even at times frightened that your allergic reactions will get out of control. It's only when we have all the information that we can help you plan the best ways to avoid your irritants. Shall we begin?"*

Focused approach: *"Mr. Haddon, I'd like to ask you some questions about your allergies so we can eventually work out a lifestyle plan that will allow you to avoid or minimize your stressful reactions to the various things that irritate you. Your chart indicates you have both food and environmental allergies. To begin, could you tell me to which foods you are allergic?"*

Thunder Stealer

It is respectful to give our clients the opportunity to offer their ideas. In our enthusiasm we sometimes jump in with our views and opinions before giving our clients a chance to speak. This can be intimidating and prevent them from expressing their real views. Clients feel hurt or angry when we share our beliefs without listening to their point of view about their own healthcare situation.

Upstaging approach: *"Well, Miss Ricco, together we have agreed on six possible steps you could take to minimize your facial blemishes. I'm interested in knowing what you think of each of these options. I know which I would recommend. Definitely get rid of any oil-based skin care products you have and start using oil-free*

products. Don't you agree that this change would prevent your pores from clogging up? And you likely agree that you should buy the special soap Dr. Best recommended, don't you? I think you should go for our second option, too."*

Considerate approach: *"Well, Miss Ricco, together we have agreed upon six possible steps you could take to minimize your facial blemishes. I'm interested in knowing what you think of each of the options."*

Multiple Choice Mix-Ups

Clients become confused if we ask many questions at once and do not know what information we are looking for or where to begin.

Bombarding approach: *"Mrs. Parker, there are some things we need to know to help you through your labor, delivery, and postpartum stay. Have you discussed what kind of delivery you prefer? Have you and your husband met with your physician and gone over all the options for analgesics or anesthesia during labor? Do you know the various types—general, spinal, perineal block? And next we need to know your plans for breast-feeding. Have you decided on that yet?"*

Clear approach: *"Mrs. Parker, there are some things we need to know to help you through your labor, delivery, and stay afterward. I'd like to review your plans for pain management during labor and for feeding your baby. Are you comfortable enough to go over these two areas now?" You pause to check out her readiness. "First, are you planning to use any type of pain medication during your labor and delivery?"*

Incomprehensible and Cryptic Codes

We become accustomed to medical terminology and develop our own jargon, which can confuse clients.

Confusing approach: *"I've come with your digoxin, Mr. Winters. Before I give it, I need to check out your apical and radial pulses and estimate your edema. Have you had any angina, palpitations, or SOB this morning? We want to prevent chemotoxicity."*

Clear approach: *"Mr. Winters, I've come with your heart medication—digoxin. Before I give it to you, I need to check your heart rate over your heart with my stethoscope and at your wrist. Have you had any chest* pain this morning?" After pausing for an answer, you ask, "Have you noticed any fluttering or fast beating of your heart this morning?" After receiving his answer, you ask, "Have you had any shortness of breath at any time this morning?"

Offensive Misuse of "Why"

Threatening approach: *A client is slamming his pillow against his bed frame: "Why are you doing that, Mr. Kent?"*

A teenager is using his crutches incorrectly: "Why aren't you weight bearing more?"

A diabetic woman is having three toes on her left foot amputated: "Why don't you take better care of your feet?"

An older woman who is widowed is sad: "Why are you letting life slip by you instead of getting back into things?"

Gentle approach: *To the client who is slamming his pillow against his bed frame: "Will you tell me what's wrong, Mr. Kent?"*

To the teenager who is using his crutches incorrectly: "What is it that prevents you from weight bearing more?"

To the diabetic woman who is having three toes on her left foot amputated: "What factors make it difficult for you to take better care of your feet?"

To the widow who is sad: "What are some of the things that keep you sad and prevent you from getting involved in things you used to enjoy?"

These questions invite the client to respond.

Misuse of Open and Closed Questions

Closed approach: *A client has just returned from the radiology department in which he underwent a barium enema, a procedure he was dreading. You ask, "Did your barium enema procedure go OK?"*

This question requires only a yes or no response and does not invite your client to elaborate further about his experience. Here is another example:

In taking an initial health history, you ask your client, "Do you eat a well-balanced diet?"

The yes or no response to this type of question will tell you little about the client's nutritional intake. Here is another example:

Your 63-year-old client is going to be transferred to an extended care facility. You ask, "Are you looking forward to going to Haven's Point?"

This approach gives your client little choice about how to answer.

Open Approach: *A client has just returned from the radiology department in which he underwent a barium enema, a procedure he was dreading. You say, "Tell me how the procedure went for you."*

In taking an initial health history, you ask your client, "What did you eat for breakfast today?"

Your 63-year-old client is going to be transferred to an extended care facility. You ask, "How do you feel about leaving here and going to live at Haven's Point?"

These three examples are open-ended questions that require your client's elaboration. The information obtained by asking these questions provides you with a better understanding of your client's perspective.

Mystery Interview

When we ask questions of our clients, they respond with the belief that, as skilled clinicians, we are sorting, sifting, and analyzing their data to contribute to their nursing care plan. It makes our clients feel connected and respected when we give them feedback on the problem-solving process.

The wrong way would be as follows:

Abrupt approach: *You have been doing an initial health assessment with a client admitted for extreme and rapid weight loss. The time allotted for the interview is over, and you say to your client, "I've got to go now. I'll see you later, and we can continue our interview then."*

Clients feel left out when we end an interview without giving them any indication of our assessment.

Clear approach: *If you must end an interview before you can complete your assessment, you can say something like this: "We've talked about your weight loss problem a fair amount today. To determine all the factors that might be contributing to your weight loss, I need to obtain more information from you at our next interview. Until we meet again this afternoon, could you think about anything you can recall, anything unusual that happened to you at the time you first started losing weight?"*

Even though this closing remark does not offer a definite summary, it does show that you are up to date with your clinical assessment of the problem. Informing clients of what is happening, including your plans and what clients can expect next, provides helpful transitions so that they can map their progress, feel included, and worry less.

Self-Care Nudge

When you are overwhelmed with stress and need a pause, breathe in to a count of four and out to a count of six. Do this several times. Teach it to your patients! Neuroscience teaches us that this elongated outbreath stimulates the parasympathetic nervous system to restore calm. The sympathetic nervous system (initiates the stress response) and the parasympathetic nervous system (restores calm) work like a see-saw, only one can operate at a time. I learned this from reading and watching videos of Rick Hanson, a psychologist and neuroscientist. Watch Daily Challenge - Day 1: Find Calm in Your Body - YouTube (also in Self-Care Exercise in Chapter 1).

CONTINUING TO BUILD YOUR SKILLS IN ASKING QUESTIONS...LESSONS LEARNED

1. End with a question that invites further disclosure. "What other questions should I be asking? Is there anything else that would be helpful for me to know?" (This question is also useful in consumer situations when you are contracting for a service or purchasing a product.)

2. Sometimes *silence is golden.* Take a moment to pause to give yourself and the other person time to think more critically, process information, and remember details lost in an anxious moment. Take a breath to center yourself and communicate your willingness to be responsive to the other's genuine concerns. When you are quiet and the other person is deciding whether to reveal important sensitive information or ask questions that might be troubling, you create sacred space by inviting deeper communication.

If you use the suggestions in this chapter, your question asking will be assertive and responsible. You will respect your right to secure the information you need to complete the nursing process yet maintain the dignity of your clients. Reflect on the questions in Box 12.2, and find your own words to help clients actively participate in their own healing journeys. Remember that clients and families will ask you questions, too. Sometimes you may need to answer the same questions and provide the same answers over and over, especially in times of high anxiety or when you work

---

> **BOX 12.2 Questions to Deepen Healing Relationships**
>
> 1. What can we do to help you?
> 2. Tell me what is on your mind just now.
> 3. You look uncertain. What is that about?
> 4. I might be wrong, but you look like you are worried. What is bothering you?
> 5. What questions do you have for me?
> 6. What do you need to feel better?
> 7. What have you already done to help yourself feel better?
> 8. What have you found helpful to make you feel more comfortable?
> 9. For the nurse working with the terminally ill, consider the need of this client to talk intimately. What do you allow your client to tell you? If someone you know and love was dying, what care would you want for her or him?

with the family of a dying person (American Association of Colleges of Nursing, 2000). You ask questions with respect, and you answer questions with respect.

> **WIT AND WISDOM**
>
> *Notice the word "communion" in communication; the two-way exchange of words, thoughts, energy, and the unspoken.*
>
> **Nance Guilmartin, 2010**

> **WIT AND WISDOM**
>
> *The one question a nurse should ask every patient at the beginning of a shift is, "What is one thing that will make today better for you?"*
>
> **Ani Burr, 2012**

Return to "Active Learning" at the beginning of the chapter and write your responses.

PRACTICING ASKING QUESTIONS

Skill Building/Reflection/Discussion: Exercise 1

What is the one question nurses should ask patients? "What one thing will make today better for you?" Reflect on this question. Take the opportunity to pose this question to several patients. Observe patients' reactions to your posing this question and to your meeting this need. Write a journal entry of your reflection, and discuss your findings with other students or coworkers.

Critical Thinking: Exercise 2

As a nurse working on an orthopedic unit, you are nursing a newly admitted, elderly female client, Mrs. Haley, diagnosed with Alzheimer's disease and a broken left hip. This evening her son and daughter-in-law and her frail, elderly husband with whom she lived before her recent admission, have come to the unit to visit your client. It is your responsibility to determine how your client fell and broke her hip.

Working on your own, choose and write down what your first three questions would be. Be able to defend them by describing the following:

- Why you chose to ask those questions
- What exactly you would ask
- How you would ask the questions
- Whom you would ask
- When you would pose your questions
- Where you would ask your questions

When you have finished writing down your three questions, compare the similarities and differences between your approach and the approaches of your classmates. This exercise focuses on your question-asking and problem-solving skills. What has this exercise taught you about the relationship between question asking and problem solving?

Appreciative Inquiry/Creative Approach to Dementia: Exercise 3

Dementia touches many lives. Appreciative Inquiry is a method of continuous improvement in organizations based on asking questions about strengths rather than weaknesses. It is based on the belief than an organization will grow in the direction of its attention. Read this article, which used the 4Ds of the Appreciative Inquiry approach: the process of Discovery; Dream; Design and Destiny, applied to a case example of a care situation that usually ends with disruption and distress. Write a reflection on your response to this approach to patient care (McCarthy, 2017).

QSEN Learning Strategy: Exercise 4

Reflective practice is the art of constantly asking yourself, "Why did I do what I did?", applying what you know from multiple perspectives, and concluding the best action to take in similar situations in the future. Applied to quality and safety competencies, reflective questioning is the basis for a spirit of inquiry that can improve practice. This constant learning from asking questions about your experience is critical in moving from novice to expert. Focus on these reflective questions in caring for your patients. How can this help focus the questions you ask them?

- *Patient-centered care:* What is the most important thing I can do right now for my patient?
- *Teamwork and collaboration:* Who needs to know the information I have about my patient?
- *Evidence-based practice:* What is the basis for my actions in caring for this patient?
- *Quality improvement:* How can I improve the outcomes of my care from actual to best practice?
- *Safety:* Where are potential safety hazards that could lead to error?
- *Informatics:* How can technology improve how I manage care?

REFERENCES

American Association of Colleges of Nursing. (2000). *City of Hope National Medical Center: The-End-of-Life Nursing Education Consortium (ELNEC) Faculty Guide, Module 9: Preparation and Care for the Time of Death*. Duarte, CA: Medical Center.

Andrews, A. (2011). *The noticer: Sometimes all a person needs is a little perspective*. Nashville, TN: Thomas Nelson.

Burr, A. (2012). *The one question nurses should ask every patient*. Scrubs | The Leading Lifestyle Magazine for the Healthcare Community (scrubsmag.com).

Carter, M. A. (2009). Trust, power, and vulnerability: A discourse on helping in nursing. *Nursing Clinics of North America, 44*(4), 393.

Cegala, D. J., & Post, D. M. (2009). The impact of patients' participation on physicians' patient–centered communication. *Patient Education and Counseling, 77*(2), 202.

Gallagher, R. S. (2009). *How to tell anyone anything: Breakthrough techniques for handling difficult conversations at work*. New York, NY: AMACOM.

Guilmartin, N. (2010). *The power of pause: How to be more effective in a demanding, 24/7 world*. San Francisco, CA: Jossey-Bass.

Judson, T. J., Desky, A. S., & Press, M. J. (2013). Encouraging patients to ask questions. *Journal of the American Medical Association, 309*(22), 2325.

Knoll, S., & Leifso, G. (2009). Asking questions—Improving practice. *Canadian Operating Room Nursing Journal, 27*(3), 6.

Matiti, M. R., & Trorey, G. M. (2008). Patients' expectations of the maintenance of their dignity. *Journal of Clinical Nursing, 17*, 2709.

McCarthy, B. (2017). Appreciative Inquiry: An alternative to behaviour management. *Dementia, 16*(2), 249–253. https://doi.org/10.1177/1471301216634921.

Nickitas, D. (2012). Asking questions and appreciating inquiry: A winning strategy for the nurse educator and professional nurse learner. *Journal of Continuing Education in Nursing, 43*(3), 106.

Plews-Ogan, M., Owens, J., & May, N. (2012). *Choosing Wisdom: Strategies and inspiration for growing through life- changing difficulties*. West Conshohocken, PA: Templeton Press.

Ryan, J. (2017). *Wait, what?: And life's other essential questions*. New York, NY: HarperOne.

Stanier, M. B. (2016). *The coaching habit: Say less, ask more & change the way you lead forever*. Vancouver, BC, Canada: Page Two Publishing.

Stoker, J. (2013). *Overcoming fake talk: How to hold real conversations that create respect, build relationships, and get results*. New York, NY: McGraw-Hill.

Sundeen, S. J., Rankin, E. A. D., & Stuart, G. W. (1998). *Nurse–client interaction: Implementing the nursing process* (6th ed.). St. Louis, MO: Mosby.

Wilkenfeld, D. A., & Campbell, G. (2021). Improving informed consent by enhancing the role of nurses. *Nursing Ethics, 28*(4), 575–584. https://doiorg.esearch.ut.edu/10.1177/0969733020956375.

13

Expressing Opinions

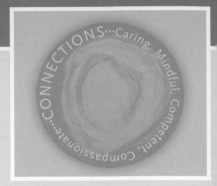

Boldness, without the rules of propriety, becomes insubordination.

Confucius

OBJECTIVES

1. Distinguish between giving advice and expressing opinions.
2. Identify strategies to express opinions in an assertive way.
3. Discuss examples of sharing positive regard for others.
4. Identify the effects on empowerment of expressing opinions.
5. Participate in exercises to build skills in expressing opinions.

INTRODUCTION

When you share your opinion, you are not telling the person what to do, rather, you are sharing the benefit of your point of view. Expressing opinions as a nurse refers to the act of disclosing what you think or feel about healthcare situations affecting your clients or colleagues, including contributions to organizational changes in which every

discipline's voice needs to be heard. In a study of Canadian hospital nurses' roles in interprofessional communication, the distinction between nurse and physician "understanding, practices, and beliefs about care was studied in examining critical incidents." The study concluded, "The value of nurses *embedded in care* work is key to supporting interprofessional team's work during formal goals of care communication" (Strachen, Kryworuchko, Nouvet, Downar, & You, 2018, p. 26). As you read, reflect on what motivates you to express your opinions and what causes hesitation. The assertive communication skills you are learning can support you as role models and change agents for other staff (Yalcin, Baykal, & Turkmen, 2021).

HOW TO DIFFERENTIATE BETWEEN GIVING ADVICE AND EXPRESSING OPINIONS

Expressing opinions or offering recommendations is an assertive behavior. Having confidence in your ability to communicate, or self-efficacy, can help prevent miscommunication, which is a significant threat to the safety of hospitalized clients (Raica, 2009). In a professional setting, your opinions are offered as additional information for clients' and colleagues' problem-solving and decision-making processes. In contrast, giving advice is a unilateral process of solving problems or making decisions for others.

Offering advice prevents clients from becoming independent and gives colleagues the idea that you might think they are incapable of self-direction.

Expressing opinions can be part of providing clients with a fuller picture to make choices about their health and treatment plans. Clients have a moral right to information, and you as a nurse have a duty to provide information. Expressing opinions is not telling others what to do but giving them the benefit of your point of view. It assists clients in their health decision making and avoids both the dependency when clients rely on their nurses and the anger and blame when the nurses' advice is rejected at some point.

WHEN TO EXPRESS YOUR OPINIONS AS A NURSE

Clients and colleagues may seek your nursing counsel when they are at a point at which they must make a decision about any of the following:

Whether to provide or withhold information: For example, clients may wonder whether they should expose information about their condition to a physician or to another family member. Colleagues may be in a quandary about whether to reveal information to clients and/or their families or to colleagues or supervisors. Fellow students may be undecided about whether to confide in their nursing instructors about personal problems.

Whether to comply with a treatment plan or resist it: Some clients may have conflicting doubts and hopes about their health problems and might be unsettled about whether to follow a treatment plan or attempt to survive without it. Fellow nurses may have mixed feelings about adhering to restrictions imposed on tasks they can perform while making a home visit. Student colleagues may face a dilemma about whether to report an honors violation.

Which strategies to implement to achieve the desired outcomes: Clients who know what expected health status they are aiming for may not be able to decide which treatment plan to follow. Colleagues at work may know exactly what outcomes they want but need help in deciding what actions they can take to most likely ensure that they reach their goals. Classmates may be lost about what approach to take to ensure that they receive a high grade on their next assignment.

Your views may be sought by clients or colleagues at any one of these decision points. Your opinions provide others with information that can be incorporated into their decision-making process.

Also, expressing your opinions can help combat burnout. Reflective debriefing sessions, implemented by social workers, were implemented for intensive care nurses to help them combat moral distress with issues such as what they

saw as the provision of nonbeneficial care. These as-needed sessions helped nurses with constructive confrontation of other staff about truth-telling in giving patients and families a prognosis, which is an example of interprofessional collaboration (Browning & Cruz, 2018). As always, we are not alone. We are in this together with many colleagues.

YOUR FEELINGS ABOUT EXPRESSING OPINIONS

Many of us feel differently about opinions we have sought than about viewpoints we did not seek. In our culture in which we place a high value on liberty and the freedom to act as we choose within the limits of the law, many of us likely feel some resentment when others take it on themselves to try to influence us without our consent. We are usually more willing to consider opinions that we have agreed to receive. This knowledge of our nature suggests a principle for expressing opinions: whenever possible, find out if your opinion is wanted. You may have strong opinions about what decision a person should make, but you are wasting your time and may be jeopardizing the relationship if you persist in expressing them without the person's consent.

In response to the previous questions, many of you will have indicated that you expect to be given opinions from someone whose counsel you have sought and that you feel cheated when denied such counsel. When we ask lawyers, physicians, and teachers for their professional opinions, we expect them to provide us with guidance, and so it is with our clients and colleagues who seek our points of view in our professional capacity as nurses. Remember that people sometimes have the right to learn from their own mistakes. It could be possible that your answer is not the best one for them anyway. When others make their own decisions, the blame or the glory is their own.

WIT AND WISDOM
Sometimes not to decide is to decide.

Author Unknown

Here are two more questions about expressing opinions:
1. How do you feel when clients (or friends, family members, or work colleagues) who have asked for your opinion do not act on the views you express?
2. How do you feel when clients (or friends, family members, or work colleagues) incorporate your opinions into their actions?

You may have no strong feelings about whether other people act on your opinions. On the other hand, you may experience pride or relief that others follow your counsel, or you may feel hurt or disappointment when they do not. The strength of your feelings may be related to how much you derive a sense of power or control over other people's actions. Consider to what extent your self-esteem as a nurse depends on your clients or colleagues doing things your way versus knowing you offered them your wisest counsel so that they had adequate information on which to base their decisions.

The degree to which we allow others the freedom to make their own decisions depends on the degree to which we value their autonomy and well-being more than we care that our opinions are revered. As nurses, we must keep in mind what expectations our clients have about seeking opinions and, more important, what agendas we carry around about offering others our viewpoints.

Self-Care Nudge
Keep a list of compliments you receive.

HOW TO EXPRESS YOUR OPINIONS IN AN ASSERTIVE WAY

As a nurse you will be called on to express healthcare opinions in your profession and in life. Because you are an educated, professional nurse, there will be innumerable times when you will be tempted to express opinions to clients, friends, or family about their healthcare. You will feel more confident about handling these situations if you have worked out some principles to follow in expressing opinions. The following section offers some guidelines.

Get the Consent before Expressing Your Opinions
To avoid generating feelings of hostility or resentment in clients, ask if they are interested in hearing your viewpoint. Here are several phrases you can use that can flow naturally into your conversation:

"A former client told me a good way to get around a situation like yours. Would you like to hear that suggestion?"

"I've read an article that had ideas on how to solve your problem. Do you want to hear what it had to say?"

"I have faced difficulties similar to yours. By trial and error, I worked things out. Would you be interested in hearing what worked for me?"

"I've seen others with a problem similar to yours. Would you like to hear what worked for them?"

"I've thought about this, and I have some opinions I'd like to express to the team if you'd like to hear them."

Although you think you may have helpful information, the other person may not necessarily want to hear it. As one friend of a psychiatric nurse once remarked, "If you know of any other developmental crisis I'm about due for, just keep it to yourself!"

Clients or colleagues from whom you are requesting permission to proceed will let you know whether they want to hear your ideas. Those who are verbal and direct will reply with a definite yes or no. Those who are less direct will send you nonverbal signals that will tell you to proceed or refrain from sharing your conclusions. If they look away, change the subject or argue that their situation is unique. Be warned and back off. If they give interested gestures, that is your cue to continue.

Make Allowances for the Uniqueness of Your Client or Colleague
We give opinions based on the knowledge that our ideas have worked in similar situations with like people and circumstances. However, it is impossible for us to know circumstances and personal factors that affect others. We should be tentative about offering our persuasions to show our consideration of others' special circumstances.

Avoiding strong phrases such as "I really think you should…," makes your views more likely to be received as useful in other people's problem-solving processes.

When offering your opinion, to offer others a fair chance to accept or reject your ideas try asking:

"Do you think this idea will help in your situation?"

Include the Rationale for Your Viewpoint
Your clients and colleagues expect you to have opinions about healthcare and work-related or school-related issues. Giving your rationale ensures that sufficient information is available for clients and colleagues to make the final decision.

Here are some phrases that you might use to include your rationale with your opinions to clients:

"In my view, options 2 and 4 would be the most likely to get the results you are looking for. Which options do you favor?"

"If you have the money, I think the clinic in Health-town is the best resource for you. If finances are strained, you might wish to consider one of the self-help groups here in town. What do you think?"

"If I were feeling as desperate as you seem to be, I think I would go for the quick-start option rather than the slower one for now. How does that plan sound to you?"

"I hesitate to suggest plan A because your social supports and family are out of town. Plan B would ensure that you get some regular supervision while you are learning the technique. What do you prefer?"

"In my clinical experience, using the prepared formula works better than the one clients have to mix from scratch. That's my recommendation. Does that help you make a decision?"

"I really don't know which way would be better for you. In my experience, there have been clients who have been happy with both treatment choices. So my advice is to choose the one you like!"

In all these examples the nurse has offered a reason for the preference and turned the final decision back to the client. If we want clients to take charge of their own healthcare, we can offer them our professional opinions yet make it clear that the final responsibility for a choice is theirs.

With your colleagues on the healthcare team, you might include your rationale in the following ways:

"Mrs. Jones is beginning to improve, so I think it would be a mistake for us to transfer her just now. Maybe Mrs. Hanes could be moved first so that Mrs. Jones would have an extra week of physical therapy. What do you think?"

"I think we should ask the instructor to go over the section on neuroanatomy one more time before the examination. It's worth 40%, and she spent only one lecture period on it. What do you think?"

"We have nursing students from two different universities on this unit this month. Even though they are on different shifts, the patients have to answer the same questions over again and have commented about it. Do you see this as a problem?"

"I think we should have a first-year student representative on the faculty curriculum committee in addition to the second-year rep. We need a student there to get our perspective across to the faculty, don't you think?"

"Since you ask, Dr. Kenson, I have been Mr. Jones's nurse for the last week and a half, and I feel strongly that he could be discharged sooner than you are recommending. His condition is stabilized, and the home care nurses could see him daily for his injection and dressing change. He is very anxious to get back to his own surroundings and begin to take up his life again. What do you think?"

These examples demonstrate how to present your opinions assertively and still consider your colleagues'

viewpoints. Giving your opinions does not mean coercing your colleagues into adopting your ideas. Providing a rationale for your point of view and inviting others' opinions makes the decision making a collaborative process.

The decision-making climate set by nurse executives and managers may influence the style of decision making used by staff nurses with their clients. The model of shared governance encourages nurses to participate in running the unit (Watson, 2002). Nurses may be organized as a council to oversee the clinical, administrative, research, and educational areas of nursing practice (Miller, 2002). Nurses who are committed to a mutual problem-solving approach with clients want the same kind of respect and collegiality in the work environment as in a participatory management structure. Nurses can influence how decisions are made by staying alert and assertively making and taking opportunities to express their opinions as another source of information for the workplace decision-making process. Become involved in setting the local, state, and national legislative agenda on issues related to healthcare, nursing, and advocacy for special client populations, such as those who are aging (Watson, 2002). At a time of change in a healthcare system, along with uncertainty comes opportunity. Nurses are positioned to become more involved in health policy and advocacy. Building skills in expressing opinions supports your role in the political arena to articulate issues you believe are important. Nurses who find this arena of nursing rewarding and exhilarating can pursue further education in advocacy and health policy (Stokowski et al., 2010).

Expressing your opinions is also assertive and responsible. It protects your right to have your point of view included in the decision-making process and respects others' rights to know what you are thinking. By including your views, you are ensuring that another piece of information is available to the decision makers.

HOW TO SHARE YOUR POSITIVE REGARD FOR OTHERS

You may notice a particular behavior of a client, family member, or colleague that, in your opinion, is noteworthy. Giving specific positive feedback is another form of expressing your opinions that can demonstrate your assertive communication style. Berent and Evans (1992) gave examples of how to compliment and commend people for their actions:

"You're always willing to help."
"You're always open to new ideas."
"I see improvement in…"
"It took a lot of courage for you to…"

Contribute your opinion of shared good work:

"We've worked hard on this."
"We came up with some good ideas."

In work groups or other successful collaborations, the sharing of humorous positive comments creates energy and goodwill:

"Are we a great team or what?"
"We are so wonderful, I can hardly stand it."
"We want a prize…we did so well."
"Just call us terrific!"

Sharing positive opinions sets the stage for others to feel comfortable in loosening up a bit and sharing their ideas in a friendly, accepting environment. This promotes creativity and teamwork, which is a noninvasive, cost-effective tool! In a climate in which professional and personal change comes at an unprecedented rate, rewarding colleagues with praise or by other methods becomes important.

SIMPLIFY AND DEEPEN

Too often we underestimate the power of a touch, a smile, a kind word, a listening ear, an honest compliment, or the smallest act of caring, all of which have the potential to turn a life around.

Leo F. Buscaglia

HOW TO MASTER THE ART OF NOT EXPRESSING YOUR OPINIONS

Some of us do not need any help expressing our opinions, but rather need an awareness of knowing when not to share and the strength not to be right. When someone tells a story in which the details are not absolutely correct, consider whether the accuracy is crucial. You hear someone say it was "100 degrees" yesterday, but you heard on the weather report that there was "a high of 99 degrees." Is your usual response to correct the person? Consider the results. The correction is experienced as a put-down comment, which does not build relationships. This is a startling concept to some of us. Just give it some thought. Exercise 5 (near the end of this chapter) will help you explore this further.

WIT AND WISDOM

The antidote to extraversion is measured words.

Julia Balzer Riley

HOW TO EMPOWER YOURSELF BY EXPRESSING OPINIONS

At times in your career you may feel powerless in the face of decisions that are made without your input or with which you disagree. You can make a choice about when to share your disagreement even if you see no choice but to comply with the decision. For example, if a new policy is to be implemented that seems unreasonable to you but not unsafe, you can say the following:

"I understand that this new policy is in place. I will comply with it, but I do want to voice my disagreement for the following reasons…I will try it this way and see how it goes, but I'll get back to you with any problems we encounter."

A teenage patient with asthma has chosen to smoke cigarettes. You might say the following:

"John, of course, your choice to smoke is your decision, but I want to express my concern for how this can affect your health. I can tell you more about how that can happen if you are willing to listen, but I can't in good conscience avoid opening up the discussion."

Sometimes just being able to voice your disagreement makes you feel more authentic and more assertive. Assertiveness is a matter of choice and is not necessary or appropriate in every situation. You may have a strong sense of fairness, but if another customer who is obviously belligerent and inebriated cuts in front of you in line at the grocery store, you would probably make a choice not to share your opinion about fairness. This does not mean you are nonassertive but that you have good judgment. You make decisions about what opinions to share, with whom, and when. Some of these decisions are based on unpleasant results from past experiences. Try to remember that everyone has to learn some things the hard way. As you learn when to take appropriate risks to express your opinion and earn the respect of clients and colleagues, you may find that your input is requested because you are viewed as an authentic person who is willing to take a stand.

Return to "Active Learning" at the beginning of the chapter and write your responses.

PRACTICING EXPRESSING OPINIONS

Critical Thinking/Reflection: Exercise 1

In your journal write about a time when you expressed your opinion and were glad you did. Write about a time when you did not share your opinion and regretted it. Reflect on what you learned from these experiences that can apply to your professional life.

Skill Building/Reflection/Discussion: Exercise 2

In your journal write your reflection on these questions, and, if you have the opportunity, compare your reflection with those of classmates.

1. How do you feel when others express their opinions to you without your seeking them?
2. How do you feel when others refrain from giving you their opinions when you have sought their counsel?

Application: Exercise 3

For 1 day, observe opportunities to express your positive opinions of others. Take the plunge and give one compliment that you would ordinarily not share. How did the person respond? Commit yourself to giving one compliment each day for a week and ask one colleague to try the experiment, too. Arrange for a specific time to sit down and share your experiences. This kind of positive energy can do wonders for the profession. Imagine if every nurse gave one compliment each day!

Application: Exercise 4

Practice not sharing your opinion. Do you ever feel the need to correct someone whose facts in your opinion are not accurate? For 1 week, note when this happens. Ask yourself if it is important that you correct the person. If it is not a life-and-death matter, try resisting the impulse to be right. This may well be a stress-reducing activity for you and others—the area of letting it go!

Creative Expression: Exercise 5

What beliefs are important to you? In your journal, use this simple format to create a poem by completing a list, each line starting with "I prefer...." Continue until you have exhausted your ideas. Some of my students comment that this is the first poem they have ever written. It is an empowering expressive arts process that I used in hospice with great success. To deepen the process, try writing to "I believe."
    Sample:

I prefer cats who sit on my lap
I prefer fall with a nip in the air
I prefer short hair to long
I prefer chocolate
I prefer handwritten letters
I prefer quiet conversation with coffee in the morning
I prefer dancing

(Riley, 2012)

Quality and Safety Education for Nurses Learning Strategy: Exercise 6

Improving safety emphasizes shared team leadership and contributions from all team members. Shared decision-making is a key teamwork and collaboration skill identified in the Quality and Safety Education for Nurses (QSEN) competencies. Each person on the team must contribute critical information from the perspective of their discipline to enable the team to make the best, most informed decision. Nurses need to practice the skill of sharing information with all members of the team.

- Patients are active members of the healthcare team. How do you balance sharing your knowledge and education with patients and at the same time provide important feedback with patients?
- Practice sharing key assessment information with another provider by organizing information using SBAR (situation, background, assessment, recommendation) as noted in the QSEN strategy in Chapter 11, Exercise 3 to further develop skills in teamwork and collaboration.
- Care should be based on evidence-based standards. How can you advocate for your patient by sharing with other team members what is important to the patient?
- As a member of a quality improvement project team, how would you share vital information that contributes to the design of quality assessment data?
- Safety depends on each of the team members speaking up about what they see and observe. How would you report what you believe to be an unsafe practice?
- Informatics offers electronic forms of communication. What are vulnerable points to ensure opinions expressed in an email are accurate and conveyed appropriately?

REFERENCES

Berent, I. M., & Evans, R. L. (1992). *The right words: The 350 best things to say to get along with people*. New York, NY: Warner Books.

Browning, E. D., & Cruz, J. S. (2018). Reflective debriefing: A social work intervention addressing moral distress among ICU nurses. *Journal of Social Work in End-of-Life & Palliative Care, 14*(1), 44.

Miller, E. D. (2002). Shared governance and performance improvement: A new opportunity to build trust in a restructured health care system. *Nursing Administration Quarterly, 26*(3), 60.

Raica, D. A. (2009). Effect of action-oriented communication training on nurses' communication self-efficacy. *Med Surg Nursing, 18*(6), 343.

Riley, J. B. (2012). *Art in small spaces: Art at the bedside*. Ellenton. In *FL: CSP*.

Stokowski, L. A., Sansoucie, D. A., McDonald, K. G., Stein, J., Robinson, C., & Lovejoy, A. (2010). Advocacy: It is what we do. *Advances in Neonatal Care, 10*(2), 75.

Strachen, P. H., Kryworuchko, J., Nouvet, E., Downar, J., & You, J. J. (2018). Canadian hospital nurses' roles in communication and decision-making about goals of care: An interpretive description of critical incidents. *Applied Nursing Research, 40*, 26.

Watson, D. S. (2002). The perfect storm (president's message). *Association of Perioperative Registered Nurses Journal, 75*(6), 3.

Yalcin, B., Baykal, U., & Turkmen, E. (2021). Why do nurses choose to stay silent? A qualitative study. *International Journal of Nursing Practice*, e13010. https://doi.org/10.1111/ijn.13010.

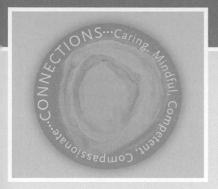

14

CONNECTIONS...Caring, Mindful, Competent, Compassionate...

Using Humor

Life would be tragic if it weren't funny.

Stephen Hawking

OBJECTIVES

1. Define therapeutic humor.
2. Distinguish between positive and negative humor.
3. Identify three criteria for the appropriate use of humor in healthcare.
4. Discuss the functions of humor in healthcare.
5. Identify strategies to implement humor in healthcare.
6. Identify three ways humor can be used to promote positive communication in healthcare.
7. Discuss creative ways to add humor and play to relieve stress, build relationships, and promote creativity.
8. Identify possible health benefits of laughter.
9. Participate in exercises to build skills in the appropriate uses of humor.

⚡ ACTIVE LEARNING

Think about how you will write your answers as you read this chapter.

What?
Write one thing you learned from this chapter.

So What?
How will this affect your nursing practice?

Now What?
How will you implement this new knowledge or skill?

Think About It ...

Self-Care Nudge

Take a breath and smile. When you smile, the brain releases neurochemicals that elevate your mood, calm the nervous system, and decrease pain. Smiling boosts immunity and supports healthy blood sugar and blood pressure.

Thakur & Sharma, 2021

INTRODUCING THERAPEUTIC HUMOR

Stephen Hawking, a theoretical physicist and cosmologist, coped with amyotrophic lateral sclerosis (ALS), or Lou Gehrig's disease, which is a progressive neurodegenerative disease, from an early age, and died at age 76. In a documentary he said, "When I turned 21, my expectations were reduced to zero. It was important that I came to appreciate what I did have…not to become angry, no matter how difficult life is, because you can lose all hope if you can't laugh at yourself and life in general" (Sears, 2018, p. 5). Nurses can use therapeutic humor to help themselves and clients cope with life's challenges. The Association for Applied and Therapeutic Humor (AATH) defined therapeutic humor as "any intervention that promotes health and wellness by stimulating a playful discovery, expression or appreciation of the absurdity of or incongruity of life's situations. This intervention may enhance health or be used as a complementary treatment of illness to facilitate healing or coping whether physical, emotional, cognitive, or spiritual" (AATH, 2000). Humor training with patients with chronic pain showed promise for the introduction of humor to reframe the challenge of chronic pain as part of a multimodal approach. The research reported increased feelings of well-being and resilience (Kugler et al., 2021). A humor therapy intervention, playing a 30-minute humorous CD twice a week for 8 weeks, documented reduced blood pressure in a study of 40 hemodialysis patients (Eshg, Ezzati, Nasiri, & Ghafouri, 2017). In Iran, a humor therapy intervention was found to be an effective nursing intervention in decreasing pain intensity of elders in nursing homes living with chronic pain (Behrouz et al., 2017).

Humor is an important part of human behavior and everyday life, providing the ability to see the amusing side of a difficult situation. Whether it is subtly woven into nursing interactions or used in a more structured way for a specific patient, humor can lead to a more personal, holistic approach, providing comforting and compassionate care (Tremayne, 2014). You don't have to tell jokes or be a comedian to use humor successfully in nursing. Yet one nurse reports that as a nursing student she could improve a child's mood. "I would make goofy faces, sing silly songs, and imitate popular characters…such as Barney" (Starr, 2009). Reflect on your own comfort with humor in the clinical setting as you read this chapter. As we begin to discuss humor, remember that the best advice is to follow the client's lead and to "dip a toe in the water" to see if humor fits the occasion (McGhee, 1998). A literature review of therapeutic reciprocity, "a genuine sharing of thoughts, feelings, and experiences between nurse and patient where mutual learning occurs and shared meanings develop," noted that patients see nurses who use humor as friendly and approachable (Marino, 2017, p. 91). Palliative care nurses use humor to cope with grief-related stressors, although other problem-focused coping strategies also were essential (Nunes, Jose, & Vapelas, 2018). Humor research in health-caring situations involving aging, crisis intervention, and disaster demonstrates similar results (Adamle, Ludwick, Zeller, & Winchell, 2008).

To be able to laugh at a tough situation provides temporary relief from fear and worry. This changes the perception of a stressful event and adds a sense of control such as the power to choose your own attitude or response. A nurse who has experienced the challenges of menopause, for example, may use her own humorous perspective to reframe or alter the view of the situation for her client. Hot flashes become "power surges." This can lead to a discussion of the positive side of the middle years.

Humor can also help nurses build relationships with clients and colleagues. Analysis of observations of client–nurse interactions in a cancer treatment unit demonstrated the importance of social exchange, trust, and humor (Lotzar & Bottorff, 2001). A study of humor between nurse and client and among staff demonstrated that nurse–client humor helped both nurse and client to cope with unpleasant procedures. When studying hospice nurses' coping

strategies, Harris (2013) found three major themes: social support, humor, and prayer/meditation. From observations and interviews in an intensive care unit and a palliative care unit, Canadian researchers concluded that humor promotes positive team relationships and adds a human dimension to support and care given to seriously ill clients and their families (Dean & Major, 2008). Humor does the following (Green, 1994):

- Invites interaction
- Puts others at ease
- Wins affection
- Helps us cope with stress and fear

If you can laugh at your own shortcomings and learn from your mistakes, you are free to be creative. Being creative means taking the risk to fail. Nurse managers who can tolerate personal mistakes create a safe environment in which staff can dare to be innovative. Healthcare staff whose managers use humor effectively and appropriately are viewed as more effective and report higher job satisfaction (Canisius College, 2008). Do you approach patients and colleagues with a smile? A genuine smile builds trust and helps create a smiling culture with colleagues (Thakur & Sharma, 2021).

POSITIVE VERSUS NEGATIVE HUMOR

Distinguishing between positive and negative humor is important. Positive humor, "constructive, empathic humor" (Fry & Salameh, 1987), is associated with love, hope, joy, creativity, or a gentle sense of playfulness. Its intent is to bring people closer together. Negative humor puts people on the defensive and makes them feel put down. It may be sarcastic, racist, sexist, or ageist, and it reinforces negative stereotypes about different cultures, age groups, or conditions. Negative humor isolates you and alienates people.

Reflect on how nurses using humor to cope may reflect negatively on the nursing profession. Dark humor or gallows humor may be shared privately in times of stress in the clinical setting among colleagues. "Nurse" humor on the Internet may not be positive even if it is funny, and it can be "an insidious erosion of nursing's ethical foundations." Consider a meme, "Nurses are like (inserted image of a nurse with her arms raised to the sky)—Thank you, Lord, that annoying family member left," or "Be nice to me…I may be your nurse someday. Just remember that catheters and needles come in sizes that I choose" (Wright, 2017). Before you hit the button to share or send, ask yourself if this is how you want your own work to be judged. "Nurses should resist not perpetuate…" negative humor that demeans patients or nurses (Wright, 2017, p. 44).

Positive humor communicates that the human condition is shared, that we all have problems, and that no one is perfect. The highest form of humor is the ability to laugh at ourselves. Follow this adage: "Take your work seriously, but yourself lightly." One nurse who volunteers as a clown in her hospice work relates an example of humor with an older man whose movements have slowed with his illness. The nurse and the client often joke about this because she admits to being slow in the mornings, too. The nurse gave her client a button that showed a turtle saying, "I may be slow, but I won the race." The client loved the gift and wears it whenever the nurse visits. Positive humor adds to your relationships with clients, families, and colleagues by eliciting cooperation (Box 14.1).

Your response to another person's humor says something about who you are. To reinforce positive humor by laughing and sharing your own humorous perspective, but to refuse to laugh at or participate in demeaning humor by remaining quiet or gently commenting, "I don't think that's funny," is an assertive statement of your belief system. Although it may be difficult to make this type of response to demeaning humor, this is a responsible way to deal with such humor and does not encourage or reinforce put-down humor as does nervous laughter. Recognize, however, that humor serves to relieve tension, and negative humor may be a coping mechanism in tough situations. The medical humor, or gallows humor, that staff use to cope is appropriate when kept among staff because it permits sharing of frustration and promotes group cohesion (Simon, 1988).

BOX 14.1   Get Creative

- Celebrate holidays; decorate your unit or office. One intensive care unit staff hung handmade paper snowflakes from the ceiling at Christmas.
- Wear decorative scrubs when appropriate.
- Enlarge and post cartoons on the ceiling over examining tables or on walls in examining rooms.
- Give stickers to adults and children after a procedure. The stickers given when people donate blood are popular.
- Blow up a glove and draw a funny face on it to make an instant balloon to cheer a child.
- Use crafts. One examining table has crocheted "booties" on the stirrups.
- Wear holiday accessories or a festive pin, earrings, or tie.

Negative humor may serve to relieve tension for the sender of the communication, but it can demean others and undermine your credibility if shared inappropriately. When information about acquired immunodeficiency syndrome (AIDS) first became public, several radio stations aired macabre jokes about the illness, and it was common to hear people repeat these jokes. People often make jokes about subjects that cause anxiety, such as sexuality, relationships, and death. AIDS is one issue that touches all three.

National tragedies, such as the space shuttle disaster, can also be the source of jokes. Humor is often used as a catharsis to provide relief. In a study of such jokes, this humor was found to serve as an "antidote to personal tension and pain" and helped "neutralize the pain of a nation" (Green, 1994).

Humor is listed as an adaptive response to terminal illness by the End-of-Life Nursing Education Consortium curriculum (American Association of Colleges of Nursing and City of Hope National Medical Center, 2000). Joy Ufema (2002), a well-known expert on death and dying, tells us that it is right to provide relief from the seriousness of being terminally ill but advises that you take your cue from the client. She writes of the courage of a woman with leukemia who agreed to be interviewed on *60 Minutes* while they were discussing funeral preparations; the client wondered if she should ask her friend, the church organist, to play. When the interviewer said she was sure that, were their situations reversed, the client would do it for her friend if asked, the client retorted that she did not think she would be asked because she could not play the organ.

Humor is highly individualized. People find different things funny. Pay attention to the subjects of your clients' jokes or humorous comments. This gives you a clue about their topics of concern. If a preoperative patient lightly says, "Well, I won't die from it," it is likely he would benefit from a little extra time to talk about these fears. Be alert for what seems like inappropriate humor in timing or subject. This is a clue that clients or colleagues may benefit from more serious discussion of the issue. Allow your clients the right to hostile or macabre humor, but do not participate in it yourself. To listen without using off-putting body language shows your ability to allow for individual coping responses. To build on this negative humor may create problems. Consider a situation in which you are upset with a relative or close friend. You make negative comments or jokes to relieve tension. If a friend or spouse joins in, you may be offended and state, "It's OK for me to joke about my mother, but not for you to!"

In humor workshops held for clients who test positive for human immunodeficiency virus (HIV), participants suggest that nurses "allow us our own form of humor. We know it is black humor. Don't take offense at it and, please, touch us more; don't act as if you can't wait to get out of the room." Although this may be seen as negative humor by nurses, it is initiated by clients as a way of coping with anxiety. Coping styles vary. What people find funny varies. What is constant is your clients' need to feel that someone understands and accepts them wherever they are along their own journey of coping with illness.

If humor should become offensive, you can change the subject or tell your clients that you appreciate their need to use humor, but that you are embarrassed by it.

> **WIT AND WISDOM**
> *Laughter is the most inexpensive and most effective wonder drug. Laughter is a universal medicine.*
> **Bertrand Russell**

CRITERIA FOR THE APPROPRIATE USE OF HUMOR

Have you heard the adage, "There is a time and place for everything"? Pay attention to timing, receptivity, and content (Leiber, 1986) in the use of intentional humor as an intervention.

Timing: When patients are admitted to an acute care setting such as the emergency department, they and their families want efficient, caring attention and treatment. Humor may be inappropriate unless initiated by patients or family members. You will be able to distinguish between banter among clients and family members to ease tension and the put-down humor or sarcasm that needs intervention. In chronic illness, humor may be a much-needed coping technique. One woman with arthritis refers to her condition as "Old Arthur."

Receptivity: Some people have been raised to believe that humor is frivolous; thus, a humorous intervention would not be appreciated. If you use humor and it offends, apologize and explain that your intentions were to be helpful.

Content: Avoid sexist, racist, or sarcastic humor. Remember, just because someone makes light of an issue such as obesity does not give you permission to joke about these personal issues. Your efforts might be interpreted as ridicule.

Nurse–client relationships may provide occasions for humor that seems less amusing when it is retold and thus taken out of context. Trust your own judgment when relating a story. Observe a colleague whose sense of humor you admire. If you have an idea about how to use humor and you question its appropriateness, check it out with a coworker.

FUNCTIONS OF HUMOR IN HEALTHCARE

Robinson (1990), dubbed the fairy godmother of humor in nursing, examined the functions of humor used in the hospital setting by studying the jokes that were told. She found that humor serves both social and psychological functions.

Social functions include the following:
- *Coping with disruptive acts of hospital custom:* Consider the banter about "air-conditioned" hospital gowns.
- *Establishing relationships:* Clients who are disfigured may have a series of one-liners they use to break the ice when someone seems shocked by their appearance.
- *Coping with social conflict:* One nurse who has good rapport with a physician was surprised by his irritability one day. Realizing that he was having a bad day but was unaware of the effect of his behavior, she retorted, "Dr. Smith, did you have nails for breakfast this morning?" He laughed and apologized.
- *Promoting group solidarity:* Two teams of nurses with separate medication carts competed to dress a stuffed animal attached to their carts with a different costume for every holiday.

Psychological functions include the following:
- *Relief of tension:* One supervisor of a telemetry unit puts on oversized clown sunglasses and strolls down the hall when staff members are irritable.
- *Release of hostility and anger:* A Nerf basketball and hoop or a Koosh ball to toss in the staff lounge is helpful.
- *Denial of reality:* Humor in the operating room that would seem offensive elsewhere helps staff diffuse tension.
- *Coping with disability and death:* Individuals infected with HIV practice their "death rattle" and laugh about it.

From my work with nurses, I find humor works in three ways:
1. *Prevention:* Using humor strategies before a crisis occurs in a work environment makes staff more willing to work together when tension is great. Have a baby picture contest for staff. Provide a candy jar labeled "Grump Beans" for a grumpy day. Get involved in a community project in which people can work together in an informal setting. Organize a community project for colleagues that could be done in conjunction with the traditional Christmas party.
2. *Perception:* Injecting humor into a situation changes the perception that the situation is so terrible that it cannot be handled. Keep a magic wand at the desk. When the pace is hectic, grab the wand and make a promise that the end of the day is in sight!
3. *Perspective:* Humor helps us to keep the big picture in view and not to take ourselves too seriously. Make light of your own idiosyncrasies. Get people to laugh with you (Riley, 2004a).

A qualitative research study of personal health resources in older women demonstrated the use of humor, beauty, and cultural activities as strategies used to maintain physical health and mental well-being. The interviews revealed these women had clear ideas about what helped them feel well even in the face of serious disease. Joking with others helped them cope with low-status jobs, pain, and marital difficulties. The researchers reported that study participants' lifelong experience as caregivers and homemakers provided special information about what can promote health, which is a wisdom that we can tap into when supporting older adults (Forssen, 2007).

Studies have shown that hospitalized children use humor, laughter, and play to deal with stressors that make them feel bad, nervous, or worried; to provide distraction from anxiety and pain; and to reduce fear of injury and chemotherapy. They respond to clowning, jokes and riddles, puppets, games such as peek-a-boo for young children, music, storytelling, and stickers from staff (Dowling, 2002). Jill Sonke, a dancer-in-residence in the Arts in Medicine program at the University of Florida, Gainesville, uses the energy of dance and movement to raise a child's spirits. Helping a child create and fly paper airplanes in his room boosted his morale and his energy. Mary Lisa Kitakis, an artist-in-residence in the same program, brought T-shirts and paint for a child on a bone marrow transplant unit. The child would stand at the window waiting for her to come (Samuels & Lane, 1998). A nurse artist offered touch drawing (Koff-Chapin, 2018) to an 89-year-old hospice client, who exclaimed, "I am having FUN!" A review of the research literature on caring revealed that humor was a part of the emotional care of clients (Watson, 2011).

NURSES AND CLIENTS…USING HUMOR TOGETHER IN HEALTHCARING

Humor can be used in healthcare settings in simple interventions that serve these functions. Pediatric staff on one unit wear customized buttons with teddy bears in addition to formal name pins. A nurse in a heart center wears a button that says, "Speak slowly, I'm a natural blonde." This pin consistently breaks the ice with patients.

When asked how they think humor works in healthcare, nurses reply as follows:
- Humor shows you care.
- Nurses are accepted better when they have a sense of humor.
- Humor shows you your clients' personalities with their defenses down.
- Humor reduces tension and helps you get on with work.
- Humor makes us equals, because we all laugh at the same things.

Clients initiate humor as an important means of self-expression. If humor has been a coping strategy throughout the client's life, then humor is likely to be even more important. Sometimes in the face of serious illness, humor may be the only personal attribute unchanged by disease and the one thing in the client's control. A study of oncology nurses' responses to client-initiated humor demonstrated that nurses were more likely to recognize and respond to spoken humor or inflection, pitch, or manner of speech than to nonverbal behavior (Adamle et al., 2008). When you recognize and respond to a client's humor, you are demonstrating an understanding of the client's perception of the illness experience. Clients using humor expect a response from you even if it is not a humorous retort. Without an acknowledgment, the client may experience embarrassment, withdrawal, or humiliation. This can become a barrier to communication and affect the "physical and psychosocial function and informally damage the trust and confidence in nurses that patients need to subsist during illness" (Adamle et al., 2008).

Clients initiate humor that shows creative coping skills. An 83-year-old woman in a rehabilitation unit of a nursing home, for example, takes great delight in wearing large, colorful earrings. She lives in southern Florida and wears her "resort" jewelry when she goes to physical therapy. Now her therapist has begun wearing wild earrings, and a nurse has gotten in on the act by presenting a pair of earrings to the client to fuel the competition. This same woman has also been given a pair of purple high-top basketball sneakers by her daughter. The client has been asked to wear shoes that help her navigate better in her wheelchair because she has weakness on one side. At the nurse's encouragement, the daughter has glued jewels to the purple sneakers. Her mother is thrilled and calls people to her room to see them. This woman clearly has a rich sense of humor that she has passed on to her daughter. Walking down the hall, you can hear them laughing and talking. The physical therapist and nurse see the use of humor and playful attitude as positive coping strategies in this family and build on them. This strengthens their working relationships and creates an environment in which the patient can talk about serious concerns with people who understand her.

A hospice client using the expressive arts for life review, such as making a legacy, worked with the process of making collages for each of the five decades of his life. He was a social worker who worked with troubled youth. His dream was to be able to share lessons learned from this work. We worked with collage words to summarize concepts in several long articles he had been unable to get published. When we put these words together, they became poems. The following, as a tribute to him, is one of these poems that illustrates his values, which included laughter and whimsy. He died shortly after the completion of his legacy work.

On Dealing with Cancer

Simple solutions?
Be thankful
Do you see emptiness
Or possibilities?
Making peace with the process…
Are you ready?
The moments you live for,
Uncertain,
Living the dream…
No kid was born bad
You're invited
to be delighted
Never give up your dream
Blessings
It's never too late
to learn
something new
Yes, you can!
When opportunity knocks
Make sure you can hear it
Life is a ride
Dare to be extraordinary
Variety is the spice of life
Off the beaten track
Belly laughs
Shades of whimsy
Love in bloom

By Roger Skinner, MSW/LCSW, July 2009;
used with permission and in hope of making
a difference in your life.

HUMOR STRATEGIES

SIMPLIFY AND DEEPEN

The word *silly* comes from the German word *selig,* meaning "blessed." Perhaps there is something sacred in being silly.

Try Gentle Banter

"A light touch may be the right touch" (Green, 1994). Humor provides comic relief from tension and worry. Banter, a playful and friendly exchange of teasing comments, sometimes works and sometimes does not, but it is worth a try when you assess it is appropriate (Bates, 2017). For example:

A client rushing onto a gynecology unit for an early morning admission was greeted by a nurse who said, "Congratulations! You win. You're the first one here."

The client laughed and talked about how "wild" her morning had been trying to get there on time.

A client was wearing a large fabric protective shoe after foot surgery. One nurse said, "I hope you got that in some glamorous way…maybe skiing in Aspen?" The client laughed and shared her story.

A home health nurse reported working with an older couple while giving insulin injections to the wife. They had a running joke about how the client could make healthy food choices at the fast-food restaurant the couple went to each day. When the nurse would leave, she would tell the wife, "No sausage biscuit today, OK?" They shared many good laughs over this. The nurse talked with pride about this couple's mobility well into their 80s. She used humor to try to teach, yet recognized that these trips to the restaurant were the highlight of this couple's days.

Let Humor Take the Lead

To Green (1994), letting humor take the lead is the "art of putting things lightly." Observe what is happening to your clients and see how you can add a light touch. Try using the "good news, bad news" approach.

"The bad news is you have to leave your room for a test. The good news is we can have a fascinating conversation on the way."

Green offers some examples of putting things lightly:

The doctor says, "Well, Mr. Saunders, you'll be able to resume your normal activities soon, but you may not be able to play shortstop for the Detroit Tigers this season."
"This injection will make you feel like a kid again—getting your first bee sting."

Being able to laugh at yourself may provide some great material. Consider all those embarrassing moments that you can use to make a real connection with a client. A hospital chaplain relates the story of another chaplain new to the hospital who was shy about approaching clients for fear of disturbing them. One day, after trying to visit a client several times, the chaplain entered the room, tripped, grabbed onto the curtains to keep from falling, swung widely, and landed face down in the bed beside the client. The chaplain looked up and said, "This certainly is an icebreaker, isn't it?" The client laughed and was able to initiate a conversation about her own discomfort at being in the hospital and how hard it was for her to talk; this was the beginning of a very human relationship!

Look for the Positive

Take the initiative to encourage a positive attitude. Ask your client, "What brings joy to your life?" or "What do you do for fun?" Ask your clients what is going well for them today. Share your own positive moments.

> *"I saw the first rose in my garden today."*
>
> *"My grandson is visiting and watched me shave this morning. His father uses an electric razor, and my grandson asked, 'Grandpa, why do you put whipped cream on your face?'" (Green, 1994).*
>
> *"There was a rainbow after the storm today."*
>
> *"I saw a hot air balloon on my way to work this morning."*

Encourage clients and staff to share their own stories. Listening for clues about your clients' interests suggests positive conversation ideas. Asking about children or grandchildren also may be well received.

COMIC VISION: HUMOR AND PLAY AND CREATIVITY

A humor kit in a colorful basket can be useful to add a light touch. A clown doll that laughs can be used when staff is tense. Wearing a clown nose adds a bit of comic relief. A magic wand might inspire a client in behavior change. Green (1994) shared the story of wearing funny glasses while visiting her father in the hospital. He loved them and used them to greet his physicians. Some hospitals have humor carts or humor rooms equipped with items to pass the time or to get a good laugh.

Being able to keep your perspective and to play with problems can lead to creative solutions. Pink (2005) delineated six skills or abilities to help us thrive in the changing work world in which he says we are moving from the Information Age to the Conceptual Age. Play, cultivating humor and valuing laughter, is one of these six skills. In the Conceptual Age, we will apply "R-directed," right brain thinking to "bring unconventional thought, emotional meaning, and esthetic style to interactions, programs, and product design" (Carlson, 2005). Carlson suggested that nurses have already evolved to the Conceptual Age. Several other skill sets he delineates that inform this conclusion are empathy, caring, and imagining the world as it seems to another. Nurses use story, understanding, communication, and self-knowledge. They create meaning and find spiritual fulfillment in their work (Carlson, 2005; Pink, 2005).

Pink (2005) wrote that play is important in our work and personal lives, manifesting itself in games, humor, and joyfulness. Sixty percent of Americans play video games (Yanev, 2023). Evidence supports that video games enhance the right brain's ability to use pattern recognition in problem solving. The use of such gaming is found in the military and in healthcare. Video games are used for health education (Thompson, 2012) and to treat phobias and anxiety disorders with virtual reality technology.

Play is diversion. Consider the process of studying for an examination or writing a paper. Try building in a plan to take a playful break to clear your mind and make your studying and writing more efficient. A student vowed to study "all weekend" for an anatomy test but found that she wasted time with so much time allowed. When she scheduled a designated time for study with the reward of seeing a movie for a break, she found she returned to study with more efficiency.

Humor is a part of play and taps the right brain's ability to put situations in context, or to see a big picture, and to explore new ways of looking at problems. Humor is a part of the emotional intelligence needed for a whole-mind worker. Humor can help clarify a situation in a team meeting. It can contribute to cohesion, decrease hostility, and improve morale. Brainstorming can often take a silly turn when off-the-wall ideas are introduced and not censoring any ideas can promote creativity. Consider the sticky notes we use for reminders and how they might have been invented. Humor and play help develop your comic vision and the ability to bring perspective and not take oneself so seriously. Box 14.2 provides strategies to develop your comic vision.

Be Creative

Each of us has different talents. Often, we separate our personal selves from our professional selves. Consider people who love and raise animals. One director of a human resource department brought his eight Dalmatian puppies to work one day for a visit. Never has staff from that department been so united in their delight on any one subject! One home health agency was forced to require a family to contain its dog before a home visit because the nurse had once been bitten and was afraid of dogs. The family sent the dog to obedience school and mailed the diploma to the agency. Grateful, the nurse delivered a bone as a graduation present for the dog.

Staff and volunteers who are clowns can share their talents by visiting pediatric or geriatric facilities. Staff who play musical instruments or sing can perform for other staff members on special occasions. Elder Clowns and

BOX 14.2   Strategies to Develop Your Comic Vision

1. Start with yourself. Laugh at yourself. Give yourself permission to be human. If you trip, laugh out loud.
2. Attend funny movies. Rent classic comedy videos.
3. Collect humorous one-liners that are "inside" jokes with your work team.
4. Laugh with others for what they do, at the incongruities in life in which we all share.
5. Pay attention to your own self-talk. Replace negative thoughts with positive ones. Focus on being someone others find pleasant company.
6. Ask yourself, "Does anyone look forward to seeing me walk down the hall toward them?"
7. Share your comic vision to make other people laugh. Laughter is CONTAGIOUS and adds much-needed joy in all our lives.

"Laughter Bosses," staff trained by an Elder Clown, provided humor interventions for geriatric residents in 35 Australian government-accredited residential care facilities, which resulted in staff reporting increased work satisfaction and enthusiasm (Chenoweth et al., 2014).

One hospital has a plant-filled atrium in its central hall. The maintenance staff in plant facilities keep a large rubber lizard among the plants and reposition him frequently. He gets a bow for special occasions. This little bit of humor provides visible relief for people who linger a moment to see something of beauty in a hospital.

To contribute to the morale of staff and clients, consider how you can use your own talents and ideas to add a little joy to your workplace. We embellish our nursing practice with our own gifts (see Box 14.1).

WIT AND WISDOM
There is no question that a playfully light attitude is characteristic of creative individuals.

Mihalyi Csikszentmihalyi

THE HEALING POWER OF LAUGHTER

Think about how good it feels to laugh. Consider a time when you just could not stop laughing, perhaps in a greeting card shop when one card after another evokes more laughter. Gelotology is the study of the physiology of laughter. Dr. William Fry is known for his research in this field and acknowledges that there is evidence of the usefulness of laughter in wellness, but there is much work to be done (Bennet, Zeller,

Rosenberg, & McCann, 2003). These studies suggested that laughter may produce:

- Stimulation of the production of catecholamines and hormones that enhance feelings of well-being and pain tolerance
- Decrease in anxiety
- Increase in cardiac and respiratory rates
- Enhancement of metabolism
- Improvement of muscle tone
- Perception of the relief of stress and tension with increased relaxation, which may last up to 45 minutes following laughter
- Increased numbers of natural killer (NK) cells that fight viral infections and some cancer cells
- Increased T cells (T lymphocytes) that fight infection
- Increased antibody immunoglobulin A (IgA), which fights upper respiratory infections
- Increased gamma interferon, which helps activate the immune system (Riley, 2004b)

Dr. Madan Kataria, a physician in Mumbai, India, created World Laughter Clubs and teaches exercises to create laughter that are practiced regularly by these groups. Dr. Kataria, a yoga teacher, found that laughter and yoga Pranayama exercises produced similar results. There are thousands of these clubs, now called Laughter Yoga clubs, worldwide (Kataria, 2019). Steve Wilson (https://www.worldlaughtertour.com) certifies laughter trainers. Kataria's purpose with these clubs is to help people be more playful and more creative. Research demonstrates that a belief in the benefits of laughter is sufficient for the body to experience positive benefits (Wilkins & Eisenbraun, 2009).

MOMENTS OF CONNECTION...
A Touch of Magic

A nurse received a magic wand at a workshop given by the author. She wrote to tell a story of its use. When visiting a friend who had just had a mastectomy, she took her several gifts, including the magic wand. The friend inquired about the use of the wand and the nurse replied it was so she would always have a nurse when necessary. About this time, the door to the room opened and in came a nurse asking if the client needed anything. The friends looked at each other and burst into laughter. Later, the door opened and another nurse entered asking if the client had called. Now they were true believers. As they talked, the friend was able to share her fears and joked that the surgeon had also taken a few nips and tucks for figure improvement. The wand had been an icebreaker, and laughing together had set the stage for comfort in sharing concerns (Riley, 1999).

HE WHO LAUGHS, LASTS

The first step along the journey is to smile a little, then a little more, then laugh, and then laugh a little more (Feeg, 2002). R. Dale Leichty (1987) delivered an address, "Humor and the Surgeon," in which he concluded:

> *Humor is an innate but fragile part of human life…and this scary world can sometimes erode it. To hold on to this gift of laughter, we must develop two faculties. The first is perspective, knowing that we exist somewhere between the tiniest and the infinite mysteries. Perspective is indeed the secret of philosophy. The second is a humorous outlook…that senses "the world is mad" … but also understands that human vanities and pretenses have made it that way. It tells us, from time to time at least, to stand back and smile or laugh at them.*

Return to "Active Learning" at the beginning of the chapter and write your responses.

PRACTICING USING HUMOR

Reflection: Exercise 1

In your journal, write five things that make you laugh.

Skill Building/Small Group Work: Exercise 2

In a small group, make a group list of 10 things to do just for FUN! Now, contract to do one fun thing within 2 weeks from this day. Complete the following: "By 2 weeks from today, I promise to _____."

Self-Assessment: Exercise 3

Recall an incident in which you were the recipient of negative humor. How did you feel? Identify someone with a rich, positive sense of humor. Describe how you feel when you are with this person.

Observation/Assessment: Exercise 4

In your clinical experiences, begin to look for times when a client may be receptive to humor. Note if the client/family/ visitors use humor and how it is received. Remember to greet clients with a smile. Pay attention to other staff's use of humor with clients and with each other. Remembering the distinctions between negative and positive humor, try using humor and reflect on the experience in your journal.

REFERENCES

Adamle, K. N., Ludwick, R., Zeller, R., & Winchell, J. (2008). Oncology nurses' responses to patient-initiated humor. *Cancer Nursing, 31*(6), E1.

American Association of Colleges of Nursing and City of Hope National Medical Center. (2000). *Module 6, Communication.* In *The-End-of-Life Nursing Education Consortium (ELNEC) faculty guide.* Duarte, CA: Medical Center.

Association for Applied and Therapeutic Humor (AATH). (2000). Official definition of therapeutic humor. *Definitions* (humormatters.com).

Bates, J. (2017). Humor: A bit of banter can lift the spirits—and it's not always annoying, opinion. *Nursing Standard, 32*(7).

Behrouz, S., Mazloom, S. R., Kooshiar, H., Aghebati, N., Asgharipour, N., & Behnam, H. (2017). Instigating the effect of humor therapy on chronic pain in the elderly living in nursing homes in Mashhad. *Iran Evidence Base Care Journal, 7*(2), 27.

Bennet, M. P., Zeller, J. M., Rosenberg, L., & McCann, J. (2003). The effect of mirthful laughter on stress and natural killer cell activity. *Alternative Therapies in Health and Medicine, 9*(2), 38.

Canisius College. (2008). *Laughter is the best medicine. ScienceDaily.*

Carlson, K. (2005). A red hat and a new mind. *Journal of Perianesthesia Nursing, 20*(6), 453.

Chenoweth, L., Low, L., Goodenough, B., Liu, Z., Bordaty, H., Casey, A. N., et al. (2014). Something to SMILE about: Potential benefits to staff from humor therapy with nursing home residents. *Journal of Gerontological Nursing, 40*(2), 47.

Dean, R. A. K., & Major, J. E. (2008). From critical care to comfort care: The sustaining value of humour. *Journal of Clinical Nursing, 17*(8), 1088.

Dowling, J. S. (2002). Humor: A coping strategy for pediatric patients. *Pediatric Nursing, 28*(2), 123.

Dutton, J. (2012). *In the lab with the world's leading laugh scientist. Mental Floss Magazine.* March issue, 2012.

Eshg, Z. M., Ezzati, J., Nasiri, N., & Ghafouri, R. (2017). Effect of humor therapy on blood pressure of patients undergoing hemodialysis. *Journal of Research in Medical and Dental Science, 5*(6), 85.

Feeg, V. D. (2002). Laugh a little—it might help. *Pediatric Nursing, 28*(2), 92.

Forssen, A. S. (2007). Humour, beauty, and culture as personal health resources: Experiences of elderly Swedish women. *Scandinavian Journal of Public Health, 35*(3), 228.

Fry, W. F. Jr., & Salameh, W. A. (Eds.). (1987). *Handbook of humor and psychotherapy: Advances in the clinical use of humor.* Sarasota, FL: Professional Resource Exchange.

Green, L. (1994). *Making sense of humor: How to add joy to your life.* Manchester: CT: Knowledge, Ideas, and Trends.

Harris, L. J. M. (2013). Caring and coping: Exploring how nurses manage workplace stress. *American Journal of Hospice and Palliative Care, 15*(8), 446.

Kataria, M. (2019). *Laughter Breathing Exercises & Its History* from Dr. Kataria (laughteryoga.org).

Koff-Chapin, D. (2018). *The center for touch drawings: Resources for creative awakening.* https://touchdrawing.com/.

Kugler, L., Kuhbandner, C., Gerum, S., Hierl, C., Munster, T., Offereins, B., et al. (2021). Evaluation of a humor training for patients with chronic pain: A randomized trial. *Journal of*

Pain Research, 14, 3121–3133. https://doi.org/10.2147/JPR. S313868.

Leiber, D. B. (1986). Laughter and humor in critical care. *Dimensions in Critical Care Nursing, 5*(3), 162.

Leichty, R. D. (1987). Humor and the surgeon. *Archives of Surgery, 122*(5), 519.

Lotzar, M., & Bottorff, J. L. (2001). An observational study of the development of a nurse–patient relationship. *Clinical Nursing Research, 10*(3), 275.

Marino, M. G. (2017). Therapeutic reciprocity: A concept synthesis. *International Journal of Human Caring, 21*(2), 91.

McGhee, P. (1998). RX: Laughter. *RN, 28*(7), 50.

Nunes, I., Jose, H., & Vapelas, M. L. (2018). Grieving with humor and professional grief in palliative care nurses. *Holistic Nursing Practice, 32*(2), 98.

Pink, D. H. (2005). *A whole new mind: Moving from the information age to the conceptual age.* New York, NY: Riverhead Books.

Riley, J. B. (1999). *From the heart to the hands: Keys to successful healthcaring connections.* Ellicott City, MD: Integrated Management and Publishing Systems.

Riley, J. B. (2004a). *Humor at work.* Ellenton, FL: Constant Source Press.

Riley, J. B. (2004b). Taking life lightly: Humor, the great alternative. In C. Eliopoulos (Ed.). *Invitation to holistic health: A guide to living a balanced life.* Sudbury, MA: Jones & Bartlett Learning.

Robinson, V. M. (1990). *Humor and the health professions.* Thorofare, NJ: Charles B. Slack.

Samuels, M., & Lane, M. R. (1998). *Creative healing: How to heal yourself by tapping your hidden creativity.* San Francisco, CA: Harper San Francisco.

Sears, D. (2018). *Humor opens nursing spaces.* June, July, August: *The Oklahoma Nurse.*

Simon, J. M. (1988). Therapeutic humor: Who's fooling who? *Journal of Psychosocial Nursing and Mental Health Services, 26*(4), 9.

Starr, C. (2009). Lighten up! *American Journal of Nursing, 109*(2), 72AAA.

Tremayne, P. (2014). Using humor to enhance the nurse–patient relationship. *Nursing Standard, 28*(30), 37.

Thakur, K., & Sharma, S. K. (2021). Nurse with smile: Does it make difference in patients' healing? *Industrial Psychiatry, 30*(1), 6–10. doi:10.4103/ipj.ipj_165_20.

Thompson, D. (2012). Designing serious video games for health behavior change: Current status and future directions. *Journal of Diabetes and Science Technology, 6*(4), 807.

Ufema, J. (2002). Communication: Lighten our souls (insights on death and dying column). *Nursing, 32*(4), 28.

Watson, J. (2011). *Nursing: Human science and human care: A theory of nursing.* Sudbury, MA: Jones & Bartlett Learning.

Wilkins, J., & Eisenbraun, A. J. (2009). Humor theories and the physiological benefits of laughter. *Holistic Nursing Practice, 23*(6), 349.

Wright, D. K. (2017). Nursing memes at odd with our values. *Canadian Nurse, 118*(2), 44.

Yanev, V. (2023). Video Game Demographics: Who plays games in 2023, Accessed 2/14/23 at Video Game Demographics – Who Plays Games in 2023? (techjury.net).

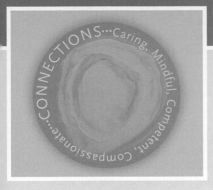

15

Embracing the Spiritual Journey of Healthcaring: Meaning Making

They say you can bear anything if you can tell a story about it.

The Mermaid Chair by Sue M. Kidd (2005)

OBJECTIVES

1. Define spiritual care.
2. Review the personal Spiritual Assessment Tool, and begin to complete it.
3. Examine the Faith and Belief: Importance, Community, and Address in Care (FICA) tool for taking a spiritual history.
4. Discuss themes of spirituality.
5. Discuss strategies to nurture the spirit.
6. Identify nursing interventions to meet the spiritual needs of the client and family.
7. Describe behaviors that the nurse can use to adopt a hopeful perspective and offer hope.
8. Discuss the role of the nurse in helping the client find meaning in illness.
9. Participate in exercises to build skills in meeting spiritual needs in health.

🛈 ACTIVE LEARNING

Think about how you will write your answers as you read this chapter.

What?
Write one thing you learned from this chapter.

So What?
How will this affect your nursing practice?

Now What?
How will you implement this new knowledge or skill?

Think About It …

DEFINITION OF SPIRITUALITY

Studies support that nurses who feel more comfortable with spirituality are better able to provide spiritual care (Cone & Giske, 2016). Spiritual care is an essential part of quality care and is associated with patient satisfaction and improved well-being (Ellington, Bilitteri, Reblin, & Clayton, 2017, p. 517). The American Nurses Association (ANA) defined spiritual care as "the practical expression of presence, guidance, and interventions, individual or communal, to support, nurture, or encourage an individual's or group's ability to achieve wholeness; health; personal, spiritual, and social well-being; integration of body, mind, and spirit and a sense of connection to self, others, and a higher power" (ANA, 2012, pp. 57–58 in Abell, Garrett-Wright, &

Abell, 2018). We value the uniqueness of each person. We understand that spiritual distress can affect the ability to cope as life's challenges threaten one's faith. We reflect on the value of spirituality in our own lives and appreciate the importance of mindfulness, the ability to be fully present in the moment without judgment (Hospice and Palliative Nurses Association [HPNA], 2021; Brooke, 2021).

This chapter invites you to envision nursing practice as coming together with patients in caring and compassion ("taking off our shoes") and standing on holy ground (O'Brien, 2021). Remember that, although it is life and clinical experience with spirituality that affect a nurse's skills and comfort with spiritual care, educating yourself helps you assess spiritual needs and feel comfortable with such conversations (Cone & Giske, 2016).

The word *spirituality* comes from a Latin word meaning "breath of life" (Brillhart, 2005). Spirituality in practice is "to demonstrate a unique capacity for love, joy, caring, compassion, and for finding meaning in life's difficult experience." Nurses' spiritual interventions "reflect the human traits of caring, love, honesty, wisdom, and imagination… a belief in a higher power, higher existence, or a guiding spirit…something outside the self and beyond the individual nurse or patient" (Dossey, 1998b). Spirituality includes "unconditional love, trust, forgiveness, hope, and imagination…a sense of awe and wonder regarding life" (Brillhart, 2005). The use of a spiritually based complementary group intervention with US combat veterans experiencing symptoms of posttraumatic stress disorder (PTSD) from the wars in Iraq and Afghanistan showed promising results (Bormann, Thorp, Wetherill, & Golshan, 2008).

> *Spirituality is good science… More than 250 studies now show that religious practice—the specific religion doesn't seem to matter—is correlated with greater health and increased longevity…some say that clinicians have no business taking on the role of spiritual guide…but we are not being asked to become spiritual counselors. We're being asked to integrate a holistic approach and extend love, compassion, and empathy…the bedrock upon which nursing has always rested (Dossey, 1998a).*

Harold Koenig, M.D., at Duke University's Center for the Study of Religion/Spirituality and Health reported on the results of more than 70 data-based, peer-reviewed published papers. Findings showed that people who attend religious services on a regular basis have better health outcomes, have stronger immune systems, have lower stress, and recover from hip fractures and open-heart surgeries more quickly than do less religious people. Older adults with religious faith seem to be better protected from cardiovascular

disease and cancer (Koenig, 1999). Spirituality has been shown to be an important variable in quality of life in persons living with human immunodeficiency virus infection (Tuck, McCain, & Elswick, Jr., 2001). In a study of persons with spinal cord injury, life satisfaction increased as spirituality increased (Brillhart, 2005). Exploring meaning in life and prayer has been associated with increased psychological well-being in breast cancer survivors (Meraviglia, 2006). Spirituality has been part of the vision of nursing since the time of Florence Nightingale (Calabria & Macrae, 1994). From his continued review of the literature and research, Koenig (2007) concluded: "Addressing spiritual issues in clinical practice can bring back life into our profession and, for many of our patients, can help them regain their lives by finding hope, meaning, and healing." The goal of practicing spiritually sensitive care is to support clients in the search for meaning and solace without injecting our own opinions or values (Lackey, 2009).

Erickson, Tomlin, and Swain (2010) believed that human beings are holistic with multiple interacting subsystems. "Permeating all subsystems are the inherent bases… which include the genetic and spiritual drive." Our "spiritual drive starts before our biophysical existence, continues through our lifetime, and culminates during transformation. It is always present, and pervades our subsystems even though we may not be consciously aware of it. It inspires us to search for our Life Purpose" (Erickson, 2006). As nurses, every interaction we share with our clients allows us to nurture and facilitate the client's spiritual essence and drive. Through this sharing of experiences, moments, and events, the nurse and client journey together to gain a better understanding of spirituality and to work toward their life purpose or reason for being (Erickson, 2006).

It is this spiritual connection that is the essence of being present with clients in moments of tragedy in which the seeds of personal triumph are planted. This discussion is not based on religious denomination but on the spiritual path to finding personal meaning and to helping the patient and family find meaning in illness and suffering (Travelbee, 1970).

BEGINNING YOUR JOURNEY OF SPIRITUAL CARE

Where can you begin? Ellington and colleagues (2017) suggested communication strategies for oncology nurses that can support the new nurse: working on our own spiritual awareness, initiating spiritual communication, and taking a spiritual history.

Take time now to begin your own spiritual assessment using Box 15.1. Review it and begin to answer the questions. Use this tool to continue to reflect on your own views

BOX 15.1   Spiritual Assessment Tool

The following reflective questions may assist you in assessing, evaluating, and increasing your awareness of spirituality in yourself and others.

Meaning and Purpose

These questions assess a person's ability to seek meaning and fulfillment in life, manifest hope, and accept ambiguity and uncertainty:

- What gives your life meaning?
- Do you have a sense of purpose in life?
- Does your illness interfere with your life goals?
- Why do you want to get well?
- How hopeful are you about obtaining a better degree of health?
- Do you feel that you have a responsibility in maintaining your health?
- Will you be able to make changes in your life to maintain your health?
- Are you motivated to get well?
- What is the most important or powerful thing in your life?

Inner Strengths

These questions assess a person's ability to manifest joy and recognize strengths, choices, goals, and faith:

- What brings you joy and peace in your life?
- What can you do to feel alive and full of spirit?
- What traits do you like about yourself?
- What are your personal strengths?
- What choices are available to you to enhance your healing?
- What life goals have you set for yourself?
- Do you think that stress in any way caused your illness?
- How aware were you of your body before you became sick?
- What do you believe in?
- Is faith important in your life?
- How has your illness influenced your faith?
- Does faith play a role in recognizing your health?

Interconnections

These questions assess a person's positive self-concept, self-esteem, and sense of self; sense of belonging in the world with others; capacity to pursue personal interests; and ability to demonstrate love of self and self-forgiveness:

- How do you feel about yourself right now?
- How do you feel when you have a true sense of yourself?
- Do you pursue things of personal interest?
- What do you do to show love for yourself?
- Can you forgive yourself?
- What do you do to heal your spirit?

These questions assess a person's ability to connect in life-giving ways with family, friends, and social groups and to engage in the forgiveness of others:

- Who are the significant people in your life?
- Do you have friends or family in town who are available to help you?
- Who are the people to whom you are closest?
- Do you belong to any groups?
- Can you ask people for help when you need it?
- Can you share your feelings with others?
- What are some of the most loving things that others have done for you?
- What are the loving things that you do for other people?
- Are you able to forgive others?

These questions assess a person's capacity for finding meaning in worship or religious activities, and a connectedness with a divinity:

- Is worship important to you?
- What do you consider the most significant act of worship in your life?
- Do you participate in any religious activities?
- Do you believe in God or a higher power?
- Do you think that prayer is powerful?
- Have you ever tried to empty your mind of all thoughts to see what the experience might be?
- Do you use relaxation or imagery skills?
- Do you meditate?
- Do you pray?
- What is your prayer?
- How are your prayers answered?
- Do you have a sense of belonging in this world?

These questions assess a person's ability to experience a sense of connection with life and nature, an awareness of the effects of the environment on life and well-being, and a capacity or concern for the health of the environment:

- Do you ever feel a connection with the world or universe?
- How does your environment affect your state of well-being?
- What are your environmental stressors at work and at home?
- What strategies reduce your environmental stressors?
- Do you have any concerns for the state of your immediate environment?
- Are you involved with environmental issues such as recycling environmental resources at home, at work, or in your community?
- Are you concerned about the survival of the planet?

From Dossey, B. M. (1998). Holistic modalities & healing moments. *American Journal of Nursing, 98*(6), 44–47.
Sources: Burkhardt, M. A. (1989). Spirituality: An analysis of the concept. *Holistic Nursing Practice, 3*(3), 69; Dossey, B. M., & Keegan, L. (Eds.). (1995). *Holistic nursing: A handbook for practice* (2nd ed.). Gaithersburg, MD: Aspen Publishers.

of spirituality to increase your comfort level with conversations with clients (Booth & Kaylor, 2018).

Initiating conversations about spiritual concerns is supported by the skills you have studied such as caring, warmth, being genuine, being present, and listening. With respect for diverse backgrounds, the nurse is open to the client's views and does not seek to impose personal beliefs. A question that can provide information about the whole person is "What do I need to know about you as a person to give you the best care possible?" This is the Patient Dignity Question (PDQ) (Chochinov, McClement, Thompson, Dufault, & Harlos, 2015, p. 972).

Taking a spiritual history supports your deepening conversation and spiritual care. See Box 15.2 and the section that follows.

FAITH AND BELIEF: IMPORTANCE, COMMUNITY, AND ADDRESS IN CARE: TAKING A SPIRITUAL HISTORY

A documented spiritual history is mandated by The Joint Commission (TJC) for clients who are admitted for care

in an acute care hospital or nursing home and those seen through a home health agency (Koenig, 2007). Beginning this conversation opens a dialogue about spiritual issues and gives the client permission to talk about spirituality with you (Koenig, 2007).

The acronym *FICA* stands for Faith and Belief: Importance, Community, and Address in Care, which is a tool developed by Christina M. Puchalski, M.D., founder and director of the George Washington Institute for Spirituality and Health. This brief tool is a good way to begin to incorporate spiritual assessment in your work. Before beginning this history taking, it is helpful to explain why you are asking these questions. Clients may find the conversation anxiety producing because they expect it might mean that they are facing a terminal diagnosis. Simply let the client know that the questions you will be asking will allow you to be more sensitive to any spiritual needs a client may have.

The Essence of the Spiritual History

A single question concerning spiritual history can be "Do you have any spiritual needs or concerns related to your health?" Sometimes the initiation of even this short history is met with the response that the client has no interest in religion or spirituality and does not use these for coping with illness. At this point, you can take a different tack and ask about other ways the client is coping: what gives meaning and purpose in the face of illness, what social supports are useful, and what cultural beliefs may influence the treatment of illness. This gets at the essence of the spiritual history (Koenig, 2007).

Knowing that in times of crisis clients may feel at a loss for coping strategies, ask if the client has ever been in a similar situation and, if so, what was helpful then; for example, "What has been a source of strength for you?" and "Who has been helpful to talk to in the past?" Such questions may stimulate problem solving about what might be helpful at this time.

THEMES OF SPIRITUALITY

Nagai-Jacobson and Burkhardt (1989) review general themes that emerge in the literature that broaden the concept of spirituality. They found that spirituality has the following characteristics:
- It is a broader concept than religion.
- It involves a personal quest for meaning and purpose in life.
- It relates to the inner essence of a person.
- It is a sense of harmonious interconnectedness with self, others, nature, and an Ultimate Other.
- It is the integrating factor of the human person.

Discussions of spirituality in nursing suggest that interactions between nurses and their clients involve the spirituality of both and that this relationship can transform them all in the search for a meaning in life. The nature of such client–nurse relationships is sacred. It is a walk on holy ground as two people meet at what Newman (1989) called *choice points* presented by health crises. These choice points or events are "opportunities to experience more fully the reality of the patterns of our lives." These are times when former ways of coping and relating to life no longer work. When a person is confronted with disability, new ways of existing, of behaving, and of finding meaning are necessary. A woman whose husband was experiencing the deterioration of Alzheimer's disease, for example, found her own health affected by the strain of being a caregiver. Unable to drive or visit with friends, she befriended a wild, stray cat who was reluctant to make physical contact. Over time, the mother cat brought her kittens to the woman. Feeding these kittens and playing with them gave this woman's life a purpose and some joy in the midst of the suffering she was sharing with her husband. "God sent me this cat," she said. "We needed each other." She slowed down and stayed focused in the present.

A qualitative research study of opportunities for enhanced spirituality in well adults revealed six themes: connectedness, relationships with "self, others, nature, the universe, or a higher power"; beliefs, such as a belief in God or in good versus bad; inner motivating factors, guides for behavior and attitude; divine providence, belief in a higher power; understanding the mystery, looking for meaning and purpose in life; and walking through, using our inner resources on life's journey (Cavendish et al., 2000). The researchers concluded that nurses need to be more aware of the significance of life events in clients' lives to make accurate nursing diagnoses and to intervene in meaningful ways. Support of clients' coping strategies, inner resources, and beliefs and an understanding of spirituality that allows nurses to foster even small changes in the spiritual aspect of their clients' lives can have a significant effect (Cavendish et al., 2000).

THE NURSE AS A SPIRITUAL PERSON AND CAREGIVER

Life is a journey. Peck (1998) suggested that we must appreciate the fact that life is complex. This means to "abandon the urge to simplify everything, to look for easy answers, and to begin to think multidimensionally, to stay in the mystery and paradoxes of life." Those who would simplify nursing practice would teach students how to do "things" such as treatments, techniques, and procedures. How easy it would be if the quality of nursing care could be quantified by how accurately or quickly procedures could be performed. Consider this: "The essence of nursing is not

doing…but being open to whatever arises in the interaction with the client. It is being fully present with an unconditional acceptance of the client's experience" (Newman, 1989). Perhaps we can think of life not as a series of problems to be solved but rather as a mystery to unravel.

SIMPLIFY AND DEEPEN

Authentic leisure implies an approach to living that allows one to relax into a level of being that deepens self-awareness, nourishes one's wholeness, and enriches connections with the Sacred Source and other people.

Burkhardt and Nagai-Jacobson, 2022, p. 141

Spiritual Care Begins with the Nurse

To be a nurse is to be given a sacred trust. Clients and families come to us fearfully in their darkest hours, in the face of their own mortality, or at the time of childbirth in the face of the wonder of creation. Burkhardt and Nagai-Jacobson (1994) spoke of a "reawakening spirit in nursing practice." To have the ability to stay connected to the experience of another, you must pay attention to nurturing your own spirit. Moore (1998) spoke of living artfully as a necessity for the care of the soul or spirit. To do so, he suggested the following:

- Pause (the opposite of being busy), stop, reflect, savor the moment, and experience wonder at the things around you, be still.
- Take time for self, people, relationships, and things—living creatures, too! To take time for relationships, even difficult ones, deepens our understanding and appreciation.
- Be mindful of, or pay attention to, what is happening all around you so that you recognize the need to stop and focus on this moment rather than thinking about the past or the future.

But how can you slow down, considering the demands of nursing? Other chapters in this volume address methods such as relaxation techniques and meditation. Practicing these techniques helps you to be in touch with your own spirit and helps you to be centered. The process of centering helps you focus on this moment. Remember the value of rest, of time to do nothing, and of playful leisure time. Focusing on the moment can mean slowing down to really enjoy the taste and texture and smells of the food you eat, taking time to stroke the fur of a cat or dog, listening to the sound of birds singing, enjoying music rather than using it for background noise, stroking the hair of a child, listening to another person without offering an opinion, hugging a friend, and listening to laughter and joining in. In a series of community classes for cancer patients and their families, one man said that cancer had changed his focus from "working for a living to the art of living." These simple suggestions are mindful activities. They are what clients tell us they do to stay connected to life in tough times. For them, these are the things that make life worthwhile. Nurses reported spiritual renewal practicing mindfulness and other spiritual self-care processes such as meditation, time in nature, yoga, and music in retreats as part of a study to support nurses' spirituality (Bay, Ivy, & Terry, 2010). Perhaps such activities can replenish your energy to do your life's work. Visit ANA's COVID-19 Self-Care Package for Nurses (Free) (nursingworld.org) (2022).

Communication is more than verbal and nonverbal behavior. The ability to stay present in the moment requires conscious effort, which is sometimes a struggle. When you feel overwhelmed, take time to return to being still and paying attention to the gifts of the senses. When you are frightened, remember the following lyrics: "When you are troubled and cannot sleep, just count your blessings instead of sheep." Emmons (2007) discussed results of gratitude research. Study participants who kept a weekly gratitude journal exercised with more regularity, had fewer physical complaints, felt better about their lives, and were more optimistic than the control group who kept journals about neutral events. Participants who kept a daily gratitude journal were more likely to offer emotional support to someone else. People who are grateful are more likely to believe in an interconnectedness of all life and demonstrate a commitment to others. Consider starting your own gratitude journal, writing a few words each day about the things for which you are grateful, or just spend a few moments before you go to sleep to say thank you for the things for which you are grateful or for the people and things in your life you appreciate.

Reflect on this mnemonic for fear when you are afraid and in spiritual distress. FEAR is:

F: Forgetting
E: that Everything
A: is All
R: Right

Offering simple strategies that work for you may be useful to your clients.

Self-Care Nudge

How do you relax? What helps you rest? Stop, breathe, consider.

Meeting the Spiritual Needs of the Client

Spiritual care is not separate from all other aspects of nursing care. In Watson's conceptual model of nursing, spirituality is central. "The human spirit is regarded as the most powerful force in human existence and the source behind striving for self-transcendence through spiritual evolutions and the achievement of inner harmony. Nurses practicing within this framework promote harmony of body, mind, and spirit, regardless of the external health problem, age, or life circumstance of the person" (Touchy, 2001).

Caring in nursing requires intention, relationship, and actions (Touchy, 2001). Spiritual care is how you do what you do. It is an attitude and an openness to the shared experience of the human condition. When you assist a patient with morning care, when you offer a bedpan or a urinal, when you take a temperature, and when you bathe a person who has soiled himself, you perform ordinary tasks; when done mindfully, they provide spiritual care. In a book on spiritual fulfillment in everyday life, Fields, Taylor, Weyler, and Ingrasci (1984) talk about performing simple daily tasks as a way to get in touch with the natural cycles of life and death.

Spiritually sensitive communication strategies identified in a qualitative research case study in home hospice care included the following: creating space for expression of emotions and beliefs about spirituality, supporting meaning making in the experience, emphasizing caregiver strengths, and reframing negative experiences (Reblin, Otis-Green, Ellington, & Clayton, 2014).

When searching for meaning, a client may have a need to explore spiritual and psychological issues and to talk about religious feelings or the lack of them. The client is not asking for advice or opinions; instead, it is a time to talk about feelings and to express doubts, fears, and anguish. Even clients with strong religious beliefs may need encouragement in crisis. You can support a client with religious beliefs by encouraging prayer or meditation (Narayanasamy, 2004). Consider the role of spirituality, religion, and culture in healthcare beliefs. Participants in a study of spiritual practices in the self-management of diabetes in African Americans used prayer, reading the Bible, listening to Christian radio and television programs, church attendance, and testimonies from people with diabetes (Casarez, Engebretson, & Ostwald, 2010). Perhaps a selection of scripture, a morning prayer, or a testimony of success about the use of spiritual practices in making better food choices is a "nudge" to make better food choices or take a walk that day, which are ways to get us to think before we choose (Donnelly, 2010; Thaler & Sustein, 2008). Clients can be very vulnerable and not comfortable sharing sensitive information such as their belief system. It is important to respect the individual's freedom of choice about a personal belief system and not to try to persuade or encourage a patient to adopt your personal point of view (Buswell, Clegg, Grout, Minardi, & Morgan, 2006).

Spiritual needs may be greater during times of illness, and a separation from routine comforting spiritual or religious practices can be a source of stress. The spiritual history and spiritual assessment may provide information that helps in mutual problem solving to find ways to meet these needs (Delgado, 2007).

Being Fully Present

The daily routine of nurses is not routine to clients. One reason it takes courage to be fully present with clients is that to be present is to understand their fear and pain. Words and procedures you will come to see as commonplace strike fear in the hearts of company presidents who find themselves in a setting they cannot control. Do not be fooled by clients who seem to be calm and confident. Assume that your clients and their families see you as a lifeline, and work from there.

"Spiritual care begins with presence...In essence, the presence of love we bring to any situation is the basic way we integrate spirituality into care" (Burkhardt & Nagai-Jacobson, 2002). It is about how we do the things we do, who we are, and how we are with one another. Each moment is new. Each moment is different. In Chapter 9, you read about the highest level of empathy, in which you recognize the other's humanity and personhood regardless of the illness, its circumstance, or its stigma. You understand that we are all connected. Consider this for a moment: Can you view all of your work as sacred and feel that you are standing on holy ground day by day (O'Brien, 2021)? What if you set that intention each day as you begin your work? Spiritual care does not take extra time. It is a part of all you do.

Offering Prayer

In a national study of more than 2000 Americans, about 75% of those responding report they pray to prevent illness and 22% report they pray to alleviate a medical condition with a high degree of perceived helpfulness (McCaffrey, 2004). Prayer "is an intimate conversation between us and God"; it is "an expression of spirit that is a fundamental way of connection with our inner self and the Sacred Source" (Burkhardt & Nagai-Jacobson, 2002); it is "an expression of the spirit...a deep human instinct that flows from the core of one's being where the longing for and awareness of one's connectedness with the source of life are blended... [and] represents a longed for communion or communication with God or the Absolute" (Dossey & Keegan, 2012). Prayer as a nursing intervention such as praying with a client, praying aloud in the presence of a client, offering time of silence for prayer, fostering a supportive environment for prayer, or praying in your own quiet time is based on an assessment of the spiritual needs of a client. Praying at the end of a time with a client or praying prematurely may be seen as dismissive, a way to escape after the content of an

---

BOX 15.3   Thoughts on Prayer

Consider...
- Not everyone is receptive to or believes in prayer.
- Prayer traditions vary.
- Clients may offer cues that they are open to prayer by verbal references or the presence of inspirational or religious reading material or religious objects.
- Prayer may help the client with feelings of isolation.
- It is appropriate to ask the client if he or she would like a prayer and for what.
- Prayer can express what the clients would pray if they were able.
- Prayer may be a brief, simple statement of the client's hopes, fears, and needs and God's ability to be with the client in difficult times.
- Prayer for the greatest good for all involved is an inclusive prayer.
- Prayer allows for "intimacy without exposure."

Modified from Bayfront Medical Center. (2002). *Pastoral care volunteer training manual: The use of prayer (handout).* St. Petersburg, FL: Bayfront Medical Center.

interaction has been emotional, or a way of cutting off conversation (Bayfront Medical Center, 2002). Consider the use of prayer in the middle of a visit, which allows time for the client to respond emotionally to the prayer if appropriate. See the thoughts on prayer listed in Box 15.3.

 MOMENTS OF CONNECTION...
Where Can I Begin?

"The foundation began in my first year of nursing, at age 21, when an experienced nurse noticed my confusion and helplessness in dealing with a dying patient one evening. I didn't ask for help; I never did. The patient had no family present, so it really was up to me. This nurse took me into the room and said, 'Hello. We're with you. You are not alone.' She was speaking to the patient and to me. It was years before I finally believed what she said. By the grace of God, I know that we are never alone, and I can share this belief now with conviction."

Being Silent

Being still, being comfortable with silence, and understanding that it is acceptable not to have answers, or even words, may come naturally to the introvert, who is a person who thinks to talk. For the extravert, a person who talks to think, such a realization may be growth. One therapist who is an extreme extravert said that the only way he could still his mind and his mouth was to learn to meditate. Yes, it is acceptable and even therapeutic to be quiet, just to be, and not to do all the time. Thirty years ago, a nursing instructor said, "If you don't know what to say, just be quiet and stay there. Try saying, 'I don't have any words to help, but I will stay with you a while.'" These words are still good counsel.

A psychologist, when talking about her experience as a patient, said, "I want the nurse to understand that I am not myself when I am ill. I'm not the person I present to the outside world. I appreciate your understanding this and not judging me or my behavior. I don't want you to try to fix my problems. All I want is for you to acknowledge my pain, even by just a kind look when you stop in to check on me."

Silence means acceptance. There are no expectations that clients or nurses must have all the answers. There is no right thing to say or perfect nursing care plan to write that can make things all better for clients. Part of the challenge for all nurses is to live with this realization.

Using "Oh...?," "Hmm...," and "Really?"

Although asking questions may seem to be a good way to encourage a distressed person to say more, questions may be experienced as attacks, intrusions, or demands (Bogia, 1985). Rabbinical pastor and chaplain Kate Fagan, in a hospital training class for pastoral volunteers, recommends the use of encouraging or questioning sounds or body language as cues that encourage the client to continue talking. Try "Oh...?" when you sense that the client has more to say and then be quiet. It is not always easy to wait, but it is essential. You can also say, "Hmm..." or ask, "Really?" again, followed by silence. These strategies may elicit further conversation more effectively than more involved verbal responses, but they need to be used with discernment and not overused.

Other strategies are useful when a client is in crisis. Try an observation about the physical facts of a situation. When a client is crying, saying "There are tears in your eyes" encourages elaboration because you have acknowledged the tears. Use an "I" statement, such as "I wonder if you have some ideas about that?" when a client presents a scenario that seems puzzling to him or her. The "seems-to-me" approach is useful; for example, "You seem to be upset." Avoid the overused question "How does that make you feel?", which may lead clients to believe you are trying to analyze them (Bogia, 1985). Remember that humor can be an element of spiritual coping as clients try to gain perspective and make meaning, and our humor can foster deeper, more trusting relationships with clients (Johnson, 2002).

Recognizing Opportunities for Moments of Connection

Martin Buber (1958) distinguished between two types of relationships, the I–It and the I–Thou. The I–It relationship can be experienced as nurses do the work of patient care. Teaching and caring can become routine and, although excellent in form, may lack substance or a real connection with the patient. The I–It is the world of "experiencing and using...a typical subject–object relationship." The I–Thou relationship can be experienced only with the whole being. The I–Thou is "characterized by mutuality, directness, presentness, intensity" (Friedman, 1966). "The It is the eternal chrysalis, the Thou, the eternal butterfly" (Buber, 1958).

Just as the world of the nurse provides the potential for a genuine relationship with the patient, the I–It can become the I–Thou in special moments of connection to the patient or to a family member in the potential crisis situation of surgery and illness.

A nurse's personal or family experience with surgery and/or illness can contribute to a deeper understanding of patient and family needs. Nursing is a sacred trust in which the patient and family agree to give up conventional constraints on behavior in exchange for acceptance of their personal response to the traumatic experience of surgery. The nurse's ability to stay connected to the pain of the human condition is one ingredient that can create I–Thou relationships. These moments of connection, however brief, sustain the patient and family throughout the crisis and provide the meaning the nurse so badly needs to revitalize in the nursing practice.

Tapping Resources

In a study in Iran, prayer reduced the pain of patients having Extracorporeal Shock Wave Lithotripsy (ESWL). This painful treatment is used to "break up" kidney stones. The test group was instructed to repeat the prayer, "peace be upon Mohammad and his descendants" (Torki, Heidari, Norian, Ravieie, & Sedahi, 2021). So that spiritual care can be provided to clients from a variety of traditions, it is helpful to take the initiative to learn about available resources. As part of a spiritual assessment, you can find out about clergy with whom the client is acquainted who may be contacted with the client's permission. Find out if your organization has access to a pastoral care department for referral, and find out what faith traditions are represented. Take responsibility for learning about rituals, sacred texts, devotional articles, prayer, and sacred music from different traditions (O'Brien, 2021). Martin (2004) recommended three strategies for enhancing spiritual well-being in nursing homes: offer religious activities in the facility; with permission, inform the local church of choice about the admission; and offer opportunities for the expression of clients' faith. Martin wrote, "Residents of extended-care facilities must give up a great deal of their former lives and possessions when they embark on this new chapter. Connection with the sacred should not be among the losses."

Family members with online access sought and received spiritual comfort using an Internet-based pancreatic cancer chat room through Johns Hopkins Hospital (Nolan et al., 2006). If you find ways to combine personal interest and skills with computers with your nursing career, you might design a website as a resource to assist clients and families in receiving information and support.

Nearing Death

As clients near death, nurses work as part of a team to provide spiritual care. When is the right time? Nurses learn to trust their intuition about the right time to talk about the client's concerns. Nurses offer a nurturing touch, silent presence, a prayer, or, if the client prefers, a chance to speak to a member of the clergy. Remember that some clients may be able to attend all or part of a religious service held in your facility. Encourage family to provide sacred music that has offered comfort to the client in the past. Some clients like to listen to recordings of sermons or sacred texts. Nurses create a climate for hope to grow and flourish (Box 15.4). The nurse can ask clients to consider special messages or special mementos for which they want to make arrangements (Piemme, 1998).

Helping in Life Review and Life Repair

Clients near death may find peace by engaging in life review and repair. You can suggest reflection through journal writing. Life review raises issues of forgiveness. There may be a need for forgiveness or acceptance of self. Recent research distinguishes between "decisional forgiveness," which is a behavioral intention to forgive, and "emotional forgiveness," which is a shift from negative, unforgiving emotions to positive, other-oriented emotions. Emotional forgiveness was found to have more positive effects on health and well-being (Horrigan, 2008). Nurses in hospice and palliative care may build open and deep relationships with clients. For nurses in such a position, the following question might assist the process of life review: "If you had your life to live over again, what would you like to be different?" (Kemp, 2001). It may be helpful to ask the client if there is unfinished business in life that he or she might now be able to address. One hospice client replied that she did not believe she had ever told her daughter how truly proud she was of her. The nurse helped her determine a good time to do this and supported the client's resolve to do it, even though talk of feelings did not come easy. After the talk, the client seemed to experience more peace. (Schachter-Shalomii & Miller, R. 2014), founder of the Spiritual Eldering Institute, now Sage-ing International, offers an in-depth process in his work and in the book *From Age-ing to Sage-ing*.

The accompanying Moments of Connection help illustrate the different forms communication may take as nurses support clients and families in these intimate times.

BOX 15.4   Notes on Hope

Hope is trust and confidence. Hope is patient. Hope brings enthusiasm and adds animation. Hope is a fuel to keep us going, a tonic to energize, a driving force to move us forward, daily bread to feed the soul. Hope is in contrast to expectation, which takes us from the present to a focus on the future; this can bring disappointment when things do not go as we planned (Brussat & Brussat, 1998). "Hope is the belief…that one can have a life in the midst of trauma and suffering. Hope that you will be able to cope with the suffering, hope that something good will come from it, hope for remission—if not a cure, hope for an extension of time, hope for the future welfare of your family, hope to keep your dignity, hope for life after life" (Hampton, 1998).

To *bring hope* you must have hope. To keep a hopeful countenance, learn to forgive yourself for your mistakes so you can take the risk of opportunities of the future; learn to leave room for the future, love yourself, laugh and keep a sense of humor, trust in God, celebrate your imagination, cherish your dreams, create visions, set goals. In the face of difficulties, remember: Within every problem there is a lesson. Embrace the lesson and release the problem. To face the uncertainty of life, consider this notion: I am uncertain about the future, but I am certain it will be positive.

To *instill hope* you show it in your face; in your kind, positive words; in your ability to truly face someone—to look into the eyes; in your presence rather than avoidance; in your presence in the face of suffering; in your openness to hear hopeless words; and in your offered prayer. Encourage clients to display cards and have family bring photographs or art from children or grandchildren. Suggest the family provide favorite music. Comment on flowers as reminders of connection in the client's life.

🌸 MOMENTS OF CONNECTION…
Having the Courage to Share a Prayer

"A patient who had been on the acute pain service three previous times during the same admission was received in the postanesthesia care unit (PACU) after an exploration of the abdomen and was in a great deal of pain as I started her patient-controlled analgesia (PCA). I told her I would stay with her until the pain was controlled. For the next 2 hours I gave her multiple boluses, but her pain was not relieved satisfactorily. During this time, I patted her forehead and moistened her lips. When I asked her what else I could do for her, she asked if I would pray with her. We were still in the PACU, and I was aware that several other nurses were rolling their eyes. We said the Lord's Prayer. She soon relaxed and appeared more comfortable."

MOMENTS OF CONNECTION...

Wishes and Dreams

"It was springtime, and she was a young leukemia patient who would probably not leave the hospital before a 'celestial discharge.' We had chatted for days about her wishes and dreams. She had never gone to a circus, seen a bluebird, or been to Disneyland. Several nurses got together. Mickey Mouse appeared in her room. I came as a clown with my 'trick' dog, bringing a video of the circus. A pet shop owner brought in two blue birds to spend the afternoon. She was laughing and crying. She said she didn't know nurses did all these things. I asked her if she was happy and content. She replied, 'The only thing I haven't seen is God, and I'll see Him soon, but I know I've seen the angels.'"

 MOMENTS OF CONNECTION...

I Clearly Felt Her Presence

"I was working as a hospice nurse with a very independent client who always wanted to be in control up in the chair each day. As her pain increased and my visits became more frequent, I took on more of a nurturing role. I am also a massage therapist, and when she became bedridden, I would frequently give her a massage. She asked to purchase a gift certificate for a massage for her sister. On the day she passed, I went into her room where her body lay cold and still. I thanked her for the opportunity to be her friend and nurse. I clearly felt her presence and love. A month later, her sister came for a massage after having been very distraught over her loss. It was a marvelous experience for both of us. She still returns monthly for a massage, and each time we remember her sister and her gift."

Finding Meaning

By understanding that meaning can come from suffering, you can be alert to times when clients or family members want to share what they have learned. Clients may give you clues that they want to talk further. Here are some things your clients might say and possible interventions to help them share their understanding of what has happened:

Client 1: "So much has happened in such a short time. I never knew I could handle so many things."

Nurse: "You've been thinking about all the things you've been through. Tell me about it."

Client 2: "Having AIDS makes me value life more."

Nurse: "Can you share how you see life now?"

Client 3: "When you lose a child, your other children become all the more precious."

Nurse: "How do you think things will change between you and your children?"

BOX 15.5   Possible Meanings of Illness and Suffering

I have learned...
- That I can love.
- That loving hurts.
- That I can survive.
- That healing occurs.
- That I have grown.
- That I can forgive.
- That I can forgive myself.
- That you taught me much.
- That I can be a receiver.
- That change is a necessary part of life.
- That I am grateful for the many things you gave me.
- That I wouldn't miss you if you hadn't been so important to me.
- That I cannot control everything.
- That I can care.
- That I can become involved.
- That I need a significant other.
- That I can reevaluate myself.
- That a new page of my life is being written.
- That I will have to change.
- That I can start again.
- That I am wiser.
- That I have discovered a new level of courage.
- That I am more open.
- That I can make new contacts on my own.
- That I can ask for support.
- That I am stronger, more independent, more joyful, and happier.
- That I have choices.
- That I am really never alone.
- The value and importance of the present.
- To fill my days in new ways.
- To appreciate this disruption in my life as motivation to grow.
- To enjoy aloneness.
- To appreciate life more.

Reprinted from Hannaford, M., & Popkin, M. (1992). *Windows: Healing and helping through loss* (pp. 77–78). Atlanta, GA: Active Parenting.

Hannaford and Popkin (1992) reported things that people have learned from loss, as listed in Box 15.5. Their book *Windows* is used as a text for a grief class that is taught to caregivers who may support clients and families during loss. They suggested questions and statements that may "encourage the griever as he turns loss into meaningful experience." Box 15.6 lists questions and statements that might be helpful, and Box 15.7 lists comments that might be harmful.

BOX 15.6 Questions or Statements that May Help

- As you look at this experience, is it possible that you have found new meaning in relationships that you were not aware of before?
- Have you considered your growth during this time, the changes in you that this loss seems to have brought?
- How has the experience changed your life?
- How has it influenced your life purpose and belief system?
- What positive action have you taken or might you take as a result of this lesson?
- You seem to have learned that there are a lot of things over which we have no control.
- You have gained a lot of self-confidence in your ability to handle a crisis.
- You seem to feel that, with all the loss, you are gaining a kind of independence that you never knew you could enjoy.
- I like to hear you laugh; it seems that you are more able to express your feelings since your recent experience.

Reprinted from Hannaford, M., & Popkin, M. (1992). *Windows: Healing and helping through loss* (pp. 129–130). Atlanta, GA: Active Parenting.

BOX 15.7 Comments that May Do More Harm than Good

- As you look at this, you have no doubt learned never to do it again.
- Life's lessons are hard, and you have certainly made this one into a hard one.
- When you make mistakes, you always have to pay.
- If you had kept in touch, you wouldn't feel so bad.
- You'll learn from this one to be kind from now on.
- I do hope you've learned your lesson.
- Everything will be all right.

Reprinted from Hannaford, M., & Popkin, M. (1992). *Windows: Healing and helping through loss* (pp. 129–130). Atlanta, GA: Active Parenting.

FINDING GOD IN THE BUSYNESS

How do you as a nurse find God for yourself with the pace you keep? Hanrahan (2006), a writer, anthropologist, and painter, speaks of "finding God in the busyness." She writes about the great longing for stillness and silence and the assumption that it is necessary to go "on retreat" to find God. She suggests that quiet and withdrawal are not necessary for spiritual health and that to be busy does not have to mean a disconnection from God. Hanrahan works with indigenous people in Canada who have always seen God everywhere and in everything. "I saw God in the face of an Elder in the Yukon and heard in the prayers we said to open our meetings. I met God in the bubbly Turkish man who drove me to the airport…and in the Mexican professor–taxi driver, a refugee from the institutional Revolutionary Party's long, hard rule, a man empty of bitterness" (Hanrahan, 2006). She felt God as her head hit the pillow in a hotel on a business trip. Her advice speaks to slowing down for a moment of gratitude or connection.

Remember that there is often nobody better placed or better qualified to provide spiritual care than the nurse (Kemp, 2001). Consider that sometimes nurturing the sacred in your own life is the best approach.

We come full circle. Spiritual care begins and ends with the caregiver. You nurture your own spirit, thus becoming open to your clients' experiences in a genuine, holistic way. Your experience with your clients nourishes your spirit and offers renewal.

Return to "Active Learning" at the beginning of the chapter and write your responses.

 PRACTICING EMBRACING THE SPIRITUAL JOURNEY OF HEALTHCARING… MEANING MAKING

Skill Building: Exercise 1

In dyads in class, take turns taking a spiritual history using the FICA tool in Box 15.2. Discuss your response, comfort level, and concerns you might have in using this tool with patients. Discuss other spiritual assessment tools used in your clinical settings.

Critical Thinking/Reflection/Intention Setting: Exercise 2

In the "Spiritual Care Begins with the Nurse" section of this chapter, suggestions are given to nurture your spirit. In your journal, create a plan to nurture your spirit, and set and write an intention to integrate this plan into your life and work.

Creative Expression/Discussion: Exercise 3

John Paul Lederach, author of more than 20 books on conflict transformation and peace building and whose wife has Parkinson's disease, is quoted in Jarem Sawatsky's book, *Dancing with Elephants: Mindfulness Training for Those Living with Dementia, Chronic Illness or an Aging Brain* (Sawatsky, 2017): Faith is also about a sense of awe that is captured in the mystery of the extraordinary gift of life and the world we were born into. Nature often brings that for me…We need a daily dose of vitamin awe. How can you put yourself "in nature" to get your daily dose of vitamin awe?

Use this poem to begin a discussion of nature as a source of spiritual connection.

Take a Quiet Walk for Me
Walk slowly
by the quiet path
And look at the trees
and the sky
by day and night…
Remembering the good times
on the lakeshore,
in the woods
Near the meadows
and the black softness
of the friendly hollows…

Copyright © Howard G. Kirkman. Used with permission.

Reflection/Discussion: Exercise 4

Sit quietly for 3 minutes and reflect on those things for which you are grateful. Identify someone living or deceased toward whom you feel great gratitude and write that person a gratitude letter. Discuss your experience of reflecting on and expressing gratitude. Might you do this more often?

Ritual and Celebration: Exercise 5

The Blessing of the Hands is a nondenominational ceremony or ritual with the intent to renew and honor nurses. It is often conducted at Nurse Week celebrations. It could also be incorporated into celebrations in a school of nursing. Research this tradition online, then, with other students and staff, discuss interest in conducting such a ceremony in a clinical setting or school of nursing celebration (Wolpert, 2010).

Quality and Safety Education for Nurses Learning Strategy: Exercise 6

Patient-centered care includes the skill of "Providing patient-centered care with sensitivity and respect for the diversity of human experience." The experience of illness is a vulnerable time for patients and their families. Understanding their values and beliefs about health and the meaning of illness is important for providing spiritual care. Asking patients reflective questions may be a way to assist patients in making sense of their illness within the context of their values, beliefs, and life circumstances.

- Guide patients in describing a time when they felt healthy and alive. It is helpful to prompt patients to describe what was happening at the time, how they felt, and who was involved.
- What contributed to their feelings of health and well-being?
- By helping patients recall times they felt at their healthiest, nurses can better understand their values and beliefs and how they frame the challenges in their current situation. By hearing their story, nurses can guide patients in identifying spiritual dimensions of care, the role of a higher power in their life, what gives their life meaning, and perceptions of threats they currently feel. By understanding patient values and beliefs, nurses can help patients explore their response to illness and help them in seeking resources to address unresolved spiritual needs that can be a barrier to active engagement in care and affect patient recovery and healing.
- Why is identifying and recognizing patient values and beliefs an important aspect of quality safe care?
- When is it important to make exceptions to evidence-based standards to honor patient values and beliefs?

REFERENCES

Abell, C. H., Garrett-Wright, D., & Abell, C. E. (2018). Nurses' perception of competence in providing spiritual care. *Journal of Holistic Nursing, 36*(1), 3.

American Nurses Association (ANA). (2012). *Faith community, nursing* (2nd ed.). Silver Spring, MD: American Nurses Association.

American Nurses Association (ANA). (2022). ANA's COVID-19 Self-Care Package for Nurses (Free) (nursingworld.org).

Bay, P. S., Ivy, S. S., & Terry, C. L. (2010). The effect of spiritual retreat on nurses' spirituality. *Holistic Nursing Practice, 24*(3), 125.

Bayfront Medical Center. (2002). *Pastoral care volunteer training manual: The use of prayer (handout)*. St. Petersburg, FL: Bayfront Medical Center.

Bogia, B. P. (1985). Responding to questions in pastoral care. *Journal of Pastoral Care, 13*(4), 357.

Booth, L., & Kaylor, S. (2018). Teaching spiritual care within nursing education: A holistic approach. *Holistic Nursing Practice, 32*(4), 177.

Bormann, J. E., Thorp, S., Wetherill, J. L., & Golshan, S. (2008). A spiritually based group intervention for combat veterans with posttraumatic stress disorder. *Journal of Holistic Nursing, 26*(2), 109.

Brillhart, B. (2005). A study of spirituality and life satisfaction among persons with spinal cord injury. *Rehabilitation Nursing, 30*(1), 31.

Brooke, W. (2021). Turning inward: Mindfulness as a gateway to presence and spiritual knowing in nursing. *Beginnings: American Holistic Nurses Association Newsletter,* June 2021, 6.

Brussat, F., & Brussat, M. A. (1998). *Spiritual literacy: Reading the sacred in everyday life*. New York, NY: Touchstone Books.

Buber, M. (1958). *I and thou*. New York, NY: Charles Scribner's Sons.

Burkhardt, M. A., & Nagai-Jacobson, M. G. (1994). Reawakening spirit in nursing practice. *Journal of Holistic Nursing, 12*(1), 8.

Burkhardt, M. A., & Nagai-Jacobson, M. G. (2002). *Spirituality: Living our connectedness*. Albany, NY: Delmar/Thomson Learning.

Burkhardt, M. A., & Nagai-Jacobson, M. G. (2022). Spirituality and health. In *Dossey & Keegan's holistic nursing: A handbook for practice* (8th ed.). Burlington, MA: Jones & Bartlett Learning.

Buswell, J., Clegg, A., Grout, G., Minardi, H. A., & Morgan, A. (2006). Ask the experts: Spirituality in care [gerontological care and practice]. *Nursing Older People, 18*(1), 14.

Calabria, M. D., & Macrae, J. A. (Eds.). (1994). *Suggestions for thought by Florence Nightingale: Selections and commentaries* (a volume in the Studies in Health, Illness, and Caregiving series). Philadelphia, PA: University of Pennsylvania Press.

Casarez, R. L. P., Engebretson, J. C., & Ostwald, S. K. (2010). Spiritual practices in self-management of diabetes in African Americans. *Holistic Nursing Practice, 24*(4), 227.

Cavendish, R., Luise, B. K., Horne, K., Bauer, M., Medefindt, J., Gallo, M. A., et al. (2000). Opportunities for enhanced spirituality relevant to well adults. *Nursing Diagnosis, 11*(4), 151.

Chochinov, H. M., McClement, S., Thompson, H. T., Dufault, B., & Harlos, M. (2015). Eliciting personhood within clinical practice: Effects on patients, families, and health care providers. *Journal of Pain and Symptom Management, 49*, 974.

Cone, P. H., & Giske, T. (2016). Nurses' comfort level with spiritual assessment: A study among nurses working in diverse healthcare settings. *Journal of Clinical Nursing, 26*, 3125.

Delgado, C. (2007). Meeting clients' spiritual needs. *Nursing Clinics of North America, 42*(2), 279.

Donnelly, G. F. (2010). Health choices and heightened awareness: The art of the nudge! *Holistic Nursing Practice, 24*(4), 179.

Dossey, B. M., & Keegan, L. (1995). *Holistic nursing: A handbook for practice (2nd ed.)*. Gaithersburg, MD: Aspen Publishers.

Dossey, B. (1998a). Body-mind-spirit: Attending to holistic care. *American Journal of Nursing, 98*(8), 35.

Dossey, B. (1998b). Holistic modalities and healing moments. *American Journal of Nursing, 98*(6), 44–47.

Ellington, L., Bilitteri, J., Reblin, M., & Clayton, M. F. (2017). Spiritual care communication in cancer patients. *Seminars in Oncology Nursing, 33*(5), 517.

Emmons, R. A. (2007). *Thanks: How the new science of gratitude can make you happier*. Boston, MA: Houghton Mifflin.

Erickson, H. (Ed.). (2006). *Modeling and role-modeling: A view from the clients' world*. Cedar Park, TX: Unicorns Unlimited.

Erickson, H., Tomlin, E., & Swain, M. A. (2010). *Modeling and role-modeling: A theory and paradigm for nursing*. Cedar Park, TX: Unicorns Unlimited.

Fields, R., Taylor, P., Weyler, R., & Ingrasci, R. (1984). *Chop wood, carry water: A guide to finding spiritual fulfillment in everyday life*. Los Angeles, CA: JP Tarcher.

Friedman, M. S. (1966). *The life of dialogue*. New York, NY: Harper & Row.

Hampton, C. (1998). Hope and healing after traumatic illness. [Paper presented to the Case Management Society of America, Georgia chapter, September 26, 1998].

Hannaford, M., & Popkin, M. (1992). *Windows: Healing and helping through loss*. Atlanta, GA: Active Parenting.

Hanrahan, M. (2006). Finding God in the busyness. The social edge: A monthly social justice and faith website. http://www.thesocialedge.com/columns/maurahanrahan/index.shtml.

Horrigan, B. (2008). Matters of note: New forgiveness research looks at its effect on others. *Explore, 4*(1), 11.

Hospice and Palliative Nurses Association (HPNA). (2021). Spiritual care. *Journal of Hospice & Palliative Nursing, 23*(6), E34–E35.

Johnson, P. (2002). The use of humor and its influences on spirituality and coping in breast cancer survivors. *Oncology Nursing Forum, 29*(4), 691.

Kemp, C. (2001). Spiritual care interventions. In B. Ferrell, & N. Coyle (Eds.). *Textbook of palliative care*. New York, NY: Oxford University Press.

Kidd, S. M. (2005). *The mermaid chair*. New York, NY: Penguin Books.

Koenig, H. G. (1999). *The healing power of faith: Science explores medicine's last great frontier*. New York, NY: Simon & Schuster.

Koenig, H. G. (2007). *Spirituality in patient care: Why, how, when, and what*. West Conshohocken, PA: Templeton Press.

Lackey, S. A. (2009). Opening the door to spiritually sensitive care. *Nursing, 39*(4), 46.

Martin, I. (2004). Nurturing that old-time religion. *Vibrant Life, 20*(5), 14.

McCaffrey, A. (2004). Prayer for health concerns: Results of a national survey on prevalence and patterns of use. *Archives of Internal Medicine, 164*(8), 858.

Meraviglia, M. (2006). Effects of spirituality in breast cancer survivors. *Oncology Nursing Forum, 33*(1), E1.

Moore, T. (1998). *Care of the soul*. New York, NY: HarperCollins.

Nagai-Jacobson, M. G., & Burkhardt, M. A. (1989). Spirituality: Cornerstone of holistic nursing practice. *Holistic Nursing Practice, 3*(3), 18.

Narayanasamy, A. (2004). The puzzle of spirituality for nursing: A guide to practical assessment. *British Journal of Nursing, 13*(19), 1140.

Newman, M. A. (1989). The spirit of nursing. *Holistic Nursing Practice, 3*(3), 1.

Nolan, M. T., Hodgin, M. B., Olsen, S. J., Coleman, J., Sauter, P. K., Baker, D., et al. (2006). Spiritual issues of family members in a pancreatic cancer chat room. *Oncology Nursing Forum, 33*(2), 239.

O'Brien, M. E. (2021). *Spirituality in nursing: Standing on holy ground* (7th ed.). Burlington, MA: Jones & Bartlett Learning.

Peck, M. S. (1998). *Further along the road less traveled: The unending journey toward spiritual growth*. New York, NY: Touchstone Books.

Piemme, J. A. (1998). Discussing end-of-life decisions. *Innovative Breast Cancer Care, 4*(1), 31.

Reblin, M., Otis-Green, S., Ellington, L., & Clayton, M. F. (2014). Strategies to support spirituality in health care communication: A home hospice caregiver. *Journal of Holistic Nursing, 32*(4), 269.

Sawatsky, J. (2017). *Dancing with elephants: Mindfulness training for those living with dementia, chronic illness or an aging brain.* Rosemary Beach, FL: Red Canoe Press.

Schachter-Shalomi, Z., & Miller, R. (2014). *From age-ing to sage-ing: A profound new vision of growing older.* New York, NY: Grand Central Publishing.

Thaler, R. H., & Sustein, C. R. (2008). *Nudge: Improving decisions about health, wealth and happiness.* London, UK: Penguin Books.

Torki, M., Heidari, H., Norian, K., Ravieie, L., & Sedahi, M. (2021). Prayer on the severity of pain in patients undergoing lithotripsy. *JRH, 8*(2), 19–27. http://jrh.mazums.ac.ir/article-1-621-en.html.

Touchy, T. A. (2001). Nurturing hope and spirituality in the nursing home. *Holistic Nursing Practice, 15*(4), 45.

Travelbee, J. (1970). *Interventions in psychiatric nursing.* Philadelphia, PA: FA Davis.

Tuck, I., McCain, N. L., & Elswick, R. K., Jr. (2001). Spirituality and psychosocial well-being in HIV+ adults. *Advances in Nursing, 33*(6), 776.

Wolpert, N. S. (2010). Blessing of the hands. *Nursing Management, 41*(5), 29.

Advanced Competencies for Communication in Nursing

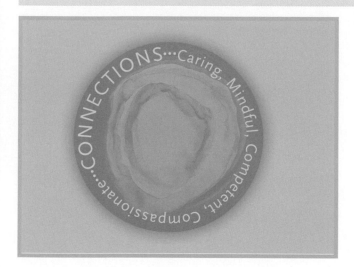

PART II

Advanced Competencies for
Communication in Nursing

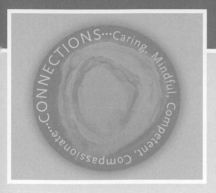

CONNECTIONS···Caring, Mindful, Competent, Compassionate···

16

Requesting Support

You create your opportunities by asking for them.

Shakti Gawain

OBJECTIVES

1. Discuss the relationship between social support and health.
2. Complete a support system assessment.

3. Distinguish between assertive, nonassertive, and aggressive requests for support.
4. Practice making requests for support in selected exercises.

Think about how you will write your answers as you read this chapter.

What?
Write one thing you learned from this chapter.

So What?
How will this affect your nursing practice?

Now What?
How will you implement this new knowledge or skill?

Think About It ...

In a study of nurses' ethical challenges caring for persons with COVID-19, "active control and planning, seeking support as well as catharsis, and staying focused," were useful coping strategies (Jia et al., 2021). How important is being able to ask for what you need?

"Own your own career," is good advice. Some nurses see themselves as just employees. Some students set goals to just "get through" nursing school. In contrast, others set their own goals to develop professionally to make the best of their time in nursing school, and, to do this, they think proactively and are not shy about asking for support. Which nurse

or which student are you? (Laskowski-Jones, 2018). In this chapter you find guidelines to make requests for support in a way that will bring the greatest likelihood of success. You will learn how to be specific about your needs and how to plan an assertive strategy. The exercises will give you the opportunity to practice assertive ways to request support.

RECOGNIZING THE IMPORTANCE OF SOCIAL SUPPORT FOR HEALTH AND WORK LIFE

The literature suggested that a positive relationship exists between the presence of social support and health and coping with illness (Komblith et al., 2001). A study of veterans demonstrated that perceived social support was associated with decreased incidence of posttraumatic stress disorder (Duax, Bohnert, Rauch, & Defever 2014). Stroke survivors with higher perceived levels of social support scored higher on a health-related quality of life instrument (Kruithof, van Mierlo, Visser-Meily, van Heugten, & Powt, 2013). In a study of the work environment of secondary school teachers, coworker support had an inverse relationship to anxiety and depression (Mahan et al., 2010). Employers are looking at ways to support nurses to reduce stress and promote recruitment and retention. The American Nurses Credentialing Center (2014) defined criteria for the selection of healthcare organizations that demonstrate sustained excellence in nursing care in the Magnet Recognition Program by supporting nurses in professional practice. Leaders are encouraged to demonstrate their own compassion and to recognize the economic benefits of institutional compassion in times of trauma.

Self-Care Nudge

Take a breath. What would it mean if you offered yourself compassion? When you are emotionally upset, Tara Brach recommends Radical Compassion to be mindfully present for yourself, and offers the acronym, RAIN: "Recognize what is going on; Allow the experience to be there, just as it is; Investigate with interest and care; Nurture with self-compassion" (Brach, 2022).

What is one way you can be compassionate with yourself as you would with a friend?

DETERMINING THE SUPPORT YOU NEED AT WORK OR SCHOOL

Support is anything that helps you work more effectively and feel better about how you are functioning. Dossey, Luck, & Schaub (2015) in *Nurse Coaching*, define support as "An environment in which assistance is perceived. This can include but is not limited to persons, equipment, faith, organization structure...etc." Conceptualizing support as cognitive, affective, and physical support (CAPS) can help you assess your needs and secure the support you require to work effectively as a nurse.

Cognitive support helps you think intelligently about your job, decide how to approach problems, and discover the how and why of doing things a certain way and provides criteria for doing your work. One method of providing nurses with cognitive support is through mentors. In a study using a mentorship model, newly graduated nurses who were mentored demonstrated a higher level of competency as evaluated by their head nurses than they did in two evaluations before the mentorship (Komaratat & Oumtanee, 2009). Group mentoring, as a cost-effective "best practice model," has been successful with novice nurses (Kostovich & Thurn, 2013). Mentoring may increase a sense of belonging, career optimism, professional growth, competence, and security (Weese, Jakubik, Eliades, & Huth, 2015). At a university in southern Ontario, senior nursing students became role models and resources for other students in relationships that were mutually beneficial (Dennison, 2010; see the section "Looking for a Mentor" later in this chapter).

Affective support is acknowledgment for the work you do and a feeling of nurturance. Nurse managers need continued support and confirmation of their important role in today's world in which nursing practices are changing, clients' conditions are more acute, and recruitment and retention are challenging issues. Mentoring for nurse managers transcends all areas of nursing (Dellasega, 2021). Respect, honor, and recognition of employees by the acknowledgment of positive performance are needed frequently and not only during an annual review. Expressing gratitude and appreciation can create feelings of goodwill and nurturance among nurses, which is a form of job gratification that makes them feel better about their workplaces, clients, and colleagues (Doherty, 2002). Mentoring can also provide affective support. In a study of a mentorship program initiated when the nurse turnover rate increased to 31%, nurses working in inpatient units, surgery, and emergency rooms who participated in a 1-year pilot program had a 0% turnover rate. Three years after the program continued and was expanded to other departments, the hospital staff turnover rate decreased to 10.3% (Fox, 2010).

Physical support is being provided with the staff, materials, and processes needed to get work done. Staffing requirements, which is an essential aspect of physical support, are discussed in the abundance of articles on retention. In this era, the belief is that the provision of adequate cognitive and affective support will attract nurses. The requirements for supplies, equipment, and environmental conveniences have likely been met in most nursing workplaces through technology, computerization, and adherence to stringent occupational hazard and safety regulations.

As nurses, we need to be assertive about securing the support necessary to function comfortably and confidently at work. The clearer we are about the support we need to do our jobs, the more likely we are to secure it. We devote a great deal of energy to attempting to improve the health status of our clients. Getting the support we need to do our work can help us maintain our own health and enhance how we feel about both our work and our coworkers.

Conceptualizing cognitive, affective, and physical components of support provides you with an organizing framework for your individual support assessment. The first step in your systematic approach is to determine whether you are satisfied with the quality and quantity of each facet of support. Quality refers to the nature or characteristics of the support; quantity refers to the amount of support.

Look at the checklist in Box 16.1. Grab a pencil and indicate the pluses and minuses in your support system.

After you have completed this checklist, take note of those areas in which you have the support you need at work or school. It is easy to take for granted the support we have, and noticing the benefits makes us more appreciative.

Next, look at those areas in which the support you would like is not available. Answer the following questions about those instances in which you are not satisfied with the quantity or quality of the support you receive:

BOX 16.1   Credits and Debits in Your Support System

For each cognitive, affective, or physical support item, ask yourself the following:
- Am I satisfied with the quality of support I get to do my job?
- Am I satisfied with the quantity of support I get to do my job?

	Satisfied with:			
	Quality		Quantity	
	Yes	No	Yes	No

Cognitive Support

1. Inspiration: You work with people whose knowledge and skill levels show how you can improve your nursing care.
2. Information: Resources (books, procedural manuals, memoranda, and online information) are available to provide clear information or instruction about relevant nursing procedures.
3. Advice: Colleagues offer expertise and show a willingness to help guide and/or direct you.
4. Challenge: Colleagues intellectually stimulate you by encouraging you to examine, question, and critique your nursing care.
5. Direction: Colleagues exhibit or freely share their philosophies and beliefs about nursing in a way that is helpful to you.

Affective Support

1. Empathy: Colleagues show interest in you and listen to you, and you feel respected and understood.
2. Recognition: Colleagues acknowledge the knowledge and skills you possess, and you are able to make independent decisions and use your talents properly.
3. Praise: Colleagues express admiration for your work and compliment you or show attention and genuine interest in your nursing.
4. Reassurance: Forgiveness for imperfections of omission or commission is offered with acceptance and encouragement for you to continue to do your best nursing.
5. Concern: Colleagues show warm, caring interest in you as a person, and you have a sense that they look forward to working with you; they are concerned for your welfare as a person (not just as a nurse or student).
6. Feedback: Honest, forthright evaluation of your work is offered or is available to you when you ask for it; constructive criticism is given in a straightforward, clear manner and is worded in such a way that you can accept it.
7. Cooperation: Colleagues share ideas with you; there is little greedy competitiveness, and nurses enjoy working together to improve client care.
8. Enthusiasm: Nurses and others are motivated, and the atmosphere is lively; creative ideas to improve nursing care are encouraged.

Physical Support

1. Adequate personnel: Staff with essential knowledge and skills is available to perform the necessary nursing functions.
2. Sharing: When circumstances dictate, colleagues share the workload and help each other; rarely do colleagues avoid helping or refuse to pitch in and lend a hand.
3. Supplies: Sufficient nursing or administrative supplies are consistently available to allow you to smoothly perform your work.
4. Equipment: Equipment on your unit is efficient, in working order, and is easily accessible.
5. Environment: The physical design and decor of your working environment allow you to work without inconvenience, hassles, or unpleasant distractions.

- What exactly dissatisfies me about the quantity or quality of the support?
- If I had a choice, how would I change things to ensure that I receive the support I need?

Be as specific as possible in answering these questions. The clearer and more detailed you can be about the gaps in your support system at work or school, the greater your chances of rectifying the situation. By answering these questions, you indicate your desired outcome.

REQUESTING THE SUPPORT YOU NEED AT WORK OR SCHOOL

The first step is to identify your needs for support. The next step is to decide if you wish to pursue the acquisition of this support. Can you manage without it, or would the presence of that support really enhance your working situation? Once you have decided to try to obtain the support, your next step is to design your strategy. You need to answer the following questions:

- Who is the best person to ask for this support?
- What is the best way to seek this support?
- How can I present my case in a way that increases the probability of securing the support I want at work or school?

THREE STORIES OF SUCCESS: READ WHAT WORKS AND WHAT DOES NOT IN SEEKING THE SUPPORT YOU NEED

Making a Request for Cognitive Support... A Student Approaches the Dean

You are a student nurse in a small college. You and other students have identified problems with writing skills. Points have been taken from papers for poor sentence structure, grammatical errors, and poor organization of content. Although the college has specific courses designated as writing intensive, no formal support is offered to help students with their writing skills. Knowing that several other colleges have writing centers, you decide to approach the dean of your school of nursing with your request.

After making an appointment with the dean, you prepare your strategy for your 20-minute appointment. You must make the dean aware of the problem, how it is affecting the students' ability to be successful in assignments, and the benefit of good writing skills for nursing practice. You want to urge the dean to explore your recommendation for support for students.

You obtain information on comparably sized schools in your region and learn that many of these schools have writing centers with writing tutors. You survey your classmates to see how many have identified a need for improved writing skills. You obtain specific information from your colleagues about how often they have had points subtracted from assigned papers for poor writing skills.

Armed with this information, you next prepare yourself for the interview with the dean. You envision yourself looking relaxed and calm. In your mind's eye, you see yourself presenting your arguments in a clear, straightforward, and assertive manner. You notice how the dean is paying attention to what you are saying and taking notes. You visualize the dean agreeing with your concerns and promising to explore the feasibility of a writing center.

Assertive Approach

The following is an example of how your interview with the dean might go if you were assertive.

Assertive you: *"Thank you for seeing me, Dr. Thomas. I want to talk to you about students' concerns about problems with writing skills and how this is affecting course performance."*

Dr. Thomas: *"Oh? Is that the case? Can you tell me any more about the situation?"*

Assertive you: *"Yes, I can. Although we have writing-intensive courses and faculty tell us writing skills are important for our success, our school has no writing center for individual assistance and for tutoring. I have checked with other schools of comparable size in this region and have a list of those with on-campus writing centers. I have surveyed the student body and have responses that indicate how many students are affected by the problem. I have made a copy of the information I have compiled that you may keep"* [hands Dr. Thomas a well-organized information packet]. *"We are excited about the quality of education we are getting here and think we have identified a resource that would help support that."*

Dr. Thomas: *"I can't argue with your facts. You have certainly done your homework. Your suggestion sounds like a good solution to the situation. I certainly want our students to have access to help with writing skills. I assure you that I will bring the matter up at the next faculty meeting. We have been talking about this and exploring online writing labs, too. Your concern and initiative on behalf of the students to get the support you need are impressive. We have a faculty meeting this week. I'll share your data and get back to you in 1 week. Thank you for bringing this important matter to my attention."*

Your assertive approach has brought the students' concerns to the dean's attention. By thanking Dr. Thomas for seeing you, you showed your respect for her busy schedule.

You reinforced your awareness by getting right to the point of your visit. Your acknowledgment of the assets of your school library indicated to the dean that you were appreciative of the positive resources available and were not just complaining. You clearly outlined the situation and respectfully offered a possible solution. Your research and approach to the dean helped you present your needs and provided data to increase the possibility that the cognitive support requested could be provided.

In contrast to this assertive approach, you could have used a nonassertive or aggressive approach with the dean. Let us examine the consequences of both of these less-effective approaches.

Nonassertive Approach

When we act nonassertively in any situation, we come across as unsure, undecided, and without confidence. These nonassertive qualities give others the message that we do not expect to receive what we are seeking. Messages of uncertainty work against us by putting doubts about our requests in the minds of potential providers. Here is an example of a nonassertive approach:

Nonassertive you: *"I appreciate your seeing me, Dr. Thomas. It's about bad grades on papers. Uh, did you know that we have trouble with our written work?"*

Dr. Thomas: *"What's this about bad grades on papers? What's the problem?"*

Nonassertive you: *"Well, I'm not the only one who has had points taken off for poor grammar and stuff. It's quite a problem, you see…I mean, I don't know what to do. I thought I could write okay."*

Dr. Thomas: *"Yes, I know some students have problems with grammar. But I don't understand what the problem is."*

Nonassertive you: *"Well, you see, that's just the problem. We get points taken off for writing skills and we think we should be able to have some help with that from someone on campus."*

Dr. Thomas: *"Well, how big a problem is this?"*

Nonassertive you: *"Well, last week I got a 'C' on a paper. Others are complaining, too."*

Dr. Thomas: *"If you want my assistance, I need to know more about how many students are affected by this problem to see if any action is necessary. I'll be happy to look into this matter when you provide me with the information to do so."*

When we are nonassertive, we are asking to have our requests for support ignored. In this example, you were not armed with the information you needed to convince Dr. Thomas of the importance of the problem. Your content was not delivered in an objective, forthright manner. Because of your style, delivery, and preparation, being nonassertive lost your case.

Let us look at an aggressive approach.

Aggressive Approach

When we are aggressive, we go after what we want in a way that is upsetting, disrespectful, or threatening to others. When we attack other people to get what we want, we create bad feelings that take considerable energy and time to overcome.

Here is an example of an aggressive approach:

Aggressive you: *"Thanks for seeing me, Dr. Thomas. You've just got to do something about our getting points taken off of papers for writing skills. I'm fed up with having no help. Other schools have tutors for students. They have writing centers. We pay a lot of tuition. It's not fair we don't get help. How would you like to be punished for something you don't know how to do?"*

Dr. Thomas: *"I can see you are upset about this, and it sounds quite important. When you have calmed down and can talk to me rationally about the problem, I'll be glad to meet with you."*

Being aggressive did not get you what you were seeking, but it did create an unpleasant relationship between you and your dean. Now there are two problems. When we are aggressive, we are often out of control and do not present our arguments in a logical, clear way. A rational, well-planned, assertive approach is more likely to secure the needed support and maintain a good relationship with the person whose help we are seeking.

SIMPLIFY AND DEEPEN

What are ways you can be more supportive to co-workers, other students, or people in your personal life? Find one way today.

Making a Request for Affective Support… A Student Approaches Classmates about Toxic Competition for Grades

You are a senior nursing student. You have noticed that as each academic quarter begins, your colleagues are becoming more and more competitive about grades. When grades are posted, students converge on the posting and hover around, checking out how each student did. Some students are very upset or depressed for days if they receive anything less than a B+.

There is less sharing of articles, ideas, and material that would help colleagues do well on assignments. Students are starting to hoard materials, hoping that another person will not do well if the material is not easily accessible. Trying to get the academic edge is the name of the game, and it has resulted in bickering, unfriendliness, and backbiting. You are aware of the loss of cooperation among your colleagues. This situation leaves you feeling isolated and bereft, and you sense it makes others feel that way, too.

You decide to try to rectify or reverse the situation. After giving the matter some thought, you decide that the best strategy is to get your closest colleagues together and raise your concerns. Having the entire group present would provide more influence than trying to reach each person individually. You decide to invite your group over for coffee, with the plan to bring up your agenda.

In preparation, you think through how you will approach the topic. You decide to allow some time for chitchat and for everyone to get reacquainted. You plan to have coffee and snacks to break the ice and get everyone mixing. You decide that the best way to broach the subject is to begin with your feelings of loss. You do not want the discussion to disintegrate into a gripe session, so you come up with several suggestions that the group could consider.

In addition to planning the content, you spend time preparing yourself emotionally for the meeting with your fellow students. You envision yourself and your colleagues looking relaxed. You imagine that when you raise the issue of lack of cooperative support, your classmates will look interested and agree with your assessment of the situation. In your mind's eye, others look eager to return to more cooperative ways of relating to each other, and there are even suggestions from the group members.

When you are prepared, you carry out your plan. The following is what an assertive approach to your request for support might be like.

Assertive Approach

After your colleagues have enjoyed getting reacquainted, you bring up your issue in the following way:

> Assertive you: *"I'm really enjoying seeing all of you again. It's like old times. Something I've noticed as we get further along in the program is that we are becoming more obsessed with grades. It's really bothering me that we don't share ideas and materials the way we used to. It's as if we are all operating in isolation—each student for herself. It's too cutthroat for me. I'd like to propose that we restart our weekly study group so that we can share our ideas and knowledge as well as our books and articles. I think we could really help each other, and*

> *it would make us feel more like we were in this thing together instead of in competition. What do you think?"*
>
> Colleague: *"I think it's a great idea. I've been feeling lonely for our shared times, but I guess I just assumed you guys were so 'nose to the grindstone' that you didn't need our group support. I'd love to start meeting again."*
>
> Another colleague: *"I think it would be a good idea to make a list of the projects that we are working on and circulate it. Then when we find articles on someone's topic, we could let the person know. It wouldn't take any more time, and it would really help us all out."*
>
> Another colleague: *"I'm house sitting for my brother, and he has a huge dining room table that we could use for our meetings."*

Your assertive strategy worked. By putting effort into setting the scene and allowing the opportunity for people to realize how much they had missed each other, you furthered your cause immensely. By expressing your feelings, you avoided blaming anyone. Including a suggestion got the ball rolling and gave others a chance to present their ideas. It is likely that your strategy has set things in motion for securing the cooperative support you were after.

Consider how things might have gone if you had chosen a nonassertive approach.

Nonassertive Approach

When we are nonassertive, at some level we are conveying the feeling that we do not have much faith in ourselves or our ideas. If we are not able to convey that we believe strongly in what we are saying, it is highly unlikely that we will convince anyone else. Being nonassertive involves little advance preparation and little visualization of positive outcomes. When we are nonassertive, we look unsure and sound hesitant.

Here is what your strategy might have been like if you had taken a nonassertive approach.

You invite your colleagues over for coffee, and sooner or later the conversation rolls around to school and grades. Soon everyone is comparing how they are doing on their assignments, and an uncomfortable atmosphere of competition surfaces. You attempt to intervene as follows:

> Nonassertive you: *"Uh, this is the kind of thing I find so disappointing…I mean, all we ever talk about anymore is grades and who's got an A."*
>
> Colleague: *"Well, it's only natural. That's what we're here for. Grades are the most important things in our lives as students."*
>
> Nonassertive you: *"Well, they are important, I agree. But so is feeling good and sharing things with friends."*
>
> Colleague: *"Yes, but when we get good grades, that's the thing that makes us feel good these days."*

Nonassertive you: *"Well, I was wondering if we could help each other out more, like we used to do. Don't you ever long to get our study group together?"*

Colleague: *"Those days were fun. Now, though, we hardly take any of the same subjects. I'm afraid it would take more time and energy than I've got to get us together and make it time well spent."*

Nonassertion got you nowhere except feeling more discouraged about the situation. By not presenting a positive, concrete solution to your complaints, you missed an opportunity to influence your colleagues' outlook on the situation. You avoided emphasizing the benefits of sharing, and, consequently, your colleagues swayed the argument to the negative aspects of meeting. Not only did you fail to obtain cooperation, but you are likely feeling disappointed in your lack of assertiveness.

Consider how the scene might change if you were aggressive.

Aggressive Approach

Although we may get what we want when we are aggressive, we lose out on the good feelings between ourselves and the other person. Sometimes the bad feelings generated by aggressiveness take extensive time to repair.

Here is one possible scenario if you were to use an aggressive approach:

Aggressive you: *"Come on, you guys, stop talking about school and grades. I've had enough of it. You've got your heads buried so deeply in the books that you can't even take time to have fun. I remember when you used to be a fun group to be with. Now I get the feeling that if anyone does well, it's like stealing points from someone else. When are you going to wake up and realize that those little numbers on your papers aren't nearly as important as having some contact as people?"*

Colleague: *"Well, you may not care about grades, but I do. I might want to go to graduate school someday, and my grades have to be good. You don't even take that into consideration."*

Another colleague: *"If you can't even see how important school is to some of us, then there's no point in getting together. I think we're on different wavelengths."*

By being aggressive, you have further ostracized yourself from your colleagues. Your demonstration of insensitivity about the value your friends put on school has cost you their cooperation. By not seeing things through their eyes, you have lost your connection to a valuable source of support.

Making a Request for Physical Support…A New Nurse Manager Needs Help

You are a new nurse manager working on a surgical unit in a general hospital. You have 20 staff members whose evaluations are due in 2 weeks. You are working to make sure staff has as much detailed feedback as possible to begin to improve work habits. Together you will need to discuss goals and plans for improvement. You share your office with several other nurse managers. You have no private space to conduct evaluations. Meeting in the cafeteria or public space does not offer respectful privacy. To successfully conduct these evaluation meetings, you need the physical support of adequate private space.

You have identified what dissatisfies you about the lack of private space; now you need to decide how you would like to see things changed. You know there is absolutely no possibility of getting a room designated for evaluations because of budget cutbacks. What would be satisfactory is a room that could be booked in advance for an evaluation and used for other purposes as well. There is a room on the unit that is designated for Dr. Gait, the physician in charge of the unit. She makes rounds each morning and occasionally uses her room then, but at other times it is not used by anyone. You decide to attempt to secure access to Dr. Gait's office for the purpose of completing employee evaluations. It is important to have the privacy, and you are certain that you and the staff can do better problem solving without distractions.

Having decided to seek support, the next step is to determine how to go about acquiring it. The interpersonal style you use to make your request will greatly influence the outcome. A meek or indirect approach leaves you open to being misunderstood or ignored. An aggressive or overly confrontational presentation will put others on the defensive and likely result in rejection. A balance of speaking up for your rights for support without hurting others is what the situation requires.

You already know that the other nurse managers agree that a private space is necessary. The lines of communication on the unit dictate that you should make your request to the head nurse. You decide that she needs some advance notice about the issue, and you approach her with a request for a meeting time to discuss the issue. Your request for a meeting is simple, straightforward, and clear:

Assertive you: *"Ms. Peters, I would like to make an appointment with you to discuss the need for some private space in which to conduct evaluations. I'm on duty for the next 3 days. Do you have about 15 or 20 minutes during that time when I can discuss this matter with you?"*

Once the meeting has been arranged, you need to plan your strategy. You have asked for about 15 minutes, during which time you must convince Ms. Peters of the importance of having a private place to interview clients. You prepare for the meeting by itemizing all the reasons you and your colleagues have concerning the need for privacy. You are well aware that you will have more success in getting your request granted if you can present a reasonable solution, so you itemize the reasons for using Dr. Gait's office.

Having secured your facts, you are now ready for your encounter with Ms. Peters. You prepare by visualizing yourself talking to her in a relaxed, confident manner. In your mind's eye, you envision her listening to you intently, nodding her head in agreement with the points you are making. You imagine yourself successfully counteracting any arguments she has against the use of Dr. Gait's office. All in all, your mental rehearsal of the meeting is successful, which increases your confidence.

Here is an example of how your meeting with your head nurse, Ms. Peters, might go if you were assertive.

Assertive Approach

Assertive you: *"Thank you for setting aside the time to meet with me, Ms. Peters. As you know, I wish to discuss the need for some private space to complete staff evaluations. I've talked to the other nurse managers, and we all agree evaluation conferences can provide valuable information for staff and leadership.*

However, there is one major problem we have encountered. There is no designated space for us to conduct the evaluations, so we end up in the corridor, the nurse's station, or the coffee shop; in all these locations, what we say can be overheard by other clients and staff. We are concerned that some staff may hold back information about themselves that might be important because of embarrassment and lack of confidentiality. We would like to have a room where we could meet in private.

A little checking shows that Dr. Gait rarely uses her office in the afternoons. The other nurse managers and I suggest that Dr. Gait's office might be a place we could use. What do you think of this idea?"

Ms. Peters: *"I can see your point about the privacy. As you know, I'm interested in having staff evaluations done as comfortably as possible, so I would like to push for a room if the privacy will mean staff will be open. In the past Dr. Gait has wanted her office off-limits to nurses because she has done her dictating and teaching to her residents in there. But from what you are saying, she doesn't use the office for those purposes anymore. I will talk to her about making her office available to*

our nursing managers in the afternoons. Thank you for your interest and your suggestions."

Your assertive strategy worked. Your reasons for needing a private room were sound. Your astute inclusion of the data about the vacancy of Dr. Gait's office added credibility to your suggestion. You ended your suggestion by respectfully asking for the head nurse's opinion. Your delivery was forthright. Never once did you beat around the bush or sound hesitant. You did not even have to rush because you had already made an appointment with your head nurse.

Here are some examples of ineffective ways to make the same request for a private room.

Nonassertive Approach

When we are nonassertive, we do not give full credit to our needs. We act shy or make light of factors that are really important to us. When we avoid expressing ourselves clearly and forthrightly, we waive control over our legitimate rights. Being nonassertive invites others to walk all over us.

In this situation, a nonassertive nurse would not likely book time with her manager but would hope that she could catch the head nurse's attention without advance notice. Nonassertive nurses would not likely plan an effective strategy in advance and would not envision themselves being successful. Verbally nonassertive approaches are limp and unclear, and they do not convey confidence or conviction. Here is an example of nonassertion:

Nonassertive you: *"Uh, Ms. Peters, do you have a few minutes?"*

Ms. Peters has no idea what you want to talk to her about nor how long it will take. If she is a typically busy head nurse, she will probably have other things planned for that moment.

Ms. Peters: *"I can see you briefly. What is it about?"*
Nonassertive you: *"Well, it's about the evaluations I have to give staff. I think it's rather hard…I mean, sometimes there are so many people around. It's hard to talk to staff when there's no privacy, do you know what I mean? Something's really got to be done, I think."*

It is possible that this approach may put Ms. Peters on the defensive. By not finishing your sentence you have given the impression that completing evaluations is difficult. You have provided no rationale for the idea that privacy is essential. By not clearly explaining your points, you are ensuring that Ms. Peters will not understand and, consequently, will not be sympathetic to your cause.

Ms. Peters: *"Well, I realize that it might be difficult to do evaluations, but it's essential that the conferences be held in a timely manner. Client care depends on effective staff."*

Nonassertive you: *"Uh, yes…it is important. It's just that, you know, it's hard to talk to staff when there are other people around. Isn't there a quiet place we could go to? How about Dr. Gait's office?"*

Ms. Peters: *"Well, you know that she needs her office to be available to her. You can always use a quiet corner of the sunroom or even ask clients to leave the room if you want to have to meet with a staff member."*

Nonassertive you: *"Yeah…I guess so. I haven't tried that yet. Maybe that'll work…I hate to ask a client to leave…but I'll give it a try."*

You have lost your case. By not being clear about what you wanted and not defending your suggestion, you have permitted your manager to overlook your suggestion and not understand your valid concerns. Had you better prepared your defense and your speech, you might have secured the support you were requesting.

Aggressive Approach

When we behave aggressively, we forget to give due respect to the other person's rights. We become so intent on getting what we want that we tend to bulldoze the other person. Here is an example of an aggressive approach to trying to secure a private place for interviewing:

Aggressive you: *"Ms. Peters, I need to see you as soon as possible about my evaluations. When can you see me? Today?"*

This rush on Ms. Peters does not give her much breathing space. You have indicated there is urgency about your need to see her that is out of proportion to the truth. In no way have you respected her own timetable or any agenda she may wish to complete. She is probably already on the defensive.

When you get to see Ms. Peters, you begin as follows:

Aggressive you: *"You've got to do something about getting us a quiet place to do these evaluations if you want them done right. It's impossible to do them when everyone can hear what you are saying. How would you like to have someone tell you your work needs improvement when every client and staff member around can hear? If you don't get us a quiet place, then they just won't be done right. Why can't we use Dr. Gait's office? This one doctor has a whole office to herself, even when she's not around."*

Ms. Peters: *"It's not up to you to dictate how the office space will be assigned on the unit. When you've learned proper etiquette and protocol, I'd be glad to discuss this issue with you. In the meantime, do the best you can. That'll be all for today."*

You have made your dissatisfaction very clear. In the process of doing so, however, you have put your manager on the defensive and created a rift between you. There are now two problems to be solved: the lack of privacy and the discord between the two of you. When you attack other people, they are likely to divert energy to their injured feelings instead of attending to the issue for which you are fighting. Using an aggressive approach diminishes the chances that you will secure the physical support you were hoping to get.

Planning an Assertive Strategy for Making Requests

The preceding examples illustrate the importance of planning and implementing an assertive strategy for seeking cognitive, affective, or physical support. If it is important for you to have the support you have identified, then it is important to invest the time and energy to secure it. As a nurse, you spend considerable energy trying to meet your clients' needs for support. If you can secure the support you need at work or school, then it is more likely that you will have the energy to extend support to your clients and colleagues. Nurses who keep on giving without adequate cognitive, affective, or physical support are draining their own reserves. We spend a great deal of time trying to get our clients to take care of their health; securing the support we need as nurses provides them with an example to follow.

Just because you use an assertive approach does not mean that you will get the support you seek. Sometimes support is not forthcoming, no matter what strategy is used. On occasion your colleagues may not have the interest or skills to support you. Other times there may not be the money or time to provide you with the support you are seeking. At those times you must decide whether you can continue to work in the system without the support. If you cannot secure the support you need from others at work or school, you may be able to get some support from friends or family to see you through. Only you can decide whether the support is adequate. Because you are the seeker and receiver, it is your perception of the support that is important.

Providing Support at Work and School

The cognitive, affective, physical support (CAPS) framework is helpful for articulating exactly what support you need at work and school. It also can be a guideline to help you determine your colleagues' need for support. Support is a nebulous concept; breaking it down into cognitive, affective, and physical components helps you to decipher your colleagues' needs for support. One way to obtain support is to offer it to others. In so doing, a bond is built between you that encourages both parties to give and take. Contributing to the effort to build a solid support system at work and school will add to your feelings of confidence and competence. It is worth the effort to learn the assertive way to make requests for the support you need.

LOOKING FOR A MENTOR

What can a mentor offer (see Box 16.2.)? McMahon (2005) described her first 6 months as a new nurse as a difficult time during which she felt she had to prove herself in a hostile environment without support. Yet when she confided in a nurse from another unit whose leadership skills she admired, she found herself in her first mentoring situation. She had expressed her thoughts and feelings and opened the door to get just the support she needed to grow into her new role. How did she do this? She identified her problem, assessed who was a safe person with whom she could discuss the issue, expressed her thoughts and feelings, and built a rapport with someone who was able to mentor her.

As a new nurse, consider trying to find a mentor through professional associations and networking at organization events. Pay attention to nurses whose work and practice you admire. In my career as a student and professional, I have consistently reached out to classmates or staff from whom I could learn and consistently offered assistance to others. As an entrepreneur, asking for what I need and joining appropriate organizations has helped me. Whenever I have moved, I searched other holistic nurses from my membership in the American Holistic Nursing Association in my community and one by one taken them to lunch. From that evolved the development of a nursing business, speaking engagements, faculty positions, and a contact that led to my expressive arts bedside work in hospice. You never know

---

BOX 16.2   What Can a Mentor Offer?

Knowledge, skills, wisdom from experience, and a love of nursing
A trusted patient relationship to support your growth
Coaching, motivation, energy, advocacy, and nurturing
Compassion and generosity
Mutual sharing of resources
Celebration of your success

---

until you ask! Make yourself known so when opportunities arise, you will come to mind.

Consider, too, what qualities you have and can develop that would make you a good mentor as you develop your professional career. Look for "teachable moments" that you can use to teach others. As you move and grow in comfort with your knowledge and skills, consider how you can offer support to new graduates or nurses new to your work setting. Invite a colleague to a professional association meeting. Share a journal article or start a journal club at work to discuss evidence-based practice or topics of mutual interest. Help another nurse submit an article or prepare a presentation for a conference (Laskowski-Jones, 2018).

Ulrich and Ulrich (2010), in their book, *The Why of Work*, challenged us to look for meaning in our work, to look for opportunities to use our talents to pursue our aspirations, and to work synergistically with others with creativity, resilience, hope, and resourcefulness in a work environment in which we can all thrive. To be able to do this, you must identify what you need to enable you to do your best work and seek the support needed. Look for ways to incorporate skills you want to grow at work and interests you have that might add value in the work setting, making it more likely colleagues will support you. Perhaps you have organization skills or computer skills that might be useful in problem solving. This process, called *job crafting,* may help you and others embellish the work with individual gifts and talents (Wrzesniewski, Berg, & Dutton, 2010). Remember, we are all in this together.

Return to "Active Learning" at the beginning of the chapter and write your responses.

PRACTICING REQUESTING SUPPORT

Video Reflection: Exercise 1

View the 3-minute video *Do Nurses Ask for Help?* for a light-hearted example that poses the real question for nurses. After you watch the video, with another student or colleague, reflect on when and why you hesitate to ask for help you need in your personal and professional life (see https://www.youtube.com/watch?v=ZuPD3m920VY).

Self-Assessment and Reflection: Exercise 2

Consider your personal support system. Make a list of people, relatives, and friends whom you might be able to ask for support. Write a journal entry about strengths and weaknesses in your personal support system. Identify what support you might need and what support you might be able to offer others. If you have difficulty asking others for help, consider a quote from a cancer patient in an I Can

Cope cancer support program. "When you refuse to ask others to help, you deny them the pleasure you get when you are able to help another."

Professional Development: Exercise 3

Identify a nursing specialty of interest to you. Search online for journals or organizations related to that specialty. Search for local chapter meetings or LinkedIn for professionals in that specialty. Consider how you can use such resources for networking.

Quality and Safety Education for Nurses Competencies: Teamwork and Collaboration; Safety: Exercise 4 QSEN

Being aware of the environment includes an awareness of your own limitations as well as recognizing the capacity of those around you. Effective teams "watch each other's backs." Mutual support is an important teamwork behavior and requires knowing our own limitations in delivering safe care and maintaining a watchful eye across the team. Write a reflective case study at the end of your clinical experience, guided by the following:

- Identify instances in which you felt you needed assistance in completing care assigned to you.
- Which team member did you ask to assist you?
- What influenced your decision to ask this person?
- How can you improve your self-awareness to recognize your limitations to provide care within a safety zone but also continue to expand your learning and expertise?
- What is your response when you notice another team member needs assistance?
- How does the concept of mutual support influence a culture of safety?

🌱 MOMENTS OF CONNECTION...
The Loss of a Cat, a Friend, a Companion

A nurse was finding it hard to concentrate at work and was often moved to tears. "I was just on overload. My husband had just asked for a divorce. I was worried about being a single parent and how I would survive financially. It was just so overwhelming. Then we had to have our cat put to sleep because of massive cancer. I knew only one person would really understand: the oncology supervisor. She responded right away when I told her about the cat. She's an animal lover, too. I made an appointment to see her on my lunch break. She listened and really knew my grief was just compounded. It's like losing a child. She didn't make fun of me. She is so special."

WIT AND WISDOM
Why Not?
Marion was a hospice client whose speech was limited after having had a stroke. One thing she could clearly say was, "Why not?" She would say it with a different voice inflection depending on what she was trying to communicate. It became almost a life philosophy. Take a risk...ask for what you want and need...allow others to have an opportunity to help you...you might just be surprised... "Why not?"

REFERENCES

American Nurses Credentialing Center. (2014). *Magnet application manual.* Silver Spring, MD: American Nurses Credentialing Center.

Brach, T. (2022). RAIN: A practice of radical compassion. https://www.tarabrach.com/rain-practice-radical-compassion/.

Dellasega, C. (2021). *Toxic nursing: Managing bullying, bad attitudes, and total turmoil.* Indianapolis, IN: Sigma Theta Tau International.

Dennison, S. (2010). Peer mentoring: Untapped potential. *Journal of Nursing Education, 49*(6), 340.

Doherty, R. (2002). Tune up your employee retention efforts. *Healthcare Review, 15*(6), 11.

Dossey, B., Luck, S., & Schaub, B. G. (2015). *Nurse coaching: Integrative approaches for health and wellbeing.* North Miami, FL: International Nurse Coach Association.

Duax, J. M., Bohnert, K. M., Rauch, S. A. M., & Defever, A. M. (2014). Posttraumatic stress disorder symptoms, levels of social support, and emotional hiding in returning veterans. *Journal of Rehabilitation Research and Development, 51*(4), 571.

Fox, K. C. (2010). Mentor program boosts new nurses' satisfaction and lowers turnover rate. *Journal of Continuing Education in Nursing, 41*(7), 311.

Jia, Y., Chen, O., Xiao, Z., Xiao, J., Bian, J., & Jia, H. (2021). Nurses' ethical challenges caring for people with COVID-19: A qualitative study. *Nursing Ethics, 28*(2), 33–45. https://doi.org/10.1177/0969733020944453.

Komaratat, S., & Oumtanee, A. (2009). Using a mentorship model to prepare newly graduated nurses for competency. *Journal of Continuing Education in Nursing, 40*(10), 475.

Komblith, A. B., Herndon, J. E., II, Zuckerman, E., Viscoli, C. M., Horwitz, R. I., Cooper, M. R., et al. (2001). Social support as a buffer to the psychological impact of stressful life events in women with breast cancer. *Cancer, 91*(2), 443.

Kostovich, C. T., & Thurn, K. E. (2013). Group mentoring: A story of transition for undergraduate baccalaureate nursing students. *Nurse Education Today, 33*, 413.

Kruithof, W. J., van Mierlo, M. L., Visser-Meily, J. M. A., van Heugten, C. M., & Powt, M. W. (2013). Associations between social support and stroke survivors' health-related quality of life: A systematic review. *Patient Education and Counseling, 93*(2), 169.

Laskowski-Jones, L. (2018). Own your nursing career. *Nursing, 48*(1), 6.

Mahan, P. L., Mahan, M. P., Park, N., Shelton, C., Brown, K. C., & Weaver, M. T. (2010). Work environment stressors, social support, anxiety, and depression among secondary school teachers. *American Association of Occupational Health Nurses Journal, 58*(5), 197.

McMahon, L. (2005). Mentoring: A means of healing new nurses. *Holistic Nursing Practice, 19*(5), 195.

Ulrich, D., & Ulrich, W. (2010). *The why of work*. New York, NY: McGraw-Hill.

Weese, M. M., Jakubik, L. D., Eliades, A. B., & Huth, J. J. (2015). Mentoring practices benefiting pediatric nurses. *Journal of Pediatric Nursing, 30*(2), 385–394.

Wrzesniewski, A., Berg, J. M., & Dutton, J. E. (2010). Turn the job you have into the job you want. *Harvard Business Review, 88*(6), 127.

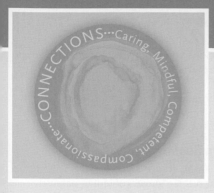

CONNECTIONS···Caring, Mindful, Competent, Compassionate···

17

Overcoming Evaluation Anxiety

Courage is fear holding on a minute longer.

George S. Patton

OBJECTIVES

1. Define evaluation anxiety.
2. Describe characteristics of evaluation anxiety.
3. Identify strategies to handle job performance appraisals assertively.
4. Discuss techniques to decrease test anxiety.
5. Identify benefits of criticism.
6. Identify assertive strategies to handle difficult situations in student performance evaluations.
7. Participate in exercises to overcome evaluation anxiety.

🔋 ACTIVE LEARNING

Think about how you will write your answers as you read this chapter.

What?
Write one thing you learned from this chapter.

So What?
How will this affect your nursing practice?

Now What?
How will you implement this new knowledge or skill?

Think About It ...

Healthcaring nursing students are presented with what can seem an overwhelming amount of content, often practice self-negligence instead of self-care, and fear harming patients if their performance is not perfect. Wadi, Yusoff, Rahim, & Lah (2022), conducting a qualitative study of factors affecting test anxiety in medical students, parallel the experience of nursing students.

DEFINING EVALUATION ANXIETY

When you are anxious, take 1 minute to take a deep breath and notice the air moving in and out of your chest. Notice your body's sensations, the air around you, and listen to the sound of your breathing (Devney, 2018). You will learn more about relaxation and guided imagery for relief of anxiety in Chapters 19 and 20.

Reflect on the old saying, "To err is human." Yes, it applies to all of us. We know this and yet we still think we have to be perfect. Students are asked to participate in simulation and role-play, which is experiential learning that can cause anxiety that interferes with critical thinking (Diaz, Panosky, & Shelton, 2014; Hutchinson & Goodin, 2013). In our competitive culture, we idolize excellence in personal performance, products, and services. Making mistakes is the antithesis of our cultural standard for excellence. Because of our preoccupation with perfection, it is difficult to believe that making mistakes is a normal part of human endeavor. We face these unrealistic expectations whenever we are in a situation in which our knowledge, skills, and behavior must be evaluated. In this chapter you will learn how to approach evaluations, test taking, and criticism in more positive ways so you can learn from them. These approaches will help you as a student and throughout your career as a nurse.

Evaluation anxiety occurs when we are upset about having our performance judged and are intimidated by the evaluation process. We cannot directly control others' responses to our work, and overvaluing the responses of others creates a kind of anxiety that interferes with

175

performing at our best. One form of evaluation anxiety is test anxiety, which has negative effects on academic performance. For nursing students, test anxiety can be evident in both written examinations and evaluations of clinical proficiency (Boggs, Shields, & Goodin, 2011). Instead of focusing on relevant parts of a task, students with high test anxiety worry about how they are performing and how well others are doing and ruminate about alternatives (Meichenbaum, 1972). High test anxiety is associated with intrusion of irrelevant thoughts such as preoccupation with feelings of inadequacy, anticipation of punishment, and loss of status and esteem.

Accompanying these cognitive aspects of test anxiety are emotionality; the autonomic arousal aspect of anxiety; and a variety of physical symptoms including increased heart rate, increased muscular tension, gastrointestinal changes, changes in breathing, and dietary and sleep pattern disturbances (Meichenbaum, 1972). These physiologic symptoms are distressing and must be alleviated just as much as negative thought processes. Learning to relax and decrease unpleasant symptoms helps diminish their negative effects.

One of the most significant and recurring problems experienced by health professionals is a fear of making a mistake and being evaluated negatively. Clinicians in practice have revealed fears about committing errors in diagnosis or treatment. Nursing students and nurses, too, fear making mistakes.

Examples of other nursing situations that engender anxiety in students are the initial clinical experience on a unit, nursing procedures, hospital equipment, patient simulators, evaluation by faculty, observation by instructors, tardiness, and conversations with physicians (Kaplan & Ura, 2010; Moscaritolo, 2010).

The two major factors underlying our evaluation anxiety as nurses are concern for client safety and concern for our own security.

> **WIT AND WISDOM**
> *No Knowing, No Growing*
> It's safe to perform
> Your tasks, do your duty.
> Look inside yourself
> And see only beauty.
> Have you the courage
> To ask for inspection?
> Can you face hearing
> You're less than perfection?
> Have you learned yet
> We're better for knowing?
> To take bad with good,
> A chance to keep growing.

Concern for Client Safety

Nursing involves caring for the health of fellow human beings. Health is a precious commodity, which makes the stakes high if a nursing error negatively effects our clients' health or pushes them into illness. This responsibility underlies our anxiety about making an error in our nursing practice.

Concern for Our Own Security

Clients are becoming more knowledgeable and critical about healthcare and its cost. No longer content to passively submit to treatment, consumers of healthcare are demanding to know the rationale for regimens and to have access to a second opinion. In extreme cases clients are suing physicians and other healthcare professionals, including nurses, for ineffective healthcare. This potential threat from clients represents a powerful source of disapproval, with implications for career advancement and public embarrassment. The loss of your job and financial assets could also result from unsafe care. Today, nurses are aware of their accountability for the nursing care provided and their vulnerability to investigations of these actions through the legal process.

Evaluation anxiety is an unpleasant, ever-lurking phenomenon that threatens nurses and other health professionals. As nurses, we are committed to making a positive difference for our clients, yet today's work environments are loaded with potential deterrents to this goal: inadequate staffing, the more acute health conditions of clients, technological complexity, information overload, and the uncertainty of healthcare reform. In its mildest form, evaluation anxiety can detract from enjoyment in the workplace; when strong, it can be overwhelming and interfere with our ability to perform competently as nurses.

As nursing students or as practicing registered nurses, we need to develop ways to minimize evaluation anxiety so that we can confidently handle clinical or written examinations, job performance appraisals, and everyday criticisms, all of which are naturally recurring events in the professional life of nurses.

Characteristics of Evaluation Anxiety

People who suffer from evaluation anxiety exhibit ways of thinking that make them feel uneasy and interfere with their ability to perform in adaptive ways. Those experiencing evaluation anxiety have been reported in the literature to have the following characteristics (Dweck & Wortman, 1982; Wine, 1982):

- *Self-focus versus task focus.* Some people spend more time thinking about their performance than they do completing the actual task. Attention to their performance detracts from the necessary attention needed to

TABLE 17.1 Constructive and Destructive Self-Thoughts

Constructive Thoughts	Destructive Thoughts
"I'm doing a good job. I can't do everything I'd like to do for my clients today because we're short-staffed, but I'll make sure I do the most important things."	"I've got to do everything for my clients or I'll feel like a failure." "If I don't do everything just perfectly, I'll be letting down my clients and the rest of the team."
"I've done the important things I can for the clients on the unit. Now I'll prepare a concise report for the evening staff."	"How can I possibly explain to the evening staff that I didn't get everything done on the day shift? They'll think I'm incompetent and disorganized."
"One thing I didn't make arrangements for was an extra load of linen for the evening staff. Now that I know you have to put your order in before 1 p.m., I won't forget in the future."	"They're going to crucify me for not arranging an extra load of linen. They'll be mad at me for days for that mistake."
"I can go home knowing I did the best I could today. It was very busy, and we were short-staffed this evening, but we gave our clients the best care we could under the circumstances."	"What a day! All I can think about is what still needs to be done. I'll be miserable mulling over how I could have done things better."

do the task adequately. Self-focused thoughts are negative and self-devaluing, and they lead to self-doubt. Not only does a focus on self versus task detract from task performance, but the focus on negative aspects of one's performance engenders feelings of anxiety.

- *Self-blame.* Some people with evaluation anxiety tend to blame themselves for their poor performance more than they blame circumstances or other external factors.
- *Worry and concern about evaluation.* People with high evaluation anxiety tend to place great emphasis on how they are doing compared with others and how the examiner is evaluating them.

Those with low evaluation anxiety react to performance evaluation with an external, situational, task-oriented focus. For those with high evaluation anxiety, failure signifies a lack of ability. Those with low evaluation anxiety generate thoughts about the task or situation that encourage solutions or completion of the task, whereas those with high evaluation anxiety give up and see themselves as the main reason for failure.

High-anxiety individuals do not fully explore options such as trying different strategies or looking for an external causative factor, which leaves them with feelings of failure and uneasiness. Mistakes are interpreted as failures and not as stepping stones in the process of discovering the best solution. People with high performance anxiety tend to attribute success to factors other than their own ability, yet they readily assume that failure is their own doing. This view leads to feelings of pressure in every new achievement situation (Dweck & Wortman, 1982; Wine, 1982). Consider, too, the effect of past negative experiences on the evaluation process. Students and nurses with previous work experience who have had a traumatic incident in performance appraisal may have so much anxiety that the process is highly emotionally charged (Marquis & Huston, 1998). It is useful to spend some time reflecting on your fears and worries to determine how realistic they are.

In our culture it is easy to berate ourselves when we make a mistake. In addition to our self-chastisement, we sometimes invent disapproval or exaggerate the disapproval of others. How we internally evaluate ourselves can be constructive or destructive.

Examples of constructive and destructive thoughts in relation to being evaluated are given in Table 17.1.

Gaining Control over Your Evaluation Anxiety

Students who are afraid of evaluation are rendered incapable of engaging with a topic of learning and seeing it from multiple perspectives due to their fear of being wrong.

Because evaluation anxiety affects cognitive, affective, and psychomotor dimensions, a multifaceted approach is needed to help overcome it, such as the following:

- You can use positive self-talk (see Chapter 21) to overcome your self-defeating internal dialogue. Making sure that your inner voice is reassuring and comforts you in your day-to-day activities and during those times when you are having an examination or a performance appraisal.
- Relaxation (see Chapter 19) helps you focus on the task and act more efficiently. You feel more at ease and overcome the negative physiologic effects of evaluation anxiety when you relax.

- Imagery (see Chapter 20) helps you picture yourself performing in a way that makes you feel good about yourself. Your positive visualizations keep you focused on performing your best and engender positive feelings that overpower the uneasiness generated by your anxiety.
- Learning how to make use of feedback from others (see Chapter 18) helps you prepare yourself for situations in which your performance is evaluated. Practice sessions with helpful colleagues can boost your confidence.

In addition to these four approaches, avoiding errors requires thinking before acting. Using the nursing process on a consistent basis helps to ensure that your nursing actions are safe, ethical, and helpful.

Handling Job Performance Appraisals Assertively

At many points in our nursing careers, we receive both formal and informal evaluations of our performance. For us, the purpose of these evaluations is to learn what we are doing well (so that we can continue to do it) and where we need to improve our work performance. For the employer, evaluations serve as a check on whether employees are fulfilling the expectations of the work contract.

Evaluations are helpful to both parties and should occur regularly. As the employee, you can take an assertive approach to evaluations, which will help ease your anxiety. The following sections describe several assertive steps you can take to prepare for an evaluation. The example given is for a nurse employed in service.

As a student nurse, apply the same preparatory procedures for evaluations at your school. It is helpful early in your course or clinical experience to carefully read the guidelines for successful completion and clarify anything you do not understand. Review clinical competencies, procedures, and behaviors expected for each clinical rotation. Keep your own documentation of the completion of specific requirements in a clinical rotation and bring this to an evaluation meeting. Pay attention to the details of assignments on course syllabi.

Before Your Evaluation

1. Find out the schedule for evaluations in your agency. Many agencies offer an evaluation for new employees after 3 to 6 months of probationary employment and yearly thereafter.
2. Find out in advance the criteria by which your employer will be evaluating you. Having this information gives you the chance to make notes about how you think you have met the standards expected of someone in your position.
3. If your employer does not have a set of standard criteria for evaluation, suggest that one be developed soon. Request that your job description or the standards of nursing care prepared by your professional nursing association be used as the reference for determining your performance level.
4. Review what you and your colleagues in similar nursing positions actually do in the workplace. Compare this time and task allotment with what your job description outlines. At your evaluation, point out any discrepancies to your employer. If job descriptions are not updated, you may find that a significant part of your daily work is not being acknowledged.
5. Prepare your own evaluation of your work performance before meeting with your employer. Go to your appointment armed with specific examples of how you have met the requirements of your job description. Be aware of where you need to improve and what support you will need from your head nurse to make the necessary changes.
6. Develop goals toward which you would like to work. Be as clear, realistic, and specific as possible in the preparation of these work objectives so that you can articulate them clearly in your performance evaluation.
7. If the date at which your evaluation should have occurred passes, request an evaluation from your employer. Evaluations protect you by providing guidelines for maintaining or changing your professional behavior. You need feedback to know if your nursing care is within the legal and qualitative expectations of your agency.
8. Prepare mentally for your evaluation interview by ensuring that your self-talk is encouraging, and visualize yourself looking and feeling calm and confident during your interview.

During Your Evaluation

1. Inform your employer that you wish to discuss your goals at some time during the interview.
2. Allow your employer uninterrupted time to comment about your work.
3. Ask for clarification of any points that are not understood. Request evidence of your employer's points so that comments are backed up with examples. These illustrations clarify the kind of behavior your employer expects.
4. Your employer may have suggestions about ways in which you can improve your performance. Agree only to those changes that are realistic, given your time and potential and the support available in the workplace.
5. Share your performance goals with your employer and ask for support for the achievement of your career plans. Ask your employer for a list of goals toward which you should be working.
6. Do not sign your evaluation until you are fully satisfied that it is an accurate and fair assessment of how you do your job.

7. Thank your employer for the supervision and the feedback you receive.
8. Come to an agreement about the date for your next evaluation.

After Your Evaluation

1. Take time to reflect on how you handled the evaluation. Praise yourself for the ways you handled yourself assertively. Make note of things you would like to do differently in your next evaluation interview.
2. Follow up on the goals you and your employer set. Take time to develop your strategy to achieve your objectives and set intermediate and final deadlines. Think about people and resources you can tap to help develop your talents.
3. Keep a diary of your work performance in preparation for your next performance evaluation.

Consider the maxim to "underpromise and overdeliver." If you are asked when you can finish a project, overestimate the time it will take. When you deliver the results before the agreed-on date, you distinguish yourself. Avoid the temptation to give a date earlier than is reasonable to look good at the moment. Nurses following this practice should not feel anxious at job appraisal time.

🌸 MOMENTS OF CONNECTION...
Beyond the Call of Duty

"A young woman with a newborn child and very poor support systems was angry at the world because of chronic pain from a neck and back injury. She would refuse treatment and medications, yet was angry that we wouldn't do anything to stop her pain. It was hard to continue to interact with her, knowing that she would be critical of everything we did. After a period of months of contact with her, just listening to her, not becoming offended by her attacks, and understanding what she was experiencing, she now relies on me as her support. In a crisis, she will call. I calm her and help her think through the situation. Although this is beyond the normal attention given to a client, it is a special connection that can assist her to build her problem-solving skills, cope, and receive the care she needs by simply offering caring and understanding."

Coping with the Anxiety of Written Examinations

Taking examinations is part of student life and part of nursing. If you experience test anxiety, remember some helpful common-sense tips:
Be prepared!
Get a good night's sleep.
Eat a healthy breakfast/healthy snacks.
Arrive early.

Keep a positive attitude, saying to yourself, "I can do this." Calm yourself through your breath. Try slowing your breathing.

The following sections describe some assertive steps you can take to make you feel better prepared and less anxious about examinations.

Before Your Examination

1. Find out all you can about what content (or skill) will be tested on the examination. This knowledge helps you narrow down the material to study.
2. Review the objectives for the course and focus on content that directly relates to these objectives.
3. Find out the format of the examination (whether it is multiple choice or essay). This information determines your study approach.
4. If you need guidance on how to study, consult your teachers, the counseling center, or a study guide.
5. Consider forming or joining a study group. Effective study groups can make preparation for examinations fun and fruitful.
6. Make a realistic timetable of study preparations for the examination and stick to it. Keeping pace with your schedule helps you integrate the material you are studying. If you are rushed, prioritize what is important to learn and cover it first.
7. Find out where the examination is being held and familiarize yourself with the room. Choose a seat in which you will be comfortable. Be sure you know the exact hour of the examination.
8. Make sure you have all the necessary tools to help you in the examination, such as a calculator with a spare battery, sharpened pencils, a watch, tissues, and your good luck charm!
9. Mentally prepare before the examination by visualizing yourself in the examination room, looking calm and smiling as you read the questions because you know the answers. As you study for the examination, be sure that your self-talk is positive. Tell yourself that you are learning and that you are covering the material in a sensible way. Encourage yourself and do not allow self-defeating thoughts about failure or mistakes to take over your internal dialogue.
10. Put yourself through a dry run of the examination. If it is a written test, obtain examinations from previous years and complete them in the specified time limits. If there are no old examinations, make up your own questions and answer them in a simulated examination situation. If you are being examined on your nursing technique, perform the procedure in front of your colleagues. Have them evaluate you using the criteria that your instructor will use.

11. Plan a postexamination reward. This treat will give you something to look forward to and will prevent you from dwelling on the examination after it is over.

During Your Examination

1. Decide in advance what time you will be arriving at the place of the examination. If you are a person who likes to talk with colleagues before the examination, then arrive early. If preexamination cramming with colleagues raises your anxiety level, then time your arrival accordingly.
2. Take time to calm down before even looking at the examination. Sit calmly and do deep breathing.
3. Maintain this focused calm throughout the examination. If you are thinking about passing or failing instead of staying focused on the examination questions, your concentration will slip. Just as athletes do not perform their best when they are thinking about winning the gold medal or breaking a record during an event, neither do you perform your best if you are thinking about anything other than the best response to the question in front of you. Thinking about anything else creates anxiety and interferes with your concentration on the questions.
4. If you are distracted by an external interference that can be stopped (e.g., noise from other candidates or the proctors or uncomfortable conditions in the room), be assertive and ask the proctor to handle the situation. If nothing can be done about the external distractions, then tell yourself to refocus, giving all your attention to the question at hand.
5. Read over the entire examination before answering any questions. This way you know what is expected of you, and you can pace yourself throughout the allotted time.
6. Before answering any question, be sure you understand what is expected so that your answers will be at the appropriate level. If you merely describe an issue when you are expected to critique it, then you will not get full credit.
7. Tackle questions to which you know the answers first. This strategy boosts your confidence.
8. Decide how much time to spend on any one question (usually determined by the number of points allotted), and stick to your timetable so that you are not rushed at the end.
9. If you finish before the allotted time, read over your answers before submitting them. This review ensures that you have answered all the questions. In addition, you may think of some points to add.

After Your Examination

1. Decide whether you wish to join your colleagues for a "postmortem." Sometimes going over an examination only increases your anxiety.

2. Follow through with your plan for celebration after the examination. Doing something fun helps to clear your mind and relax you after all the hard work you did.
3. After you get your results, check to see where you did well and where you need to improve. Find out whether you need to study the content more or whether you need experience in interpreting the questions. This information will help you prepare for future examinations.

Self-Care Nudge
Try experimenting with hand massage with lotion and/or lavender preparations 15 minutes before an examination. Aromatherapy is complementary therapy that nurses can use for themselves and in clinical practice. Consult clinical protocols before clinical use (Sayed et al., 2020).

WIT AND WISDOM
The enemy of the good is the better.
Unknown

Dealing with Criticism

Many people feel anxious about receiving criticism. Here are some perceptions on criticism that shed a more positive light on the issue:
- Think about criticism as a gift instead of bad news. Criticism offers you the chance to reevaluate your performance. People who take time to criticize you are often interested in you or the job you are doing.
- Seek more information from the person who is criticizing you. Use negative inquiry, which is an assertiveness technique. Ask for specific facts about the particular behavior for which you are being criticized. This information helps you determine the validity of the criticism.
- You are not obliged to agree with all criticism you receive. Take time to review the criticism, extract what fits your self-assessment, and discard what does not fit.
- If you receive criticism you have heard before, take note of it. There is likely some truth to criticism you hear repeatedly.
- Reply to unjust or aggressive criticism; do not let it pass without speaking up. You will feel better about yourself if you confront or correct the person who is unfairly criticizing you. Some people deliver destructive criticism to make themselves feel more powerful or superior. You do not have to accept the criticism. You can assert yourself.
- Reply with civility. Incivility or rude or discourteous behavior violates the desired climate of mutual respect (Clark, Farnsworth, & Landrum, 2009).

- Realize that criticism does not mean there is something wrong with you. You may be accurately criticized for doing something ineffectively or incorrectly, but that in no way means you are a bad or stupid person.

Assertively Handling Difficult Situations in Nursing Student Performance Evaluations

Some situations increase our evaluation anxiety. We need to prepare ourselves for uncomfortable situations such as those in which an evaluator is aggressive, we are given an evaluation without time to prepare, or serious allegations are made without evidence. Several examples of difficult evaluation situations follow, with suggestions for handling them assertively.

Harshly Delivered Criticism

Your clinical instructor tells you that your charting is fine and your treatments are performed superbly, and she compliments you on your effective sterile technique. She also points out that your organization is poor. She notes that your rooms look disheveled and cluttered. "How can you or your clients find things you need in that confusion? Half the time your beds aren't made until after noon, and the room is a mess. This is a disgrace to the nursing profession."

You know that these comments are legitimate, even though they are delivered in an aggressive way. You tend to be disorganized and messy at home as well. Here is an assertive reply to this evaluation:

Assertive response: *"Thank you for the feedback on my nursing skills. I don't know what to do about my organization. It's a bad habit I've had for years, even before I came into nursing. I always admire nurses who can do things well and keep their workspace uncluttered at the same time. I don't know where to begin. Can you give me some suggestions about how I can improve?"*

This reply acknowledges both the compliments and the criticisms from your instructor. Your openness to improve your organization is demonstrated by your request for help. If you really want to improve, you will follow through with some of the suggestions your instructor provides.

Unexpected Aggressive Criticism

You have been assigned to a telemetry unit in a general hospital for the past 7 weeks. It is your last week on the unit, so you decide to stop at the head nurse's office to thank her for the help she has given you during your practicum.

Without having requested it, the head nurse gives you this piece of advice: "I'm glad you enjoyed your time with us. Here's some advice I'd like to give you before you leave us: Improve your charting. It's a mess to read. I spent 10 minutes trying to decipher one of your notes the other day.

You'll never make a good nurse if you can't communicate to the rest of the world what you have done."

Assertive response: *"I am aware that my charting is too long and difficult to read. Miss Jameson, my clinical instructor, has also pointed out my need to improve. Do you have any suggestions to help me learn how to improve my charting?"*

This reply acknowledges the feedback from your head nurse. Although her feedback is aggressive, you maintained an assertive stance in your response. Your request for guidance invites her to contribute to your development in a more positive way.

Allegations without Evidence

Your clinical instructor is giving you your final evaluation on your performance on the obstetric unit where you have been working for the past 3 weeks. She has made several negative comments about your handling of the babies and your interactions with the new mothers. However, she has given no examples to support her comments and has never observed you directly. You believe that your performance is acceptable and that it meets the standards set out in the procedural manual. You reply in the following way:

Assertive response: *"My own assessment of my handling of the babies and my interactions with the mothers is that I treat them both with respect and care. I would appreciate your providing me with more concrete evidence of any rough handling, because this charge has serious implications for my career. I have worked closely with Ms. Green in the nursery and Mrs. Nuthers on the unit. Both these staff nurses could provide you with a thorough assessment of my performance. I would like to have a joint meeting with you and these nurses to discuss my performance. I will not sign this evaluation form until this meeting has taken place."*

This assertive response lets your instructor know that you intend to protect your reputation. You have made a reasonable request for another evaluation. Your straightforward manner, which is neither insulting nor disrespectful to your instructor, increases the likelihood of having another evaluation.

MOVING FROM REACTIVE TO PROACTIVE BEHAVIOR

The ability to seek out opportunities for evaluation sets you apart as a person who has vision and wants to improve rather than hide in hopes that no one will notice your mistakes.

Consider beginning the process of reflective journal writing after each clinical day to gain insight into your actions, reactions, biases, and values. Lasater and Nielsen (2009) conducted research on a model for reflective journal writing as a student assignment with faculty input. You can use this process on your own as a proactive strategy, including entries such as a description of the situation, your previous experience, what you noticed, how you interpreted your observations, how you responded and set goals for the client's care, your reflection on the effectiveness of the interventions, and lessons learned. Covey (2004) suggested that "being proactive" is the first of seven habits of highly effective people. According to Covey, being proactive means that "we are responsible for our own lives." Proactive people "do not blame circumstances…for their behavior." For a student nurse, a proactive behavior is being prepared for a clinical assignment and open to questions and dialogue about the client's care. The reactive person blames other people and specific situations for problems. To be evaluated can be experienced as criticism and can evoke a natural tendency to look for excuses. As your skills improve and your confidence increases, you should find yourself moving from being reactive to being proactive, seeking out evaluation. You give your permission for others to give you feedback. You take responsibility for corrective action without having your feelings hurt.

SIMPLIFY AND DEEPEN

They cannot take away our self-respect if we do not give it to them.

Mahatma Gandhi

Return to "Active Learning" at the beginning of the chapter and write your responses.

PRACTICING OVERCOMING EVALUATION ANXIETY

Skill Building: Exercise 1

Practice the 4-7-8 breath for relaxation. This is a simple strategy for you and your client. Give yourself the gift of practicing it **once** now. Follow the video at www.drweil.com.

Video: Dr. Weil's Breathing Exercises: 4-7-8 Breath (drweil.com)

Skill Building: Exercise 2

Your colleague in the school of nursing has an important physiology test coming up in 2 days. Over coffee in the cafeteria, she says the following:

Nervous Nina: *"I'm terrified about this examination. Everyone says Dr. Capitell is such a hard grader. I did OK on the first test, but the stuff we've covered since then is a lot more complicated. I can't fail because it will put my course selection out of sequence. I've put so much time into studying this stuff that I'd better pass. I'll be glad when it's over."*

How would you intervene to help minimize your friend's evaluation anxiety? Prepare your suggested strategy, and then work with classmates in groups of four to compare your suggestions.

Skill Building/Small Group Work: Exercise 3

You are a staff nurse working in the operating room of a general hospital. A student doing her clinical practicum in the operating room is talking to you during a coffee break. This is what she says:

Anxious Anita: *"Tomorrow's going to be awful! I've got to scrub for Dr. Shark, and I've seen how he yells at students if they don't do exactly what he wants. And, to top it off, my clinical instructor chooses tomorrow to evaluate me! I'll be a wreck by 4 o'clock tomorrow."*

How would you help this student nurse cope with her evaluation anxiety? Prepare your own response, and then work in groups of four to compare and share strategies.

Creative Expression/Reflection/Journal Entry/ Photo Collage: Exercise 4

Create a collage depicting yourself as you want to be: confident and accomplished. To do this, collect several magazines that appeal to you, a background (use a piece of colored art paper, mat board, or even cardboard), scissors, and a glue stick. Set a goal of creating a full picture of you being your best self professionally and personally. Without a lot of thought, select images and words or phrases that appeal to you. Create a collage by gluing these to the background. When you finish, take a few minutes to write your thoughts and feelings about your expressive art. Set the collage in a place where you will see it frequently and hold these images.

An alternative to making a concrete piece of art is to arrange pictures and words, take a picture with your phone, and refer to it there when you need a boost.

REFERENCES

Boggs, C., Shields, D., & Goodin, H. J. (2011). Using guided reflection to reduce test anxiety in nursing students. *Journal of Holistic Nursing, 29*(2), 140.

Clark, C. M., Farnsworth, J., & Landrum, R. E. (2009). Development and description of incivility in nursing education. *Journal of Theory Construction and Testing, 13*(1), 7.

Covey, S. R. (2004). *The 7 habits of highly effective people.* New York: Free Press.

Devney, A. M. (2018). Rapid anxiety reduction tools for nursing staff, faculty and students. *COJ Nursing & Healthcare, 2*(5), 1–2.

Diaz, D. A., Panosky, D. M., & Shelton, D. (2014). Simulation: Introduction to correctional nursing in a prison setting. *Journal of Correctional Health Care, 20*(3), 240.

Dweck, C. S., & Wortman, C. B. (1982). Learned helplessness, anxiety, and achievement motivation. In W. H. Krohne, & L. Laux (Eds.), *Achievement, stress, and anxiety*. Washington, DC: Hemisphere Publishing.

Hutchinson, T. L., & Goodin, H. J. (2013). Nursing anxiety as a context for teaching/learning. *Journal of Holistic Nursing, 31*(1), 19.

Kaplan, B., & Ura, D. (2010). Use of multiple patient simulators to enhance prioritizing delegating skills for senior students. *Journal of Nursing Education, 49*(7), 371.

Lasater, K., & Nielsen, A. (2009). Reflective journaling for clinical judgment development and evaluation. *Journal of Nursing Education, 48*(1), 40.

Marquis, B. L., & Huston, C. J. (1998). *Management decision making for nurses: 124 Case studies*. Philadelphia, PA: Lippincott-Raven.

Meichenbaum, D. H. (1972). Cognitive modification of test anxious college students. *Journal of Consulting and Clinical Psychology, 39*(3), 370.

Moscaritolo, L. M. (2010). Interventional strategies to decrease nursing student anxiety in the clinical learning environment. *Journal of Nursing Education, 48*(1), 17.

Sayed, A. M., Morsy, M., Tawfik, G. M., Naveed, S., Minh-Duc, N. T., Hieu, T. H., et al. (2020). The best route of administration of lavender for anxiety: A systematic review and network meta-analysis. *Journal of General Hospital Psychiatry, 64*, 33–40. May-June. 10.1016/j.genhosppsych.2020.02.001.

Wadi, M., Yusoff, M. S. B., Rahim, A. F. A., & Lah, N. A. Z. N. (2022). Factors affecting test anxiety: A qualitative analysis of medical students' views. *BMC Psychology, 10*(8). https://doi.org/10.1186/s40359-021-00715-2.

Weil, A. (2018). Breathing exercises: 4-7-8 breath. Video: Dr. Weil's Breathing Exercises: 4-7-8 Breath (drweil.com).

Wine, J. D. (1982). Evaluation anxiety: A cognitive-attentional construct. In W. H. Krohne, & L. Laux (Eds.), *Achievement, stress, and anxiety*. Washington, DC: Hemisphere Publishing.

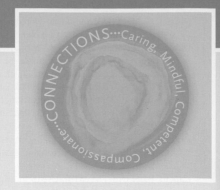

Working with Feedback

I think it's very important to have a feedback loop, where you're constantly thinking about what you've done and how you could be doing it better.

Elon Musk

OBJECTIVES

1. Discuss the importance of feedback in communication.
2. Identify strategies for giving feedback.
3. Discuss steps for receiving feedback to promote self-growth.

4. Practice seeking, giving, and receiving feedback in selected exercises.

> **💡 ACTIVE LEARNING**
>
> Think about how you will write your answers as you read this chapter.
>
> **What?**
> Write one thing you learned from this chapter.
>
> **So What?**
> How will this affect your nursing practice?
>
> **Now What?**
> How will you implement this new knowledge or skill?
>
> **Think About It …**

WHY FEEDBACK IS IMPORTANT

Have you ever heard the statement, "feedback is a gift"? Consider this as you read this chapter. An extensive literature review concluded that evaluative feedback, novel in nursing education, which included dialogue, reflection, and self-assessment, supported the development of evaluation of clinical practice (Ilangakoon, Ajjawi, Endacott, & Rees, 2022).

As you read this chapter, be patient with yourself. Receiving even constructive feedback is not a guarantee that you will absorb it and change immediately. Robinson-Walker

(2017) is a nurse coach who wrote about learning spirals and that sometimes we have to keep coming back to our behavior, getting feedback more than once, as we work on self-awareness and personal and professional growth.

Giving constructive feedback, not an innate skill for most (Blatchley, 2017), is intended to "promote improvement or development of the person receiving feedback" (Duffy, 2013). It is focused on behavior that can be changed, not on personality that cannot (Greenfield, 2014). Discussions about how to give feedback distinguish between positive and negative feedback, and either one can be regarded as a gift. Consider the two parts of the word, "feed" and "back." In one sense of the word, *feed* implies to nourish, even to comfort, or to meet another's needs. *Back* in this context is the return of something to another. When these two notions are combined, feedback means the returning of nourishment to another person. In this sense, feedback is something positive—a gift for the other person. The gift that is given is one person's thoughts and feelings about another person's behavior. When you take a positive approach to giving or receiving feedback, this creates a comfort zone for others and "turns negative feedback into productive dialogue…fosters a learning environment… and turns criticism into pure gold" (Gallagher, 2009). Cultivate positive people in your life by giving specific praise about colleagues, especially in front of people important to them (Anderson, 2002). Giving immediate positive feedback is best when possible (Blatchley, 2017). This chapter invites you to use the technique of reframing, which is seeing or describing a situation from a different perspective.

Feedback helps us see our behavior from another person's perspective. This reflection indicates how someone else is reacting to our communication. This picture helps us decide whether to continue acting in the same way or to change. Viewed in this way, feedback is a springboard for self-growth. Feeling happy with ourselves is one of the most joyous experiences in life. This contentment is an acknowledgment of what we like about ourselves, and it solidifies our self-concept. Contemplating a change in our way of behaving is really envisioning a new self-concept. Feedback has the potential for expanding our development as human beings. To be most effective, feedback on our progress toward goals must be frequent and specific (Eisenberg & Goodall, 2001). Consider the nursing process as an example of a feedback mechanism. Assessment, planning, and intervention can change based on feedback from the client in the evaluation phases and on additional information obtained in continuing assessment. Improving care based on feedback has been a part of nursing since the days of Florence Nightingale. Continuous quality improvement, which is really just data-driven problem-solving, examines processes in the delivery of care to improve service and depends on regular feedback for excellence. The 360-degree feedback, or multisource performance approval data, is used as a staff development tool because feedback is drawn from peers and subordinates to supplement direct observation by the manager (Watkins & Leigh, 2009).

Giving feedback differs from giving advice. Giving feedback is merely a reflection of how another person's behavior has affected us; it is not advice about how a person should change. After receiving our feedback, clients or colleagues may wish to make changes in their behavior. One thing we may be asked is, "What do you think I should do to change?" Often, we have advice to give, but a note of caution is in order.

To avoid hurting the feelings of others and to ensure that we are being respectful, options we may offer should be made as suggestions for the other person's consideration. We can never know what changes will be comfortable or suitable for another person because each of us must decide what suits our personal style and priorities. Our suggestions will be more readily received if they are offered tentatively, as in the following:

"Something I've tried is this."
"Perhaps adding this change will help you."
"When I was trying to change in the same way, my sister-in-law suggested I do this…It worked for me, and maybe it will work for you."

These examples allow the receiver the final option of accepting or rejecting your advice.

For feedback to be integrated, it must be delivered in a way that is receivable, and the receiver must be open to considering the feedback. The following sections discuss some steps you can take to increase the probability that your feedback will be accepted.

HOW TO GIVE FEEDBACK

First, check your reason for wanting to give feedback. What is motivating you to give feedback? What do you hope to accomplish by delivering feedback? Any reasons based on the belief that your feedback will benefit the other person by increasing the opportunities for self-growth are in agreement with the intention of feedback. There are many reasons for giving feedback that are unacceptable in a caring, therapeutic relationship. Feeling irritable and wanting to lash out at another as a way of obtaining revenge, wanting to display your superior knowledge to discredit another, or wanting to rigidly control the behavior of clients or colleagues because of intolerance are not good reasons for giving feedback.

Gain Permission to Give Feedback

The next step is to gain permission from your client or colleague to give feedback so the individual will be more open to your input (Ambrose & Moscinski, 2002). Permission may be requested verbally by simply asking if the other person would like the feedback, or the request can be made through nonverbal checking.

The following example includes verbal and nonverbal ways of obtaining permission to give feedback.

You have been teaching a new father to bathe his newborn, and he has given a return demonstration.

"I noticed how securely you have been holding your baby daughter—I'm sure it makes her feel safe and secure. It looks like she's enjoying the bath you are giving her and especially how you are talking to her. I'd like to point out one suggestion for improvement."

Here you pause and look at the father, who nods his approval for you to continue.

"When you allow your daughter's umbilical cord to get wet, it increases the chance that she'll get an infection. I've got some suggestions, if you'd like to hear them, for how you could keep her cord dry."

Again, you make eye contact with the father and do not proceed until he conveys his interest in hearing your suggestions.

"Some ways to keep the cord dry are to fill the tub with less water and hold her at about a 45-degree angle. Also, you can squeeze out the washcloth so that water doesn't accidentally drip on her cord."

Be Specific

Giving feedback to clients or colleagues is not your chance to bombard them with everything about their behavior that you like or dislike. To give your feedback impact, you must focus on specific, observable behavior. The following situation between two nurses illustrates how to be specific when giving feedback.

You are on the evening shift and are still relatively new to the procedures on the unit. Before the night shift comes on, you always have last-minute charting to do and tying together of loose ends for your report. For the past four nights, one of the night nurses has come on duty 30 minutes early and tried to engage you in a social conversation. Your hints that you do not have time to talk at that moment have been ignored, and she has persisted in bending your ear about her date or how she slept that day. You approach her with the following:

"Rhonda, I'd like to talk to you about how your coming in early and talking to me is affecting me."

At this point you wait until she's agreeable to discuss the issue and proceed as follows:

"I'd love to talk with you, but when you try to capture my attention at the end of my shift, it agitates me because I'm trying to tie up so many loose ends and get things in order for the night shift. I find myself getting so tense that I can't pay enough attention to what you are trying to tell me, and I don't get my work completed the way I'd like to. Do you understand what I'm saying?"

Here you must pause and give Rhonda a chance to respond. You might proceed as follows:

"I've got a suggestion that will allow me to get my last-minute work done and still give us a chance to visit before I leave. Want to hear it?"

Restricting your feedback to observable behavior prevents you from blurting out something cruel such as, "Can't you wait till your shift starts to talk my ear off?" or "I can't stand you bugging me like this!" Being specific helps you keep feedback realistic and acceptable.

Convey Your Perspective

When you give feedback, you must remind yourself that you are reporting your view of things. Nothing is innately or objectively right or wrong about your perspective; it is simply how you see the world. Because every relationship you have with colleagues and clients has significance and influence for both parties, however, your reactions are important to others.

When looking in the mirror after getting your hair cut in a new style, you might smile with approval, blush with embarrassment, or feel reluctant to pay for such an outrageous coiffure! The hairdresser might glow with pleasure at your sophisticated new image, and your friends may look ambivalent about the new you. Any of these reactions is legitimate, and none is better than the other. Each reaction is feedback based on the viewer's frame of reference. When you are giving feedback, you need to keep in mind that, as important as your views are, the receiver may not agree with your perspective.

To ensure that you give feedback respectfully, you can couch your comments with phrases such as these:

"As I see it…"
"I felt happy (sad) when you clapped (did not applaud)."
"From my perspective…"
"The way I see things is…"

Using the first person to convey your thoughts and feelings prevents you from accusing or labeling another person's behavior.

Because I am responsible for customer service training in a hospital setting, it is my job to give feedback when I observe poor customer service. When I am in the role of client, I am in a good position to assess the quality of service. When I give feedback, I share my perspective of someone who has "been there." When I went to the laboratory to have my blood drawn, a woman came into the room, did not identify herself, and was wearing no name tag. When I asked her about it, I learned she was a student. A staff member came in to help, and I learned that students were not routinely given name pins. I shared this information with the manager and indicated how uncomfortable it made me as a patient to not know who was working with me. She agreed and arranged to provide the students with name tags. It is not always easy to give feedback if it requires correction, but it may help others. In this case we were able to upgrade the image of the staff as professionals.

Use This Formula to Give Assertive Feedback

In difficult situations in which you need to tell others how their behavior is affecting you and request a behavior change, the following formula, often used in assertiveness training, is one method that is helpful (Carr-Ruffino, 2001):

1. When you… (describe the behavior without judging it)
2. The effects are… (describe concretely how it affects your life in a practical sense)

3. I feel… (describe your feelings without blaming; the "I" statement implies ownership of your own feelings)
4. I prefer… (describe what response or change you would like or, if possible, give the other person a chance to come up with a solution)
For example:
1. "When you speak in a loud voice when I am trying to listen to someone on the telephone…"
2. "I cannot hear, and I must ask the caller to repeat the message."
3. "I feel embarrassed that the patient might think the unit is in chaos."
4. "How can we handle this?" or "I would prefer you to speak more softly or finish the conversation away from the telephone."
Let us try this with the name pin issue:

"When you don't wear a name pin, I can't call you by name and I don't know who to ask for if I need to talk with you later. I don't feel as if I'm in a setting in which people are professional, and I can't even be sure you work here. Were you given a name tag? No? In that case, I'd like to check into this because I think wearing name tags might make other patients feel more comfortable, too. Would that be all right with you?"

Invite Comments from the Receiver

Because the feedback you give is from your perspective, it is important to keep in mind how others might feel when receiving your comments. One way to do this is to check out their reactions by using phrases such as "What do you think about my comments to you?" or "Could you tell me your reaction to what I've just told you?" Giving feedback requires consideration. You never know how others will respond to your feedback, and you must allow them to express their reactions. People need time to grasp what you are saying, mull it over, ask for more information, and express their feelings and thoughts about what you have said.

Be Genuine

It warrants saying that those who give feedback should be honest when expressing their views. If you do not mean it, do not say it! When you are sincere in giving feedback, you build trust. If you are verbalizing something positive but the frown on your face indicates displeasure, then the receiver of your feedback gets a mixed message. It is important to keep your verbal and nonverbal behavior congruent.

Check Out How Your Feedback Is Being Received

If you can honestly say that the feedback was given in the best interest of the receiver, if you gained permission before proceeding with your feedback, and if you were specific in your comments and gave them tentatively, then you know that you have given feedback in a caring way.

In addition to your self-assessment, you can also pick up clues from your clients or colleagues about whether your way of giving feedback is acceptable. If they indicate that they understand what you are saying and verbally and non-verbally indicate that they would like you to continue, then you know that your manner of giving feedback is respectful. If they become embarrassed or angry or move away from you, they may be indicating that they are not yet ready to receive any feedback from you or at least not in the dose you are administering. When you receive clues that your clients or colleagues are becoming defensive about your comments, it is important to pause and check with them on how to proceed. You might stop altogether or choose gentler and more receivable words.

HOW TO RECEIVE FEEDBACK

Feedback is an opportunity for self-growth, therefore, knowing how to get the most out of the experience is worthwhile. Clearly, giving feedback requires risking another person's feelings and the relationship you have. Knowing about that risk has implications for how you can act when one of your clients or colleagues takes a chance on giving you feedback.

Get Focused

It is important to be focused when receiving feedback. This means not thinking or worrying about some other issue but attending to the feedback and listening respectfully. Remember that feedback can help you develop your clinical and interpersonal skills, build your self-confidence and self-esteem, and motivate you to continue to learn more about yourself (Clynes & Raftery, 2008).

Arrange to Have Enough Time to Receive the Feedback

Being unrushed when feedback is being given is also important. If you know you are hurried, say that you value learning others' ideas and would like to schedule another time to hear them. Making another appointment is important because it indicates that you respect other people's opinions and intend to follow through. You could say the following:

"I'm touched that you have gone to the effort of preparing some feedback for me on the in-service I gave. Could we schedule a convenient time to go over your views? I want to hear what you have to say when I'm not as pressed for time as I am today, so I can take it all in."

Make Sure You Understand the Feedback

Let feedback givers have the floor long enough to clearly state their views and then ask questions about anything that was unclear.

After your nursing instructor has given you feedback on your sterile technique, for example, you might respond as follows:

"I think I understand your comments. You noticed that I opened the tray before washing my hands and then I left the tray exposed to the air while I washed them. I also had the client's furniture placed in my way so I had to lean over the sterile field and I almost contaminated it. I think those were the main areas in which I need to improve, weren't they?"

It is not only respectful to repeat the feedback to ensure that you understood it, but it is also a way of outlining the points once more as a reminder to yourself.

Request Guidance on How to Change

If you would like to make changes in your behavior because of the feedback, then ask for directions for change—if you genuinely want to hear them. Consider this example:

Your student nurse colleague has given you feedback about your leadership style during your first week as team leader. Most of her comments were positive, but she also indicated that she occasionally felt slighted or put down when you unilaterally made decisions about the nursing care for her clients.

You are surprised to hear her reaction because you had assumed that it was up to you as team leader to take charge, but you feel bad that your leadership style may cause your team members to feel unimportant or left out. You want to change to a more respectful leadership style, so you could respond to your colleague as follows:

"Thank you for your comments. I'm pleased about the areas in which I seem to be doing well, but I really want to overcome being so autocratic. What could I do differently as team leader to make you feel more included in the decision making for your clients?"

Show Appreciation for the Feedback

Thank others for their feedback. Even if you are not going to change, it has likely been of benefit to hear another person's point of view about your behavior, and you can express your gratitude for this information. Here is an example:

One of your nursing instructors tells you that she fears your habit of taking only half the allotted time for lunch

will wear you out, and she worries about your health. You respond as follows:

"Thanks for your concern, Mrs. Brown. I find that the physical nursing care on this medical floor demands much more of me than the care on the ear, nose, and throat floor I just came from, where I had more than enough time. I'm slowly getting more accustomed to the pace in the 9 days I've been here, and I'm sure I'll soon be organized and relaxed enough to take the full break at lunchtime."

Think About the Feedback You Receive

You are the one who benefits from thinking over any feedback you have been given. Take the opportunity to consider the implications of feedback you receive. Here is an example:

One of your patients, uncomfortable because of her pain, often lashes out at others. As you start her bath one morning, she snarls at you:

"Oh! It's you! Miss Sugary Sweet Nancy Nurse! Your smile is sickening, and your cheeriness is just too much to take this morning! Go away and find someone else to gush over!"

Your first reaction may be one of feeling hurt. Or you may brush off her comments and rationalize that she spoke because of her pain and did not really mean them. As time passes, you might find yourself recalling her words and wondering if perhaps you are too cheery and bubbly with your clients; as a result, you might begin to keep your distance and not allow yourself to reach out to their sadness or fear. To be fair to yourself, you should really check out the answer to your concern about your possible insensitivity.

By reevaluating your ability to be warm and compassionate with your clients, you can learn about your strong points and areas in which you could be connecting more humanly with them. By making use of the feedback you receive, you can grow and develop, both personally and professionally.

SIMPLIFY AND DEEPEN

Criticism may not be agreeable, but it is necessary. It fulfills the same function as pain in the human body. It calls attention to an unhealthy state of things.

Winston Churchill

HOW TO SEEK FEEDBACK

As you become comfortable with receiving feedback, you may wish to seek out feedback from others before they offer it. To seek out feedback is to publicly announce that you are ready for self-growth; it implies that you have the confidence to look at your strengths and explore areas in which you could make improvements.

Be Sure You Are Ready to Receive Feedback

Before seeking feedback, check to see that you are really ready to receive it. When you are not fully open to receiving feedback, you convey that message either verbally or nonverbally. Verbally, you may become angry, get defensive, or make excuses to rationalize your behavior. Nonverbally, you may physically tune out feedback by losing eye contact, turning your body away, or folding your arms to create a barrier against the penetration of the feedback. Both verbal and nonverbal responses are disrespectful to the person from whom you are asking for feedback.

Self-Care Nudge

Be kind to yourself and recognize that there are times when we are simply not ready to hear feedback. In those cases, we should protect ourselves and not seek out others' reactions until we are confident enough to examine them. Receiving feedback with implications for change when we feel shaky or unconfident may serve only to make us feel worse about ourselves. It is a risk to ask for feedback; when we are ready to receive feedback, then it has great potential for enhancing self-growth.

 MOMENTS OF CONNECTION...

Put It in Writing

One nurse manager, when asked for suggestions on how to build staff skills, talked about writing thank-you or acknowledgment cards for staff when they were observed doing something extra for clients, family, or coworkers. During Nurse Week, this manager sends each staff member a card thanking the person for his or her contributions and mentioning at least one specific thing about that person. Staff report saving such cards and notes and reviewing them in tough times.

Be Specific in Your Request for Feedback

Clarify the aspects of your behavior about which you want feedback. Delineating those areas helps your clients and colleagues focus, and it ensures that you receive the information you want to hear. For example, after you complete a preoperative teaching session with your surgical client, you ask him the following:

"What did you think about the session?"

This request for feedback is vague and does not help your client to address any particular area. The following request would help your client to focus his comments:

"I included this brochure, which I will leave with you. It reviews what you can expect to happen immediately after surgery. What other questions do you have at this time?"

Use Feedback as Caring Communication

If you follow the guidelines for giving, receiving, and seeking feedback outlined previously, your feedback behavior will be assertive. Clearly, feedback is a responsible process because it allows participants to make use of all the information available. As you care for your clients you are part of an ongoing "cycle of exchange and interconnection" (Jasmine, 2009), giving and receiving feedback, and with each interaction striving to create a balance between a varied set of nursing functions and caring behaviors (Jasmine, 2009). Commend clients for progress you see in their goals, and encourage them to feel pride in their accomplishments and in their ability to cope and heal. Behavioral science tells us that whatever behavior we reward will be strengthened or repeated. Remember to take time to comment on what your colleagues do that makes your day easier, like nurse managers' specific, positive feedback and saying thank you offering support and encouragement. In your development of interpersonal communication skills, feedback is a crucial factor.

Return to "Active Learning" at the beginning of the chapter and write your responses.

 PRACTICING WORKING WITH FEEDBACK

Reflection/Discussion: Exercise 1

Reflect on the last time you were given feedback on your performance. What were your thoughts and feelings about the way in which it was provided? Identify what could have been improved (Duffy, 2013).

Being Curious: Exercise 2

Question your own assumptions by exploring 15 surprising facts about feedback at The psychology behind better workplace feedback (15 surprising facts) (cognology.com.au) (Windust, 2019). Each "fact" offers a reference for further study.

Skill Building/Dyads: Exercise 3

Work with a partner, with one of you as listener and the other as speaker. The speaker chooses any topic and talks about it for 5 minutes. The listener conveys interest in the speaker's topic and uses the communication behaviors learned in earlier chapters.

After 5 minutes, the listener makes a specific request to the speaker for feedback on his or her listening skills. The speaker responds by giving feedback on the specific points requested by the listener. If appropriate, the speaker offers to give additional feedback on the abilities of the listener. The listener responds to the feedback given by the speaker.

After you have finished this exercise, take a few minutes to answer these questions.

As the speaker:

1. Was the listener's request for feedback specific?
2. Did the listener look as if he or she were open to receiving feedback from you?

As the listener:

1. How specific was your request for feedback on your listening skills to your speaker?
2. How openly did you respond to your colleague's feedback?
3. Was the speaker's feedback to you specific, clear, and tentative?

After you have answered these questions, switch roles and repeat. Discuss what you learned about seeking, receiving, and giving feedback.

Quality and Safety Education for Nurses Learning Strategy: Exercise 4 (QSEN)

Learning to incorporate feedback is essential to improve quality of care. Gain experience through this exercise with your clinical group or class.

Sleep deprivation is a human factor that influences safe delivery of care. To practice the skills involved in accurately collecting information for feedback and discussing it with the team, maintain a sleep diary for 1 week. Record the number of hours you slept each night, your time to bed and time awakened, and contextual factors that influenced when you went to sleep each day and when you awakened. Use database searches to determine the evidence base for the appropriate amount of sleep for your age. Put the information into a graph. Present the project to your group, and ask for feedback to determine how effectively you have collected and presented these data.

- Reflect on the experience.
- How well did you document and communicate your data?
- How did you feel as you were receiving feedback?
- How effective was the group in providing detailed feedback in a constructive manner?
- How can you apply the lessons from this experience to communicate information more effectively?
- What steps would you take based on the feedback to improve the project?
- From a quality improvement standpoint, how well did you measure against the evidence-based sleep standard? What steps can you take to improve your sleep patterns?

REFERENCES

Ambrose, L., & Moscinski, P. (2002). The power of feedback. *Healthcare Executive, 17*(5), 56.

Anderson, K. (2002). Don't worry, be happy. *Nursing, 32*(1), 69.

Blatchley, A. (2017). A nurse manager's guide to giving effective feedback. *Nurse Leader, 15*(5), 331.

Carr-Ruffino, N. (2001). *The promotable woman: Advancing through leadership skills.* New York, NY: Career Press.

Clynes, M. R., & Raftery, S. E. C. (2008). Feedback: An essential element of student learning in clinical practice. *Nurse Education in Practice, 8*(6), 405.

Duffy, K. (2013). Providing constructive feedback to students during mentoring. *Nursing Standard, 27*(31), 50.

Eisenberg, E. M., & Goodall, H. L., Jr. (2001). *Organizational communication: Balancing creativity and constraint.* New York, NY: Bedford/St. Martin's Press.

Gallagher, R. S. (2009). *How to tell anyone anything: Breakthrough techniques for handling difficult conversations at work.* New York, NY: AMACOM.

Greenfield, J. (2014). Why every practice nurse should have an annual appraisal. *Practicing Nurse, 44*(9), 32.

Ilangakoon, C., Ajjawi, R., Endacott, R., & Rees, C. E. (2022). The relationship between feedback and evaluative judgement in undergraduate nursing and midwifery education: An Integrative review. *Nurse Education in Practice, 58.* https://doi.org/10.1016/j.nepr.2021.103255.

Jasmine, T. (2009). Art, science, or both? Keeping the care in nursing. *Nursing Clinics of North America, 44*(4), 415.

Robinson-Walker, C. (2017). Learning spirals. *Nurse Leader, 15*(5), 298.

Windust, J. (2019). The psychology behind better workplace feedback (15 surprising facts) (cognology.com.au).

Watkins, R., & Leigh, D. (2009). *Handbook of improving performance in the workplace: Selecting and implementing performance interventions.* Vol. 2. San Francisco, CA: Pfeiffer.

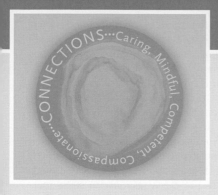

19

Using Relaxation Techniques to Become More Mindful

Nursing school made me realize how well I handle stress…Said no one ever.

Someecards

OBJECTIVES

1. Define mindfulness.
2. Discuss the hungry, angry, lonely, and tired (HALT) approach for resiliency and stress management.
3. Discuss the importance of relaxation skills for the nurse.
4. Identify stressors in nursing.
5. Describe guidelines for beginning to practice meditation to elicit the relaxation response.
6. Identify the steps of progressive relaxation for deep relaxation.
7. Identify brief, practical strategies for immediate relaxation.
8. Identify brief stretching exercises to promote relaxation.
9. Practice relaxation techniques to become more mindful.

❓ ACTIVE LEARNING

Think about how you will write your answers as you read this chapter.

What?
Write one thing you learned from this chapter.

So What?
How will this affect your nursing practice?

Now What?
How will you implement this new knowledge or skill?

Think About It …

AN INTRODUCTION TO MINDFULNESS TO SUPPORT PRESENCE IN NURSING CARE

To come to the bedside whole, present for our patients, we strive to be present for ourselves. Anxiety, which is fear of the unknown, is a common experience for students and, for some, throughout their lives. This chapter offers ideas and strategies to help you relax so that you can "show up" ready to embrace our work as being "all about the patient." Relaxation strategies help us be more mindful. John Kabat-Zinn (2017), founder of the Center for Mindfulness in Medicine, Health Care, and Society at the University of Massachusetts Medical School, who teaches mindfulness-based stress reduction (MBSR), defined mindfulness as a "means paying attention in a particular way: on purpose, in the present moment, and nonjudgmentally." Eckhart Tolle said that being present is infinitely more powerful than anything you can say or do (Tolle, 1999). A study using mindfulness breathing meditation with nurses showed improvement of psychological well-being (Ibrahim, Komariah, & Herliani, 2022). To promote resilience in nurses, a study was conducted in which, in an eight-week program, six resilience factors (cognitive flexibility, coping, self-efficacy, self-esteem, self-care, and mindfullness) were addressed with positive results (Janzarik, Wollschlager, & Lieb, 2022).

Patricia Arcari (2017), PhD, RN, Integrative Medicine at the Dana-Farber Cancer Center in Boston, believed that mindfulness can be a natural process that can fit into anyone's daily routine; emphasizes awareness, bringing your attention to your breath and to what is happening in the moment; and practices appreciation, which she calls a

BOX 19.1   To Begin a Mindfulness Practice

To begin a mindfulness practice:

1. Sit up straight in a chair, feet flat on floor, with arms and legs uncrossed.
2. Pay attention to your breath, doing nothing special but noticing the air coming into and out of your nostrils.
3. Do not judge any thoughts that come into your mind; notice your mind has wandered and return your focus to your breath.
4. Start with the 5-minute script or audio *Breathing Meditation* (5:31 min) at http://marc.ucla.edu/mindful-meditations (UCLA Health, 2022). This is the script I used to begin my classes with nursing students.
5. Take the opportunity to practice mindfulness as you walk to a patient's room. Consciously bring your attention to this moment and to your breath and set the intention to be present with your patient, without judgment of what is happening.

Modified from Sheridan, C. (2016). *The mindful nurse: Using the power of mindfulness and compassion to help you thrive in your work.* Buffalo, NY: Rivertime Press; Torney, D. (2017). *Mindfulness for emerging adults: Finding balance, belonging, focus and meaning in the digital age.* Duluth, MN: Whole Person Associates.

natural by-product of mindfulness. In Ponte and Koppel's (2015) pilot program on mindfulness, nurses reported less stress and improved connections with patients and families. A study of mindfulness training with Bachelor of Science in Nursing (BSN) students suggests students have stress relief, better concentration, time management, and study and test-taking skills (Foster, 2018). To get started, see Box 19.1 and see Exercise 8 in this chapter for a free resource for in-depth, online mindfulness training.

HALT!

Do you ever feel overwhelmed? If I were to ask my nursing students to list their stressors, we would all be overwhelmed, but help is available to you, and it is important to build relaxation skills early in your student or work career to help you be successful (Jameson, 2014). Relaxation skills, a mainstay in complementary medicine in recent years, are tools for effective stress management that are a part of a proactive approach to taking responsibility for coming to your work strong and feeling emotionally and physically well (Lee & Yeo, 2013). Resilience is the ability to adjust to change or to "bounce back." Relaxation strategies work best when you are not totally depleted. HALT is an acronym for hungry, angry, lonely, and tired and was introduced in

Alcoholics Anonymous to remind us of vulnerabilities that make us less resilient (Friedmann et al., 2003). To make the best use of relaxation skills, pay attention to your own self-care needs. Choose nutritious foods. Go off the unit to take lunch times and breaks, which are your allotted times to refresh yourself. Deal with fear, frustration, and hurt, which are emotions that lead to anger. Nurture relationships with others by scheduling time to be together, recognizing that, although we may be connected electronically, we may become isolated. Research about how women respond to stress shows that a woman's response is to "tend and befriend," in contrast to men's response to stress that is known as "fight or flight." Research demonstrated that women tend to nurture their children and seek out companionship, especially with other women; this is related to the hormone oxytocin (Taylor et al., 2000). Ironically, women may judge these behaviors as less worthy than completing their to-do list, ignore healthy ways of dealing with stress, and put time with other women friends at the bottom of their list of priorities. Commit to getting 8 hours of sleep when possible and allow yourself time to just rest!

SIMPLIFY AND DEEPEN

There is no need to go to India or anywhere else to find peace. You will find that deep place of silence right in your room, your garden, or even your bathtub.

Elisabeth Kubler-Ross

IMPORTANCE OF RELAXING YOUR BODY

There is no quick fix to manage stress because stress is a result of "an interaction between a negative environment, unhealthy lifestyles, and self-defeating attitudes and beliefs" (Micozzi, 2014). Exposure to noise and artificial light can be stressors for nurses and contribute to job dissatisfaction (Applebaum, Fowler, Fiedler, Osinubi, & Robson, 2010). Interruptions in the work environment of nurses can have a significant effect on client safety (McGillis Hall, Pedersen, & Fairley, 2010). Injuries can occur when we are "just not thinking." Consider a time when you were driving and suddenly realized that your mind was not on your driving and you do not remember how you got from one place to another. Geller (2010) used mindfulness exercises in his work with job safety analysis (JSA) to promote prompt reaction to prevent industrial accidents. This chapter encourages you to develop a habit of daily relaxation, a letting-go technique to eliminate the negative buildup of stress in your body and on preparing your body to relax during your workplace interactions. Physical stress that builds up can have long-term negative effects on the body. Relaxation brings relief from tension anxiety and fear and contributes to a general sense of well-being.

Chronic tightened muscles, tension headaches, or digestive disturbances reflect your "disease" and register diminished well-being. Built-up stress reactions steal valuable energy and put you at risk of holding back or closing off in your interpersonal relationships and interfere with focus needed for learning and for patient care.

Self-Care Nudge

Stand up now and stretch. Take a few moments to do this before you go into the clinical setting.

> **WIT AND WISDOM**
> *For fast-acting relief, try slowing down.*
>
> **Lily Tomlin**

STRESS OF NURSING AS AN OCCUPATION

Occupational stress is a major health issue for nurses. Contact with death, patients, and their families; conflicts with coworkers and supervisors; and uncertainty about effectiveness of care "affect nurses' health-related quality of life negatively, while it can also be considered as an influence on patient outcomes" (Sarafis et al., 2016, p. 56). As a nurse, you navigate several organizational structures to ensure client well-being, including the nursing hierarchy, the medical hierarchy, and the agency's bureaucracy. To survive this organizational maze, you need effective interpersonal communication techniques and efficient management skills. Increased acuteness of clients' conditions and a shortage of personnel contribute to increased stress. In addition to expertise in your own profession, you need to be proficient in interprofessional communication.

One of the most frequently cited sources of stress in nursing is the excessive workload, which gives nurses the feeling that they are always in a hurry, as if in a race with time. This factor is intensified by nurses' day-to-day encounters with distressing and anxiety-provoking situations, as well as insufficient resources in these times of healthcare restraint. As helping professionals, each of you has a vision of what your workplace, colleagues, and clients will be like, and these images may not prepare you for the reality you encounter. This chapter invites you to empower yourself by taking charge of your individual resourcefulness for increasing your relaxation response.

We help clients by reviewing the basics of health promotion, such as eating nutritiously, exercising regularly, securing adequate sleep, engaging in supportive social encounters, and making time for solitude and/or spiritual contemplation. When we practice these ourselves, we have an enhanced sense of well-being and readiness to handle the stress of working as a nurse. This chapter invites your work to become more mindful through meditation, progressive relaxation, and on-the-spot relaxation exercises. These techniques are designed to relax your body, putting it in a state in which the fight-or-flight response or the defense-alarm syndrome of arousal is greatly diminished or eliminated so that your energy is available for communicating effectively (Luskin & Pelletier, 2005).

MEDITATION AS A WAY TO AUGMENT YOUR RELAXATION RESPONSE

Meditation is a "mind body practice with many methods and variations…rounded in the silence and stillness of compassionate, nonjudgmental present-moment awareness. Although contemplative meditation practices are largely rooted in the world's spiritual traditions, the practice of meditation does not require belief in any particular religious or cultural system" (Fortney & Taylor, 2010). Meditation has become a general term that includes a variety of practices to relax the body and still the mind. The word *meditation* comes from the root word *meditari*, which means to "consider" or "pay attention to something" (Fontaine, 2014). Meditation is an experiential exercise you do by yourself and for yourself to benefit from the subjective sense of deep relaxation of the body's musculature; an added benefit is that you may possibly come to know yourself more fully. Meditation is psychologically and physically refreshing and energy restoring (Luskin & Pelletier, 2005).

Empirical study has confirmed that the meditative process relieves nervous system stress more efficiently than either dreaming or sleeping. Marked physiologic alterations accompany meditation, such as a reduction of the metabolic rate, a reduction of the breathing rate to four to six breaths per minute, an increase in the number of alpha waves in the brain (waves of 8–12 cycles per second), the appearance of theta waves in the brain (waves of 5–8 cycles per second), and a 20% reduction in the blood pressure of hypertensive patients (Luskin & Pelletier, 2005).

The regenerating effects of meditation are experienced during the meditation itself and have a carryover effect into your daily activities (Luskin & Pelletier, 2005). Once you have learned the low arousal effect during the meditation practice, you can maintain this state of neurophysiologic functioning in response to stressful situations. It is impossible to be relaxed and tense at the same time, and your enhanced ability to maintain relaxation during the day in the face of stressful interpersonal situations is what will help minimize the effects of stress on you. With practice you will be able to call on your low arousal state as needed during your working day. By itself this mechanism is helpful, and your heightened feelings of being able to cope with the pressures of everyday life will augment your good feelings (Luskin & Pelletier, 2005). When you learn to diminish your reaction to stressors, you free yourself to deal with aspects of the interpersonal situation more worthy of your energy. Being able to shift focus from being tight or nervous to feeling calm and in charge allows you to communicate more effectively.

Mindfulness is an aspect of meditation that "reflects the basic and fundamental human capacity to attend to relevant aspects of experience in a nonjudgmental and nonreactive way, which in turn cultivates clear thinking, equanimity (composure under stress), compassion, and openheartedness" (Fortney & Taylor, 2010). Mindfulness, which is developed through meditation, enables you to maintain a fluid awareness in a moment-by-moment experiential process that helps you disengage from a strong attachment of beliefs, thoughts, or emotions; this results in a greater sense of emotional balance and well-being. This evidence-based practice holds the potential for many health benefits, including challenges such as increasing healthcare costs, chronic lifestyle-induced illness, healthcare provider burnout, client dissatisfaction, and stress in clients and caregivers (Chiesa & Serretti, 2009; Deyo, Mirza, Turner, & Martin, 2009; Eckleberry-Hunt et al., 2009; Fortney & Taylor, 2010; Ludwig & Kabat-Zinn, 2008; McCray, Cronholm, Bogner, Gallo, & Neill, 2008; Paul-Labrador et al., 2006). Meditation teaches you to fix your attention firmly on a given task for increasingly protracted periods of time, overcoming the habit of flitting from one subject to another. I once heard a chaplain working in a hospice setting make this remark about meditation: "When you are trying to still the mind, if a thought comes into your head, you need not invite it to tea."

Once you have truly tried to quiet your mind or to allow images to run through it without letting any particular one become distracting, you will understand why practice and perseverance are necessary if you are to be successful. Have you noticed how your thoughts seem to wander or race? It is not easy to still the mental chatter. When you attempt to become quiet, your mind may jump from one thought or concern to another. This is expected. Think, "Oh well, a thought," and let it go. Begin with 10 minutes of meditation and increase it to 20 minutes at a time. Experiment to determine the best approach for you. You will find it gets easier to be still and be present for yourself. At this point, the subtle benefits of meditation become more pronounced (Luskin & Pelletier, 2005).

GUIDELINES FOR BEGINNING TO PRACTICE MEDITATION

The following guidelines are for a nonreligious form of meditation. It has a very simple form, requiring that you sit comfortably in a quiet place, that you focus your attention on the word *one*, and that you adopt an accepting and unconcerned attitude. These conditions will help you experience what is called the *relaxation response*, a state that research shows is associated with reduced physiologic activity. That means the heart rate will become slower and the blood pressure will fall. You will notice that you feel calmer than usual, and the entire sensation will be a pleasant one. At no time will you lose consciousness or be controlled by an outside force. The state you reach is one that you will have induced in yourself (Benson & Proctor, 2010; Payne & Donaghy, 2010). There are other forms of meditation, and you may wish to read about them or even take a course or individualized instruction in meditation.

> **WIT AND WISDOM**
> *Meditation is simplicity itself. It's about stopping and being present. That is all.*
> **Jon Kabat-Zinn**

Make Time to Meditate

To experience benefits from meditation, it is desirable to meditate for 15 to 20 minutes at least once a day. This commitment means consistently setting aside that time.

Many individuals say that they have an extremely busy schedule and simply do not have the opportunity to sit for such a long period of time each day. Very often a realistic examination of a person's schedule indicates that in fact there is sufficient time if the individual is conscientious and serious in his or her efforts. To some extent, the minor life reorientation necessitated by meditative practice may be responsible for its success. It involves a reordering of life priorities and behavioral patterns (Luskin & Pelletier, 2005).

Set the Climate to Meditate

Find a quiet place in which you will not be disturbed. Turn off your cell phone or silence the ringer on your telephone for the time you are meditating. Tell others that you do not wish to be disturbed for a specified length of time and assure them that you will be available after your meditation. Taking these precautions frees you to relax instead of tensing at sounds in your environment. Many people find it best to meditate first thing in the morning when their home is quiet and the world has not yet started to intrude. For nurses doing shift work, other arrangements can be made. Some people choose a quiet place outside their home, such as the hospital chapel.

Secure a Comfortable Position for Meditation

Find a position that is truly comfortable for you in which your body is supported by minimal muscular work.

Support your back and feet if necessary. If possible, adjust the room temperature so that you are comfortable. If you are warm enough, you are more likely to stay relaxed and not be distracted.

Develop a Passive Attitude

Distracting thoughts are likely to occur during your meditation, especially at first when you are learning to focus. Let these thoughts pass without becoming worried about their intrusion or your ability to meditate.

Select a Mental Device

To help you shift away from logical, externally oriented thoughts, select a mental device, such as a phrase, a word, or a sound, that you can repeat while you meditate. Repetition of this sound, called a *mantra,* assists in breaking the stream of distracting thoughts. Some suggestions for a mental device are single-syllable sounds or words such as *in, out, one,* or *zum,* which can be repeated silently or in a low tone while meditating. Select a mantra that is not emotionally charged and is soothing to you. Make up a word if you prefer (Benson & Proctor, 2010; Payne & Donaghy, 2010), or use a word that is rooted in your belief system. A nonreligious person might use a word such as *one, peace,* or *love,* whereas a person from the Christian tradition might use the opening words of a comforting prayer, such as "The Lord is my shepherd..." from Psalm 23. A person of the Jewish tradition might use the word *shalom* (Micozzi, 2014).

Relax Your Body

When you are ready to begin your meditation, start by relaxing your body with a body scan. Begin with the muscle groups in the head and work down to the feet. Say to yourself: "Relax your face; now allow your neck muscles to thaw; let your head relax; take the tension out of your shoulders; let your chest muscles loosen; allow your abdomen to soften; let your back muscles unfreeze; take the tension out of your thigh muscles; let your calves melt; allow your feet to rest, comfortably supported." As you tune into the difference between relaxation and tension in your muscles, you will be able to quickly release the tightness in your body in preparation for your meditation times. Wearing comfortable, loose-fitting clothing helps you assume a posture that is relaxing.

Focus on Your Breathing

Breathe through your nose and focus on, or become aware of, your breathing. This awareness helps you relax. Breathe easily and naturally, allowing the air to come to you on each inhalation (Benson & Proctor, 2010; Payne & Donaghy, 2010). Exhale slowly, allowing all the air out of the lungs. You will find that this focus on your breathing is very peaceful. When you are stressed, your breathing is quicker; by slowing your breathing and appreciating its rhythm, you begin to relieve tension. Remember not to control your breathing; you do not want to become light-headed. Just breathe easily and naturally.

While you are first focusing on your breathing, you can repeat your mental device silently on inhalation and exhalation. You can try saying to yourself as you inhale, "I am breathing in peace and calm." On exhalation, try thinking, "I am blowing out tension and negativity."

Meditate for 10 Minutes

Start by meditating for 10 minutes, then increase the time to 15 or 20 minutes as you gain experience in being still. Close your eyes during your meditation if this helps you focus on your breathing and on your mantra. Do not think of things or try to solve problems during this quiet time. Your meditation time is time out from running your life, managing time, controlling events, and performing as an adult in your hectic world. In this quiet time, for 10 to 20 minutes, you are free to just sit and breathe. Do not expend energy judging your thoughts or criticizing any distractions; simply let them pass by and remain focused on the present, on your breathing, and on your mental device.

Allow your images and thoughts to flow freely. Your mantra will come back to you. While you are meditating, you do not need to expend a great effort or concentrate. Enjoy this quiet, peaceful experience. If you need to open your eyes to check the time, arrange to have a clock in view so that moving is unnecessary.

Experience Your Unique Meditation

There are no rules or "shoulds" for what you experience in your meditations. Enjoy the peaceful break in which you can unwind and experience the sensation of relaxation. You may discover sensations in your body that you were previously too busy to notice. It may happen that, in addition to peacefulness, you achieve a level of stillness in which you might be overwhelmed with joy and a sense of unity with life. This powerful feeling is described as dissolving all fear, including the fear of death, and creating an inundation of warmth, joy, and harmony (Luskin & Pelletier, 2005).

Transcendental meditation (TM), one form of meditation, has been found to be an effective tool for the following (Sheikh, 2002):

- Changing your time orientation to the "here and now"
- Increasing your behavioral motivation to be more inner directed
- Developing sensitivity to personal needs and feelings
- Improving your ability to express feelings spontaneously

- Increasing your self-acceptance
- Raising your level of self-actualization

Such effects add to the nurse's ability to learn and maintain the perspective necessary to be able to stay connected to clients and family without becoming personally overwhelmed. A variety of relaxation and guided-imagery techniques are useful with children (Allen & Klein, 2000; Klein & Holden, 2001). In a qualitative study of the lived experience of graduate nursing students practicing TM, Perkins and Aquino-Russell (2017, p. 163) reported that students found themselves "authentically present and balanced with enhanced job performance."

End Your Meditation Peacefully

When it is time to end your meditation, pause before standing up and moving. It may be soothing to sit for a brief moment with your eyes closed before slowly opening them. Do not rush away, but rather gently leave your meditation and enter your world refreshed and relaxed.

WIT AND WISDOM

Those who seek the truth by means of intellect and learning only get further and further away from it. Not til your thoughts cease all their branching here and there, not til your mind is motionless as wood or stone, will you be on the right road to the Gate.

Huang Po

PROGRESSIVE RELAXATION

Progressive relaxation is a method of decreasing muscular tension to promote the relaxation response. This process of progressively tensing and relaxing muscle sets in a systematic way can be useful for you and for your clients (Box 19.2). A study of the use of progressive muscle relaxation with music, showed a reduction of stress and fatigue in intensive care nurses (Ozgundondu & Metin, 2019). A study combining progressive muscle relaxation and music therapy decreased stress before nursing school examinations and improved academic results (Gallego-Gomez et al., 2019). This technique helps clients with chronic tension become aware of the difference between a muscle that is tense and one that is relaxed (Fontaine, 2014). Progressive relaxation training has produced favorable results for conditions such as anxiety, hypertension, insomnia, asthma, dyspnea, and anxiety in chronic pulmonary disease, pain, and chronic tension headaches (Payne & Donaghy, 2010; Yilmaz & Kapucu, 2017; Gopichandran et al., 2021).

BOX 19.2   Sample Progressive Relaxation Exercise Script

- Find a quiet room with soft light where you are unlikely to be interrupted.
- Sit in a comfortable chair, feet flat on the floor, arms supported at your sides.
- Slowly begin to take several deep breaths, focusing on your breathing.
- Tense your facial muscles, close your eyes tightly, and hold your mouth closed.
- Relax your face, making the muscles feel as though they are sagging.
- Clench your right fist and tighten the muscles in your right arm.
- Open your right fist and relax the arm muscles, making your arm feel loose and heavy.
- Clench your left fist and tighten the muscles in your left arm.
- Open your left fist and relax the arm muscles, making your arm feel loose and heavy.
- Tighten the muscles in your right leg and squeeze the toes on your right foot.
- Relax your right leg muscles and toes.
- Tighten the muscles in your left leg and squeeze the toes on your left foot.
- Relax your left leg muscles and toes.
- Tighten your buttocks.
- Relax your buttocks.
- Relax your entire body. Allow it to feel free and heavy. You are in a state of total relaxation.
- Stay in this relaxed state for about 5 minutes. Pay attention to how your body feels in this state.
- Gradually open your eyes and slowly stretch. Experience this relaxation.

Adapted from Eliopoulos, C. (1999). *Integrating conventional & alternative therapies: Holistic care for chronic conditions.* St. Louis, MO: Mosby.

ON-THE-SPOT RELAXATION EXERCISES TO RELIEVE TENSION CAUSED BY AN INTERPERSONAL STRESSOR

Meditating on a daily basis will make you more relaxed and vital at work or school. Even with this new peacefulness, however, there will be times when a distraught client, an enraged family member, or an agitated colleague can raise your tension level. It would be ideal, but probably impractical, if you could leave the unit for some quiet time when clients and colleagues upset your peacefulness. What can help are some on-the-spot ways to regain your relaxation response. Techniques such as meditation or prayer can help you learn to maintain your perspective in the face of the complex demands of nursing. This chapter offers you creative techniques on which you can call to cool down when the heat is on. Some things you can do to relax your body when the unit is understaffed, the client population is on overload, and you are encountering interpersonal stress, presented next.

STRATEGIES FOR RELAXING YOUR BODY WHEN YOUR STRESSOR IS IMMEDIATE

Some stressful situations occur with no warning. In these instances, it helps to have on-the-spot methods for relaxing your body in your repertoire. Start by practicing a few abdominal breaths. Breathe in through your mouth, focusing on making your stomach bigger; breathe out through your nose, pushing your stomach in toward your spinal column. When working with pediatric patients, nurse researcher Sharlene Weiss (1998) called these "belly breaths" and asked children to imagine blowing up a balloon in their tummies. She explains that this simple exercise halts the sympathetic nervous system's response during stress by stimulating the parasympathetic nervous system. Try a few abdominal breaths now and notice how you feel after in contrast to before the exercise. Stop reading now and try it. Many people report feeling light-headed. Did this happen to you? We are more accustomed to shallow breathing. More oxygen to your brain can provide quicker problem-solving responses!

Each of the following brief relaxation exercises can be done on a moment's notice with no need for privacy or special equipment. Each can be done as you walk down the corridor, ride on the elevator, or stand up to face the person who is stressing you.

Exercises to Help Cope with an Unexpected Stressful Interpersonal Encounter

Imagine that it is noon on the orthopedic unit, on which you are in your third week of clinical work. The lunches have not arrived, and the clients are hungry. You are hungry. A physician strides out of the elevator, spies you, and heads in your direction. Her forceful walk, scowl, furrowed brow, and finger pointed in your direction give you clues that she is irate about something, and because you are the only nurse in the vicinity, you will likely bear the brunt of her aggression.

The following are some ideas about what you can do to relax your body before tension tightens your muscles in a fight-or-flight response. These techniques can be done in the moment while you are awaiting the approach of the

irate physician (your stressor) and even while you are communicating assertively in the face of this threat.

Sprinkling Shower

The spray from an imaginary shower nozzle is above your head, and you feel the water trickling through your hair, warming your shoulder muscles on its way down your back. Your hunched shoulders sag with relief from the warmth. You feel the warm soapy water caressing your muscles and heating your skin. The soapy lather massages your skin as it flows over you, warming your legs and feet before disappearing down the drain. As you lift your face to the nozzle, you are pelted with a clear stream of fresh water. Someone has adjusted the nozzle; you sense a firm staccato pressure on your face and over your neck and shoulders. You notice that this beating of water is simultaneously comforting and invigorating. You feel regenerated. The comforting relief you experience from the water surrounding your body makes you sigh deeply. The pressure of the water eases up to a refreshing sprinkle. As the shower turns off you are suddenly dry, and you feel warm and refreshed. As you relax, say to yourself, "This is relaxation. This is how it feels to be loose. This is what I want."

Sunbeam

Picture a radiant ball of light just above your head creating a field of bright rays vibrating in a protective pyramid around your body. Feel its protective glow encircling your body to a diameter of 4 feet. Notice that the light feels warm, and, as it envelops you, you are comforted by its penetrating rays. You find yourself raising your face to bask in the heat of the radiant sun. You can actually feel the light infiltrate your body, permeating your cells. This experience is comforting, and to your surprise you can actually feel the warmth from the light circulating from your head to your toes. Now you notice that the light is twinkling, and as it touches your skin you feel unusually invigorated. The sparkling sunbeams dance over your skin, dissipating any tension you were feeling. Your energy opens up in response to the warmth and tingling. As you relax, your muscles are overwhelmed with a feeling of profound comfort and safety in the rays of your own special sunbeam. As you relax, say to yourself, "This is relaxation. This is how it feels to be loose. This is what I want."

Safety Shield

Picture a clear plexiglass shield that rises up to surround you when you sense danger. Your protective shield is about 2 feet away from your body, and it allows you to move freely while it protects you on all sides. You can see quite clearly into the outside world, as if the shield were invisible. Inside your shield, the air is fresh and makes your skin tingle as it circulates around your body. This is your personal air supply and, when you breathe, you notice that the air penetrates your lungs, invigorating your cells as it circulates throughout your body. You feel energized and nourished by this special supply of air in your protected space. You also notice that you feel calm and well defended inside your shield because you realize that the shield deflects tension away from you. You are relaxed and free from any tensions outside your shield, and you feel this assurance in your body. You notice your breathing is slowing down with the nourishing air, and you feel that your muscles are loose and fluidly mobile. You relax because you know you are safe. As you relax, say to yourself, "This is relaxation. This is how it feels to be loose. This is what I want."

Sweeper

A magic broom comes out of nowhere to sweep the tension from your body. It rakes through your hair, leaving your scalp tingling as the circulation is invigorated. Your head feels warm and free of tension after this stimulation. You notice that your neck moves easily and is relaxed instead of stiff. As the broom sweeps the stress from your shoulders, they relax and feel lighter. You stand less rigidly and notice that your back is free from any tension. This broom is powerful and thorough in its ability to brush the stress off and away from your body. You can feel its bristles brush away the tension from your abdomen and the fronts and backs of your legs. When your feet are swept, you feel lighter and more mobile; this sensation is energizing. You know you are tension free, and you feel safe when the stress is swept into a pan and thrown far away from your body. Without the encumbrance of stress and tension, you feel ready to handle anything. The sweeping has regenerated your batteries and renewed your energy. Your feet are moving with renewed energy, and you are tempted to get up and dance on the balls of your feet. You feel alive and free! As you relax, say to yourself, "This is relaxation. This is how it feels to be loose. This is what I want."

Massage

A pair of powerful hands comes out of nowhere and lays itself across your shoulders. These large but gentle hands are unusually warm and radiate heat to your upper back. The motion is soothing, and the heat penetrates deep inside. You rotate your shoulders easily after these comforting hands have massaged away the tension. No effort is needed to stand or move. You are relaxed. The hands move up to knead the knots in your neck muscles. The touch is magical, as if by merely being there, the hands can dissipate tightness from built-up tension. Before moving on, the hands shake the tension away from your body so that it is no longer a threat. Next, the hands move to your lower back

and massage the tightness out of your spine. The pressure is firm, and with each small circular stroke you notice that your breathing gets more relaxed; it slows down, and you are totally soothed by the comfort and compassion emanating from the hands. You can feel the muscles in your neck, shoulders, and back filling with blood, becoming warm and supple under the gifted touch of the hands as they massage away fear and tightness. You feel release and a sense of freedom. You feel warm and protected. As you relax, say to yourself, "This is relaxation. This is how it feels to be loose. This is what I want."

Advantages of On-the-Spot Relaxation Exercises

Each of these brief but powerful relaxation strategies takes about a minute to experience. In that short time, you can shift from tightness and fear to relaxation and a feeling of competence. Using these calming strategies will give you inner self-confidence. As you become aware of when your body is relaxed, you will become even more skilled at calming yourself in the face of tension. Relaxation is a skill, a coordination of mind and muscles, and it can be learned by anyone who wants to do so and is willing to spend the time and effort (Percival, Percival, & Taylor, 1977).

STRETCHES TO CREATE RELAXATION IN PREPARATION FOR A STRESSFUL INTERPERSONAL ENCOUNTER

If you have more warning about an upcoming stressful interpersonal encounter, you can add soothing stretches to augment the benefits of meditation and on-the-spot exercises. Before encountering a stressor, or at any time during your hectic day, break away from the busy pace of the unit and find a quiet place in which to relax your muscles for a minute or so. Find some privacy in the bathroom or an empty office. Here are some stretches you can do that take little space and can be done from a standing position without any equipment.

These exercises involve tensing and relaxing the muscles until you feel the difference between the two sensations and learn to consciously relax any tense muscle. As your muscles learn the difference, they will develop a relaxation response (Percival et al., 1977).

High Stretch and Relax

Stand erect and stack your hands on top of your head. While taking a deep breath, reach high overhead, lifting your chest and moving your head back slightly. Stretch slowly until your hands are as high as they will go. Hold this for 3 seconds. Now exhale, letting the air out with a long, easy sigh while dropping your arms slowly to your sides.

Let your shoulders sag, your head fall forward, and your knees go loose and slightly bent. Remain in this relaxed position for 3 to 5 seconds. Allow all the tension to seep out of your neck, arms, shoulders, and chest muscles. Repeat this a few times before returning to work (Percival et al., 1977).

Shoulder Rotation

The shoulder rotation stretch improves shoulder flexibility and relaxes your shoulder girdle. Stand with your feet comfortably apart. Raise your elbows to shoulder height, allowing your forearms and hands to dangle loosely. Rotate elbows forward in large circles at a medium pace, keeping your hands and arms loose throughout. Move the shoulders in as large an arc as possible for about 20 rotations (Percival et al., 1977).

Shoulder Shrug and Relax

The shoulder shrug relaxation exercise can be done even while you are talking on the phone. Stand with your feet comfortably apart. As you take a deep breath, shrug your shoulders up to your ears and moderately tighten the muscles throughout your body. Hold for 3 to 5 seconds. Now exhale with a long, deep sigh, letting your shoulders drop down and your muscles go loose so that your knees bend slightly and your head drops forward to your chest. Repeat this several times (Percival et al., 1977).

Arms Out, Up, and Relax

Stand erect with your feet comfortably apart. Lift your arms out to your sides and up over your head, simultaneously pulling your stomach in and lifting your chest. When you have reached as high as you can, let your arms drop loosely down. Allow your head to sag so that your chin touches your chest and your knees go soft. Try to get as loose and limp as you can. Feel the tension drain out. Repeat this several times before returning to work (Percival et al., 1977).

 MOMENTS OF CONNECTION...

Take Time

> When asked how nurses can revitalize their practice, one nurse responded: "Take time to listen, to care, to share. Take time for yourself, especially. Life is too short to put it all into work. You have a lot to gain for yourself and can give more to others when you have energy and a meaningful life of your own."

With practice you will be able to call on your relaxation response at any moment. Being able to relax gives you the power to release tension in your muscles, reclaiming that energy for dealing with interpersonal stressors in your life. In the next few chapters, you will learn ways to change your mind-set to handle difficult situations in your relationships with clients and colleagues.

Return to "Active Learning" at the beginning of the chapter and write your responses.

PRACTICING USING RELAXATION TECHNIQUES TO BECOME MORE MINDFUL

Skill Building: Exercise 1

Refer to Box 19.1 to begin a mindfulness practice. On your own, listen to the audio or download the script and practice reading it slowly, taking turns (see Guided Meditations - UCLA Mindful Awareness Research Center - Los Angeles, CA [uclahealth.org]).

Discuss your experience. UCLA Mindful is an app available for Apple or Android devices that has the same meditations. Look for the 5-minute "Breathing Meditation" in "Basic Meditations."

Breathing Exercises: Exercise 2

Try these breathing exercises for yourself, and then introduce them to a patient in need of calming.

A. Brief breathing activity for patients: Guide your patient in a deep-breathing exercise. Repeat, "I am relaxed." I am (inhale), relaxed (exhale) to help focus and slow a patient's breathing (Sheridan, 2016).

B. The 4-7-8 breath: (For important details, be sure to watch the brief video referenced.) Andrew Weil, MD, an integrative medicine physician, in the video linked below advises practicing this technique of breathing for 4 cycles twice a day and recommends it whenever something that causes anxiety occurs. He suggests it to help you sleep and even to combat food cravings. It is helpful for mild to moderate anxiety. It is something you can use as another tool for self-care that is cost-effective, without side effects, and readily available (3-minute video demonstration at https://www.drweil.com/videos-features/videos/breathing-exercises-4-7-8-breath/). Weil calls this a natural tranquilizer that is subtle but more powerful with practice, and he recommends starting with only four breaths at one time to avoid feeling lightheaded:

1. With your mouth closed, inhale to a mental count of 4.
2. Hold your breath to a mental count of 7.
3. Exhale through your mouth to a mental count of 8.

Skill Building/Walking Meditation: Exercise 3

Dance and movement are being explored as part of the expressive arts in healing movement. Reflect on your own experience with dance and movement and how these are related to your ability to relax. Try a walking meditation. Walk silently for 10 minutes by yourself and without music, paying attention to all your senses. Reflect on differences in your state of relaxation before and after the walking meditation. Experiment with moving to music you enjoy as another way to add to your repertoire of relaxation strategies, especially when you cannot quiet your mind enough to use more mental strategies.

Skill Building: Exercise 4

Give the on-the-spot relaxation visualizations a try over the next few days. Notice when you get distracted and design a way of refocusing on your soothing internal technique. Note when you are able to distinguish the change from tension in your muscles to letting go in a relaxation response. As you practice, this will get easier, and you will be able to relax more quickly.

Skill Building: Exercise 5

In clinical, take a moment to try out one of the relaxing stretch–release exercises. Time yourself to see how long it took to find a spot and complete a few relaxing stretch–releases. Stretching and releasing remind your body to relax, and you will be more focused when you return to the unit.

Smart Phone Resources: Exercise 6

Both Apple and Android platforms offer applications with music for relaxation and sleep. Search for your own and ask others for recommendations.

Internet Resource: Exercise 7

Visit http://palousemindfulness.com/selfguidedMBSR.html to access a free 8-week Mindfulness-Based Stress Reduction course. Explore the course, note the audio and videos referenced, and open Graduate Readings for excellent short articles. Identify clients for whom this would be a useful reference. In your career as an adult learner, such resources may support you without the cost of travel or conference admission. Consider taking this free course as a gift to yourself.

REFERENCES

Allen, J. S., & Klein, R. J. (2000). *Ready, set, relax: A research-based program of relaxation, learning and self-esteem for children*. Watertown, WI: Inner Coaching.

Applebaum, D., Fowler, S., Fiedler, N., Osinubi, O., & Robson, M. (2010). The impact of environmental factors on nursing stress, job satisfaction, and turnover intention. *Journal of Nursing Administration, 40*(7/8), 323.

Arcari, P. (2017). *6 Ways to practice mindfulness. [Infographic]* | Dana-Farber Cancer Institute.

Benson, H., & Proctor, W. (2010). *Relaxation revolution: Enhancing your health through the science and genetics of mind body healing*. New York, NY: Scribner.

Chiesa, A., & Serretti, A. (2009). Mindfulness based stress reduction for stress management in healthy people: A review and meta-analysis. *Journal of Alternative and Complementary Medicine, 15*(5), 593.

Deyo, R., Mirza, S. K., Turner, J. A., & Martin, B. I. (2009). Overtreating chronic back pain, time to back off? *Journal of the American Board of Family Medicine, 22*(1), 62.

Eckleberry-Hunt, J., Lick, D., Boura, J., Hunt, R., Balasubramaniam, M., Mulhem, E., et al. (2009). An exploratory study of resident burnout and wellness. *Academic Medicine, 84*(2), 269.

Fontaine, K. L. (2014). *Complementary & alternative therapies for nursing practice*. Boston, MA: Pearson.

Fortney, L., & Taylor, M. (2010). Meditation in medical practice: A review of the evidence and practice. *Primary Care, 37*(1), 81.

Foster, D. (2018). *Effects of mindfulness training on perceived level of stress and performance-related attributes in BSN students. Nursing Education Research Conference 2018 (NERC 2018)* (nursingrepository.org).

Friedmann, P. D., Herman, D. S., Freedman, S., Lemon, S. C., Ramsey, S., & Stein, M. D. (2003). Treatment of sleep disturbance in alcohol recovery: A national survey of addiction medicine physicians. *Journal of Addictive Diseases, 22*(2), 91.

Gallego-Gomez, J. I., Balanza, S., Leal-Llopis, J., Garcia-Mendez, J. A., Oliva-Perez, J., Domenenxh-Tortosa, J., et al. (2019). Effectiveness of music therapy and progressive muscle relaxation in reducing stress before exams and improving academic performance in nursing students: A randomized trial. *Nursing Education Today, 84*, Article 104217. https://doi.org/10.1016/j.nedt.2019.104217.

Geller, S. (2010). Industrial Safety and Hygiene News: Are you mindful or mindless when working? Are you mindful or mindless when working? *Industrial Safety and Hygiene News*.

Gopichandran, L., Srivastsave, A. K., Vanamail, P., Kanniammal, C., Valli, G., Mahendra, J., et al. (2021). Effectiveness of progressive muscle relaxation and deep breathing exercise on pain, disability, and sleep among patients with chronic tension-type headache. *Holistic Nursing Practice*. doi:10.1097/hnp.0000000000000460.

Ibrahim, K., Komariah, M., & Herliani, Y. K. (2022). The effect of mindfulness breathing meditation on psychological well-being. *Holistic Nursing Practice, 36*(1), 46–51. doi:10.1097/HNP.0000000000000464.

Jameson, P. R. (2014). The effects of a hardiness educational intervention on hardiness and perceived stress of junior baccalaureate nursing students. *Nurse Education Today, 34*, 603.

Janzarik, G., Wollschlager, D., & Lieb, K. (2022). A group intervention to promote resilience in nursing professionals: A randomized controlled trial. *International Journal of Environmental Research and Public Health, 19,* 649. doi:10.1097/HNP.0000000000000464.

Kabat-Zinn, J. (2017). Mindfulness: 3 definitions of mindfulness that might surprise you. *Psychology Today Australia,* Posted November 1, 2017.

Klein, N. C., & Holden, M. (2001). *Healing images for children: Teaching relaxation and guided imagery to children facing cancer and other serious illness.* Watertown, WI: Inner Coaching.

Lee, E. O., & Yeo, Y. (2013). Relaxation practice for health in the United States: Findings from the National Health Interview Study. *Journal of Holistic Nursing, 31*(2), 139.

Ludwig, D. S., & Kabat-Zinn, J. (2008). Mindfulness in medicine. *Journal of the American Medical Association, 300*(11), 1350.

Luskin, F., & Pelletier, K. (2005). *Stress free for good: Ten scientifically proven life skills for health and happiness.* New York, NY: HarperOne.

McCray, L. W., Cronholm, P. F., Bogner, H. R., Gallo, J. J., & Neill, R. A. (2008). Resident physician burnout, is there hope? *Family Medicine, 40*(9), 626.

McGillis Hall, L., Pedersen, C., & Fairley, L (2010). Losing the moment: Understanding interruptions to nurses' work. *Journal of Nursing Administration, 40*(4), 169.

Micozzi, M. S. (2014). *Fundamentals of complementary and integrative medicine.* St. Louis, MO: Saunders.

Ozgundondu, B., & Metin, Z. G. (2019). Effects of progressive muscle relaxation combined with music on stress, fatigue, and coping styles among intensive care nurses. *Intensive & Critical Care Nursing, 54,* 54–63. https://doi.org/10.1016/j.iccn.2019.07.007.

Paul-Labrador, M., Polk, D., Dwyer, J. H., Velasquez, I., Nidich, S., Rainforth, M., et al. (2006). Effects of a randomized controlled trial of transcendental meditation on components of the metabolic syndrome in subjects with coronary artery heart disease. *Archives of Internal Medicine, 166*(11), 1218.

Payne, R. A., & Donaghy, M. (2010). *Payne's handbook of relaxation techniques: A practical guide for the health care professional.* Edinburgh, UK: Elsevier.

Percival, J., Percival, L., & Taylor, J. (1977). *The complete guide to total fitness.* Scarborough, Ontario: Prentice Hall.

Perkins, J. B., & Aquino-Russel, C. (2017). Graduate nurses experience the sacred during transcendental meditation. *International Journal for Human Caring, 21*(4), 163.

Ponte, P. R., & Koppel, P. (2015). Cultivating mindfulness to enhance nursing practice. *American Journal of Nursing, 115*(6), 48–55.

Sarafis, P., Rousaki, E., Tsounis, A., Malliarou, M., Lahana, L., Bamidis, P., et al. (2016). The impact of occupational stress on nurses' caring behaviors and their health related quality of life. *BioMed Central, 15,* 56.

Sheikh, A. A. (Ed.). (2002). *Healing images: The role of imagination in health.* New York, NY: Baywood Publishing.

Sheridan, C. (2016). *The mindful nurse: Using the power of mindfulness and compassion to help you thrive in your work.* Buffalo, NY: Rivertime Press.

Taylor, S. E., Klein, L. C., Lewis, B. P., Gruenewald, T. L., Gurung, R. A. R., & Updegraff, J. A. (2000). Behavioral responses to stress in females: Tend-and-befriend, not fight-or-flight. *Psychological Review, 107*(3), 411.

Tolle, E. (1999). *The power of now: A guide to spiritual enlightenment.* Novato, CA: New World Library.

Torney, D. (2017). *Mindfulness for emerging adults: Finding balance, belonging, focus and meaning in the digital age.* Duluth, MN: Whole Person Associates.

UCLA Health. (2022). Guided Mediations. Guided Meditations - UCLA Mindful Awareness Research Center - Los Angeles, CA (uclahealth.org).

Weiss, S. (1998). Using relaxation imagery with children. In *Paper presented at the 22nd annual seminar of the Florida Association of Pediatric Tumor Programs.*

Yilmaz, C. K., & Kapucu, S. (2017). The effect of progressive relaxation exercises on fatigue and sleep quality in individuals with COPD. *Holistic Nursing Practice, 31*(6), 369.

20

Incorporating Imagery in Professional Practice and Self-Care

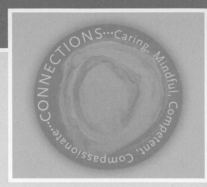

Your imagination practice is equivalent to an actual experience in so far as your nervous system is concerned.

Dr. Maxwell Maltz

OBJECTIVES

1. Define imagery or visualization.
2. Practice imagery using the tart lemon exercise.
3. Discuss the history of the use of imagery.
4. Identify uses of imagery in clinical practice.
5. Identify brief imagery exercises to cope with stressful situations.
6. Discuss the use of imagery techniques to improve communication skills.
7. Participate in selected exercises to build skills in using imagery in professional practice and self-care.

⚙ ACTIVE LEARNING

Incorporating Imagery in Professional Practice and Self-Care
Think about how you will write your answers as you read this chapter.

What?
Write one thing you learned from this chapter.

So What?
How will this affect your nursing practice?

Now What?
How will you implement this new knowledge or skill?

Think About It ...

DEFINITION OF IMAGERY

An *image* is defined as a mental picture (Merriam-Webster Online Dictionary, 2022). The term *visualization* is interchangeable with the term *imagery*. To visualize is to see or image mentally (Merriam-Webster Online Dictionary, 2022).

We use the term to mean creating an image of something invisible, absent, or abstract. As you read this chapter, begin to create an image of yourself as a confident, successful nurse, communicating assertively, gaining respect, and becoming a dedicated patient advocate. Boehm and Tse (2013) recommended guided imagery for new graduates to reduce stress and to increase proficiency by mental rehearsal.

Imagery or visualization is a process of mentally picturing an event we wish will occur in the present or future. It is a process of actually experiencing a picture that we hold in our mind's eye. In visualizing our picture, we may incorporate our senses to taste it, smell it, and feel it, and imagine the sounds and emotions associated with it. For example, when we visualize a freshly baked apple pie, we can actually smell it, taste the apples, and visualize eating the pie. We might evoke an image in vivid sensory detail of an absent loved one for extra emotional comfort. We might mentally rehearse a nursing procedure before performing it. As part of our fitness training, we might mentally rehearse running a 5K race, envisioning successfully completing the run and being at the finish line.

Try This Experiment: The Tart Lemon

Close your eyes and imagine that you are in your home. Picture yourself walking into your kitchen and looking at the refrigerator. In your mind's eye, see the refrigerator. Open it and pull open the fruit and vegetable drawer. You see a large, bright, yellow lemon. Pick it up and notice the yellow, shiny, bumpy surface. Feel the weight of the lemon in your hand. Now take the lemon to a cutting board. Squeeze the lemon before you cut it. You can already smell the citrus scent. Cut the lemon and inhale its fragrance. Open your mouth. Now squeeze a few drops of the cold, tart lemon juice onto your tongue. Open your eyes. Did your mouth pucker? Could you see the lemon, smell it, taste it?

WIT AND WISDOM

Go confidently in the direction of your dreams. Live the life you imagined.

Henry David Thoreau

NOTE

Not everyone uses imagery the same way. Some people report being actively involved in the scene. Some see it as actors on a stage. Others get sensory impressions but not a clear image. Do not be concerned if you cannot "see" things. Practice helps. This experiment helps you understand the behavioral applications of imagery.

When we visualize ourselves communicating, such as by listening actively, we can hear ourselves articulating empathic words; feel ourselves being warm, genuine, and natural; and enjoy observing a positive interaction between ourselves and our clients or colleagues.

Imagery is like a directed, deliberate daydream with purpose. It is much more than mere fantasy. The key to successful visualization is to be clear about what you want and then commit to that course of action in your imagery. This is a crucial step for producing successful results. In your mind's eye, there need be neither limitations nor constraints.

How does imagery work? Research shows that the neurophysiology of the brain does not distinguish between an image and the experience of the imagined place or situation as demonstrated through dimensional brain studies (Sternberg, 2010). "The body does not know the difference between what one is thinking and what is actually happening. The image or thought is experienced with one or more of the senses with an associated emotion linking the mind with a feeling state and the body with a resulting physiologic change" (Reed, 2007). For example, beginning to worry about an examination, thinking about being unsuccessful, and thinking about

the consequences cause the body to respond with a cascade of chemicals of the stress response (adrenaline and cortisol) interfering with immune function and our ability to cope (Reed, 2007).

This chapter focuses on how you can use imagery to positively influence your interpersonal communication. You will learn the steps required to formulate a clear image of how you want to communicate with your clients or colleagues. You can then use that visualization to help you actualize your vision in reality.

Imagery has been used in physical healing for a long time. You may be interested in the history of visualization in medicine.

Self-Care Nudge

Drink water! How much water have you drunk today? When your body is not hydrated you may feel as if you are tired for no reason. Some people are really thirsty and not hungry. It's ok to start small. How about substituting water for at least one other beverage today?

HISTORY OF IMAGERY

Imagery may be the oldest healing technique used by humans. Early records of this technique have been found on cuneiform tablets from Babylonia and Samaria. Greek, Egyptian, Asian, and ancient Indian civilizations used visualization.

In all of these cultures, disease was seen as a supernatural force that had incorporated itself into the ill person's being. The shaman, or physician-priest, would heal through rituals or ceremonies by confronting the disease-causing demon with a positive force and exorcising the demon from the patient. The shaman derived his power from visualization of a higher authority, god, or spirit. At that time, medicine was controlled by religion, mysticism, and magic (Johnston, 2002).

Paracelsus, a Renaissance physician, is known as the father of scientific medicine and modern drug therapy. A man opposed to the notion of separating the healing process from the spirit, he said, "The spirit is the master, imagination the tool, and the body the plastic material. The power of the imagination is a great factor in medicine. It may produce diseases in man and in animals, and it may cure them…Ills of the body may be cured by the physical remedies or by the power of the spirit acting through the soul" (Hartmann, 2007). The views of Paracelsus differed from those of the early shamans because Paracelsus believed that people's own thoughts, as well as gods and spirits, could be healing (Samuels & Samuels, 1975).

The mind–body dichotomy was first conceived during the Renaissance. The French philosopher Descartes helped establish the split with his attempts to free scientific questions from arguments concerning God. Scientists could then be concerned about the body without theological debate, and the philosophers and theologians were left to study the spirit and mind (Fontaine, 2014).

After the Renaissance, techniques of healing were divided into two systems: scientific and religious. Our Western society has adopted scientific healing—surgery and drug therapy. With increasing scientific investigation and medical specialization, the body–mind–spirit split continued into the 20th century. By 1900, however, a number of medical scientists had begun investigating how the mind affects the body and healing (Samuels & Samuels, 1975).

Jacobson (1942), searching for effective methods of relaxation, demonstrated that the imagery we use in thought processes produces a muscular reactivity that resembles what occurs during the actual performance of the imagined act. In other words, if we imagine ourselves in our mind's eye as running, the muscles we normally use when we run contract slightly.

Many scientists, as well as members of the medical profession, have continued to accept that the autonomic nervous system is unconscious, automatic, and not within conscious control. In the late 1960s, physiologists DiCara and Miller demonstrated that parts of the autonomic nervous system can be conditioned and controlled. They determined that rats could learn how to alter their stomach acidity, brain wave patterns, blood pressure, and blood flow (Miller, 1969). Furthermore, in their work with humans, scientists have verified that yogis have the ability to control specific processes of the body such as metabolic rate and heart rate (Lauria, 1968).

Groundwork laid by these scientists has been revolutionary in the current shift away from the body–mind–spirit split to body–mind integration. The implications of these findings for nursing and medicine are extraordinary and exciting!

APPLICATION OF IMAGERY IN HEALTHCARE

In a randomized clinical trial, Kermani, Aghebati, Mohajer, & Ghavami (2020) demonstrated the benefits of guided imagery and breathing relaxation to promote the quality of sleep of elderly patients following abdominal surgery. Patients receiving radiation for breast cancer shifted from feelings of fear to a sense of strength and calmness after nurse-guided imagery sessions (Serra, 2012). "Imagery creates a bridge between mind and body, linking perception, emotion, and psychological, physiological, and behavioural

responses" (Apostolo & Kolcaba, 2009). Helms (2006) described guided imagery as a complementary intervention to help the mind "see" positive images of desired outcomes to influence health and well-being, part of the content in the development of the NCLEX-RN®. Imaging positive results can have the opposite effect of the stress response, promoting relaxation, helping control blood pressure, helping to control pain and anxiety, facilitating the action of medication and treatments, minimizing side effects, promoting coping with chronic illness, optimizing healing, and promoting comfort during and after procedures (Lewandowski, Good, & Draucher, 2005; McCaffrey & Taylor, 2005; Reed, 2007; Riedel, 2012; Wynd, 2005). Imagery techniques include end state, which involves the image of a healed state; process, which involves imaging step-by-step to a goal, such as successful, comfortable completion of a procedure; receptive, which involves images for healing that arise from the person's own mind; active, which involves a conscious choice of a healing image, such as a healing white light directed to the affected area; and anatomic, such as imaging of the opening of constricted vessels (Schaub & Burt, 2013). Here is a specific example. A client with excessive gastric secretions was asked to gaze at the dryness and texture of blotting paper while imagining absorbent dryness. Tests indicated that, after 10 days of performing these visualizations, the client's excessive secretions normalized (Luthe, 1969). The use of imagery empowers the client to promote wellness when disease produces a sense of loss of control.

One hypothesis is that the feelings of hope and anticipation are recorded by the limbic system in place of hopelessness and despair. Psychoneuroimmunology is the study of the "multidirectional interactions among behavioral, neuroendocrine, and immunologic processes of adaptation. Thoughts, emotions, and information are reciprocal stimuli to sensory and motor neurons, glandular tissues, and immune cells via chemical transmitters" (Giedt, 1997). Clients who are enthusiastic about feeling better using imagery and who explicitly follow instructions show dramatic relief of their symptoms and marked improvement in their conditions.

There is evidence that visualization can influence a person's heart rate, blood flow, immune response, and total physiology. Visualization is a noninvasive, cost-effective intervention. Given this, what then are the implications of imagery?

IMPLICATIONS OF IMAGERY

How does the knowledge that it is possible to voluntarily affect the autonomic nervous system using visualization influence us in our nursing care? First, we as nurses can adopt a holistic philosophy of body, mind, and spirit integration. A holistic perspective emphasizes the interrelationship of the parts that make up the whole person. It acknowledges that the mind affects the body and vice versa. Accepting this notion of interdependence means understanding the power that exists within our whole body–mind–spirit beings to heal ourselves. This internal power can be used to maintain and increase our level of wellness, either alone or in conjunction with an external source of healing (Samuels & Bennett, 1974). The American Holistic Nurses Association offers a forum for the discussion of the research and practice of holistic nursing, and nurses in other states conduct workshops on interventions such as therapeutic touch. At the San Francisco State University, a large urban, public university, nursing students reported personal and professional benefits from both live and video instruction and practice of guided imagery as a complementary therapy (Windle, Berger, & Kim, 2021). A simple application of imagery in nursing is the use of alternative language when performing procedures, which is language that, although still truthful, suggests a different sensation than anticipated. When giving an injection, suggest, "You may feel a stick." This language decreases anxiety and shifts the pattern from response to "pain" to response to "a stick." The use of imagery is also gaining increasing acceptance in the areas of corporate finance and sports. Researchers have discovered, for example, that a frequent characteristic of executives of major US corporations is that "these people knew what they wanted out of life. They could see it, taste it, smell it, and imagine the sounds and emotions associated with it. They prelived it before they had it. And that sharp, sensory vision became a powerful driving force in their lives" (Mayer, 1984).

In an experiment that was conducted at the University of Western Australia, one basketball team practiced 20 minutes longer a day, whereas a second team used these 20 minutes to imagine themselves playing the game and mentally correcting themselves each time they missed a basket. After a period of weeks, the group that physically practiced the game improved 24%, and the group visualizing themselves as practicing improved 23% (Mayer, 1984).

Professional golfer Jack Nicklaus uses visualization to improve the muscle memory and motor skills involved in golf. Nicklaus has said that good golf requires one-half mental rehearsal and one-half physical coordination. He never hits a shot without first seeing a sharp, clear picture of that shot in his mind's eye (Mayer, 1984).

Imagery has been used in medicine, athletics, and business. It is a process that can be applied by people in various walks of life to achieve success in whatever they value. We now look at how imagery can be used by nurses to improve their interpersonal communication skills.

RELATIONSHIP BETWEEN IMAGERY AND INTERPERSONAL COMMUNICATION

If we are clear about what is important to us and if we are committed to creating what we value, imagery is an invaluable tool for self-direction (Mayer, 1984). This idea is the key to how imagery can be used by nurses to improve their interpersonal communication skills. If you are clear that it is important to be an effective communicator and you are committed to creating that outcome, then imagery can help you achieve that goal. Silk and Norwood (2002–2003) used the term *mental holography* to refer to the creation of mental images to enhance communication. They state that a hologram is "a manipulation of light from different sources to create a very realistic, three-dimensional image of a person or object that is not physically present…the study of holograms is 'holography.'" They suggest that when speakers learn to create sharp, vivid images in their minds, they can better communicate this image via language and body language.

As a professional nurse, you want to implement the interpersonal communication skills you are learning in this book in a way that is beneficial to your clients, your colleagues, and yourself. Imagery grants you a visualization of yourself implementing these skills in a helpful and effective way. It provides you with a picture of yourself as a nurse who can handle a variety of interpersonal situations confidently and competently. These images act like a beacon, beckoning you to achieve the goal of being a competent communicator. Having a mental hologram of yourself that envisions how you want to act and be seen supports your success in projecting this image.

As you read about each of the interpersonal communication behaviors, you learn the correct way to implement each one with your clients and colleagues. You develop a vision of yourself executing the communication behavior you are studying. When using imagery, some people experience themselves participating, whereas others observe themselves as actors on a stage. Some people get impressions without clear images. Some clients report better success with the use of the word *pretend* rather than *imagine*. Your perception may be fuzzy and vague at first. It is essential that you work at making this image of yourself as clear as possible. You need to create an image that envisions you communicating in a positive, effective, and competent manner. The more detailed and specific you can make your visualization, the more effective it will be to guide your actual communication.

Imagining yourself being successful is much like a rehearsal. This mental dry run helps cement an image of yourself performing the skill correctly. When the dress rehearsal goes well, it gives you confidence that your live performance will also be positive. You may find that the actual visualization process takes you 1 minute or less. The more you use this process, the more proficient you will become.

Seeing yourself perform the way you want to is just one more step toward successfully carrying out your performance in public. Having an image of yourself communicating well makes the future reality of such an event a viable possibility. Imagery helps you become familiar with your desired outcome so that you start accepting the notion that achieving your ideal is possible and forthcoming. Imagery makes you believe that you can achieve your goals.

Imagery can be influential in helping us communicate in a way that is in keeping with our goals as a nurse. If golf scores and management strategies can be improved through visualization, so can nurses' interpersonal communication skills.

Consider, too, the use of imagery to explore how mental models, which are deeply ingrained, can negatively influence the nurse's performance. Krejci (1997) helped students examine their images in response to words such as *nurse, doctor, power,* and *caring.* Sometimes these mental models are outdated and can affect the ability of nurses to grow professionally. Krejci cited the example of students' imagery about the word *power,* which often depicts a female nurse as a bystander watching a male figure wielding power. By reflecting on the importance of the caring and advocacy roles of the nurse, nurses can reframe their views of power and claim the power of their role.

Brief Imagery Exercises to Cope with Stressful Situations

Consider one of the following brief images when you take a moment to put distance between yourself and the strong emotions of a situation that you want to face calmly. An intense emotional situation may impair your judgment and make you speak before you think. Being relaxed and focused will better enable you to respond rationally rather than react emotionally. Imagine one of the following that most appeals to you. Pay attention to all your senses as you mentally experience:

- A leaf floating downstream
- Clouds moving across the sky
- Helium-filled balloons rising
- Bubbles being blown away (Payne & Donaghy, 2010)

Brief audio-guided imageries are useful strategies for stress relief. A study of guided imagery for treating compassion fatigue and anxiety in mental health staff showed promising results (Kiley et al., 2018). Guided imagery was one of the contemplative practices added to the NCLEX-RN preparatory course. Students found such activities useful and said they would use them again (Fiske, 2017; see Exercise 1 in this chapter for online samples).

USE OF IMAGERY TO IMPROVE YOUR ABILITY TO COMMUNICATE

Here are some of the essential points of effective imagery. First, imagery requires discipline, which is the willingness to briefly stop what you are doing and undertake the visualization process. Imagery is most effective when you are relaxed, so begin your imagery with three deep breaths to facilitate relaxation. (Refer to Chapter 19 for other relaxation exercises.) Relaxation helps you let go of the thoughts swimming around in your head. This enables you to focus on becoming clear about what you want to create with your imagery. Once you are clear about your goal or purpose, commit to creating it with no reservations and with complete faith that your goal or purpose will be attained. Using all your senses, allow yourself to feel the experience of your goal being attained as though it were happening at the very moment of your visualization.

Although this may sound complex at the outset, with practice you will be able to go through these steps quickly and effectively.

You might think that the practice of visualization is quite abstract because it occurs unseen inside your head. On the contrary, there are concrete and specific things you can do to ensure that your visualization influences your future performance in the way you intend. The following are some systematic steps you can take to make sure that your visualization has the desired results.

MOMENTS OF CONNECTION...
Just Imagine...Offering a Peaceful Pause for the People You Serve (You Can Try It, Too!)

A nursing student, already an RN going back to earn a Bachelor of Science in Nursing (BSN) degree, wanted to begin to integrate guided imagery into her work in intensive care. She remembered the practical language her instructor had offered to help her clients use imagery in a simple way. Remind the client, "Your body stays here while you are in the hospital, but you can go anywhere you want in your mind. Think of a place you would rather be, a place of comfort, beauty, or a time, a memory which you would like to revisit." *When the nurse offered this suggestion, her client, a grandmother said she would prefer to be baking cookies with her grandchildren, so the nursing student suggested she imagine being in her kitchen, evoking all her senses: feeling the heat from the oven, smelling the scent of cookies, seeing her grandchildren, and listening to her grandchildren's laughter. She reported noticing no discomfort from the procedure the nurse performed.*

Be Clear about Your Desired Outcome

Before you envision how you will communicate, you must be clear about what you want. Do you want to be warm and comforting? Do you want to obtain specific information from your client or colleague or get you point across? It helps to be clear about what you want to happen. The more your mental rehearsal is tailored to reality, the more positive an influence it will have on your subsequent performance. It might be helpful for you to compare a poorly articulated goal with a clearer, more detailed one.

Barb and Jane are both nurses working on a burn unit. Both nurses are concerned about Mrs. Charter, who has become withdrawn and tearful in the past 48 hours. Each nurse decides on her own desired outcome for an intervention.

Barb makes it her goal to help Mrs. Charter overcome her blue mood. This goal is not as clear as it might be, because it does not provide Barb with many clues about how to proceed. Not only is it not specific, but it is unlikely that it is a logical place to begin without more data.

Jane's aim is to determine whether Mrs. Charter is aware of what might be causing her mood change and to discuss what might help. Her aim is to put Mrs. Charter at ease so that she can talk more freely about her feelings. This clearer desired outcome provides Jane with some guidelines on how to proceed.

SIMPLIFY AND DEEPEN

Your imagination is your preview of life's coming attractions.

Albert Einstein

Mentally Outline the Entire Interaction from Beginning to End

You will feel more prepared for your interaction if you mentally outline it in your imagery. For instance, if you are going to be teaching a client to care for a colostomy, do not limit your visualization to the time when you will be talking. Bring into your vision your preparation time, postsession time, and the direct teaching time. When you visualize your preparation, you will anticipate all the equipment you will need and, consequently, will have it ready. You might become aware that you fear embarrassment in discussing the hygienic and sexual aspects of colostomy care with a male client. This awareness will prompt you to discuss your concerns with an experienced colleague before the session.

When imagining the teaching session, consider the beginning, middle, and end. Find out how much time you have and imagine yourself using the time productively.

Envision the conclusion of the lesson: Will you want time to debrief and discuss the session with a colleague afterward? Is it likely that you will have follow-up assignments after the session for which you must allow time, such as making referrals, writing records, or securing information for the client? By mentally going through the entire encounter, you will be much better prepared.

Concentrate on Visualizing Details

Envision the most ideal environment for your encounter and take in all its details. In reality, try to approximate this environment in terms of privacy, lighting, warmth, accessibility to equipment, or whatever other criteria are important.

Visualize how you would like to be dressed for your interaction. If it is a play session with the children on the pediatric medical unit, you will likely envision yourself in brightly-colored scrubs. If you are preparing yourself for your job performance interview with your manager, envision yourself wearing clothes in which you feel your best. Pay attention to your posture and facial expressions. If you want to be business-like with a serious middle-aged client, then picture how you will move to convey your intentions. If you wish to appear relaxed and confident as you present your case at your first nursing rounds, mentally see and feel yourself confident. Imagine seeing others responding favorably, listening, taking you seriously, and interested.

In addition to visual imagery, use your other senses. For instance, listen to what you are saying and how you are saying it. If what you are saying does not come across in the way you intended, then roll back the reel and replay it.

Envision how you want to feel during your communication, and be sure to concentrate on the positive. Evoke feelings of calmness, confidence, competence, or compassion. It is important to pause and actually experience these good feelings in your rehearsal so that you will be more likely to recognize them and allow them to surface in the real situation. Additionally, visualize your client or colleague having feelings that are appropriate for the situation.

Using your wide-angle lens, see the entire interaction going as you planned. For example, your bereaved colleague feels relieved to have shed a few tears with you after the death of her long-term client, your skeptical supervisor seems positively impressed with your suggestion for a new staffing schedule, and your once-worried client is able to drop off to sleep after your reassuring preoperative teaching session.

Envision the Best and Plan for the Unexpected

There are times when we are concerned about an interaction with a client or colleague. Envisioning a positive rehearsal helps relieve some of that worry. Envision unexpected turns of events you might encounter, and practice how to cope with them. For example, if it is the first time you will be teaching prenatal classes and you are afraid of questions about labor and delivery you can't answer, imagine saying, "I don't know…but I'll find out for you," or an angry colleague might unnerve you with her hostility. If you visualize anger in advance, you can prepare yourself with effective ways to respond.

Rehearse Repeatedly When Necessary

Each of us has interpersonal situations in which we lack confidence. Some of us shudder at having to interact with angry, hostile people, whereas others remain calm and empathic with volatile clients and colleagues. Some of us dread taking charge of teaching sessions, whereas others love that opportunity. Some of us believe we relate better on a one-to-one basis, and others prefer groups. For those interpersonal situations in which you feel uncomfortable, repeat your positive visualization several times. A single visualization may not be enough. Repeating the scene in your mind's eye will prevent you from being caught off guard in the actual event, and you will be able to respond instead of react.

When we are worried, we can either lapse into expecting the worst or choose to concentrate on seeing a positive picture. A positive visualization attracts like a magnet, getting you closer to your goal. If you repeat your positive visualization enough times, you will perform well in reality.

Review Your Live Performance and Update Your Visualization

After you have completed your interaction, take time to evaluate how the session went. If there were parts of your interaction with which you were less than pleased, consider how you could improve your next exchange and visualize that happening. For example, envision how you could rephrase your words, arrange the room differently, or include gestures such as touch. This rehearsal will prepare you for the next time.

Do not put yourself down for your errors. Instead, give yourself credit for your improvements. Remember that you are learning and consider that each practice will get you closer to the way you want to communicate to clients and colleagues. Think back to your rehearsal and notice where you met or even surpassed your ideals. Visualize congratulating yourself on your successes.

Return to "Active Learning" at the beginning of the chapter and write your responses.

 PRACTICING INCORPORATING IMAGERY IN PROFESSIONAL PRACTICE AND SELF-CARE

Skill Building: Exercise 1

Access the following link from Dartmouth College's Student Wellness Center to sample brief guided-imagery exercises and choose one. In class you can choose different ones to use and discuss your experiences (see https://students.dartmouth.edu/wellness-center/wellness-mindfulness/relaxation-downloads/guided-imagery-visualization).

Imagineering Your Success: Exercise 2

What if you could tell your story of success before it happened, to hold it in your mind and heart to guide you? Using your imagination and what you learned about guided imagery, write a brief story about your best self 5 years from now in a setting that is ideal for you. Do you see yourself as a staff nurse working with children in an intensive care unit or as a manager, an anesthetist, faculty, midwife, nurse practitioner, informatics nurse, travel nurse, or director of nurses? Who might you become with your strengths and interests you learned about in Chapter 3, Starting with YOU? Robert Olen Butler says, "story is a yearning meeting an obstacle." One approach is to use these story prompts and write for 10 minutes. *Once upon a time…/Every day… But one day…/Because of that…/Because of that…/Because of that…/Until finally…/Ever since then…* Have fun with the assignment as you dare to dream.

Self-Assessment: Exercise 3

In this chapter, the following images are offered as distancing strategies to help you relax and center. Imagine your stressors released one at a time as a leaf floating downstream, clouds moving across the sky, helium-filled balloons rising, and bubbles being blown away. Take a few minutes now to experience each to identify which works best for you. Practice it often so it will be a readily available strategy when you need it. These are useful with adult and pediatric patients.

Self-Assessment: Exercise 4

McKim (1972) has adapted a psychological test to help assess the vividness of your images. Rate the following items using the criteria rating: C = clear, V = vague, and N = no image at all:
- Face of a friend
- Rose
- Playful puppy
- Full moon
- Sound of rain on a window

- Taste of pepper
- Smell of peppermint
- Sound of fingernails scraping on a chalkboard
- Smell of coffee brewing
- Feeling of stretching to reach for an item on a tall shelf

Skill Building: Exercise 5

McKim (1972) suggested that it is even more important to be able to control imagery than to evoke clear pictures. Rate your ability to control the following images using the criteria rating: C = controlled the image well, U = unsure, and N = not able to control the image:

- Rose unfolding into full bloom
- Flat rock skipping across the surface of a lake
- Pinwheel spinning clockwise, then reversing
- Car racing forward, then running backward
- Sofa moving unaided up to the ceiling and back to the floor
- Balloon drifting up into the sky and then returning to the ground
- Wave crashing onto the shore and then reversing itself
- Yourself sitting down in a chair and then standing
- Words appearing on a computer screen and then disappearing as if deleted
- Cake rising as viewed through a glass oven door and then going back to uncooked cake batter

McKim (1972) cautioned you not to be disappointed if you do poorly but to repeat the exercises after you have practiced imaging. View this visualization as a pretest that is administered before you learn the course content.

Skill Building: Exercise 6

Take the opportunity to use imagery to help you communicate more effectively with others. If you would like to invite a classmate to go shopping with you, visualize how you would like to extend the invitation and envision an enthusiastic response. Prepare yourself for a refusal by hearing the classmate extend regrets and watch yourself respond smoothly. You may have an upcoming test of your nursing care practice. Take time to see yourself successfully completing each part of the test and imagine your instructor giving you top grades.

Visualize yourself successful! With practice you will discover imagery does not require much time and can be done anywhere such as in the shower, as you walk to your meeting, and at the nurses' station. Imagery emphasizes taking control of your thinking to create positive, self-enhancing pictures of yourself for confidence. As you learn each of the communication behaviors in this book, visualize yourself using them correctly to build confidence and integration of skills into your communications repertoire.

Reflection and Creative Expression: Exercise 7

In the opening paragraph of this chapter, you were asked to begin to visualize yourself as a successful nurse. Take a few minutes to draw this image of yourself, write a journal entry describing yourself with the characteristics and behaviors of a successful nurse, or write a poem about yourself in this successful role.

Quality and Safety Education for Nurses Learning Strategy: Exercise 8 (QSEN)

The Quality and Safety Education for Nurses (QSEN) learning strategy in Chapter 12 includes a brief description of reflective practice. Reflective practice provides a structure for incorporating imagery in professional practice development and self-care by using reflective practices. Self-care is an important part of a healthy work environment and the basis for organizational safety culture. Use the principles of appreciative inquiry to imagine how you can improve self-care that is important to contribute to a healthy work environment. Appreciative inquiry is valuing the best (appreciate) and asking questions about how to make the best the norm (inquire):

- Reflect on a time when you felt alive and felt deep meaning in your clinical experience.
- Describe the experience. What was happening? What about the experience made you feel successful?
- Imagine this as the daily reality. What do you need to do for this to happen?
- Consider the threats you need to overcome and how you might manage.
- Visualize what success would look like.

Healthy work environments are part of a safety culture; self-care is a key part of developing healthy relationships critical for a safe, quality culture.

WIT AND WISDOM

The debt we owe to the play of imagination is incalculable.

Carl Jung

REFERENCES

Apostolo, J. L. A., & Kolcaba, K. (2009). The effects of guided imagery on comfort, depression, anxiety, and stress of psychiatric inpatients with depressive disorders. *Archives of Psychiatric Nursing, 23*(6), 403.

Boehm, L. B., & Tse, A. M. (2013). Application of guided imagery to facilitate the transition of new graduate registered nurses. *Journal of Continuing Education in Nursing, 44*(3), 113.

Fiske, E. (2017). Contemplative practices, self-efficacy, and NCLEX-RN success. *Nurse Educator, 42*(3), 159.

Fontaine, K. L. (2014). *Complementary & alternative therapies for nursing practice*. Boston, MA: Pearson.

Giedt, J. F. (1997). A psychoneuroimmunological intervention in holistic nursing practice. *Journal of Holistic Nursing Practice, 15*(2), 112.

Hartmann, F. (2007). *Paracelsus: Life and prophecies*. Whitefish, MT: Kessinger Publishing.

Helms, J. E. (2006). Complementary and alternative therapies: A new frontier for nursing education? *Journal of Nursing Education, 45*(3), 1117.

Jacobson, E. (1942). *Progressive relaxation*. Chicago, IL: University of Chicago Press.

Johnston, S. L. (2002). Native American and traditional and alternative medicine. *Annals of the American Academy of Political and Social Science, 583*(1), 195–213.

Kermani, A. R., Aghebati, N., Mohajer, S., & Ghavami, V. (2020). Effects of guided imagery along with breathing relaxation on sleep quality of elderly patients under abdominal surgery. *Holistic Nursing Practice, 34*(6), 334–344. doi:10.1097/HNP.0000000000000415.

Kiley, K. A., Sehgal, A. R., Neth, S., Dolata, J., Pike, E., Spilsbury, J. C., et al. (2018). The effectiveness of guided imagery in treating compassion fatigue and anxiety of mental health workers. *Social Work Research, 42*(1), 33.

Krejci, J. W. (1997). Stimulating critical thinking by exploring mental modes. *Journal of Nursing Education, 36*(10), 482.

Lauria, A. (1968). *The mind of a mnemonist*. New York, NY: Basic Books.

Lewandowski, W. A., Good, M., & Draucher, C. B. (2005). Changes in the meaning of pain with the use of guided imagery. *Pain Management Nursing, 6*(2), 58.

Luthe, W. (1969). *Autogenic therapy*. Vol. II. New York, NY: Grune & Stratton.

Mayer, A. J. (1984). *Visualization. En Route, 48*(50), 30.

McCaffrey, R., & Taylor, N. (2005). Effective anxiety treatment prior to diagnostic cardiac catheterization. *Holistic Nursing Practice, 19*(2), 70.

McKim, R. H. (1972). *Experiences in visual thinking*. Monterey, CA: Brooks/Cole.

Merriam-Webster Online Dictionary. (2022). Image Definition & Meaning – *Merriam-Webster*.

Merriam-Webster Online Dictionary. (2022). Visualize Definition & Meaning – *Merriam-Webster*.

Miller, N. (1969). Learning and visceral and glandular responses. *Science, 163*, 434.

Payne, R. A., & Donaghy, M. (2010). *Payne's handbook of relaxation techniques: A practical guide for the health care professional* (4th ed.). Edinburgh, UK: Elsevier.

Reed, T. (2007). Imagery in the clinical setting: A tool for healing. *Nursing Clinics of North America, 42*(2), 261.

Riedel, S. L. (2012). *Effects of guided imagery in persons with fibromyalgia. ProQuest Dissertations*, 515538.

Samuels, M., & Bennett, H. Z. (1974). *Be well*. Toronto, Canada: Random House.

Samuels, M., & Samuels, N. (1975). *Seeing with the mind's eye*. New York, NY: Random House.

Schaub, B. G., & Burt, M. M. (2013). Imagery. In B. M. Dossey, & L. Keegan (Eds.), *Holistic nursing: A handbook for practice*. Burlington, MA: Jones & Bartlett Learning.

Serra, D. (2012). Outcomes of guided imagery in patients receiving radiation therapy for breast cancer. *Clinical Journal of Oncology Nursing, 16*(6), 617.

Silk, G., & Norwood, M. S. (2002–2003). Mental holography: The power of imagery in communication. *Journal of Imagination in Language Learning and Teaching, 7*.

Sternberg, E. (2010). *The science of healing with Dr. Esther Sternberg*. PBS DVD.

Windle, S., Berger, K., & Kim, J. E. F. (2021). Teaching guided imagery and relaxation techniques in undergraduate nursing education. *Journal of Holistic Nursing, 39*(2), 199–206. https://doi.org/10.1177/0898010120938558.

Wynd, C. A. (2005). Guided imagery for smoking cessation and long-term abstinence. *Journal of Nursing Scholarship, 37*(3), 245.

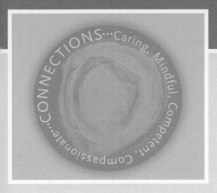

21

Incorporating Positivity into Life and Work

Man is disturbed not by things but by the views he takes of them.

Epictetus

OBJECTIVES

1. Define positivity.
2. Define self-talk and its influence on behavior.
3. Discuss the relationship between self-talk and interpersonal communication.
4. Discuss the use of affirmations as a strategy to create positive self-talk.
5. Practice positive self-talk to develop confidence in communication skills and nursing practice.

🔑 ACTIVE LEARNING

Think about how you will write your answers as you read this chapter.

What?
Write one thing you learned from this chapter.

So What?
How will this affect your nursing practice?

Now What?
How will you implement this new knowledge or skill?

Think About It …

POSITIVITY

How can bringing attention to situations and words bring positivity to your life and work? A broad discussion of positivity underpins the strategy of positive self-talk as a self-care strategy that promotes healthy communication with yourself and others.

Positivity is "the practice of being positive in your attitude and focusing on what is good in a situation" (Oxford Advanced Learner's Dictionary, 2022). More than optimism, this is an active practice of seeking out and savoring positive experiences. Rick Hanson, a psychologist and neuroscientist, teaches that our brains are hard-wired with a negativity bias, an early human survival process. Negative experiences stick to us like Velcro, whereas positive experiences slide off us like Teflon. We ruminate over mistakes and shrug off a compliment. Hanson's Book, *Resilient*, teaches us to savor even small positive experiences, to linger with them and reflect on them as a repeated practice, including bringing them to mind when we are discouraged; this changes the brain. He calls this activation and installation, learning that makes changes in the brain, neuroplasticity. Hanson teaches the HEAL process: (1) Have a beneficial experience, notice one or create one; (2) Enrich it, feel it, stay with it; (3) Absorb it, take time to savor it; and (4) Link it, bring it to mind to soothe painful thoughts (2018).

Frederickson (2009), in her book *Positivity*, delineates 10 forms of positivity (joy, gratitude, serenity, interest, hope, pride, amusement, inspiration, awe, and love) and offers a series of questions to identify each of these in your life. She suggests creating a portfolio for each. Christopher (2019) discussed the implementation of joy strategies in healthcare as a good business practice. See Chapter 30 for an exercise to create your own "joy box." Consider these books to build these practices. Positive Psychology "uses scientific understandings and interventions to help people achieve a more satisfactory life." It helps us become more resilient, productive, and engaged (American Nurse, 2015). Battie (2020) advises nurses to identify and focus on a few things that went well at the end of each day and embrace uncomfortable situations as learning opportunities. Ervine (2021) suggests choosing to be around positive people and engage in positive self-talk.

Self-Care Nudge

Pause and bring to mind something in nature that brings you joy. Perhaps a flower, the ocean, a sunrise, or your pet will come to mind (a beneficial experience). Imagine it with all your senses (enrich it). Take a few moments to savor it (absorb it). Remind yourself of this image next time you need a boost (link it) (Hanson & Hanson, 2018).

DEFINITION OF SELF-TALK

Before we explore your use of positive self-talk as a student, consider recent reports of the power of self-talk. In a clinical study of 78 patients with chronic pain, their anxiety and depression were decreased by the use of positive self-talk, distraction, and ignoring the pain (Miller-Matero, Chipungu, Martinez, Eshelman, & Eisenstein, 2017). Self-talk was part of psychological skills training for emergency care providers (Lauria et al., 2017).

Now it is your first day on a new clinical unit, and you are a bit anxious. What thoughts run through your mind? Have you noticed ongoing internal dialogue? We speak to ourselves, and we listen to ourselves. Self-talk is not unlike the conversation that occurs between two people. We would seldom talk to others the way we talk to ourselves. Self-talk is also known as inner thought, inner speech, self-instruction, or that "little voice" in your head that forms a self-communication system. The American Nurses Association published a self-care book that identifies positive self-talk as a stress management skill (Richards, Sheen, & Mazzer, 2014). Self-talk can be rational, based on reasoning, logic, or facts, or it can be irrational. It can be positive, offering encouragement or praise, or it can be negative, offering discouragement and criticism (Mayo Clinic Staff, 2009). What you tell yourself can affect your health. In a study by Levy, Slade, Kunkel, & Kasl (2002), people who said they had positive views about aging lived an average of 7.6 years longer than those who had negative views.

A familiar childhood story tells us that this skill is time tested. Remember *The Little Engine That Could*? It is the tale of an old train that was being replaced by a shiny new model. The new train refused to climb a steep hill to deliver toys to the children (Piper, 1998). The old train met the challenge with positive self-talk. He repeated, "I think I can…I think I can…I think I can," and sure enough, he was successful. This well-loved children's story goes back to 1910. We have been encouraging our children to use positive self-talk for many years.

Casual remarks made unintentionally by those around us can become self-prophecies. In response to the book, *What to Say When You Talk to Your Self*, which sold more than a million copies, thousands of letters were sent to the author by readers who related that they had believed something totally false about themselves throughout their lives based on something someone else had said (Helmstetter, 2011).

Cognitive psychologists have learned that internal dialogue has a powerful influence on our behavior. Our thoughts are our interpretations of the world, our judgments about our own behavior, and our assumptions about others' reactions to us. Our feelings are directly influenced by our thoughts, and how we construe our world provides the blueprint for our actions. It is not what is happening to us that is so significant, but how we interpret what is happening to us and what we do under the influence of these thoughts.

For any situation or interpersonal encounter we have, our self-talk determines the following:
- Our attitude toward the situation
- What we see, hear, and attend to
- How we interpret what we take in
- What we think the outcome will be
- How we act (including what we feel, say, and do)
- How we appraise the consequences of our actions

Our internal dialogue can be constructive or destructive. Take as a simple example a person whose mother has always told her that she is clumsy. Because she believes it to be so, the woman's self-talk is not positive. She says, "I'm so clumsy. I'm always bruising myself." She finds that she truly seems to be clumsy. When she changes her self-talk to "I am graceful and move easily and carefully," however, her awkwardness decreases.

Clinical Examples of Positive and Negative Self-Talk

As you read the examples, think about their possible effects on the nurses in the situation.

Tanya and Deirdre are senior nursing students. As they anticipate their forthcoming clinical placements in a public health department, these thoughts go through their minds:

Tanya: *"I've heard that the new director of the agency is a tyrant. I hate people like that. They have miserable dispositions that grate on my nerves. I'm not going to like working with her. Team conferences will be a pain. She's sure to pick on me, and, knowing me, I'll probably make some blunder that'll be a red flag for her to show me up. I'll be glad when this rotation is over."*

Tanya has set herself up for a difficult clinical placement. This negative self-talk is destructive. Thinking the way she does, Tanya will likely act defensively and be on edge that she will make a mistake. Her attitude will probably isolate her from friendly sources of support from the staff.

Deirdre: *"I've heard that the new director is a real stickler for good nursing care and demands a lot from her staff. It's great that I get to go to a health department in which the home care is so good. I'll learn a lot. I'm looking forward to making home visits and seeing nursing care there. I'm also nervous because this is new and I don't know what we'll face, but I know I'll have the best teachers and get a lot out of the experience. Too bad it's only a brief rotation."*

Deirdre has mentally prepared herself for a rewarding clinical experience. Her interpretation of the excellence of the nursing care makes her eager to observe and learn from the nurses. Her positive self-talk sets her up to expect positive interactions with staff, and she will most likely get a lot out of the experience.

Our self-talk goes on continuously in our heads and is so automatic that we have to listen carefully to hear whether it is exerting a negative or positive influence. If we want to have control of this habitual process, we need to listen to our thoughts, decide how we want to change, and consistently convert our thinking so that it influences our behavior positively.

As you read the next scenario, put yourself in the position of the student nurse and write down your reactions. You are a nursing student just entering your senior year after summer vacation. To date, your clinical experience has been on the specialty units of your hospital, such as the ophthalmology, gynecology, and the day-stay surgical unit. You are assigned to the intensive care unit and will be working with more complicated equipment. You are sure the patients will think you are clumsy, and you are afraid you'll make a terrible mistake. You hear that the staff is discouraged because they have to cut back hours temporarily because of budget problems. You know the unit has a full census of clients, and you fear the staff will not have the time or energy to help you. Your clinical instructor told you the staff is looking forward to having the students because last year's seniors were so eager to learn.

After you have written your reactions, put the list aside for the moment and review the following example of Suzanne's negative self-talk as she encounters the same situation.

Suzanne: *"I'll never cope! Who can ever have enough experience to prepare for intensive care? I hear the patients are all so sick that most of them die. I can barely think of all the scary equipment. What about the families? They won't want a student when their family member is so sick. I'm nervous already thinking about it. I feel nauseated. Why did I ever come into nursing? I don't want to be compared with last year's seniors. I'll be feeling panicky the whole time. I'll go home depressed because of the deaths. I'll feel so inadequate."*

Suzanne's self-talk is destructive. It escalates her anxiety and focuses on things that could go wrong. This is catastrophic thinking. With a mind-set like hers, she will be tuned into anything negative and may force a self-fulfilling prophecy. Her self-talk undermines her confidence and creates anxiety before and during the experience.

Take a moment to write down a constructive internal dialogue that Suzanne could use in the same situation.

Here is an example of positive self-talk for Suzanne. Compare your suggestions with this example.

Suzanne: *"This is going to be hard. There's a lot of new equipment to learn, but since I plan to work in critical care, I need to learn this. This experience might help me get a good recommendation. Everyone has to learn something new sometime. I'm bright, and I'll just make it a point to let the staff know I'm eager to learn. This is the best time to learn to deal with dying patients. These nurses have so much experience. I'm sure they can give me some help if I ask them how they cope. I know I can do this. The staff know that I'm a student and will not expect miracles from me. They will be glad for the contribution I can make to the unit. I must find out more about the unit from Betty so that I can prepare myself as much as possible for the experience."*

This self-talk is constructive. Suzanne's internal dialogue in this example is realistic and hopeful. By acknowledging her assets, Suzanne will go onto the unit feeling confident. She is likely to approach the staff in a friendly way, eager for new opportunities. Thinking about her situation as a challenge provides Suzanne with a positive goal for her career as a nurse. By deciding to seek out information beforehand, she is increasing her chances of success.

Now review your own internal dialogue that you generated earlier in this exercise. Determine whether it is positive or negative. Does your self-talk work in your best interests, or is it potentially destructive?

Positive Self-Talk: Assertive and Responsible

The previous examples demonstrate how self-talk can be harmful or helpful to us. Positive self-talk emphasizes our strengths and ability to handle the situations facing us. Mental preparation makes us feel hopeful and confident. We have the right to feel good about how we handle situations we encounter, and we can use positive self-talk as one technique to accomplish this. It is assertive to keep our internal dialogue positive.

Positive self-talk is not unrealistic or wishful thinking. It involves an accurate assessment of our abilities and the situation. Not having the knowledge or skills to effectively handle an interpersonal situation is no reason to think less of ourselves or to put ourselves down. It is being responsible to admit our lack of experience, acknowledge our willingness and ability to learn, and realistically prepare to handle the situation.

Butler (2008) warned us that when our self-talk is negative, we create our own toxic environment. Negative self-talk is harsh and judgmental, demanding super heroic achievements, chastising us for failing, and generally making us feel tense and dissatisfied with ourselves. Butler encouraged us to develop a positive, supportive way of talking to ourselves to cushion us from negative events. Chapman (1992) commented that "positive people are far more likely than others to face up to problems, make tough decisions, and refuse to look back." He says that those with a positive outlook are often mistaken for people who just let things happen as if by fate. "Not so! Positive people often have more problems, because they take more risks and live life more fully."

🌿 MOMENTS OF CONNECTION...
A Nursing Student Practices Self-Talk

Using self-talk has really helped me when I get anxious. By being less hard on myself, my self-esteem grows and I'm able to see the people around me. Today, walking to statistics class, I used self-talk. This lifted my spirits, allowing me to be more open, friendlier, and more approachable by classmates.

Changing our self-talk starts with an assessment. Butler (2008) suggested we ask ourselves the following questions:
- What am I telling myself?
- What negative thoughts am I generating that are destructive to me?
- What positive thoughts am I generating that are constructive for me?
- Is my self-talk helping me?
- How can I change my self-talk so that it is more positive?

The next step is to specify how we need to change our internal dialogue so that it is more positive. At first this planning requires considerable effort, but then it will become part of our awareness, enabling us to tune in to

internal dialogue and adjust to it quickly. Later in this chapter, you will get experience in reformulating self-talk.

Relationship Between Self-Talk and Interpersonal Communication

In Part I of this book, you learned about behaviors that are essential for caring communication. Parts of your self-talk will be about your ability to implement these behaviors with your clients and colleagues. How you construct your internal dialogue can enhance or diminish your skill level.

Here are examples involving the communication behaviors of empathy and confrontation.

EXAMPLE 1: SELF-TALK ABOUT EMPATHY

Here is what one nurse said to herself about empathy:

> *I can't be empathic and sound natural. My colleagues will laugh at me if I change my style and try to be empathic. I don't think I can think up an empathic response fast enough in a real conversation to make it sound sincere. I'll look and feel awkward trying to be empathic.*

Examine this nurse's self-talk:
1. *What is she telling herself?* She is telling herself that she will feel uncomfortable, silly, and unnatural if she attempts to be empathic. She is convincing herself that friends will not admire her attempts and that she will lose their respect.
2. *What negative thoughts are destructive?* She is convincing herself that she will not be effective in her use of empathy. She expects that she should be perfect the first time she is empathic. She is not permitting any failure, nor is she hopeful that her colleagues will support her.
3. *What positive thoughts is she generating?* This nurse is not generating one positive thought that might give her the hope and encouragement to try being more empathic.
4. *Is her self-talk helping her?* This self-talk will likely stop her from including empathy in her communication strategies. These thoughts will make her feel bad on two counts: She will miss providing the benefits of empathy to others, and she will feel disappointed in her lack of willingness to try. She is left feeling convinced that neither she nor her colleagues have confidence in her ability. Her thoughts are nonassertive and irresponsible, and they are not in any way helpful to her.
5. *How can she change her self-talk so that it is more positive?* Here is an example of how her self-talk could be more positive: I'm going to try to use empathy, even if I am a little stilted and awkward at first. I am convinced empathy is important and know that my colleagues and clients

will appreciate my efforts to show them that I understand, even if my attempts aren't perfect. Some colleagues may tease me. When I try to be more empathic, I will not let them deter me from including empathy in my communication. It may take a while to find the right words, but that's OK. It will likely seem longer to me than to the other person. I want to improve my communication, and I know that something new takes time. I can be patient with myself until empathy comes more naturally.

This positive self-talk is assertive and responsible. It emphasizes the importance this nurse places on being empathic and gives her encouragement to try being more understanding. It is not a glib dialogue; rather, it is a realistic assessment of her ability to practice and fine-tune a new skill.

EXAMPLE 2: SELF-TALK ABOUT CONFRONTATION

Here is one nurse's self-talk about confrontation:

I think it's better to keep peace by not saying anything to the boss about his abrasive manner to me these past few days. If I confront him, he'll think I'm being too sensitive, and he'll be wary of me after this. He'll pull rank on me and get angry if I confront him. The more I think about it, the crazier it seems for me to be upset about his manner; he's probably got something on his mind and doesn't realize he's taking it out on me. What if I get all upset and mix up my words? I'd really look like a fool then.

Examine this nurse's self-talk:

1. *What is she telling herself?* She is convincing herself that she would be better off not to confront her boss about an issue important to her. She is arguing that her feelings are not as important as those of her boss.
2. *What negative thoughts is she generating that are destructive?* This nurse is denying her own feelings by deceiving herself that it might be better to let this episode pass. This self-deception undermines her judgment. She is creating bad feelings about herself by suggesting that being sensitive or expecting to be treated politely is undesirable. She attempts to frighten herself with the assumption that her boss will get angry and, furthermore, that she would not be able to handle his anger. She imagines the worst scenario and tries to convince herself that she is likely to fail.
3. *What positive thoughts is she generating?* This nurse's self-talk is entirely negative and contains nothing positive for her.
4. *Is her self-talk helping her?* This negative self-talk would only deter her from standing up for something that is

important to her, which is her desire to be treated with respect. This approach makes her doubt her ability to confront and to handle one possible consequence of a confrontation: her boss's anger. Her negative self-talk is nonassertive and irresponsible in that she is allowing herself to be mistreated and refuses to accept her responsibility for letting the behavior continue.

5. *How can she change her self-talk to make it more positive?* Here is an example of how her self-talk could be more positive: I don't like to confront my boss, but I don't like to be treated disrespectfully, so I will confront him. I know I can make my points clear to him without seeming like a whiner. My boss may become angry or hostile when I confront him, but I can handle this reaction without backing off or becoming defensive. I have practiced confrontation and feel confident that I can carry it off. If my confrontation isn't perfect, it doesn't matter; that I make my point as clearly as possible is what counts. Just because he's my boss is no reason for him to treat me so badly. I have the right to be treated with respect. He is more likely to respect me in the future if I set limits now.

This positive self-talk is assertive and responsible. It encourages the nurse to stand up for herself, and it takes into account her ability to handle several possible outcomes. It is encouraging and supportive, and it would give this nurse the comfort and confidence to carry out her confrontation.

Later in this book you will learn how to communicate assertively and responsibly in the following situations in which nurses are known to have difficulty:

- When clients' or colleagues' behaviors are challenging
- When clients or colleagues demonstrate bullying or incivility
- When there is team conflict
- When evaluation anxiety is experienced

In all these situations, positive self-talk is important. Examples of self-talk in two of these situations are presented next.

EXAMPLE 3: SELF-TALK WHEN COLLEAGUES ARE DISTRESSED

Here is one nurse's self-talk when encountering a colleague who is distressed and crying:

I hate it when colleagues cry; I mean, with clients it's OK, I expect them to be upset. I don't know what to do when staff at work cry. Whenever anyone at work cries, I get tearful, too, and I'm useless to them. If anyone cries, I don't know what I'll do. I just can't cope when grown people cry. I don't know what to do to make her feel better. What if she won't stop crying? If I can't help her to calm down, then I'm not much good.

Examine this nurse's self-talk:

1. *What is she telling herself?* This nurse is telling herself that staff members do not have the same feelings and reactions as clients. She is telling herself that a great deal is expected of her and that if she does not perform adequately by calming her upset colleague, then she is not an effective person. She is convinced that if she also cries, then it will be detrimental to her colleague.
2. *What negative thoughts is she generating that are destructive?* She is putting considerable pressure on herself to perform in the only way that she thinks is acceptable. She is assuming that she will not be helpful to her colleague and gives no credit to herself. Her denial of a normal range of feelings in her colleagues prevents her compassion from surfacing in a way that would be helpful. Her impending sense of failure if she does not perform perfectly is likely making her tense.
3. *What positive thoughts is she generating?* This nurse is not saying anything comforting or encouraging to herself.
4. *Is her self-talk helpful?* Her self-talk is nonassertive because it downplays her potential to be helpful. It is not responsible because it distorts reality. Her self-talk would hinder her ability to reach out to her colleague and communicate in a helpful way. The restrictions imposed by this negative thinking would leave her feeling inadequate.
5. *How can she change her self-talk so that it is more positive?* Here is an example of how her self-talk could be more positive: Everybody gets upset, and staff are no exception. I may not be able to stop her from crying, but I think I can comfort her. I always cry when any other staff member cries; but that's OK. It just shows how compassionate I am. My crying doesn't interfere with my ability to be helpful. She may not respond to my efforts to calm her down, but that doesn't mean I'm a bad nurse. Each of us has someone special to whom we can relate when we are upset. I don't have to do a lot to be helpful. Often, just listening and being there is enough.

These inner thoughts are reassuring and confidence building. They are responsible because they do not distort the reality of the situation. They are assertive because they acknowledge the nurse's desire and ability to help. This positive self-talk is helpful.

EXAMPLE 4: SELF-TALK WHEN THERE IS TEAM CONFLICT

Here is an example of one nurse's thinking about a conflict situation on her nursing unit:

All I want is a peaceful place to work. Wherever I go there are power struggles, and I hate it. I just know this conflict is going to drag on; I wish I worked in Dr. Session's office. They never have any conflicts there. Maybe I should apply for a position in another office; I can't do anything about the conflicts between the support and clinical staff. I thought we had dealt with this conflict once and for all; I just hate these drawn-out disagreements. Whenever we discuss upsetting issues, my stomach gets in a knot, and I feel like I'm going to explode; I don't know how much more I can take. I'm useless when there's conflict. I just let it tear me apart, and that's no good. I'm afraid I'm going to give the office manager a piece of my mind. She should get this conflict under control.

Examine this nurse's self-talk:

1. *What is she telling herself?* This nurse has the erroneous notion that conflict is brief, easily resolved, and nonrecurring. The false expectation that there are some places in which conflict does not occur is self-defeating. She is trying to convince herself that there is little she can do about the conflict. She believes that the office manager or the doctor should magically control the conflict.
2. *What negative thoughts is she generating that are destructive?* Her unrealistic ideas about the nature of conflict are causing her grief. Her image of herself as someone with little control in conflict situations makes her feel hopeless and ineffective. Her anticipation of unpleasant physical signs and symptoms in conflict situations initiates her anxiety at the slightest indication of conflict.
3. *What positive thoughts is she generating?* There is nothing reassuring and hopeful about her thinking.
4. *Is her self-talk helpful?* Her self-talk is nonassertive because it does not grant her any power to contribute to the resolution of the conflict. Her distorted perception about her lack of influence to effect change is irresponsible. These thoughts are not helpful because they immobilize her and increase her tension about the conflict.
5. *How can she change her self-talk so that it is more positive?* Here is an example of how her self-talk could be more positive: Every office staff has conflict; it is an unavoidable part of working with others. Sometimes creative and effective ways of handling situations can come out of conflict. Maybe there are some positive benefits to this conflict. I can keep my cool to express my feelings about the conflict on our unit. My ideas will have more impact if I remain calm. Each thing I do to diminish the conflict goes a long way toward resolving our problems. No one person can eliminate the conflict alone, but each contribution is significant. I get anxious when there's conflict on the unit, but it is not overwhelming. I can keep it under control.

This positive self-talk is assertive and responsible. Admitting that conflict is a normal part of working with others removes the sting of disagreement and makes her more apt to tackle the problem. Believing that whatever steps she takes to manage the conflict are significant promotes positive action on her part. Putting her anxiety in perspective allows her to function without being ashamed or overwhelmed. She is responsible in her assessment of the situation and her ability. This positive internal dialogue is assertive in its acknowledgment of her desire to handle situations effectively.

Bach and Torbet (1986) asserted that we have two voices in our inner life: our "inner enemy" and our "inner ally." Our inner enemy keeps a running inventory of our weaknesses; maintains a certain misery level; and keeps all joyless, negative information on file to display at a moment's notice. Our inner ally is interested in action, growth, and change, and it prevents us from getting bogged down in doubts and fears. Our inner ally reassures us of the benefits and rewards of success, as well as the pleasures of trying, encouraging us to take risks that will help get us where we want to go. When we make mistakes, it is our inner ally that comforts us and helps us view our mistakes in perspective.

As you practice enhancing and augmenting your interpersonal communication skills, focus on what your inner ally tells you. Allow comforting and realistic thoughts to support and encourage you while learning.

Consider using the skill of positive self-talk as you grow your career when preparing for an interview, when you are going back to school, and when you are preparing for public speaking (McConnell, 2009; Schaeffer, 2006).

USE OF POSITIVE SELF-TALK TO ENHANCE YOUR INTERPERSONAL COMMUNICATION

Positive self-talk can help you at three phases of interpersonal communication: before, during, and after.

Before your interaction with a client or colleague, you can take control of your thoughts and focus on realistic and encouraging inner dialogue that will make you feel more confident about your forthcoming encounter. This preparation makes you focus on your strengths rather than worry about potential catastrophes. When you feel prepared, you will likely act more competently.

For some encounters you have hours or days to prepare your positive self-talk. At other times you get little preparation time. Even for surprise encounters, however, you can quickly tune in to your internal dialogue (it is continuously active) and talk to yourself in encouraging ways.

For example, when you take a call from an angry family member, you can say these words to yourself:

Positive self-talk: *The unit secretary tells you there is a call from an angry family member. Tell yourself, "He's impatient and angry, and it could get me upset.*

But I will stay calm and collected." Slow down, relax your breathing, and loosen up your shoulders. You will find out what is troubling him and be able to handle it. Haste makes waste, so just remain steady and pay attention to each thing he says.

This preparation primes you to handle this aggressive client situation calmly and effectively.

During your conversation you can tune in to your inner voice and concentrate on supportive dialogue. For example, if the caller's voice is getting louder and his language is getting more hostile, you can say the following to yourself:

Positive self-talk: *"He's getting angry. That's OK. I can handle his outburst. I will remain calm and find out what is so upsetting for him. My breathing is regular, my posture is relaxed, and I will keep my voice steady. There's no point in getting upset. I can take this professionally, not personally!"*

This positive self-talk reminds you to stay in control and handle the situation effectively. The comfort provided by your own supportive thoughts helps you to act the way you want.

After an encounter you can use positive self-talk to constructively review your performance. Noting your successes and the areas in which improvement is needed are both important. This example of a constructive review may be helpful:

Positive self-talk: *"I thought I controlled my fear of his hostility really well. I actually remained calm and kept my voice tone on an even pitch. I think what I said to him helped to calm him down, but next time I'd like to achieve a relaxed body posture. My fists were clenched and my shoulders were pretty tight, and I could feel that my knees were locked. When I can relax my body, that will be one more positive message going out that I am in control and confident."*

AFFIRMATIONS AS A STRATEGY TO CREATE POSITIVE SELF-TALK

Affirmations are self-talk statements of what you want, written in the positive tense, as if they have already happened. Affirmations can help you to take an optimistic point of view about your life and work. People who are optimistic hold generalized favorable expectations of the future. Optimism versus pessimism (negative expectations about the future) has been related to a better sense of well-being in the face of life challenge, higher levels of coping,

BOX 21.1   How to Create and Use Affirmations

1. *Use the present tense:* You want your mind to know it has already happened.
2. *Be POSITIVE:* Avoid negative words. For example, "I choose healthy foods" rather than "I do not eat high-calorie foods." "There is always enough time" rather than "I will not be late."
3. *Write them down:* Keep them short and very specific.
4. *Believe:* Always believe that what you are saying is happening.
5. *Repetition:* Being repetitive and persistent helps to set them in your unconscious and conscious mind.
6. *Time:* Have a specific time set aside daily for your affirmations or link the affirmation to an activity you do each day. This will help set a pattern.

BOX 21.2   Examples of Affirmations

I am at peace with my life.
I love and accept myself.
I feel energetic and enthusiastic today.
I love and care for my body.
I am healthy.
I respect my abilities and work to my full potential.
I spend money wisely.
I am a forgiving and loving person.
I am worthy of love.
Centered and poised in the presence of God, I move through the activities of the day easily and gracefully.
I am in the right place, at the right time, doing the right thing, in the right way.

health promotion behaviors, and more success in interpersonal relationships (Carver, Scheier, & Segerstrom, 2010) (Boxes 21.1 and 21.2).

When nursing students in a holistic self-care course write a plan for one behavior change to be worked on throughout the semester, they include one or two affirmations. For example, a student who contracts to run for 30 minutes three times a week, writes, "I look forward to running three times each week and accomplishing it easily" (Riley, 2014).

SIMPLIFY AND DEEPEN

Know that joy is rarer, more difficult, and more beautiful than sadness. Once you make this all-important discovery, you must embrace joy as a moral obligation.

André Gide

A FINAL THOUGHT

Consider how you name your experiences. Could you reframe a "life crisis" into a "life challenge?" Many people find that difficult times offer the most possibility for growth in life. Reflect on your own life and the times of the "dark night of the soul." How would your life change and how could you change the way you partner with clients on their healing journeys if you could make this shift? Consider this affirmation: "Within every problem there is a lesson. Release the problem and embrace the lesson." Positive self-talk—the attitude you choose—is a tool you carry with you and is available at a moment's notice. When you have yourself on your side, you are never alone and you always have an encouraging supporter on whom to call.

Return to "Active Learning" at the beginning of the chapter and write your responses.

PRACTICING POSITIVE SELF-TALK

Critical Thinking/Mindfulness: Exercise 1

In your journal reflect on forms of negative thinking to see if you have experienced them:

- *Filtering:* magnifying negative parts of a situation and minimizing the positive parts
- *Personalizing:* blaming yourself when something goes wrong even if you had nothing to do with it
- *Catastrophizing:* expecting the worst and dramatizing a small setback as the "end of the world"
- *Polarizing:* seeing things only in black or white with no middle ground

A mindfulness practice to support you is to recognize a negative thought, take a breath, and allow the thought without judging it. Return to the breath (Sockolov, 2018).

Try these strategies to increase your positive self-talk:

- Look for the humor in life's difficult situations.
- Choose to be around positive people.
- Do not say anything negative to yourself that you would not say to someone else.

Self-Assessment/Skill Building: Exercise 2

Monitor your own self-talk for one day. Keep track of the number of times you have negative self-talk. Select a recent upsetting experience, describe it briefly, and ask yourself if it could be given a positive spin. Reframe it with humor or compassion; for example, "This is a learning experience." Try a humorous approach; for example, "Another example of God's great sense of humor." Mother Teresa used this strategy. She said, "I know God will not give me anything I cannot handle. I just wish he didn't trust me so much."

Skill Building/Online Resource: Exercise 3

Identify a challenging situation you face, such as the first day of a new clinical rotation. Write one positive self-talk statement to prepare yourself for a good start. Refer to Boxes 21.1 and 21.2. Write the statement in your journal and practice saying it to yourself at the beginning and middle of the day. Visit https://www.freeaffirmations.org/become-a-nurse-positive-affirmations for a list of affirmations written for nurses (FreeAffirmations.org, 2018).

Quality and Safety Education for Nurses Learning Strategy: Exercise 4 **QSEN**

Emotional intelligence is a developmental process that helps build confidence through improving self-awareness and how our actions affect others. By reflecting on our experiences, we can learn from them. Teamwork behaviors are dependent on our awareness of how our actions affect others. The stories we tell ourselves become our reality. How can we use stories of our success to improve self-awareness and confidence?

- Write an example of a time you felt your actions were successful.
- Describe the event. What steps did you take?
- What about the event made you feel successful?
- How can you apply these same strategies to have confidence when you face future challenges?
- How does "confidence" in your "competence" influence quality and safety?

WIT AND WISDOM

The greatest weapon against stress is our ability to choose one thought over another.

William James

REFERENCES

American Nurse. (2015). The power of the positive - American Nurse (myamericannurse.com) July 7, 2015.

Bach, G., & Torbet, L. (1986). *The everyday slow torture of self-hate*. New York, NY: Berkley Publishing Group.

Battie, R. (2020). The practice of positivity. *Association of Perioperative Registered Nurses Journal, 112*(2), 17–18. https://doi.org/10.1002/aorn.13157.

Butler, P. E. (2008). *Talking to yourself*. New York, NY: BookSurge Publishing.

Carver, C. S., Scheier, M. F., & Segerstrom, S. C. (2010). Optimism. *Clinical Psychology Review, 30*(7), 879.

Chapman, E. N. (1992). *Life is an attitude: Staying positive during tough times, how to control your outlook on life*. Menlo Park, CA: Crisp Publications.

Ervine, H. S. (2021). The power of positivity. *Association of Perioperative Registered Nurses Journal, 114*(2), 115–117. http://doi.org/10.1002/aorn.13479.

Fredrickson, B. L. (2009). *Positivity: Top-notch research reveals the upward spiral that will change your life*. New York: Three Rivers Press.

FreeAffirmations.org. (2018). Become a nurse positive affirmations. https://www.freeaffirmations.org/become-a-nurse-positive-affirmations.

Hanson, R., & Hanson, F. (2018). *Resilient*. New York, NY: Harmony Books.

Helmstetter, S. (2011). *What to say when you talk to yourself*. New York, NY: Park Avenue Press.

Lauria, M. J., Gallo, I. A., Rush, S., Brooks, J., Spiegel, R., & Weingart, S. D. (2017). Psychological skills to improve emergency care providers' performance under stress. *Annals of Emergency Medicine, 70*(6), 884.

Levy, B. A., Slade, M. D., Kunkel, S. R., & Kasl, S. V. (2002). Longevity increased by positive self- perceptions of aging. *Journal of Personality and Social Psychology, 83*(2), 261.

Mayo Clinic Staff. (2009). Positive thinking: Reduce stress and enjoy life more. http://www.mayoclinic.com/health/positive-thinking/SR00009.

McConnell, C. R. (2009). Effective oral presentations: Speaking before groups as a part of your job. *Health Care Management, 28*(3), 264.

Miller-Matero, L. R., Chipungu, K., Martinez, S., Eshelman, A., & Eisenstein, D. (2017). How do I cope with pain? Let me count the ways: Awareness of pain coping behaviors and relationships with depression and anxiety. *Psychology, Health, & Medicine, 22*(1), 19.

Oxford Advanced Learner's Dictionary. (2022). Positivity noun - definition, pictures, pronunciation and usage notes, *Oxford Advanced Learner's Dictionary* at OxfordLearnersDictionaries.com.

Piper, W. (1998). *The little engine that could*. New York, NY: Grosset & Dunlap.

Richards, K., Sheen, E., & Mazzer, M. C. (2014). *Self-care and you: Caring for the caregiver*. Silver Spring, MD: American Nurses Association.

Riley, J. B. (2014). *Nursing 430: Holistic self-care: Complementary and alternative therapies for professional self-care and practice*. Tampa, FL: University of Tampa.

Schaeffer, K. (2006). Facing down the fear factor in interviews. *Wall Street Journal*, December 12.

Sockolov, M. (2018). *Practicing mindfulness: 75 essential meditations to reduce stress, improve health and find peace in the everyday*. Emeryville, CA: Althea Press.

22

Learning to Work Together in Groups

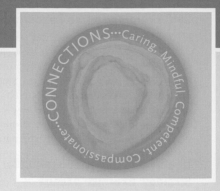

Coming together is a beginning; keeping together is progress; working together is success.

Henry Ford

OBJECTIVES

1. Identify three essential conditions for group effectiveness.
2. Identify four stages of group development.
3. Examine how different mental processes affect behavior in groups.
4. Identify maintenance roles of group members.
5. Identify task roles of group members.
6. Identify individual roles of group members that impede group progress.
7. Apply the concept of emotional intelligence to groups.
8. Discuss why meetings are important.
9. Identify examples of virtual meetings.
10. Identify tools to promote effectiveness in meetings.
11. Discuss characteristics of effective groups.
12. Describe strategies to organize a committee.
13. Participate in exercises to build skills in working together in groups.

"Nurses must have the capacity to skillfully collaborate and effectively communicate across interprofessional teams to provide the highest quality of patient care" (Stucky, Wymer, & House, 2021). Progress in full practice authority for nurse practitioners during the COVID-19 pandemic and more effort to place nurses on executive boards have elevated the nursing profession as a whole (Stucky, Brown, & Stucky, 2021). As you continue to work in groups and teams, this chapter helps you identify different personalities and behaviors that can affect team cohesiveness and have broad implications for interprofessional collaboration for positive patient care outcomes and efficient use of healthcare system resources (McTighe & Donovan, 2017; Ryan, 2017). Health Canada funded a study to identify competencies for collaborative practice. Two perceived competencies from interviews with 60 healthcare providers from varied disciplines were identified: "understanding and appreciating professional roles and responsibilities and communicating effectively" (Suter et al., 2009, p. 41) can inform our work in multidisciplinary groups. You have read about interprofessional work

in Chapter 4. Lessons from COVID-19 report that "some teams working in the context of a pandemic may maintain stable membership, but experience increased stress, others may have rotating membership, requiring teams to reestablish norms and build trust frequently" (Traylor, Tannenbaum, Thomas, & Salas, 2021, p. 4).

Consider you have just been assigned to a new work group. What can you do to set the stage to be heard and to be seen as a valuable member? Research demonstrates there are competence cues. Galinsky and Kilduff (2013) studied the effects of a temporary mind-set that helps you be more proactive in groups, such as focusing on your aspirations or goals or on happiness. Study participants were asked to write a few paragraphs on their ambitions and what they hoped to achieve in life or to write about a time when they were excited or joyful before going into a meeting. These psychological states "reduce the stress hormone cortisol and increase optimism and confidence" (Galinsky & Kilduff, 2013). Try these writing exercises on your smart phone or a piece of paper before your next group project.

We have experience with groups in many arenas in our lives. A group is two or more people coming together to pursue common goals and/or interests (Halter, 2013). Nurses have many opportunities to work in groups: staff meetings; patient care conferences; committees; project teams, such as quality improvement teams; multidisciplinary research teams (Weaver, 2008); and patient groups, such as support groups that are either motivational or educational (Touhy & Jett, 2013). In a community setting, nurses may serve on boards or task forces as volunteers or political appointees. Nurse managers convene groups to actively involve staff in problem-solving to provide safe, competent, compassionate care (Roussel, 2011). Psychiatric nurses may lead therapy groups. This chapter focuses on the dynamics of people working together in groups rather than on insight-oriented therapy groups, although some principles apply to all groups. Reynolds (2005) suggested that nurses need more education about group dynamics and that we cannot rely on working in groups just being common sense.

 ACTIVE LEARNING

Think about how you will write your answers as you read this chapter.

What?
Write one thing you learned from this chapter.

So What?
How will this affect your nursing practice?

Now What?
How will you implement this new knowledge or skill?

Think About It …

Communicating assertively in groups requires an understanding of group dynamics. This information can help you understand and modify your own behavior and help you to be a responsible group member. As you read, think about your own experience in groups as a student, as a practitioner, and as a community member.

THREE CONDITIONS FOR EFFECTIVE GROUP DEVELOPMENT

Research demonstrates that three conditions must be met for effective group development: Group members must trust one another; a sense of group identity must be present; and there must be a sense of group efficacy, which is a belief that the group can and will perform well and that the group as a whole performs better than individuals working on their own (Druskat, 2001; Gundry & LaMantia, 2001;

Rosenthal, 2001). For these conditions to be met, the group must achieve high levels of participation, cooperation, and collaboration. Communication in groups is a blending of communication styles that may conflict or agree. Alessandra (2001) wrote that a genuinely productive team "fully understands and savors its members' styles." Individuals must work together with a sense of belonging, yet each must still retain a sense of self, of a person with a personal history and story. Because obstacles exist to smooth communication in groups, it is important that there is a common purpose that is clear. As you learn more about the dynamics of people working together in a group, whether it be a team, a committee, or another form of group, consider that the group may be bigger in scope, intention, and power than the individuals of whom it is composed.

FOUR STAGES OF GROUP DEVELOPMENT

Four stages occur in the development of a group or team, although there is no set time for these stages, and it may seem that members move back and forth among the stages. Understanding these stages promotes longevity of groups. The stages are forming, storming, norming, and performing (Stuart, 2012; Tuckman, 1965). Think about individual development and consider how these stages compare: Forming is like childhood, storming is like adolescence, norming is like young adulthood, and performing is like adulthood (Box 22.1).

BOX 22.1 Stages of Group or Team Development

- In the *forming* stage, people are polite yet impersonal and unsure of their commitment. The team is figuring out team goals and beginning to obtain a clear idea of the work to be done. Members are testing group relationships to see how the work will get done and may want a dependent relationship with the leader or other group members.
- In the *storming* stage, overt or covert conflict may be evident. People may be hostile, engage in power struggles, be apathetic, and not be willing to work. They are resisting the process of teamwork, are resisting cohesion and collaboration, and do not have a commitment to the team. A hazard here is early termination of the group or committee when conflict surfaces and it is not understood as a healthy stage of building a cohesive group.
- In the *norming* stage, the group is getting organized, figuring out necessary rules and standards to get the work done, confronting problems and issues in a constructive way, and giving feedback. Members clarify

BOX 22.1   Stages of Group or Team Development—cont'd

the goals of the team; adopt new roles; define the tasks and procedures for the work to be done; and move into cohesion, collaboration, and commitment. The norms might be to turn off cell phones and beepers during the meeting, to arrive on time, to begin and end on time, to allow only one person to speak at a time, and to follow the agenda.

- In the *performing* stage, the work is getting done. People are open, can collaborate, are flexible, and are productive. They begin to do quality work, respect and support one another, motivate others by group achievement, and become flexible in their roles.

Modified from Tuckman, B. (1965). Developmental sequence in small groups. *Psychological Bulletin, 63*, 384; Stuart, G. W. (2012). *Principles and practice of psychiatric nursing* (10th ed.). St. Louis, MO: Mosby.

EFFECT OF PERSONAL MENTAL PROCESSES ON BEHAVIOR IN GROUPS

People have preferences for and are most comfortable with certain styles of mental processing. These styles include extroversion versus introversion and intuitive versus sensing modes of perceiving. Group conflict may be a reflection of differences in the way people process data. As you read, consider how these differences can be gifts to the functioning of a group.

People characterized by extroversion talk to think: Extroverts think out loud and get their energy from fast-paced conversations with quick exchanges of partially formed ideas. They get excited about their ideas and do their best work when they have time to talk them through to a logical conclusion. These people are comfortable sharing an idea just to get others' reactions. This does not mean that they necessarily believe what they say.

People characterized by introversion think to talk: Introverts prefer to contemplate their ideas before sharing them. They use fewer measured words and prefer not to share their ideas until their ideas are fully formed. They are less likely to respond quickly to questions because they wait to give their best answer.

WIT AND WISDOM

For the Extrovert

It has been said we have somewhere between 15,000 and 50,000 thoughts per day. As an extrovert, I remind myself, there is no need to express all of them. My one-liner is, "The antidote to extroversion is measured words."

WIT AND WISDOM

For the Introvert

The giraffe can reach the tender leaves only by sticking its neck out.

Take a moment to consider whether extroversion or introversion sounds like your style. If group members are not aware of these different styles of thinking and sharing ideas, the people who talk to think, extroverts, may appear always to lead the discussion and to receive no help from those who think to talk. The extroverts resent the lack of participation of the quieter members, or perhaps they never even notice. The quieter members, the introverts, may believe their opinions are not wanted and stop trying. To honor these differences, the extroverts can practice their listening skills, understanding that silence may be needed for processing and that it does not necessarily mean consensus. They can consciously slow down and ask only one question at a time, allowing time for a response. The introverts can understand this and allow the extroverts time to process their ideas aloud. They can ask for a moment to think and take the initiative to make sure they are heard. With this knowledge, a group can avoid misunderstanding each other's styles and confront this issue to continue to get the best of people's gifts. Some organizations provide staff with training in personality preferences, using a personality preference profile such as the Myers–Briggs Type Indicator (MBTI) and/or trained facilitators to promote richer problem solving that honors the different styles people bring to groups (Balzer Riley, 1997; Kroeger, Thuesen, & Rutledge, 2002).

People with an intuitive style of perceiving see the big picture: Intuitive individuals look for the end product and anticipate it. They may skip steps on the way to the solution, thinking "A,…oh, yes, D." In solving problems, they use and trust their intuition.

People with a sensing style collect data: Sensors want to know how many, how big, when, what, where, and who. They think "A,…B,…C,…, and then D." They solve problems by collecting facts.

Big-picture people may present what seem like unrealistic, fantastic ideas. They may jump to conclusions without careful consideration of all the practicalities involved in implementing their ideas. These big-picture people, or intuitives, if they can laugh at themselves, will understand the one-liner, "The possibilities are endless." Data collectors, or sensors, may have trouble making a decision because they can never obtain all the data they would like. If these people can laugh at themselves, they will understand the one-liner, "Analysis paralysis."

To honor these differences, big-picture people (intuitives) can listen to the detail people (sensors) to avoid making hasty decisions. They can be more patient with the necessary process of attention to details. Big-picture people can focus on the current issues to be resolved before a solution can be implemented. Data collectors (sensors) can give others time to express their ideas without rapid dismissal so that the creativity may be harnessed. They can understand that all the little pieces fit together to make the big picture (Kroeger et al., 2002).

To apply these concepts to group decision making, consider these two kinds of thinkers as divergent thinkers and convergent thinkers. Divergent thinkers want to express their views and broaden the discussion; this approach is characterized by the generation of options, free discussion, and gathering of diverse opinions. Convergent thinkers want to move toward conclusions; this approach is characterized by the evaluation of options, summarization of key points, and sorting of ideas into categories (Kaner, 2014).

TASK, MAINTENANCE, AND INDIVIDUAL ROLES IN GROUPS

In groups, people assume roles that can facilitate or impede the work of the group. Table 22.1 lists maintenance and task roles that help build group success. As you read, consider what roles you have played in groups and those you

TABLE 22.1 Group Roles

Role	Function
Maintenance Roles	
Encourager	To be a positive influence on the group
Harmonizer	To make/keep peace
Compromiser	To minimize conflict by seeking options
Gatekeeper	To determine the level of group acceptance of individual members
Follower	To serve as an interested audience
Rule maker	To set standards for group behaviors
Problem solver	To solve problems to allow the group to continue its work
Task Roles	
Leader	To set direction
Questioner	To clarify issues and information
Facilitator	To keep the group focused
Summarizer	To state the current position of the group
Evaluator	To assess the performance of the group
Initiator	To begin group discussion

Modified from Stuart, G. W. (2012). *Principles and practice of psychiatric nursing* (10th ed.). St. Louis, MO: Mosby.

TABLE 22.2 Individual Roles that Impede Group Progress

Role	Description
Aggressor	Annihilates other group members; destroys other member's self-esteem
Nonconformist	Finds something wrong with almost everything; very negative
Conformist	Agrees with everything
Recognition seeker	Wants to be the shining star; concerned with personal achievements
Self-confessor	Tries to use the group for therapy sessions; shares personal life
Silent one	Does not contribute
Know-it-all	Knows something about everything
Playboy/ playgirl	Lacks interest and involvement; is not committed
Latecomer	Shows lack of respect for the group and wants to be seen as important

Modified from Stuart, G. W. (2012). *Principles and practice of psychiatric nursing* (10th ed.). St. Louis, MO: Mosby; Balzer Riley, J. (1997). *Instant tools for health care teams*. St. Louis, MO: Mosby.

might be willing to assume. Table 22.2 describes roles that can hinder the progress of groups. Consider which of these behaviors you have observed in groups and honestly evaluate which roles you have played that you would be willing to reexamine and change.

EMOTIONAL INTELLIGENCE IN GROUPS

Reflect on your results from examining your own emotional intelligence in Chapter 4. Emotional intelligence, which is a concept usually applied to individuals, is the ability to access, manage, and use one's feelings in relationships and is identified as the ingredient that distinguishes the most successful leaders in business (Goleman, 2000). In healthcare, technology may help us become more efficient, but it also can lead to isolation and alienation in staff as we depend on electronic forms of communication. Using your knowledge about emotional intelligence can be useful in face-to-face meetings and lead with the application of concepts of emotionally building staff cohesion. Group emotional intelligence is about bringing emotions to the surface, understanding how they affect the team's work, and behaving inside and outside the group in ways that build relationships to strengthen the group's ability to face challenges. It is about small human acts in relationships that make a difference,

---

BOX 22.2 Norms that Foster Emotional Intelligence in Groups

- Use icebreakers to help group members get to know each other, have members share their thoughts and feelings in the group, and relieve stress with levity.
- Have a brief "check-in" from each member at the start of the meeting to see how everyone is doing and acknowledge a shift in group mood.
- Ask if each member agrees with a decision.
- Validate the contribution of members.
- Encourage members to help each other focus on the purpose or mission of the group.
- Build the expectation that the group can use humor to intervene in difficult group behaviors and encourage "inside" humor that evolves naturally from the group's history.
- Keep the group focused on problem solving, not blaming.
- Encourage team members to ask each other what they need.
- Anticipate and prepare for difficulties in the group's work.
- Periodically evaluate group effectiveness and individual member satisfaction.

Modified from Druskat, V. U. (2001). Building the emotional intelligence of groups. *Harvard Business Review, 79*(3), 81; Balzer Riley, J. (1997). *Instant tools for health care teams.* St. Louis, MO: Mosby.

such as saying "thank you" for extra effort from an individual (Druskat, 2001). See Box 22.2 for other suggestions for building group emotional intelligence for success.

IMPORTANCE OF MEETINGS

Small groups come together frequently in our work world to provide information, plan, problem solve, give feedback on performance, and make and evaluate decisions. If you spend 4 hours in meetings each week, that is more than 9000 hours, or more than 365 days, of your life. Middle managers may spend as much as 35% of their work week in meetings (Doyle & Straus, 1993).

Self-Care Nudge

When you are adding a meeting to your schedule, work to be aware of needing breaks between meetings. Do not over-schedule. Remember, "back-to-back" virtual meetings can be more exhausting than you expect. We speak of "Zoom fatigue" from virtual meetings.

To Meet or Not to Meet

A meeting is the best tool when face-to-face communication is needed. An email memo and responses are no substitute for the timeliness of communicating in person and the ability to observe and respond to nonverbal behavior. The synergy of a group of people can produce creative solutions, and objections or problems can be addressed immediately. Staff meetings can create excitement and enthusiasm, which is more possible when people meet face to face (Overgaard, 2010). People who are involved in making a decision are more likely to support it. Successful meetings can increase a sense of belonging and build team spirit (Doyle & Straus, 1993). Research of nursing students working together in groups to study family health indicated higher critical thinking skills scores than those in a routine educational program (Khosravani, Manoochehri, & Memarian, 2005). Law students traditionally form study groups to prepare for classes.

There are instances in which a meeting is not the best use of time. Although it is common for a hospital to have large informational meetings on policy changes, there is no guarantee that people's minds are engaged when their bodies are present. Following up with written material may be helpful.

When one employee demonstrates a problem behavior, such as lateness to work, it is tempting for a manager to convene a staff meeting and address the "problem" of lateness. A more appropriate course, although sometimes uncomfortable, is to confront the employee with the problem to offer counseling, coaching, and eventually a reprimand if the problem is not resolved. To present this situation as a group problem creates anger and resentment.

If a decision has already been made or no option exists, it is inappropriate to call a meeting as if an employee group had the power to make the decision. If you have only blue paint, do not ask the staff what color they would like the lounge to be painted.

VIRTUAL MEETINGS

In the spring of 2020, in the face of a pandemic, meeting via a virtual platform became a necessity for students. Healthcare professionals began to think creatively about the use of such platforms to support patients and colleagues. A palliative care team offered family conferences via telemedicine (Kuntz et al., 2020). Virtual healing retreats for respite and renewal were developed to support nurse leaders so they could be of more support to staff and patients (Geradi & Lawson, 2021). Schools of nursing turned to platforms such as Zoom when face-to-face classes were not possible. Strategies for virtual nursing education were implemented (Bourgault, Mayerson, Nai, Orsini-Garry, & Alexander, 2022).

Tools to Promote Effectiveness of Meetings

Provide an agenda for a meeting as an organizing framework and a template for the work to be accomplished. Distribute the agenda several days before the meeting so members can prepare their best thoughts and ideas on the issues to be discussed. Distinguish between action items, discussion items for future decisions, and informational items (Orlikoff & Totten, 2001). Include the amount of time available for discussion if appropriate.

Choose a person to function as a recorder for the meeting. The recorder takes notes on a flip chart, overhead transparency, whiteboard, or other memo board of what happens in the meeting. The recorder may abbreviate but does not paraphrase a contribution. The recorder may be someone who is not a member of the group, is an appointed group member, or is a volunteer member. This position might rotate among members. The record may include names of members present, members absent, and even members arriving late to draw attention to the importance of timely attendance. These notes become the basis for the minutes or meetings notes that are kept as an ongoing record of the work of the group.

Consider the use of a facilitator, such as those in a quality improvement team. The facilitator's function is to focus on content issues; to keep the group on task; to point out process issues, or how a group works together (Schwarz, 2002); to summarize; to test for consensus; and to deal with problem behaviors that may impede the group's work if no facilitator is designated or if group members do not share the task role of facilitator. For example, to deal with the behavior of the latecomer, the facilitator might acknowledge the person: "Tom, glad you could come. You can catch up with where we are by looking at the recorder's notes." A facilitator can approach the person after the meeting and simply ask why the person was late. The facilitator can ask what would make the meeting important enough to come on time. To deal with someone who interrupts another member, the facilitator might immediately say, "Just a minute, Jane, let's let Sam finish before we hear your point." Asking the person who interrupts to assume the role of recorder may help the person to listen better and capture the energy of involvement (Doyle & Straus, 1993).

SIMPLIFY AND DEEPEN

If you want others to be happy, practice compassion. If you want to be happy, practice compassion.

The Dalai Lama

CHARACTERISTICS OF AN EFFECTIVE GROUP

Members of an effective group follow the strategies listed in Box 22.3. Halvorson (2014) suggested that a compelling shared mission supports effective work groups. Huckman

BOX 22.3 Members of an Effective Group…

- Assume responsibility to share ideas and opinions and refuse to shut down. They participate willingly and communicate effectively.
- Negotiate and build consensus. They see an issue more than one way, share and value different ideas, and consider other viewpoints.
- Give and receive feedback even when it is difficult. They demonstrate a willingness to delay judgment and tolerate the confusion of a group working out its issues. They know that what seems like confusion might be a prelude to creativity.
- Commit to team goals to achieve the best outcome. They work to find a solution to which all group members are willing to commit rather than seek a quick compromise that may not receive the full support of members. They are willing to support the team's decision, knowing they have made their opinions known or chosen to support others' opinions.

Modified from Harrington-Mackin, D. (1994). *The team building tool kit: Tips, tactics, and rules for effective workplace teams.* New York, NY: AMACOM; and Kaner, S. (2014). *Facilitator's guide to participatory decision-making.* Hoboken, NJ: Jossey-Bass Business & Management Series.

and Staats's (2013) research suggested that keeping working teams intact promotes effectiveness through familiarity. They cited an interesting example of an orthopedic surgeon well known in the field of knee replacements who took 20 minutes to replace a knee while others took 1 to 2 hours. The surgeon performed more than 550 knee replacements annually (2.5 times as many as the second-most productive doctor in his hospital), with better outcomes. He accomplished this by arranging to have two dedicated teams, one each in two adjoining rooms, with nurses who had worked with him for 18 years. He reported that few of the methods he pioneered would be practical without the easy familiarity of working with the same staff each day.

MOMENTS OF CONNECTION…
A Nursing Student Reflects

I am glad we took the MBTI for class. I learned I am an introvert, but I had no idea of the actual meaning of it. Introverts draw their energy from within. They think to talk. They need to recharge when they get home. Understanding this makes me feel so much more normal. I feel like I am finally starting to look honestly at myself. I need to take a breath, figure out what I want to say, and value my thoughts and opinions enough to speak up in a group.

STRATEGIES FOR BUILDING SUCCESSFUL COMMITTEES

Understanding about working together in groups is essential to successful committee work. Pay attention to the movement of committees through the stages of group development and remember that the stage of storming is a time when committees may run into problems if group dynamics are not understood. See Box 22.4 for strategies for building a successful committee.

BOX 22.4 Strategies to Build a Successful Committee

Select the Best Members
- Select staff who want to contribute to this particular task, such as a policy and procedures committee, and who have the energy and time.
- Select staff with appropriate work experience and education.
- Select an effective chairperson.

Select a Workable Number
- Six to eight is a good number.
- Clearly outline work.
- Communicate the tasks and responsibilities of the committee; how the committee's work is to be reported; and deadlines, if any.

Set Expectations about Assignments
- To accept an assignment means to report on the work at the next meeting or on another designated date.

Provide a Written Agenda for Each Meeting
- The agenda should be distributed several days before the meeting.

Compile Written Records of Each Meeting
- Assign the role of recorder or obtain the commitment of a volunteer.

Provide Adequate Meeting Space
- Reserve a room with enough space, and, if possible, use the same room for the duration of the committee.

Consider Meeting by Video Conferencing
- Provide access to training on the video platform you are using.
- Open meeting early to allow time for troubleshooting for video and audio access.
- Have access to technical support.
- Follow etiquette of video conferencing, such as use of the mute function.

Return to "Active Learning" at the beginning of the chapter and write your responses.

 PRACTICING WORKING TOGETHER IN GROUPS

Knowledge Assessment: Exercise 1

Match the following descriptions with the four phases of group development:

_____	1. Forming	a. Resistance and conflict are expected now; there is little or no evidence of group cohesion or team commitment
_____	2. Storming	b. The work gets done; team members feel good about their achievements and are flexible in their roles to meet team goals
_____	3. Norming	c. Team members clarify group goals and figure out the rules necessary to get the work done
_____	4. Performing	d. Team members are polite, begin to identify group goals, and test relationships

Note: Answers are at the end of the exercises in this chapter.

Application: Exercise 2

Review Table 22.1. Identify a group of which you are currently a member or one in which you have been a member. List the task and maintenance roles you have seen in this group and the functions they fulfilled in the group. Share your responses with another student.

Application: Exercise 3

Review the individual roles listed in Table 22.1. Write an example of a role or roles you have played in a group and of others you have observed. Discuss this with another student.

Synthesis: Exercise 4

You are a nurse who is responsible for organizing the Nurse Week celebration committee. Outline the steps you will take to create an effective committee using the guidelines in this chapter, and write a proposal for the creation of the committee.

Synthesis: Exercise 5

In a small student or staff group, plan a renewal activity, an outing together, or a potluck event. Pay attention to how your work together illustrates the content of this chapter. These skills would translate well to renewal of spirit in the workplace. Discuss how such an activity could be held in a virtual setting.

Quality and Safety Education for Nurses Learning Strategy: Exercise 6 QSEN

Teamwork and Collaboration is a key competency to improve outcomes of care and forms the basis for a culture of safety. Interprofessional learning helps to break down silos of healthcare providers and offers the opportunity to experience teamwork behaviors that can improve how health professionals work together. There are four domains that explain interprofessional experiences: values and ethics to be able to respect and understand each other; roles and responsibilities to clarify what each team member contributes; teamwork, which defines the behaviors that characterize effectively working together; and communication to accomplish skills and attitudes for sharing critical information and building relationships.

- Reflect on a patient you have cared for recently.
- Who was part of the healthcare team?
- What were the roles and responsibilities of each provider? Were the roles clearly identified to the patient?
- Describe evidence of how each team member valued and respected others on the team, as well as the patient and family.
- Identify teamwork behaviors you observed. How could these be improved to accomplish the patient's care and monitor safety?
- Write the communication you observed among the team members. What are characteristics of effective communication? Rewrite the team communication to reflect skills and attitudes of effective communication.
- What was the impact of the team working together on the patient and family?
  Answers to Exercise 2: 1. *d*; 2. *a*; 3. *c*; 4. *b*.

REFERENCES

Alessandra, T (2001). Team meetings. *Executive Excellence, 18*(12), 17.

Balzer Riley, J. (1997). *Instant tools for health care teams.* St. Louis, MO: Mosby.

Bourgault, A., Mayerson, E., Nai, M., Orsini-Garry, A., & Alexander, I. M. (2022). Implications of the COVID-pandemic: Virtual nursing education for delirium care. *Journal of Professional Nursing, 38,* 54–64.

Doyle, M., & Straus, D. (1993). *How to make meetings work.* New York, NY: Berkley Books.

Druskat, V. U. (2001). Building the emotional intelligence of groups. *Harvard Business Review, 79*(3), 80.

Galinsky, A. D., & Kilduff, G. J. (2013). Be seen as a leader. *Harvard Business Review, 91*(12), 127.

Geradi, D., & Lawson, C. (2021). Coaching in community: Fostering resilience for nurse leaders during the COVID-19 pandemic. *Nurse Leader, 19*(3). https://doi.org/10.1016/j.mnl.2021.04.001.

Goleman, D. (2000). *Working with emotional intelligence.* New York, NY: Bantam Doubleday Dell.

Gundry, L., & LaMantia, L. (2001). Dream teams. *Executive Excellence, 18*(10), 13.

Halter, M. J. (2013). *Foundations of psychiatric mental health nursing: A clinical approach* (7th ed.). St. Louis, MO: Saunders.

Halvorson, G. (2014). Getting to "us." *Harvard Business Review, 92*(9), 38.

Huckman, R., & Staats, B. (2013). The hidden benefits of keeping teams intact. *Harvard Business Review, 91*(12), 27.

Kaner, S. (2014). *Facilitator's guide to participatory decision-making.* Hoboken, NJ: Jossey-Bass Business & Management Series.

Khosravani, S., Manoochehri, H., & Memarian, R. (2005). Developing critical thinking skills in nursing students by group dynamics. *Internet Journal of Advanced Nursing Practice, 7*(2), 1.

Kroeger, O., Thuesen, J. M., & Rutledge, H. (2002). *Type talk: The 16 personality types that determine how we live, love, and work.* New York, NY: Dell.

Kuntz, J. G., Kavalieratos, D., Esper, G. J., Ogbu, Jr, N., Mitchell, J., V., Ellis, C. M., et al. (2020). Feasibility and acceptability of inpatient palliative care E-family meetings during COVID_19 Pandemic. *Journal of Pain and Symptom Management, 60*(3), e28–e32. https://doi.org/10.1016/j.jpainsymman.2020.06.001.

McTighe, A. J., & Donovan, S. (2017). Group dynamics in healthcare settings: A strategic framework for cohesion. *Research in Psychology and Behavioral Sciences, 5*(2), 30.

Orlikoff, J. E., & Totten, M. K. (2001). How to run effective board meetings. *Trustee, 54*(4), 12.

Overgaard, P. M. (2010). 7 steps to highly effective staff meetings. *Nursing Management, 41*(3), 54.

Reynolds, F. (2005). *Communication and clinical effectiveness in rehabilitation.* Edinburgh, UK: Elsevier.

Rosenthal, M. J. (2001). High-performance teams. *Executive Excellence, 18*(10), 6.

Roussel, L. (2011). *Management and leadership for nurse administrators.* Burlington, MA: Jones & Bartlett Learning.

Ryan, S. (2017). Promoting effective teamwork in the healthcare setting. *Nursing Standard, 31*(30), 52.

Schwarz, R. M. (2002). *The skilled facilitator: Practical wisdom for developing effective groups.* San Francisco, CA: Jossey-Bass.

Stuart, G. W. (2012). *Principles and practice of psychiatric nursing* (10th ed.). St. Louis, MO: Mosby.

Stucky, C. H., Brown, W. J., & Stucky, M. G. (2021). COVID 19: An unprecedented opportunity for nurse practitioners to reform healthcare and advocate for full practice authority. *Nursing Forum, 56*(1), 222–227.

Stucky, C. H., Wymer, J. A., & House, S. (2021). Nurse leaders: Transforming interprofessional relationships to bridge healthcare quality and safety. *Nurse Leader, 20*(4), 375–380. https://doi.org/10.1016/j.mnl.2021.12.003.

Suter, E., Arndt, J., Arthur, N., Parbosingh, J., Taylor, E., & Deutschlander, S. (2009). Role understanding and effective communication as core competencies for collaborative practice. *Journal of Interprofessional Care, 23*(1), 41.

Touhy, T. A., & Jett, K. F. (2013). *Ebersole and Hess' gerontological nursing & healthy aging* (4th ed.). St. Louis, MO: Mosby.

Traylor, A. M., Tannenbaum, S. I., Thomas., E. J., & Salas, E. (2021). Helping healthcare teams save lives during COVID-19: Insights and countermeasures from team science. *American Psychologist, 76*(1), 1–13. http://dx.doi.org/10.1037/amp0000750.

Tuckman, B. (1965). Developmental sequence in small groups. *Psychological Bulletin, 63*, 384.

Weaver, T. E. (2008). Enhancing multiple disciplinary teamwork. *Nursing Outlook, 56*(3), 108.

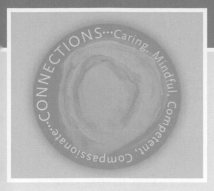

23

Navigating the Complex World of Digital Communication*

Kathleen Sitzman, PhD, RN, CNE, ANEF, FAAN

As the world becomes a more digital place, we cannot forget about the human connection.

Adam Neumann

OBJECTIVES

1. Discuss practical strategies to convey and sustain caring in digital settings.
2. Discuss three ways that social media impacts nursing.
3. Describe organizational policies to support the safe use of smartphones in healthcare.
4. Name three clinical applications that are beneficial to professional nursing practice.
5. Name several ways to appropriately use nonclinical applications in the clinical setting.
6. Describe three types of digital learning used in nursing.
7. Name one reputable search engine for digital research of nursing topics.
8. Discuss the benefits of clinical documentation utilizing an electronic health record.
9. Describe the dangers of digital communication and how to avoid them.
10. Discuss the nursing implications of increased healthcare consumer use of the Internet.

ACTIVE LEARNING

Developing Road-Worthy Practices along the Journey: Navigating the Expanding World of Digital Communication

Think about how you will write your answers as you read this chapter.

What?
Write one thing you learned from this chapter.

So What?
How will this affect your nursing practice?

Now What?
How will you implement this new knowledge or skill?

Think About It ...

* With contributions from Kathy Hribar, RN-BC, MSN; Cindy Carter, MSN, BSN, RN, IBCLC, RLC.

CARING AS THE FOUNDATION FOR ALL FORMS OF DIGITAL COMMUNICATION

Deliberative, authentic caring is a core function of professional nursing. This caring foundation encompasses caring for self, patients, colleagues, students, groups, communities, the environment, the earth, and beyond in both face-to-face and digital settings. Extensive knowledge development in nursing validates the need to consciously convey and sustain caring in digital settings wherever nurses practice (Sitzman & Watson, 2017; Sitzman & Watson, 2018). In this chapter, digital communication, as it relates to nursing practice, is described and analyzed in terms of best practices, professionalism, personal/professional safety, privacy, and baseline skills and knowledge that nurses must know wherever they work. In the midst of exciting and sometimes daunting technological developments related to digital communication, it is critical that nurses maintain a firm and ongoing intent to care in *every* digital setting they encounter. Here are some examples of what caring looks like in digital settings:

- *For self:* Exercise informed caution when interacting with strangers on social media platforms to protect physical, emotional, professional, and fiscal safety.
- *For patients:* Diligently protect patient privacy by only sharing patient information using agency approved platforms and procedures.
- *For colleagues and students:* Carefully and thoughtfully respond to digital communications from colleagues or students promptly, professionally, and compassionately, especially in situations where there is tension or ambiguity.
- *For groups, communities, and organizations:* Use digital information to become knowledgeable about how to create healthier, safer, kinder, and more productive environments in groups, communities, and organizations.
- *For the environment and the Earth:* Use digital communication strategies to reduce or eliminate the unnecessary use of paper to protect the environment.

Digital caring is embedded in carefully chosen language, pacing, and nuance. This means that timing, words, punctuation, length and rhythm of messages, choice of font, emojis, and other embellishments have the power to convey caring and also un-caring. It is important to choose carefully and thoughtfully how you create messages and how you respond to others. Conveying and sustaining caring in digital settings may be facilitated by doing the following: If there is tension, ambiguity, or strong emotions involved, it is best to pause and re-read what is written by self and/or others and take a few mindful breaths before originating a message or sending a response.

1. Consciously cultivate a firm resolve to authentically care for self and others every day in both face-to-face and digital settings.
2. Accept the fact that misunderstandings can occur; acknowledge and ask for forgiveness when this happens, and then move productively forward with compassion for yourself and others.
3. Treat each digital interaction, no matter how small or insignificant it may seem, as an opportunity to care. Everything matters, often in ways that we will never know.

It can be difficult to know how to say and/or write/text/email/post things in a caring manner while still maintaining a professional demeanor. Sitzman (2016) & Sitzman and Watson (2017) offered suggestions for what to say in commonly encountered situations. These suggestions, paraphrased here, can be tailored to meet personal style and situational needs:

- I am here to help and I want you to be successful.
- My thoughts are with you.
- I have received your message and will reply to you by date/time.

- I will do my best for you/the group/my colleagues as we work through this initiative/project/problem together.
- I would like to connect via video call. Can I send an invitation to you?
- You are important to me.
- Your work is valuable to me.
- Your observations resonate with my own.
- I would appreciate the opportunity to provide additional clarification if needed.
- Is everything okay? I want to make sure I am not missing something.
- Please tell me what you envision for this situation/project/meeting.
- Is there anything I can do to help you right now?
- I will listen carefully to your ideas and respectfully share my own as we work toward common goals.

SOCIAL MEDIA...THE BIG PICTURE

According to the American Nurses Association (ANA) Code of Ethics for Nurses, "Social media is forms of electronic communication such as websites for social networking and blogging in which users create online communities to share information, ideas, personal messages, and other content" (ANA, 2015). Within this definition are two different terms: *social media* and *social networking*. Let us consider a distinction between social media and social networking. Fraser (2011) looked at social media as a broad term for digital tools to share and discuss information, saying that the term *social media* combines new media and social networking. Social media refers to forms of digital communication that support gathering, communicating, and collaborating (Kubheka, 2017). Now, with social media, there is the potential to use an online blog as an active research journal and share comments and seek input from readers (Table 23.1). For example, Fraser (2011) shared that a colleague working on a policy update for a hospital used Twitter to learn how nurses checked nasogastric tubes at their hospitals; 25 nurses responded within minutes. This chapter introduces the progress of digital communication and invites participation with careful thought and respect for its appropriate application within professional boundaries (Box 23.1).

In *The Nurse's Social Media Advantage: How Making Connections and Sharing Ideas Can Enhance Your Nursing Practice,* Fraser (2011) challenged nurses to understand how to use social media to shift their thinking and to begin using digital tools appropriately to educate clients and colleagues; to build an online professional profile, reputation, and network; to locate others who share their interests; and to become an active part of online communities. A 2014 study of American nurses across 43 states found that

TABLE 23.1 Internet Communication Basics

Type	Description	Timing	Access
Blog	A web journal to share thoughts, information, or simply convey interests	Asynchronous; view when desired	Search for topics of interest, then subscribe to the blog or follow the author
Email	Formal communications sent to specific individuals using email addresses and email account provider	Asynchronous; sender and receiver do not need to be online together	Directed to a specific recipient or a specific group of recipients
Text	Short comments, often using shortened word forms, sent to specific people via their phone or messaging accounts	Real-time access meant for immediate communication	Directed to specific individuals using phone numbers or messaging services
Tweet	Character-limited comments, observations, or questions sent to a general group of followers	Real-time communications and feedback/comments	Follow authors on Twitter to receive alerts when authors post and comment as desired
Vlog	Video journal depicting topics of interest, educational focus, or life in general	Asynchronous; access when desired	Subscribe to vlog or search YouTube channels for topics of interest
Skype, Zoom, and many others	Free service for video communication with individuals or groups	Real-time face-to-face video and audio communications	Communicate with others who have access to the Skype application
Apps	Online applications that offer information, tools, entertainment, or other specific functions	Asynchronous; access when desired	Download apps to smartphones, tablets, or personal computers for use when and where they are needed

94% of the participants indicated that they regularly used social media, whereas fewer than 1% of the participants reported that they did not know how to use social media. Among those who use social media, social networking sites (90.33%) and podcasts (76.24%) were the most popular, followed by social question and answer sites (37.86%), blogs (31.85%), Twitter (19.06%), and SlideShare (9.92%) (Kung & Oh, 2014). A key consideration to best utilizing social media tools is knowing how to make wise decisions regarding personal presence and the confidentiality and privacy of patients, colleagues, and employers. Just as we are called to manage our face-to-face relationships, so too are we called to manage our online presence with clear judgment and caution (Fraser, 2011). It is imperative to learn and abide by your employer's policies and expectations for the use of social media (International Nurse Regulator Collaborative [INRC], 2016).

As you read this chapter, consider how you can use technology to enhance your knowledge, skills, abilities, and understanding to connect with individuals and build relationships that create community and inspire people to make a difference in the world through both personal and professional action (Fraser, 2011).

NURSES AND DIGITAL COMMUNICATION

You may already be deeply immersed in the world of digital communication or just sampling it for the first time. The nursing profession has changed dramatically and, like all of healthcare, continues to evolve rapidly. The tools to optimize performance and growth in this role are also quickly evolving. Keeping up with advancements requires a different strategy than that used by previous generations of nurses. Some of you may be reading this text through an electronic reader, or you may be taking an online course. Just as the practice of nursing is changing, so too is the delivery of nursing education.

The way information is being received has changed, and so has the way information is being transmitted. Statistics published by Finances Online (2022) at the close of 2021 estimated 4.66 billion active Internet users. In January 2017, the Pew Research Center (2018) reported 77% of

BOX 23.1   Professional and Responsible Use of Social Media

1. *Respect client confidentiality and privacy:* Follow Health Insurance Portability and Accountability Act guidelines and organizational policies. Do not share any information on social media sites that could in any way identify a patient or might lead to identification, such as diagnosis, nickname, or location/room number. Never post photos of patients, even if they give you verbal approval. There is no such thing as privacy on the Internet. Even content that has been removed can be discoverable in a court of law.

2. *Maintain privacy:* Set and maintain privacy settings on social networking accounts to limit access to personal information, and understand that even with the highest settings, people can copy and share your information without your permission. Never post photos or use language that might reflect badly on you; remember, there is no true privacy online.

3. *Respect professional boundaries:* End relationships with patients professionally at the end of service. Make it your policy not to accept client "friend" requests on your personal social media accounts. Objectivity and the professional relationship are lost. If social media is used with clients, create and use a professional account in accordance with the policies of your organization. Do

not contact patients or families using a personal phone or provide patients with your personal phone number.

4. *Protect personal and organization integrity:* Use professional channels to handle workplace disputes, and do not air your grievances online. Even "liking" a disrespectful comment reflects badly on you. Just as it is unprofessional to speak negatively about your organization or colleagues face to face, it also is unprofessional online.

5. *Maintain a professional image:* Take time to think before you blog, post, or tweet. An angry email may make you feel better now, but the consequences may be embarrassing later. Consider carefully posting or sharing political statements, images, or humor that you would not want a prospective employer to see. Keep your personal and professional life separate with different accounts.

6. *Keep your use of social media and Internet access in healthy life balance:* Be aware of the stress of information overload. Try to avoid interrupting class or work to make or receive personal texts or calls. Build in daily quiet, digital-free time. If this is hard to do, consider that you may be exhibiting signs of cell phone addiction and that it may be time to readjust priorities.

Adapted from National Council of State Boards of Nursing (NCSBN). *National Council of State Boards of Nursing (NCSBN): A Nurse's Guide to the Use of Social Media.* (2011). https://www.ncsbn.org/NCSBN_SocialMedia.pdf; International Nurse Regulator Collaborative Position Statement: Social media use: common expectations for nurses, 2014.

American adults had a smartphone, and the fastest growing group of smartphone users was reported to be the population aged 50 and older. With this rapid increase in mobile communication access, especially in the aging population, it is important for nurses to develop and master digital communication skills. The ability to type and computer literacy are considered baseline skills for all nurses.

Simpson (2007) stated that the changing healthcare environment "will demand nurses for whom technology use is as inherent as critical thinking." According to the Quality and Safety Education for Nurses (QSEN) Initiative, informatics skills are vital for future nurses, and, as such, QSEN calls nursing informatics one of the six pillars of safe and effective nursing care, recognizing this competency as one of the required knowledge, skills, and attitudes (KSAs) needed to promote patient safety. According to its definition, nurses should be able to use information technology (IT) to communicate, manage knowledge, mitigate error, and support decision making (QSEN Institute, n.d.). It is recommended that these KSAs be part of simulations during nursing

education to allow the student to begin to practice these core competencies demanded by the nursing profession; as a result, they have found their way into the core curriculums of many universities and colleges. According to QSEN, registered nurses are now required to be knowledge workers, system thinkers, and complex adaptive system managers, all of which require excellent communication skills in a dynamic, interactive, and ever-changing practice.

The Technology Informatics Guiding Education Reform (TIGER) initiative has delineated three nursing informatics competencies: basic computer competencies, information literacy, and information management (Sensmeier, Anderson, & Shaw, 2017). The Agency for Healthcare Research and Quality (AHRQ) has created several toolkits for Health Information Technology (HIT) to facilitate the process of assisting all healthcare providers (HCPs) in becoming competent in HIT (AHRQ, 2015).

Technology is not just for the entry level practitioner. Leadership skills required of nurses to appropriately respond to emerging technologies include being able to use technology to facilitate, communicate, and build relationships; having expertise in knowledge and information acquisition and distribution; and understanding and using complex technologies such as genetics and genomics in nursing (Huston, 2013).

Because of the growth and challenges within the digital side of healthcare in the past few decades, a new professional role has been established: the nurse informatician. According to *Nursing Informatics: Scope and Standards of Practice,* 2nd edition (ANA, 2014), nursing informatics is defined as "a specialty that integrates nursing science with multiple information and analytic sciences to identify, define, manage and communicate data, information, knowledge and wisdom in nursing practice" (ANA, 2014). As an advanced practice nurse with education and experience on both the clinical side of nursing and in IT, the nurse informatician focuses on supporting nursing workflow from their advanced IT knowledge and from the clinician end-user point of view. Rather than having the nurse adjust his or her work processes to meet the limitations imposed by technology, nurses in this role work to ensure that the technology supports the optimized workflows, finding opportunity for practice improvement within the process of customizing the tools and systems needed to support nursing practice. According to Roy Simpson (2007), a pioneer among nursing informaticians, "information technology can transform nursing tasks into nursing knowledge." The world of digital communication has changed healthcare forever.

Tools to Support Data Management

Extracting data from the health information system to support research or clinical practice requires a clear presentation of data for the viewer's full understanding. If pursuing a personal or educational project, an investment in a professional software package like Microsoft Office or Pages will help produce professional appearing products that are more universally accessible to the intended audience. Graphical data presentations and multidimensional dashboards are the standard in quickly conveying large volumes of information to a busy clinical audience.

Whatever type of document, spreadsheet, or presentation you create, one of the most important steps is how you save your work. Saving should begin when you open a document by creating a unique title and saving the work on your computer's hard drive. Adopt a naming convention that will help you track the desired content and version, such as "Informatics draft-1 or Cardioversion Stats 3-18." Inclusion of the draft or date will help you avoid opening numerous files to find what you want or wondering if this is the most up-to-date information. Document storage options include CD, DVD, or memory stick (*flash* or *jump drive*) in addition to the computer hard drive and the *cloud.* Organization

policy may prohibit downloading patient-specific information, and organizational network devices may block the use of flash drives, CDs, or email attachments. It is crucial that you are aware of and abide by organizational policies, Internal Review Board (IRB) requirements, and federal regulations such as the Health Insurance Portability and Accountability Act (HIPAA), when accessing patient data, even if the data do not include personal identifiers.

Tools to Support Learning

According to an Australian study, being computer savvy with social networking and communication does not necessarily translate into a preference for learning in the same manner. Even members of the "Net Generation," the so-called digital natives, were found to prefer less digital communication when it applied to learning and more hands-on and traditional face-to-face sessions (Kennedy, Judd, Churchward, Gray, & Krause, 2008). Studies report variance in learning preferences based on age, experience, and level of coursework. To be successful, all teaching methodologies, but especially those online, need to be varied and support a variety of learning styles and preferences (Hampton, Pearce, & Moser, 2017). Bennett, Moqton, & Kervin (2008) also reported on the same phenomenon, finding that even the most computer-literate students appreciate variety in the teaching methods of online classes or a hybrid blend of online and face time, because learning digitally is not felt to be the same as digital socializing.

The most successful online courses incorporate digital caring strategies in addition to actively engaging learners through the inclusion of a variety of synchronous and asynchronous techniques meant to support inclusion and varied learning styles. Online courses may be synchronous (real time) or asynchronous. Podcasts or webinars represent one way to communicate digitally and can be a part of higher education course delivery or a way to provide professional continuing education credits. In a podcast, the presenter is in a specific physical location and typically is using some type of multimedia presentation. The presentation may have in-class participants, but it is also being recorded and broadcast to one or more locations simultaneously. The recorded podcast is then placed in the organization's intranet for access by participants as needed. Personal mobile devices, tablets, smartphones, and computers can be programmed to access podcasts for watching later. Virtual meeting applications such as Skype or Zoom also allow synchronous face-to-face interactions. Whether used for communication with friends or as part of a class, this type of digital communication allows for connections that are synchronous and face-to-face.

Digital communication also enables learners to take review courses and examinations totally online. From college classes to certification examinations to the National

Council Licensure Examination (NCLEX®) licensure, accessing this type of structured online assessment is the norm. The Computerized Adaptive Testing (CAT) approach used by the National Council of State Boards of Nursing (NCSBN) for the NCLEX licensure examination improves the precision of the examination process by applying algorithms that evaluate the test taker's level of knowledge based on correct responses. The algorithm will offer questions until reaching a 95% confidence level on passing or until reaching the maximum amount of time or number of questions. In this manner, each candidate's experience can be different, varying in number of questions, time commitment to complete the examination, and specific content questions presented (NCSBN, n.d.).

Asynchronous learning opportunities, such as discussion boards, also enrich online course delivery. Normally, the instructor posts assignments that require a response, and each student answers online over the course of several days. The responses can be as a group, each student contributing to a shared online discussion, or individually, with student content only seen by the instructor. The instructor responds to posted comments to keep the group conversation on track, to clarify content, and to stimulate further thought and discussion. Thoughtful reflection and critical thinking skills are often revealed as the students explore various topics together. Another type of asynchronous activity in a learning community is blogging (i.e., using a web journal for collective sharing). Many professional nursing organizations offer blogs with links to their social networking sites for comments and communication related to the content presented.

Tools to Support Professional Practice: Really Simple Syndication Feeds

How do you currently get your news? Do you watch the nightly news on television? Do you start your morning by browsing through on online newspaper? Or are you one of the people who now gets a really simple syndication (RSS) feed to their digital device presenting focused news items as they occur? RSS feeds are a quick and effortless way to access news. RSS feeds on diverse nursing topics are offered by the *American Journal of Nursing and Nursing Outlook* and news from more focused nursing specialties like the American Association of Critical Care Nurses or the National Institute of Nursing Research. Whether it is from the national media or the most current nursing journal, we have an enormous amount of information at our fingertips, and it is part of the nurse's job to stay abreast of developments in healthcare and to assess the quality of the information being shared (Box 23.2).

Tools to Support Lifelong Learning: Digital Journals/Books

Digital textbooks combine the ease of online access with tactile study tools such as electronic highlighting and

> **BOX 23.2   MedlinePlus Evaluating Internet Health Information: A Tutorial from the National Library of Medicine (March, 2018)**
>
> Here are nine quick steps from the tutorial to consider when accessing health-related information on the Internet:
> - Who runs the site?
> - Why have they created the site?
> - What do they want from you?
> - Who is paying for the site? Does the site's information favor the sponsor?
> - Is the information reviewed by experts?
> - Where did the information come from?
> - Does the site make unbelievable or unsubstantiated claims?
> - Is the site up-to-date?
> - Do "they" want your personal information? What will "they" do with it?

MedlinePlus offers a free online tutorial to teach care providers and patients how to evaluate digital health information (https://medlineplus.gov/webeval/webeval.html).

organizing. Most publishers offer these tools as a part of their e-book collections in which a student's personal changes are saved into an account. This type of cloud computing in which your changes within the textbook are stored not on your home computer but in cyberspace, is commonplace. In addition, digital readers or tablets offer features like backlighting and font size adjustments to address the concern of eye strain.

Learning through the creation of traditional nursing care plans on paper is a thing of the past as more instructors are sending students to digital nursing care plan constructors. These tools mimic the online care planning offered in the advanced electronic health record (EHR) systems, offering suggested diagnoses based on assessment data, a library of evidence-based best practice interventions, and recommendations for reevaluation criteria. As in the practice of nursing, the nursing student may need access to numerous data sources such as a state department of health website, which can provide information on community assessments, health program goals, educational programs, and opportunities for community needs research. A number of valuable websites are included in Table 23.2.

Most research journals are offered digitally with an option for print journals in many but not all cases. Students and practicing professionals regularly access valid search engines, enter the desired key topics, and immediately access links to specific publications. Another added benefit of digitally searching for articles is the ability to limit

TABLE 23.2   Websites with Information Relevant to Healthcare and Nursing

Website	Address
Government Sites for Healthcare Professionals	
Agency for Healthcare Research and Quality	https://www.ahrq.gov
Centers for Disease Control and Prevention	https://www.cdc.gov/
PubMed Central/NCBI/NLM/NIH	https://www.ncbi.nlm.nih.gov/sites/entrez?db1pmc
US National Library of Medicine/National Institutes of Health	
Medline Plus	https://www.nlm.nih.gov/medlineplus
US National Library of Medicine	
National Guideline Clearinghouse	https://www.guideline.gov
Agency for Healthcare Research and Quality's National Guideline Clearinghouse of evidence-based clinical practice guidelines	
US National Library of Medicine	https://www.nlm.nih.gov/
Landing site for several online databases	
Office of the Surgeon General	https://www.surgeongeneral.gov/
Healthy People 2030	https://www.health.gov/healthypeople/
Office of Disease Prevention and Health Promotion	
Government Sites for Healthcare Consumers	
Healthfinder: US Department of Health and Human Services consumer health information and resources	https://www.healthfinder.gov
National Institutes of Health	https://health.nih.gov/
California Department of Healthcare Services	https://www.dhcs.ca.gov/Pages/default.aspx
One of many accessible state health departments	
President's Council on Sports, Fitness & Nutrition	https://www.fitness.gov/
US Department of Health and Human Services	https://minorityhealth.hhs.gov/
Office of Minority Health	
Information about clinical research studies	https://clinicaltrials.gov/
US National Library of Medicine	
National Women's Health Information Center	https://womenshealth.gov/
US Department of Agriculture nutrition information	https://www.nutrition.gov/
US Consumer Product Safety Commission	https://www.cpsc.gov/
Sites for Older Adults	
Sage-ing International: nonprofit organization focused on meaning making in the second half of life	https://sage-ing.org/
National Institute on Aging	https://www.nia.nih.gov/
Private Sites for Healthcare Consumers	
Mayo Clinic health information site	https://www.mayoclinic.com/
Cleveland Clinic health library	https://my.clevelandclinic.org/health
Harvard University Medical School health information site	https://www.health.harvard.edu/
American Heart Association	https://www.americanheart.org/
American Diabetes Association	https://www.diabetes.org
American Cancer Society	https://www.cancer.org/
Sites about Government Agencies and Resources	
US gateway to all government information	https://www.usa.gov/
Library of Congress	https://loc.gov
Nursing Organization Sites	
American Nurses Association	https://www.nursingworld.org/
American Holistic Nurses Association	https://wwws.ahna.org
National Council of State Boards of Nursing	https://www.ncsbn.org/
American Nursing Informatics Association	https://www.ania.org/

searches to specific authors, publications, or dates. Google Scholar is one of the quickest and simplest ways to look for journal articles. Begin your search using scholar.google.com to access scholarly research-based information rather than the general resources found in a google.com search. The Cumulative Index to Nursing and Allied Health Literature (CINAHL) is an excellent resource available through public libraries or a paid subscription service that focuses specifically on nursing and healthcare journals. PubMed is also a favorite with HCPs because it houses most interdisciplinary professional journals from all types of medicine, nursing, and pharmacology, and it is easily accessed through an Internet connection. Access to article abstracts and citations is typically free, although full text articles may require a fee if the user is not affiliated with a medical library or university.

Another important part of digital communication is knowing how to reference the information that you gather. The professional world of nursing recommends using the American Psychological Association (APA) form of citation. Many online references include an APA formatted citation for use in writing. The APA offers online access to an APA style blog with questions and guidance on how to correctly document sources. One standard way to describe a reference is through the International Standard Book Number (ISBN). This 13-digit number is issued on publication and identifies each book edition and variation published. Another online identifier for digital content is a digital object identifier (DOI), which is a way to both identify and directly link to a digital document. The DOI is a persistent number that is tied to a uniform resource locator (URL), allowing online access of the desired resource. The correct citation of references is crucial both in professional and educational projects, and the use of the DOI or ISBN identifying information is a rapid and accurate way to document and retrieve online content.

One cautionary note on searching the Internet for reliable references for scholarly and professional papers: Wikipedia, begun in 2001, is not considered reliable because it is not a peer-reviewed source. Wikipedia is a collection of contributions from thousands of people who have chosen to share their personal definitions on one site. As such, the content can represent opinion, incorrect facts, or misinterpretations, and it can change over time. Consumers are increasingly using basic searches and finding sites like Wikipedia for health-related concerns. It is an easy place to start one's research; however, clearly it is not the best source of healthcare information for professionals or consumers. As healthcare professionals, we need to guide clients to the best sources aligned with their health literacy level and needs. Peer-reviewed journals publish articles that have been evaluated by scholars within the same profession who have

confirmed that the information presented is valid and appropriate. Many healthcare delivery organizations, for example, The Cleveland Clinic or Shriners Hospitals for Children, and disease-based organizations, such as the American Heart Association (AHA), have websites that offer solid, factual, and understandable resources for the healthcare consumer. We need to continue to be open, yet discerning, in our own use and recommendations of resources and discover those that best support client and clinician needs for information.

Digital Communication in Support of Learning

Digital communication has changed the speed at which information is shared. No longer does a great idea have to be shared individually for years before it can catch on. A group of nursing students who have found a unique way to memorize the steps of a certain procedure can share it with the world on YouTube. The phenomenon of YouTube and other online video-sharing resources have enabled rapid information-sharing related to professional, educational, creative, social, and personal endeavors.

Professional video conferencing and online meetings such as Zoom, Microsoft Teams, GoToMeeting, or SKYPE take the video communication concept one step further, providing live cyberspace applications such as audio, visual, and software applications at the same time. In this way, participants at various locations can see and hear one another and can view a digital presentation such as a PowerPoint at the same time and contribute to shared documents, polls, and digital whiteboards. Organizations and hospitals often use these applications for intradepartmental meetings to allow participation from off-site locations. Many of the required continuing education courses that organizations offer for nurses are now conveniently available in online modules to ensure the ability to participate in a timely and cost-effective manner.

Another effective company-based digital communication tool is Microsoft SharePoint. In many ways it is similar to a discussion board for an online college course, only with increased capabilities. At SharePoint sites, employees can post documents, pictures, diagrams, and so forth for their department. Others in the department can access the documents, make changes, and then repost. It is a wonderful way to communicate and collaborate on projects remotely among several people in a department, as well as to keep one project calendar for the department. Because nurses often work in a shared-governance type of atmosphere, such sites are very useful for their profession. An online Wiki, like Wikipedia, is a shared web page in which groups can contribute to a project asynchronously. Access to edit and update content can be limited to specific individuals, allowing real-time updates but ensuring only the right personnel can make changes to content.

Simulations or simulation-based learning is another application of technology to support hands-on skills practice, such as cardiopulmonary resuscitation (CPR) or intravenous (IV) line insertion. Complex simulation mannequins can be programmed to support scenarios to assess performance skills, decision-making, delegation, and team work. The AHA published results of a study demonstrating that frequent simulation-based training improved CPR proficiency among hospital staff as opposed to the standard yearly instructor-led training approach (AHA, 2016).

Mobile Devices

Smartphones have become a ubiquitous part of everyday life in the United States. According to the Pew Research Center, 96% of those aged 18 to 29, 95% of those 30 to 49, 83% of those aged 50 to 64, and 61% of those aged 65 and over own and regularly use a smartphone (Pew Research Center, 2019). Nurses are increasingly relying on mobile devices. According to the Wolters Kluwer Nurse Mobile Study, "65% of the 5000+ nurses surveyed currently use a mobile device for professional purposes at work and 95% of healthcare organizations surveyed allow nurses to consult websites and other online resources to access clinical information" (Wolters Kluwer Health, 2014). The challenge of balancing allowable smartphone use for access to needed research and online tools is highlighted by a hospital in Dublin, Ireland. The issue came about when they sought to ban the use of personal mobile devices. Leadership quickly discovered that the pharmacy had created a smartphone application to replace the printed formulary for drug reference information. The app had become the clinicians' main source of safe drug administration data (Our Lady's Children's Hospital, Crumlin [OLCHC], 2014). Rather than banning the use of smartphones, leadership then developed a strong, well-researched policy that included guidelines in the appropriate use of mobile devices. So, what is the proper use of mobile devices or cell phones in the workplace, especially in nursing? Employers typically create specific policies about cell phone use during work hours and whether employees may keep phones with them throughout their shift. There is good reason for this. One recent study correlated the number of interruptions a nurse has during the process of medication administration with an increase in medication errors (Westbrook, Woods, Rob, Dunsmuir, & Day, 2010). Patients depend on a focused nurse who can provide safe and effective care. Additionally, it is reported that cell phones are a major source of contaminants, and, if used and carried throughout the workplace, these can become an infection control risk (The Cleveland Clinic, 2015). Smartphone policies should include expectations regarding sanitation of the device and hands after use (Box 23.3).

> ### BOX 23.3 Cell Phone Use at Work
>
> **If Cell Phones Are Permitted in Your Workplace**
> Respect patients and staff by keeping phones on silent or do-not-disturb mode in patient care areas. Never access social networking sites during work hours. Do not call or text friends or family except on breaks, and do so in an allowable location. Abide by organizational policies for data protection, access of external sites, and email or texting. Do access the tools, sites, and apps supported by your organization to help you perform your job. Be aware of how using your phone may appear to patients and families, even if you are accessing work-related sites or tools. Be cognizant of the potential contamination of your phone and hands when handling your phone.
>
> **If Cell Phones Are Not Permitted in Your Workplace**
> Abide by organizational policies for storage of phones and appropriate use only during breaks.

The appropriate use of social media is a positive avenue for professional presence and development. Social networking has moved into the mainstream as a form of digital communication. It is important to remember that everything said in a social media format becomes a part of the permanent record somewhere in cyberspace. For healthcare, the social media explosion has led to policies to prevent and sanction online privacy violations of HIPAA. How will the additional capabilities of Internet-based digital communication affect you and your ethical, safe nursing practice? The NCSBN published a brochure in 2011 with guidelines to define the ethical and unethical use of digital communication. It describes that disclosure of "individually identifiable information included any information that relates to the past, present, or future physical or mental health of an individual, or provides enough information that leads someone to believe the information could be used to identify an individual. Breaches...can be intentional or inadvertent" (NCSBN, 2011). Such information can be as simple as a first name, diagnosis, or room number. Always consult your organization's social media/social networking policies before posting.

Social Media and Internet Networking Capabilities

Within the healthcare environment, many health-related websites are available for patients, families, and professionals. The US Department of Health and Human Services offers an extensive listing of online support groups from "living with asthma" to "quitting smoking" (Mental Health America (n.d.). CaringBridge offers the opportunity to create a personal website to document one's health journey (CaringBridge, 2021). Such sites offer a positive way to disseminate information quickly among a large number of friends, family, and peers, which can save time for patients or family members trying to provide updates to others in the midst of their treatments. Friends can post notes of encouragement on the site. Some sites offer online support group discussion boards for patients based on their illness, injury, or need. Social media can be an effective tool to support patients' interactions and support of each other.

For nurses, a business site, such as LinkedIn, can be used to promote your career, with a place for resumes to be uploaded and a posting board to highlight your education and other accomplishments and interests. Other web-based services allow you to create a digital portfolio, holding word processing–type data and scanned copies of your college diplomas, awards, certificates, professional presentations, and so on all in one concise format. Once it is all stored, you, as the owner, can update your data regularly and provide access to other interested parties, such as a potential employer. A number of continuing education tracking applications are offered for managing continuing education units (CEUs) needed for certification and licensure.

Healthcare Apps

Software applications, or *apps,* are another example of cloud computing and may be free or may charge a licensing fee or a one-time purchase price. To understand the prevalence of apps, consider that more than 180 billion apps were downloaded from Apple's App Store from July 2008 to June 2017 (Statista, 2017). A quick investigation using one of the app stores or an Internet search engine searching for nursing apps will reveal thousands of healthcare applications for smartphones and tablets. From radiology to laboratory, medical terminology to an eye chart, clinicians can now have almost unlimited references instantly at hand. As a patient advocate, a nurse can lead patients who are technologically savvy to use such apps to help keep up with data concerning their health issues.

ELECTRONIC HEALTH RECORDS/ELECTRONIC MEDICAL RECORD

The EHR system is a software application that can be loaded onto the hard drives of multiple computers within the healthcare setting, accessed through the Internet, hosted by a vendor, or loaded on a private network or intranet. The EHR stores information about healthcare encounters in real-time. Timely charting is important in the EHR because an HCP could be remotely accessing the patient's chart from their office, making decisions, and entering orders according to the information viewed. The

ability to access current vital signs, laboratory results, and intake and output data, for example, could affect the order for a diuretic.

The evolution of the EHR and federal regulations intended to support the use of EHRs have paralleled in development. The Merit Based Incentive Payment System incorporates several programs with the intent of improving quality, engaging patients and families, improving the coordination of care, and maintaining the security of the electronic record. Incentives are based on demonstration of quality as opposed to simply installing an EHR system (HealthIT.gov, 2017). Payments are tied to demonstration of advancements like proactively sharing information with other clinicians or the patient in a comprehensive manner. This may include sharing test results, visit summaries, and therapeutic plans of care to support patient-centered care and coordination of care between providers (US Department of Health and Human Services, n.d.).

Electronic communications are also being used in unexpected ways within the EHR. In days past, a nurse would document a pressure ulcer or possible abuse case by hand-drawing the approximate size and area of a wound onto a paper-based figure of a human body and placing it in the chart. Today, nurses often use digital cameras to document pressure ulcers or abuse injuries and upload the visible evidence into the patient's EHR. One caution in this practice is to ensure protection of patient privacy by following designated protocols and using the correct equipment. Quality reviews and risk management practices are also being taken to a new level with the use of an EHR for documentation in the hospital setting. Key data elements such as date/time stamps on data input prompted follow-up assessments for pain medication effectiveness, and required documentation of quality indicators support robust quality reporting.

Computerized provider order entry (CPOE) allows the direct input of orders by the provider with real-time interaction alerts or duplicate warnings for the provider and immediate communication to the required departments. The electronic medication administration record (e-MAR) and the use of barcode scanning for bedside medication verification dramatically changes the medication administration process. The two-dimensional (2D) or three-dimensional (3D) barcode label on the medication identifies the drug, dosage, and route form, and by scanning, it matches this with the patient identification bar code and CPOE order. If all aspects are correctly matched, the medication can be safely administered. If any discrepancies exist, the system will alert the nurse of the mismatch. This type of delivery of medication is guided by the EHR to prevent medication errors. It is noteworthy that these systems should be used to support nursing professional judgment and critical thinking and not to replace them.

In addition to aligning the administration of medications to the specific orders, the drug interaction software found within the EHR can promote increased patient safety by assessing pertinent patient parameters and data. The EHR alerts the staff to possible negative reactions to medications based on abnormal laboratory results, such as nephrotoxic drugs, or physiologic parameters affected by medications, such as slowing the heart rate or lowering the blood pressure, even if the medication is correctly ordered and ready for administration. The EHR can track cumulative doses of medications and alert the clinician if defined maximum doses are reached, even if administration is within the ordered parameters.

Clinical decision support systems are tools that provide data, ideally at the exact point in the workflow in which the data are needed, to expedite a clinical decision (Box 23.4).

The Institute of Medicine reports that "about 20% of the United States population lives in rural areas, but only 9% of physicians practice there" (Effken & Abbott, 2009). Telehealth or telemedicine, providing remote care for underserved populations through e-visits, has grown due to the need to enhance care for rural patients and later due to the COVID-19 pandemic when face-to-face healthcare visits were contraindicated due to the need to maintain social distancing in an effort to avoid disease transmission. The EHRs make successful telehealthcare increasingly possible by integrating data, assessment tools, and communication devices. Telehealth systems provide high definition visual and auditory input, integrate compatible monitoring devices for physiologic information, and pull needed current and historical data from the EHR to support remote assessment and treatment. Often, the nurse is the caregiver at the patient's side, helping to guide the examination and data collection by use of digital stethoscopes and other tools. Nurses and physicians continue to increasingly provide primary care via telehealth due to continuing infectious disease transmission concerns in addition to the need to meet the needs of rural clients.

According to Demiris et al. (2008), HIT can also empower patients to move from a passive to an active role in their healthcare. When a patient begins to use patient-centered healthcare apps or when a patient reviews the literature and illness-specific information on the Internet, the patient becomes involved in the decision-making process, opening communication channels between the HCP and the patient. Many health information systems include a patient portal that offers secure access to the patient's own healthcare data, communication to care providers, and links to recommended health information resources. Patient monitoring tools and mobile devices have been developed to further provide digital communication of data to the HCP for evaluation, such as continuous blood glucose monitoring for diabetics or daily weights, heart rate, and oxygenation levels for patients with congestive heart failure (CHF).

EHRs change a nurse's documentation workflow, so it is important for nursing end-users to be involved when IT decisions are made. Without adequate input into the system design, nurses often resort to creating workarounds in which a nurse figures out a way to bypass the system requirements to develop an easier or quicker way to get the job done. These workarounds negate intended safety steps and processes and prove to be costly to the staff, facilities, and patients. This is another reason for the rise in the role of the nursing informatician whose job it is to provide the professional nurse's viewpoint and create EHRs that correctly accommodate nursing workflows and focus on needed quality outcomes and care delivery.

BOX 23.4 The Agency for Healthcare Research and Quality Five Rights of Clinical Decision Support

The CDS Five Rights model states that we can achieve CDS-supported improvements in desired healthcare outcomes if we communicate:

1. The *right information:* evidence-based, suitable to guide action, pertinent to the circumstance
2. To the *right person:* considering all members of the care team, including clinicians, patients, and their caretakers
3. In the *right CDS intervention format:* such as an alert, order set, or reference information to answer a clinical question
4. Through the *right channel:* for example, a CIS such as an EMR, PHR, or a more general channel such as the Internet or a mobile device
5. At the *right time in workflow:* for example, at time of decision/action/need

CDS, Clinical decision support; *CIS,* clinical information system; *EMR,* electronic medical record; *PHR,* personal health record.
From https://healthit.ahrq.gov/ahrq-funded-projects/current-health-it-priorities/clinical-decision-support-cds/chapter-1-approaching-clinical-decision/section-2-overview-cds-five-rights.

WIT AND WISDOM
Information is not knowledge.

Albert Einstein

DANGERS OF DIGITAL COMMUNICATION

Without the benefit of nonverbal clues and body language, the written word can be more easily misunderstood. Be sure your professional digital communications, whatever form they may take, come across as professional. Basic tips include rarely using the option to "Reply All" because too many emails bog down other email accounts and the option increases your risk of sending something inadvertently to a recipient you did not intend. Another important but often overlooked tip is not to trust every website. If you are sending information that needs to be secure (e.g., a credit card number for an online order), look at the hyperlink address. Instead of an "http://" address, it should be an "https://" address. The extra letter "s" in this case stands for a data-secured site.

Viruses, worms, malware, and hackers are real dangers in the world of digital communications. It is wise to invest in a good antivirus program for your personal access devices. Do not open emails with attachments that look suspicious. Perform a system check on your home computer on a regular basis.

Passwords can be a hassle, especially the type within a school or work account that require specific combinations of characters and change every 2 or 3 months. However, passwords are for your safety and the protection of both personal and patient information. They are important in the healthcare environment, and your protected password guarantees that you and you alone will be documenting under your name. Because your name in an EHR is your legal acceptance of what was documented, this becomes even more important. *Never* share your password with anyone or allow others to document anything, even transcribing vital signs, under your password. The temptation to simply offer a password to speed the process of high-risk medication witness or blood administration should be avoided and safety procedures followed in every detail. Most organizations hold strong policies regarding the use and sharing of passwords, and noncompliance can result in punishments as harsh as job loss.

"Stranger danger" is as real in the digital communication environment as anywhere else. Be careful with whom you share information. Common interests do not guarantee common goals or the same belief system. Be careful what you share on the Internet. Safety rules for social media include not listing your home address or phone number to prevent someone from tracing your web presence to your physical address. In addition, be aware that once a picture is posted on a social media site, access to it is free to those who want it by simply right-clicking it and saving it to their computer.

Another danger with the Internet occurs when clients (and professionals) are defrauded by faulty or misleading information. Because more and more people are turning to the Internet for health information, it is important for nurses not only to be advocates, teaching patients how to seek credible Internet information, but also to become healthcare leaders in the realm of digital communication (see Box 23.2 for specific information on evaluating websites).

Reliance on digital communication creates a new world indeed. When thoughtfully combined with professional nursing practice, it has the potential to increase our time for direct patient care in a safer environment. However, as with many new skills, proper utilization of digital communication has a steep learning curve. For those who are willing to thoughtfully participate, the long-term benefits far outweigh the short-term inconvenience.

Self-Care Nudge

Do you find yourself amazed at how much time you have spent scrolling through social media?

Challenge yourself to set your cell phone aside and do something else you have wanted to do for fun for yourself yet never find the time to do. My students reported they were surprised at how relaxing this was.

SIMPLIFY AND DEEPEN

Disconnection leads to connection. Five Reasons to Take a Break from Your Cell Phone (theodysseyonline.com).

OUR NEW CONSUMER

According to the Pew Survey of Americans' Online Health Habits (California Health Foundation, 2013), Americans are increasingly turning to the Internet for information about health. Examples include the following: people with chronic illness (interestingly, having a chronic disease increases the chance they will take advantage of social media to share their experience); individuals using mobile device apps to track weight, diet, exercise, and symptoms, as well as to find health information; family caregivers searching the Internet for health information outpaced others on the health topics surveyed; and in peer-to-peer health, people are using networks to expand contact with others, especially those with rare diseases. Not only has nursing been forever changed by digital communication, now our clients may come armed with information or misinformation about their health. Increasingly, clients search online to see what their symptoms might mean. After diagnosis, they may research their condition for more information. We teach clients how to access online resources, find digital support systems, and join virtual communities using our knowledge on how to access credible information. We need to cautiously evaluate how we offer caring support to those whose anxiety is increased by information overload or misinformation. An informed client is better able to be a true partner in patient-centered healthcare. We are called to support patient-centered care by empowering clients to assume increasing responsibility for their own health in responsible ways, leveraging the power of digital communication.

Wit and Wisdom
Man is still the most extraordinary computer of all.

John Fitzgerald Kennedy, 35th President of the United States

 MOMENTS OF CONNECTION...

Digital Communication

I teach college level courses and massive open online courses (MOOCs) on a regular basis and always try to consciously connect with my students in the cyberspace. Several years ago, a student made a comment I never forgot. It illustrates the importance of demonstrating caring in digital settings—small things make a big difference. She said, "*I was forced to complete baccalaureate education for my work. I had to complete an online program because I could not travel to a face-to-face school and still hold down a job to support my family. The whole process felt very isolating and I did not expect to enjoy it. I felt like teachers in an online program would not care about me. Then I had this instructor who provided feedback on my assignments and responded to my discussion board postings in ways that assured me she was actually reading and understanding my work. I felt cared for and understood, like I was a part of something important. I felt seen, appreciated, and heard. Every day when I would come home from work, I would throw my bags on the couch and run to my computer to see if she had said anything to me online that day, and it made me so happy when she did. This one teacher changed my whole educational experience.*"

Return to "Active Learning" at the beginning of the chapter and write your responses.

PRACTICING DIGITAL COMMUNICATION

Skill Building: Exercise 1

Visit https://www.senate.gov/ and find the webpages for the two senators from your state, or use http://www.google. com to find an official website for the government of your country. Write one paragraph about what you learned.

Application: Exercise 2

Select a chronic illness to research on the Internet. Review Table 23.2 and search appropriate sites for useful information. Try using the search engine https://www.google.com to search for basic information about the illness. Compare your results when searching using google scholar (https://scholar.google.com). Create a list of resources you would recommend for clients. Then, for the same chronic illness, search for support groups or chat rooms that might be useful to clients with this illness. With another student or in a group, discuss the benefits and liabilities of such support via the Internet.

Lifelong Learning: Exercise 3

Visit https://www.coursera.com, which is a website that partners with universities and organizations to provide universal access to education at no charge. Review the courses offered and create a list of at least three courses that might be useful to you for pursuit of lifelong learning. Search for topics you are personally interested in, that apply to your work setting, or that could help you support friends and family.

Ethical Practice: Exercise 4

Search online for the NCSBN brochure *A Nurse's Guide to the Use of Social Media*. Read the brochure and discuss the example of Maria, a hospice nurse, and how she violated patient confidentiality. Discuss possible consequences of the inappropriate use of social and digital media by determining the policies and repercussions for any sites or employers you are working with (refer to Box 23.3).

Quality and Safety Education for Nurses Competency—Informatics: Exercise 5 **QSEN**

Competency in informatics crosses all other quality and safety competencies. The KSAs that comprise competency in informatics help nurses locate and evaluate evidence-based information, use decision support tools in making care decisions, record information, manage information confidentially, and communicate among the many disciplines involved in a patient's care via the EHR. Use the following questions to assess how informatics is integrated throughout the unit. At the end of a clinical learning experience, discuss the questions in small groups to identify ways that informatics is a part of nursing practice on a daily basis and can be used to improve quality and safety:

1. *Patient-centered care:* Patients and families often search for information about their illness using the World Wide Web. How can you help guide them in using appropriate sites and evaluating the information found?

2. *Teamwork and collaboration:* When handing off a patient from one caregiver to another, there is an increased opportunity for errors and missed information that can be critical for making care decisions. Describe how automated checklists and summary data views can be used to ensure that accurate and complete information is shared in the handoff between caregivers.

3. *Evidence-based practice:* Why do we do what we do? Can you cite the evidence for the care you deliver? Demonstrate the use of a database search to investigate a question or practice you encountered in delivering care to your patient, and describe the evidence-based care guidelines you discover.

4. *Quality improvement:* Demonstrate how you would access sites that publish and share quality care standards. What digital quality improvement tools are used to measure the outcomes of care on your unit? Compare these tools with the industry standard.

5. *Safety:* Ask if there are automated safety alerts embedded in the EHR on your unit to notify staff of a possible error. What are the benefits and challenges of having automated safety alerts? How does the EHR present data to support safer care?

6. *Informatics:* Review the five rights of clinical decision support. Define decision support tools used to help staff make informed decisions. What decision support is available to the staff on your unit? How does it meet the five rights (see Box 23.4)?

REFERENCES

Agency for Healthcare Research and Quality (AHRQ). (2015). *Clinical decision support*. Agency for Healthcare Research and Quality. (ahrq.gov).

American Heart Association (AHA). (2016). AHA News: Frequent simulation-based training may improve CPR proficiency among hospital staff. https://medicalxpress.com/news/2016-11-frequent-simulation-based-cpr-proficiency-hospital.html.

American Nurses Association (ANA). (2014). *Nursing informatics: Scope and standards of practice.* Silver Spring, MD: Publishing Program of the American Nurses Association.

American Nurses Association (ANA). (2015). Code of ethics for nurses. Nursing Informatics: Scope and Standards of Practice | ANA (nursingworld.org).

Bennett, S., Maqton, K., & Kervin, L. (2008). The "digital natives" debate: A critical review of evidence. *British Journal of Educational Technology, 39*(5), 775.

California Health Foundation. (2013). Pew Survey of Americans' Online Health Habits - California Health Care Foundation (chcf.org).

CaringBridge Staff. (2021, April 26). What is caring bridge? Retrieved February 20, 2023, from https://admin.caringbridge.org/resources/what-is-caringbridge/.

Demiris, G., Afrin, L., Speedie, S., Courtney, K. L., Sondhi, M., Vimarlund, V., et al. (2008). Patient-centered applications: Use of information technology to promote disease management and wellness. A white paper by the AMIA Knowledge in Motion Working Group. *Journal of the American Medical Informatics Association, 15*(1), 8.

Effken, J. A., & Abbott, P. (2009). Health IT–enabled care for underserved rural populations: The role of nursing. *Journal of the American Medical Informatics Association, 16*(4), 439.

Finances Online. (2022). Number of Internet Users in 2022/2023: Statistics, Current Trends, and Predictions - Financesonline.com.

Fraser, R. (2011). *The nurse's social media advantage: How making connections and sharing ideas can enhance your nursing practice.* Indianapolis, IN: Sigma Theta Tau International Honor Society of Nursing.

Hampton, D., Pearce, P., & Moser, D. (2017). Preferred methods of learning for nursing students in an online degree program. *Journal of Professional Nursing, 33*(1), 27–37.

HealthIT.gov. (2017). Meaningful use. HealthIT.gov.

Huston, C. (2013). The impact of emerging technology on nursing care: Warp speed ahead. *Online Journal of Issues in Nursing, 18*(2), 1.

International Nurse Regulator Collaborative (INRC). (2016). Position statement. Social media use: Common expectations for nurses. incr-social-media-use-common-expectations-for-nurses.pdf (cno.org).

Kennedy, G., Judd, T., Churchward, A., Gray, K., & Krause, K. (2008). First year students' experiences with technology: Are they really digital natives? *Australasian Journal of Educational Technology, 24*(1).

Kubheka, B. (2017). Ethical and legal perspectives on the medical practitioners' use of social media. *South African Medical Journal, 107*(5), 386–389.

Kung, Y. M., & Oh, S. (2014). Characteristics of nurses who use social media. *Computers, Informatics, Nursing, 32*(2), 64.

Makam, A. N., Lanham, H. J., Batchelor, K., Moran, B., Howell-Stampley, T., Kirk, L., et al. (2014). The good, the bad, and the early adopters: Providers' attitudes about a common, commercial EHR. *Journal of Evaluation in Clinical Practice, 20*(1), 36–42.

Mental Health America. (n.d.). Find Support groups. Mental Health America (mhanational.org).

National Council of State Boards of Nursing (NCSBN) (n.d.). *Computerized adaptive testing (CAT).* NCSBN.

National Council of State Boards of Nursing (NCSBN). (2011). *National Council of State Boards of Nursing (NCSBN): A nurse's guide to the use of social media.* NCSBN_SocialMedia.pdf.

Our Lady's Children's Hospital, Crumlin (OLCHC). (2014). In Policy on the use of SMART/personal mobile phones for nursing staff.

Pew Research Center. (2021). Mobile fact sheet. https://www.pewresearch.org/internet/fact-sheet/mobile/.

QSEN Institute. (n.d.). QSEN competencies.

Sensmeier, J., Anderson, C., & Shaw, T. (2017). International evolution of TIGER informatics competencies. PubMed (nih.gov).

Simpson, R. L. (2007). Information technology: Building nursing intellectual capital for the information age. *Nursing Administration Quarterly, 31*(1), 84.

Sitzman, K. (2016). Mindful communication for caring online. *Advances in Nursing Science (ANS), 39*(1), 38–47.

Sitzman, K., & Watson, J. (2017). *Watson's caring science in the digital world: A guide for caring when interacting, teaching, and learning in cyberspace.* New York: Springer.

Sitzman, K., & Watson, J. (2018). *Caring science, mindful practice: Implementing Watson's human caring theory* (2nd ed.). New York: Springer.

Statista. (2017). *Cumulative number of apps downloaded from the Apple App Store from July 2008 to June 2017 (in billions).* Statista.

Personal Cell Phones on the Nursing Unit Can Impact Infection Control Programs – Consult QD (clevelandclinic.org).

US Department of Health and Human Services. (n.d.). Merit-based Incentive Payment System (MIPS) Overview - QPP (cms.gov).

Westbrook, J. I., Woods, A., Rob, M. I., Dunsmuir, W. T., & Day, R. O. (2010). Association of interruptions with an increased risk and severity of medication administration errors. *Archives of Internal Medicine, 170*(8), 683.

Wolters Kluwer Health. (2014). Wolters Kluwer Health Survey finds nurses and healthcare institutions accepting professional use of online reference & mobile technology. (prnewswire.com).

24

Learning Confrontation Skills

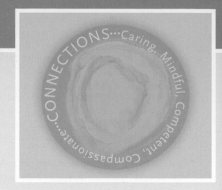

Unless you stop the crack, you will rebuild the wall.

African Proverb

OBJECTIVES

1. Identify the benefits of confrontation skills.
2. Discuss the steps of the Clarify, Articulate, Request, Encourage (CARE) model of confrontation.

3. Identify the relationship between confrontation skills and empowerment.
4. Practice confrontation in selected exercises to build confidence in the skills.

❓ ACTIVE LEARNING

Think about how you will write your answers as you read this chapter.

What?
Write one thing you learned from this chapter.

So What?
How will this affect your nursing practice?

Now What?
How will you implement this new knowledge or skill?

Think About It ...

DIFFERENT KINDS OF CONFRONTATION

"No matter what you do or who you do it with, you will experience conflict…. Communication is often the cause and can be the resolution for conflict…" (Boothe, Frasier, Weaver, & White-Kiehl, 2018). What words come to mind when you hear the word confrontation? Are they positive or negative? In this chapter you will learn how caring confrontation can support safe, competent patient care (Algieri, Torlaschi, Faraco, Wasielewsky, & Ferrante, 2014; Vertino, 2014). This text teaches skills for assertive

communication. In a study of burnout in novice nurses, training in these skills promoted coping with the stress of the workplace (Suzuki et al., 2021). The Clarify, Articulate, Request, Encourage (CARE) confrontation model in this chapter is an assertive communication approach.

Come to this work fully present and with a mindset of curiosity and caring (Sofer, 2018). Confrontation skill is "being able to identify and to respond—communicate—provide feedback—regarding those discrepancies in another person's behavior in such a manner that the other person can grow" (Tindall, 2008). It is setting feelings aside and focusing on problem solving, using a calm approach, and inviting cooperation (Gallagher, 2009; Northam, 2009). Patterson, Grenny, McMillan, and Switzler (2005) said that to confront is to hold someone accountable, to offer an opportunity to solve problems and build relationships. Their research demonstrated that leaders throughout an organization were successful because they held colleagues, coworkers, and bosses accountable. One type of confrontation is a nurse's deliberate invitation to clients and colleagues to examine incongruities or distortions between feelings, beliefs, attitudes, and behavior (Egan, 2013). This type of confrontation, designed to make others aware of incongruity, can be offered by nurses when clients or colleagues are saying one thing and doing another or obviously feeling one way and exhibiting the opposite emotions. Pointing out these discrepancies can be an invitation to expand their self-awareness. This dimension of confrontation is a gift of feedback, which is covered in Chapter 18.

Here is an example of a confrontation to expand self-awareness. John tells you that he smokes only a few cigarettes a day. He has yellow stains on the fingers of his left hand, smells of smoke, and wheezes on inspiration. His wife says he smokes two packs a day.

> Nurse: *"John, I'm concerned about conflicting information concerning your smoking. The stains on your fingers, the smell of smoke on your clothes, and the sound of your breathing indicate that you smoke more than a few cigarettes a day."*

Self-Care Nudge

Color to reduce your anxiety. During the COVID-19 pandemic, nursing students found coloring mandalas, a circular design, reduced their anxiety (Toulouian, 2021). Search online for "mandalas to color" or try coloring any design. My students reported they relaxed into the "flow" of creativity and had fun.

SITUATIONS IN WHICH CONFRONTATION IS APPROPRIATE

Confrontation has two parts: first, making others aware of the destructiveness or lack of productiveness of their behavior, and second, making a suggestion about how they could behave in a more constructive or productive way. Two situations warrant confronting clients or colleagues: when their behavior is unproductive or destructive to them and when their behavior invades our rights or the rights of others. In confronting others, we are attempting to get them to change in a way that protects their self-interests or is more considerate of others. One note of warning: Be aware that the problem belongs to the other person, and it is not our role to "fix" others.

Some nurses are reluctant to confront and do not want to discuss their differences. We think about people we know who have a tendency to be argumentative when confronted. We are concerned about the impression others will have if we confront them about an issue (Shih, 2002). Yet confrontation can be a time-saving strategy (Davidhizar & Cathon, 2002) and a matter of patient safety and quality of care (Cassity, 2017).

To avoid being labeled aggressive, we often refrain from saying anything about others' unproductive or destructive behavior. Later, we watch our clients or colleagues get into trouble, and regret we did not take the opportunity to speak up. When we do not confront those who have violated our rights or the rights of others, we feel angry because we are

frustrated and feel helpless. The next time you hesitate to confront others when you believe it needs to be done, remember this: short-term gain, long-term pain. Being nonassertive may get you off the hook for now, but in the long run, the problem will only escalate.

Patterson et al. (2005) wrote about crucial confrontations to avoid silence or violence. Neither of the two extremes, nonassertion or aggression, is acceptable to nurses who want to feel confident and act competently. There is a way to confront others that makes you feel as if you are effectively doing something about troublesome behavior. People can be confronted in such a way that they are unlikely to be offended. Moreover, they may appreciate your perspective and opinions.

🌸 MOMENTS OF CONNECTION...
A Nursing Student Practices Confrontation

Consider that, sometimes when you confront a person, you grow the relationship and become closer. My mom was expecting me home for a holiday and I just had too much work to do. She was very upset because she had been looking forward to the holiday. When I explained how stressful travel would be, that I was afraid of failing a test, and just would be distracted all weekend, she understood. We realized we both wanted the same thing: a good relationship in which we could be honest with each other. Conflict is a challenge, but it is worth it to become closer and to build bridges instead of burning them.

SIMPLIFY AND DEEPEN

You cannot change what you refuse to confront.

Source Unknown

THE CARE (CLARIFY, ARTICULATE, REQUEST, ENCOURAGE) CONFRONTATION

Elements of the CARE Confrontation

When you confront your clients or colleagues, it is important to do so in a caring way that shows concern for both your feelings and theirs. The following CARE approach is a caring way to confront others. (The format for this comprehensive confrontation is adapted from Bower & Bower, 2009.)

- **Clarify** the behavior that is problematic. Be specific about the aspect of your client's or colleague's behavior that is self-destructive or destructive to others. The behavior to be changed should be the focus so that it is clear that you are attaching no hurtful labels to others.

- Articulate why the behavior is a problem. Your articulation may include how the behavior is likely to hinder the person or irritate others or how it makes you feel.
- Request a change in your client's or colleague's behavior. Your suggestions should be offered tentatively and respectfully.
- Encourage your clients or colleagues to change by emphasizing the positive consequences of changing or the negative implications of failing to change.

Also, remember not to expect a negative response, to use neutral words without blame, and to stay open to the person's response rather than jumping to conclusions (Ryan, Oestreich, & Orr, 1996). Respect that the clients' values may be different from yours.

Examples of CARE Confrontations

The three situations outlined in the following sections demonstrate how you can confront someone assertively.

Situation 1

Your roommate leaves clothes strewn around the bedroom you share. His notes and textbooks are laid out all over the apartment. Although he does a major clean-up about every 2 weeks, things begin to pile up again, and this makes you hesitant to invite friends over. You confront your roommate with the following.

Clarify. John, you have your clothes spread out over the bedroom, and all your notes and articles for your paper are strewn around the living room and on the kitchen table.

Articulate. I'm feeling annoyed that you are messing up the shared space in our apartment.

Request. I'd like you to keep your personal belongings in your area of our den.

Encourage. That way it'll be more spacious for both of us in the apartment, and I'll feel free to invite friends over without worrying about whether the place is a mess.

Presented with this respectful and assertive confrontation, John will most likely comply and change his behavior. If such a confrontation does not result in the desired behavior change, you have the option of indicating a negative consequence, such as, "If you don't become neater, I will…" (and give a possible consequence, such as hire a cleaning service and charge him, find another roommate, or move out).

Situation 2

You are a nurse manager. Staff have been complaining that Susan sends reply emails to the entire group copied on the email when her comment is only addressed to one recipient. This means other staff member's time is wasted reading unnecessary email. You understand this is easy to do but is a time waster for others.

Clarify. Susan, it has come to my attention that you are sending replies to "all" on a group email when you are commenting to only one person.

Articulate. I know this can happen, but with all the essential emails staff receives, this clutters their email and I have been getting complaints.

Request. I ask you pay attention to this when your response is to only one recipient.

Encourage. I appreciate your attention to the email memos, and your thoughtful responses often clarify misunderstandings. I just wanted to share the feedback so we can save time.

This approach acknowledges the benefit of Susan's response but saves her from being resented by other staff or seen as unprofessional in her use of email.

CONFRONTATIONS WITH CLIENTS OR COLLEAGUES

We can often see how other people's behavior is not safe or in keeping with their goals. Each of us has blind spots about how some of what we say or do is predisposing us to emotional or physical harm or is incongruent with our professed values or attitudes. As nurses we can offer an objective perspective on how others can change and act in a way that will serve their best interests. The following examples use CARE confrontations to offer clients and colleagues ways to enhance their goals and avoid emotional or physical dangers.

Situations in Which Your Client's Behavior Is Self-Destructive or Unproductive
Situation 1

John, an 18-year-old client, has just had a torn Achilles tendon repaired. After his lesson on using crutches, you notice John is bearing too much weight on his affected leg, increasing the chance of his sutures weakening and putting strain on his tendon, preventing healing. You confront John as follows:

> When you put any weight on your injured leg, you are risking further injury to your tendon. If you weaken your tendon, you may not recover full use of your leg. I'd like you to practice using your crutches so that you place weight only on your good leg. That way you'll ensure maximum healing of your injury. Will you try that, please, John?

Situation 2

On the medical unit in your hospital, you and Judy have been working together on the evening shift for the past three evenings. Judy has been complaining of a strained back, which she has attributed to turning, positioning, and transferring the heavy clients on the unit. You have noticed that Judy takes few or no precautions to protect her back. After you have received her permission to express your views, you decide to confront her about her negligence in the following way:

> *Judy, it sounds as if your back is bothering you quite a bit. I've noticed that when you are turning our heavy patients, you tend to take the clients' full weight on your own without help from one of us or the Hoyer lift. I think you could save your back from a lot of discomfort and injury if you took the precautions of getting help and using protective devices. What do you think?*

Note the different order of elements in this CARE confrontation. The reordering makes it sound more natural in this case, yet it still contains the essential components.

Situation 3

Your classmate, Toni, has not been achieving the grades to which she has been accustomed on her nursing examinations. Toni is complaining about the severity of the examinations and the tough grading of her instructors. You are aware that Toni has not been studying as much since she began dating two men at the same time and that she has been going out almost every night. She asks you what she should do. You decide to confront her about her recent unproductive behavior:

> *Toni, I know you always do well even if the teachers are tough. It's just since you've been dating on weeknights that your grades have been lower. I'd have the same problem if I couldn't have extra time to review my class notes. It's a tough call. You know that when we go over the notes several times, we see a difference in the test grades. Maybe if you took a few minutes after classes to review, you'd see a difference, but that's not easy to do when it's tempting to go out. What do you think?*

In each of the situations presented so far, the client or colleague has been confronted about something he or she is doing or not doing that is causing physical or emotional problems. The confrontation points out the specific behavior that is problematic and proposes a clear alternative, which is checked out with the client or colleague.

Let us examine some situations in which the skill of confrontation is used to deal with behavior that violates your rights or the rights of others.

Situations in Which Your Client's or Colleague's Behavior Is Bothersome to You or Others

Mr. Wars is a 53-year-old cardiac client who has been aggressive in the three days he has been on the unit. He has complained about the food, the room, and the other clients, and today he has been angry and abusive with you in the corridor. He complains that you are the slowest nurse he has ever encountered and that you don't know what you are doing. He has picked on your appearance, questioned your credentials, and repeatedly insulted your nursing care. His aggressiveness is embarrassing, time consuming, and unpleasant for you. You recognize that he is feeling out of control and assess that a referral to the psychiatric clinical nurse specialist might be of help to you and to him. You confront him when you are in the privacy of his room:

> *Mr. Wars, we need to talk about how things are going for you. I know you are not happy with your care, and I want to talk about what we can do. I would like to help you be as comfortable as possible during these tough times for you. It upsets me to be unable to make things better for you. We have a nurse we can call whose job it is to evaluate such situations. She could spend some time with you to help you sort things out. I hope you are willing to let me call her so we can work together to turn things around for the better. How does that sound to you?*

Miss Debris is a colleague with whom you share an office. She often moves your paperwork and leaves the desk in disorder. Yesterday, you could not find any pens or the stapler. Today, Miss Debris has left a dirty coffee cup and the wrapper from her sandwich on the desk. She is about to leave without cleaning it up when you confront her:

> *When you leave the desk we share cluttered, I have to search for the things I need to do my work. I know you get busy, but this time I see trash, too. If we both are aware of keeping the work space clear, it will be ready when each of us needs it. How about taking a few seconds to dump the trash and make sure the papers and supplies are handy? It would make it easier for me to face my work, and I would appreciate it. Does that sound fair?*

Situations in Which Your Colleague's Behavior Is Unpleasant for You or Others

You have been working the night shift for the past five nights. In the three previous mornings, your nurse relief has been about 15 to 25 minutes late. You are not free to leave the unit until she arrives because there is only one nurse on duty. Her lateness leads to your being late getting home to see your family before they head off to school and work. You decide to confront her:

> Rena, I want to speak to you about your coming in 15 to 25 minutes late in the mornings. Since I can't leave until you get here, I've been getting home too late in the mornings to see my family. I would like you to arrange to be here, ready to receive report, at 7:00 a.m. when the shift begins from now on so that I can report without being too rushed and still get home on time. Can you do that?

Margaret is a new graduate working on a psychiatric unit with you. You notice that each time Margaret has an interview with a client, she goes into the session with coffee only for herself and then puts her feet up on the desk. You know this casual behavior makes clients feel insulted and not respected and gives them the impression that Margaret is less than interested in their cases. Because the clients have not had the nerve to challenge Margaret, you decide to say something to her about her behavior.

> Margaret, I couldn't help but notice that when you interview some of the clients, you have a very casual style, with a coffee cup in your hand and your feet up on the desk. I think your manner may give the impression to some clients that you aren't taking them seriously. We don't wear uniforms, so it is important that our behavior sends a clear message that we are caring professionals. Because I know you are interested in your work and like to do a good job, I thought you'd want to know if your behavior might be misinterpreted. (Await approval from Margaret before continuing.) Perhaps if you offered your clients a cup of coffee, too, and didn't put your feet up, you would show your clients your real interest in them. What do you think?

The CARE confrontation provides a way of approaching others when either their best interests or yours are threatened. CARE confrontations allow you to take action in a calm, controlled, assertive way. They prevent you from being immobilized in a situation in which you want to be confrontive but not aggressive.

Wit and Wisdom
You get what you tolerate.

Bumper Sticker

THE MAGIC OF A LITTLE WORD

Try using the word *and* instead of *but* when offering criticism or a differing opinion. The word *but* may put the person on the defensive. Berent and Evans (1992) gave some examples of the use of this style when offering advice or criticism:

- "I appreciate the intensity of your feelings about this, and I think if you were to hear my side of it you might feel differently."
- "I can understand your reasons, and I think my reasons for doing it differently are also understandable."
- "That's an interesting idea, and here's another way to think about it."

CONFRONTATION AS ONE PART OF EMPOWERMENT

Confrontation is an important skill to learn and is one aspect of many that you will use as you move forward as an empowered professional nurse. (Did you notice the use of *and* rather than *but*? Using *but* would have diminished the importance of the skill of confrontation.) As you feel more confident with your own nursing skills, the necessity for the skills of confrontation will be more obvious. Murphy (1994) admonished nurses not to be doormats and discusses the personal responsibility of nurses who want to be more effective in conflict resolution. Dealing with conflict constructively helps us create the work environment we want (Cox, 2005). Nurses need to do the following:

- Make self-improvement a priority
- Pay attention to feelings of anger and fear as signals to deal with a situation
- Speak up respectfully and before an angry blow-up occurs
- Commit to treating others respectfully
- Be honest and confront colleagues when friction first occurs rather than letting it escalate
- Practice self-care skills such as exercise, relaxation, and recreation

Later chapters discuss self-care skills that help you to be responsive, rather than reactive, to colleagues and clients. This means being able to take time to sort out which situations require confrontation and which can be tolerated or are simply an overreaction caused by fatigue or personal stress. Noddings (1994) concluded that "everywhere—in personal, social, political, and even professional life—people misunderstand one another." Confrontation takes thought, energy, and a caring attitude. In nursing, "in the caring orientation, we are more concerned with connecting, feeling—with responding positively to expressed needs, and understanding ourselves well enough to be able to summon the attitude of caring."

Return to "Active Learning" at the beginning of the chapter and write your responses.

 ## PRACTICING CONFRONTATION SKILLS

Application/Skill Building: Exercise 1

For each of the following situations, attempt a CARE confrontation. After you have prepared a response, get together with your classmates as a group and discuss your different approaches. Compare your suggestions with those at the end of this exercise.

1. Mr. Steiger, your 38-year-old client, suffers from chronic bronchitis. You have noticed him smoking outside the building before he comes for his clinic visits, and as you enter the examining room, you notice his clothes smell of smoke. Your nursing knowledge tells you that his smoking is self-destructive. How would you confront him?

2. Your client, 60-year-old Mrs. Cantor, has severe pitting edema of the ankles. She has been taught to raise her legs on a chair when sitting and to wear elastic stockings from toe to midthigh. You have observed that Mrs. Cantor is not wearing her stockings, and each time you have seen her in the chair, her feet have been on the floor. How would you confront her about her self-destructive behavior?

3. You and Jane started working in an emergency center six months ago, after your graduation from nursing school. Jane confides in you that she feels she does not have the respect of her team members and that she believes others do not listen to or act on her opinions. You have noticed that Jane takes a passive stance: She is overly cautious about her suggestions and speaks quietly. When she presents an idea, she often puts it down first. You are reasonably certain that some of her non-assertive behavior accounts for the fact that her ideas are not being considered by the team. How would you confront her about her unproductive behavior?

Suggested CARE Confrontations

1. "Mr. Steiger, I have observed you smoking on several occasions in the past few days. Smoking causes you to produce more phlegm, and that makes you cough more and become short of breath. I would like to give you some information about help available to you should you choose to stop smoking. If you were able to do this, your lungs would have a chance to clear and your breathing would become easier. If you don't stop smoking, then you are at risk for a serious lung infection. I know it is tough, but I think you'd be surprised to hear

about the successful outcomes of people using a nicotine patch. May I tell you more about it?"

2. "Mrs. Cantor, I notice that you aren't wearing your elastic stockings and your feet are on the floor instead of being raised on the stool. Wearing your elastic stockings helps prevent blood clots from forming. I strongly recommend that you wear your stockings and raise your legs on a stool so that you can prevent any more serious complications of your heart disease."

3. "Jane, I think you have some sound ideas about how we can be more efficient. I notice that when you present your ideas, you seem to hesitate and speak softly and uncertainly about your views. When you start off by saying, 'This idea may not work,' it's almost as if you've set the team up to discount your suggestions before the members have heard them. I think your suggestions might be considered if you would present your ideas in a more positive way. Then you and the team would both benefit."

Skill Building: Exercise 2

Identify a situation in which you would have liked to confront someone but did not or a current situation in which you want to prepare for approaching someone you need to confront. Write the dialogue for the confrontation using the CARE format.

Take the opportunity to practice confrontation in real life, whether at school, on the units, or in social situations. How effective are you at making CARE confrontations? Have you discovered that by using this format, you avoid both aggression and nonassertion? Do these guidelines for confronting people provide you with more confidence?

Creative Expression: Exercise 3

Reflect on a time when you did not confront someone and you were not pleased with that decision. Close your eyes and imagine the situation and the resulting emotion. Think about that feeling as if it had color, line, shape, and form. Open your eyes and, using colored markers or crayons, draw the image in your journal. Now close your eyes again and imagine successfully confronting this person and the resulting emotion. Again, think of an image that reflects the emotion and draw it. Look at your art and write a reflection about it in your journal, including differences you might see in yourself if you risked a caring confrontation. (For more expressive arts invitations for self-discovery, see Riley (2021).

Quality and Safety Education for Nurses Learning Strategy: Exercise 4 **QSEN**

Safety is a shared responsibility among all team members. How should you respond when you observe a team member engaging in unsafe behavior? The CUS communication technique is an easy-to-remember method to raise the team's safety awareness with three statements. When all members of the team are taught to use CUS, it can be used to help "get everyone on the same page" and also "stop the line" to clarify actions. Uncertain actions can lead to error when the team is not clear on the goals. Assume someone is about to change a dressing without first washing his or her hands. Practice using CUS communication:

C: I am concerned…
U: I am uncertain…
S: I feel safety is at risk…

REFERENCES

Algieri, R. D., Torlaschi, C. R., Faraco, R. L., Wasielewsky, G., & Ferrante, M. S. (2014). Interpersonal conflicts management and organizational consciousness in general surgery residency. *Journal of the American College of Surgeons, 219*(4). e155.

Berent, I. M., & Evans, R. L. (1992). *The right words: The 350 best things to say to get along with people.* New York, NY: Warner Books.

Boothe, A., Frasier, N., Weaver, C., & White-Kiehl, J. (2018). Resolving conflict: What does the giraffe say? *Nurse Leader, 16*(2), 121.

Bower, S. A., & Bower, G. H. (2009). *Asserting yourself: A practical guide for positive change.* New York, NY: Da Capo Press.

Cassity, M. (2017). When confrontation is needed. Reflections on Nursing Leadership Sigma Theta Tau (sigmanursing.org).

Cox, S. (2005). Taking the "con" out of conflict. *Nursing, 35*(12), 57.

Davidhizar, R., & Cathon, D. (2002). Strategies for effective confrontation. *Radiologic Technology, 73*(5), 476.

Egan, G. (2013). *Skilled helper: A problem-management and opportunity-development approach to helping.* Independence, KY: Cengage Learning.

Gallagher, R. S. (2009). *How to tell anyone anything: Breakthrough techniques for handling difficult conversations at work.* New York, NY: AMACOM.

Murphy, S. Z. (1994). Don't be a doormat: Personal empowerment in nursing. *Revolution, 2*(2), 66.

Noddings, N. (1994). Learning to engage in moral dialogue. *Holistic Education Review, 7*(2), 5.

Northam, S. (2009). Conflict in the workplace, part 2. Strategies to resolve conflict and restore collegial working relationships. *American Journal of Nursing, 109*(7), 65.

Patterson, K., Grenny, J., McMillan, R., & Switzler, A. (2005). *Crucial confrontations: Tools for resolving broken promises, violated expectations, and bad behavior.* New York, NY: McGraw-Hill.

Riley, J. B. (2021). *Art in small spaces…art at the bedside* (2nd ed.). Ellenton, FL: CS Publications. Contact. julia@constantsource.com for more information.

Ryan, K. D., Oestreich, D. K., & Orr, G. A., III. (1996). *The courageous messenger: How to successfully speak up at work.* San Francisco, CA: Jossey-Bass.

Shih, C. (2002). Confrontations: When does counterargumentation occur and when do people's thoughts predict their actions? *Dissertation Abstracts International A, The Humanities and Social Sciences.*

Sofer, O. J. (2018). *Say what you mean: A mindful approach to nonviolent communication.* Boulder, CO: Shambhala.

Suzuki, E., Takayama, Y., Chiaki, K., Asakura, C., Tatsuno, H., Machida, T., et al. (2021). A causal model on assertiveness, stress, coping, and workplace environment: Factors affecting novice nurses' burnout. *Nurs Open, 8,* 1452–1462. https://doi.org/10.1002/nop2.763.

Tindall, J. (2008). *Peer power: Book one, becoming an effective peer helper and conflict mediator, workbook.* New York, NY: Routledge.

Toulouian, A. C. (2021). Mandalas in the nursing classroom. *Online Journal of Complementary & Alternative Medicine, 6*(2). doi:10.33552/OJCAM.2021.06.000632.

Vertino, K. A. (2014). Evaluation of a Team STEPPS initiative on staff attitudes toward teamwork. *Journal of Nursing Administration, 44*(2), 97.

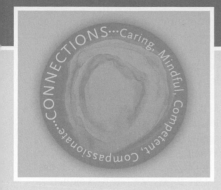

25

Refusing Unreasonable Requests

It is a mistake to look at someone who is self-assertive and say, 'It's easy for her, she has good self-esteem.' One of the ways you build self-esteem is by being self-assertive when it is not easy to do so. There are always times when self-assertiveness requires courage, no matter how high your self-esteem.

Nathaniel Branden

OBJECTIVES

1. Discuss the importance of the right to refuse unreasonable requests from clients and colleagues.
2. Distinguish between assertive, nonassertive, and aggressive refusals.
3. Participate in exercises to build skills to refuse unreasonable requests.

❓ ACTIVE LEARNING

Think about how you will write your answers as you read this chapter.

What?
Write one thing you learned from this chapter.

So What?
How will this affect your nursing practice?

Now What?
How will you implement this new knowledge or skill?

Think About It …

DEFINING UNREASONABLE REQUESTS

Speed, Goldstein, and Goldfried (2018) highlighted the benefits of assertiveness in increasing self-esteem, building relationships, and managing anxiety. In the face of the COVID-19 pandemic, Ayhan and Oz, believing that assertiveness skills would help nurses adapt more quickly in

extraordinary situations, compared face-to-face assertiveness training of nursing students with hybrid training. Both groups had increased self-esteem and assertiveness (Ayhan & Oz, 2021). The ability to refuse an unreasonable request is an assertive communication skill. As nurses, we receive requests from others for information, emotional support, and assistance. Daily, we are asked to perform activities that help our clients and colleagues. Each request seems reasonable to the person making the request. In most instances, requests from our clients and colleagues seem legitimate when we think about the request in an objective way. When a request is made of you, however, you must consider how it affects you personally as the person being asked to fulfill the request. You need to determine whether a request is reasonable. A nursing student shared an example: "This week I was able to apply what I learned in this chapter. As students, we are not able to "waste drugs" or push drugs intravenously. On a few separate occasions, nurses have told me, 'It's OK. I won't tell anyone.' That statement alone makes me uncomfortable. I respectfully declined and showed my own personal integrity and morals."

A request may be unreasonable if it affects your right to provide nursing care in a way that is consistent with your

251

ethics, values, or beliefs. Unreasonable requests are ones that escalate your negative feelings and encroach on your right to feel good about the work you are doing. For example, nurse practitioners may face patients who demand antibiotics or other treatments that may not be appropriate (Buitrago, 2013). You may be asked to perform tasks that are disrespectful of your safety or physical capabilities. It is unreasonable to respond to requests that put you in the position of hurting yourself, such as physically and emotionally stretching yourself to a point at which you feel stressed, overloaded, or irritable. However, it is important to note that sometimes you choose to fulfill a request even though you would prefer to decline. You may be asked to work an extra hour because of an emergency situation. A friend may ask a favor that is inconvenient. In these cases, you make your own decision as to whether to comply. In other cases, a request may seem unreasonable to you, and yet complying with it seems prudent. You may ask yourself not whether the request is reasonable, but whether it may be reasonable to fulfill the request.

Consider the effect on your health from the stress of saying yes when you say yes to too much. "Saying yes too often, you run the risk of over-commitment, overwork, under-achievement…under-socialization, under-enjoyment, failure to deliver on your commitments, and burnout" (Oxman & Sackett, 2013). With assertive communication skills, an important part of personal resilience for nurses (McDonald, Jackson, Wilkes, & Vickers, 2013), you learn how to refuse requests, but you choose whether to refuse the request, depending on the situation.

SIMPLIFY AND DEEPEN

The way we communicate with others and with ourselves ultimately determines the quality of our lives.

Anthony Robbins

As nurses, we have the right to work in a way that allows us to give our best nursing care to our clients; promotes positive relationships with our colleagues; and gives us feelings of satisfaction, safety, and comfort in doing our jobs. In Chapter 1, basic assertive rights were introduced. Chenevert (1997) put our rights as nurses in perspective: "Nurses are responsible people. We have dwelled so long and so hard on our responsibilities that we are often surprised at the prospect of having rights ourselves." Review your basic assertive rights listed in Box 1.2.

When you consider these rights, you need to use common sense. Of course, if you are a new graduate and your manager instructs you to give a pain medication at once, it would be inappropriate to say that you prefer to bathe another client first. If you refuse a request, you may need to provide a rationale for the refusal.

Requests for our information or ideas, attention or affection, or physical power or skills all take time, energy, and commitment to fulfill. We need to check our resources before agreeing to any request. When we take on a request that overtaxes us, we lose out because we become overloaded, and others lose out because we are ineffective when we are feeling burdened. Before saying yes to a request, we need to check to see if it is reasonable for us to accept it. If we decide it is unreasonable, then we must refuse. It is far better to refuse than to capitulate and risk a serious error (Chenevert, 1997). Recognize that sometimes people use manipulative skills to get us to say yes, such as bullying, trying to make us feel guilty, whining, or complimenting us (Levine, 2010). Reflect on your experiences with being unable to say no and learn to trust your own judgment.

SAYING NO ASSERTIVELY

The skill in saying no is to refuse the request in an assertive manner rather than in an aggressive or a nonassertive way. Paskin (2005) advised to begin by staying calm, realizing that your first reaction to an unreasonable request may be outrage. By being assertive, we protect ourselves by declining a task we cannot comfortably handle and respect the other person's rights by refusing in a polite, matter-of-fact manner. Our desire to help our clients and colleagues and our wish to be seen as helpful nurses often interfere with our ability to say no clearly and simply.

Ellis and Powers (1998) discussed irrational beliefs that keep us from acting in our own best interests. Review the irrational beliefs listed in Box 1.3. Consider two such beliefs: "I must be approved of at all times," and "If I don't do everything people ask of me, they will reject me." Beliefs like these escalate to *awful-izing:* "It would be awful, and I couldn't stand it if someone thought I considered my own needs," or "They would think I am selfish" (Ellis & Powers, 1998). Get the idea? It sounds like an exaggeration, but sometimes we base our decisions on such faulty thinking. Assertive communication is based on a consideration of both parties' needs and recognizes that we have the right to set our own priorities for our actions and time allocation. This is difficult for some people. Jokingly, workshop participants are told that they can be taught how to say no but that they will have to get counseling like everybody else to deal with the guilt (Balzer Riley, 2002). You may at some time consider counseling if you have difficulty acting in your own best interests and find that this difficulty interferes with your ability to feel good about your work and yourself.

We sometimes fumble with weak excuses in attempts to avoid accepting a request. This nonassertive behavior makes us feel guilty and helpless, and we offend the asker with our irrelevant attempts to justify our refusal. A simple no would suffice and save both people embarrassment.

Sometimes our unnecessary or irrational guilty feelings about saying no make us refuse a request in a hostile, defensive manner. This aggression makes us feel ashamed that we have behaved unprofessionally, and the other person feels put down or hurt by our explosive response. Clearly, refusing a request in a nonassertive or aggressive way does not protect our interests or those of our clients or colleagues. The assertive refusal to an unreasonable request is the only way to show respect for ourselves and others.

Saying no to unreasonable requests is a way of saying yes to yourself. Just as clients are unique individuals and you struggle to consider their individuality when providing nursing care, when you protect your rights by refusing unreasonable requests, you are respecting your own uniqueness. You are saying yes to your values, yes to your style of doing things, yes to your ways of perceiving situations, and yes to your ways of judging and deciding. It is freeing to refocus your energy, shifting it from unreasonable requests to an investment in your visions and goals.

Self-Care Nudge

Setting boundaries and maintaining them is an act of self-love. Consider these types of boundaries: physical, sexual, mental, emotional, material, time, and spiritual. Ask yourself, "Are there unreasonable requests in my life that I need to refuse for my own well-being" (Meagan, 2021)?

Examples of Refusing Requests Assertively

Here are several examples of effective, assertive ways of saying no contrasted with ineffective aggressive and nonassertive ways.

Example 1

It is Tuesday. Your colleague Elsa asks you to be on call for her this weekend. Your in-laws are coming to visit, and you have made plans to take them on a tour of the excellent countryside restaurants. Your family has been looking forward to this visit, and it is unreasonable for you to work on this particular weekend. In the past, Elsa has been on call for you.

An assertive refusal:

Elsa: *"Could you please be on call for me this weekend? Rob phoned long distance, and he's invited me to go to New York to spend the long weekend with him. I'm so excited! Can you do it?"*

Assertive you: *"No, Elsa. I'm not able to switch this weekend. My in-laws are visiting from out of town and we've made reservations to do things. I hope you can find someone to switch with. I can see you're really looking forward to going to New York to visit Rob."*

This refusal is direct and clear. You are definite, yet you soften the refusal with the inclusion of the explanation for your refusal and your empathic hope that she can secure a replacement.

Elsa is determined, however, and persists in her attempt to persuade you to switch.

Elsa: *"I know you've got company coming, but they're just in-laws and you get to see them often. I haven't seen Rob for 3 months. I know it's last minute, but Rob just found out he could be free and he called me as soon as he could. Oh, please, won't you be on call for me?"*

Assertive you: *"No, Elsa. I'm not available to switch with you this weekend."*

You continue to be clear and definite. Elsa is pleading and trying to make you feel guilty so that you will give in to her. Your response successfully protects your rights to have a weekend with your family and attends to her rights to be treated respectfully.

Elsa does not stop. She wants you to switch so she plies you with more guilt.

Elsa: *"Remember, I switched weekends with you in the spring when you wanted to go to your cousin's wedding? You agreed then that you owed me one. Well, now I'm collecting! I need you to pay me back this weekend."*

Assertive you: *"Elsa, I'm unable to help you this weekend."*

This response continues to be clear and unwavering so that Elsa is given a definite, matter-of-fact answer that is congruent with your desire to avoid becoming hostile or weakened. Although you hope Elsa will find a replacement, it is unreasonable for you to be that person this weekend.

Elsa is starting to get your assertive message.

Elsa: *"OK, OK. I see you've got plans you can't break. It's just that I'm desperate. I'll ask one of the other nurses if she can switch with me."*

By being assertive, you have prevented yourself from doing two things you did not want to do: be on call this weekend and come across as defensive or indecisive to your colleague Elsa.

A nonassertive refusal:

Elsa: *"Could you please be on call for me this weekend? Rob phoned long distance, and he's invited me to go to New York to spend the long weekend with him. I'm so excited! Can you do it?"*

Nonassertive you: *"Gee, Elsa. I don't think so…I'm sorry."*

This response does not sound convincing. Elsa gets the message that you are not really sure you cannot switch with her. It sounds like you are still debating with yourself, and Elsa will likely try to convince you to switch.

Elsa: *"I haven't seen Rob for 3 months. I know it's last minute, but Rob just found out he could be free and he called me as soon as he could. Oh, please, won't you be on call for me?"*

Nonassertive you: *"Gee, Elsa, I don't think I can. I'm sorry. I've got my in-laws coming and we've made plans. I don't think so, Elsa."*

You still have not given a definite no, and Elsa will likely keep asking you as long as she believes that there is hope.

Elsa: *"Remember, I switched weekends with you in the spring when you wanted to go to your cousin's wedding? You agreed then that you owed me one. Well, now I'm collecting! I need you to pay me back this weekend."*

Nonassertive you: *"Yes, that's true. I guess I owe you one. OK, I'll switch with you for this weekend."*

By being nonassertive and indefinite, you have agreed to a request that is unreasonable for you to take on. Giving in will most likely leave you feeling angry, and your in-laws will be disappointed you have let them down. When we are nonassertive, we forfeit our rights.

An aggressive refusal:

Elsa: *"Could you please be on call for me this weekend? Rob phoned long distance, and he's invited me to go to New York to spend the long weekend with him. I'm so excited! Can you do it?"*

Aggressive you: *"Don't you know I've got my in-laws coming to visit this weekend? There's no way I can switch with you."*

This abrasive, offensive reply shows no understanding of Elsa's predicament. Whereas a simple refusal would have sufficed, this response makes you appear unfriendly and inconsiderate.

Elsa is not put off and continues to try to convince you to change your mind.

Elsa: *"I haven't seen Rob for 3 months. I know it's last minute, but Rob just found out he could be free and he called me as soon as he could. Oh, please, won't you be on call for me?"*

Aggressive you: *"I can't help it if you haven't seen Rob for 3 months. That's your problem. I've got my own problems with my in-laws coming."*

Elsa: *"I know you've got company coming, but they're just your in-laws and you get to see them often."*

Aggressive you: *"They are just as important to me as your absentee boyfriend is to you. Maybe if you got together more often, you wouldn't be so desperate now."*

Your insensitivity to Elsa's predicament and your judgmental, accusatory remarks will considerably damage your relationship with your coworker. Aggressive responses are often disproportionate and fired by our irrational anger and guilt.

Elsa persists!

Elsa: *"Remember, I switched weekends with you in the spring when you wanted to go to your cousin's wedding? You agreed then that you owed me one. Well, now I'm collecting! I need you to pay me back this weekend."*

Aggressive you: *"I gave you plenty of notice—not 3 days like you're offering me. If you think I can drop my plans, you're crazy!"*

Elsa: *"Well, I'll never do you a favor again. Some friend you are."*

You may have won the battle by refusing an unreasonable request, but you have lost the war of conducting yourself in a considerate and professional manner. If the bad feelings created by being aggressive can ever be resolved, it will take an inordinate amount of energy and time.

Example 2

You are making a home visit to a client who has right-sided weakness. You are late in visiting two clients to whom you must give extensive diabetic teaching. Your child needs a ride home from school, and you think you can just make it on time. Mr. Gowers, your 70-year-old client, is right-handed and has not been very successful using his left hand to write. As you are about to leave, he asks you to write a letter for him to his nephew.

An assertive refusal:

Mr. Gowers: *"Could you help me write a letter to my nephew tonight? I just remembered it's his twentieth wedding anniversary, and I want to let him know I'm thinking of him. He is like a son to me. I'd do it myself, but I can't get the hang of using my left hand."*

Assertive you: *"Mr. Gowers, I won't be able to help you to write your letter today because I'm running behind schedule. I can see it is important for you to get your best wishes off to this special nephew of yours in time for his anniversary. I saw your neighbor outside. How about if I ask him to come over and write the letter?"*

This definite response makes it clear to Mr. Gowers that you are unable to do what he wants. Your expression of understanding about his urgency and your suggestion of an alternative solution would make him aware of your concern. You have protected your rights not to take on a task when you are already overloaded, and you have shown your client you are interested in his situation.

A nonassertive refusal:

Mr. Gowers: *"Could you help me write a letter to my nephew tonight? I just remembered it's his twentieth wedding anniversary, and I want to let him know I'm thinking of him. He is like a son to me. I'd do it myself, but I can't get the hang of using my left hand."*

Nonassertive you: *"Uh…well, um, I'm not sure I can, Mr. Gowers. I'm pretty busy today, but I'll try. Maybe I can come back here on my lunch hour."*

You know that you are so busy that you will be lucky to get the teaching done and pick up your son. You know you should not take on this extra task, and you are already feeling more tense because it is one more thing on your long list of things to do. You have not protected your rights for a reasonable workload, and you have conveyed a lot of ambivalence to Mr. Gowers, perhaps leaving him feeling that he is imposing on you.

An aggressive refusal:

Mr. Gowers: *"Could you help me write a letter to my nephew tonight? I just remembered it's his twentieth*

wedding anniversary, and I want to let him know I'm thinking of him. He is like a son to me. I'd do it myself, but I can't get the hang of using my left hand."

Aggressive you: *"If you think I've got time to sit down and take dictation, Mr. Gowers, you're mistaken. I'll be lucky to get my real work done today."*

This hostile rejoinder protects you from doing an unreasonable assignment, but it leaves Mr. Gowers feeling devastated. He is likely feeling guilty for asking you and embarrassed at your angry refusal. Neither of you wins with an aggressive refusal.

Example 3

A physician arrives late to the afternoon prenatal clinic. Today is especially busy because more expectant mothers have kept their appointments than usual. One of your nurses is ill, which leaves you short-staffed. In addition, you are responsible for all the prenatal teaching. The physician tells you he has missed his lunch and asks you to get him something to eat.

An assertive refusal:

Dr. Watts: *"Will you go across to the deli and pick me up a salami on rye? I missed lunch because I was so busy this morning."*

Assertive you: *"No, Dr. Watts, I can't go to the deli to get you lunch. Like you, today I am swamped with the workload."*

This assertive response clearly conveys your refusal. It is polite and matter-of-fact. You have upheld your rights to do your job and treated your colleague respectfully.

A nonassertive refusal:

Dr. Watts: *"Will you go across to the deli and pick me up a salami on rye? I missed lunch because I was so busy this morning."*

Nonassertive you: *"Um…uh, well, Dr. Watts, we're kind of busy here today, but, well, I suppose if I do it fast, it won't take too much time. Do you want it toasted or plain? Pickles? Mustard?"*

Being nonassertive is probably leaving you feeling pretty angry and disappointed in yourself. It is clear to everyone that you do not wish to get your colleague's lunch. Being nonassertive this way means you lose time and lose face.

An aggressive refusal:

Dr. Watts: *"Will you go across to the deli and pick me up a salami on rye? I missed lunch because I was so busy this morning."*

Aggressive you: *"Nurses aren't handmaidens anymore, Dr. Watts. You'd better get with the times. We're all busy, yet we managed to get our own lunches. I'm not being paid to go and fetch food for you."*

Wow! You protected your rights with this response, but in the process, you were rude to a colleague by overreacting and attacking him. Such accusatory aggressiveness only serves to escalate bad feelings. A simple refusal would have been in order.

SAYING NO EFFECTIVELY

Do:

- State your refusal very near the beginning of your reply so that your requester hears a clear, direct answer right away
- Indicate concisely the reason for saying no if it strengthens your refusal
- Communicate your understanding so that the requester realizes that you are aware of the predicament even if you cannot solve it
- Suggest an alternative source of help if it seems appropriate
- Think about your response, then speak in a forthright, calm, polite manner
- Maintain a matter-of-fact, consistent way of refusing in the face of an aggressive requester

Don't:

- Begin your refusal with a list of lengthy excuses against which an aggressive requester will argue so logically that you will be forced to concede
- Stammer, pause, hem and haw, hesitate, or burst out your refusal; this will reveal that you are unsure of your response
- Lose eye contact for lengthy periods, shift uncomfortably, or convey other nonverbal discomfort that reveals your hesitancy
- Raise your voice or give other bodily clues of being enraged; it is your right to refuse, and you do not need to become hostile to protect this privilege

DARING TO HOLD FAST TO YOUR PRINCIPLES

Sometimes it is difficult to find just the right words to express your refusal even when you are convinced of your

> **BOX 25.1   Examples of Client Assertiveness in Their Own Advocacy**
>
> *Buying time to learn more:* Gastric bypass surgery has been recommended for weight loss. "Surgery sounds so drastic to me. Can you refer me to some other people who have had this procedure, or is there a support group I could attend to learn more?"
> *Getting a second opinion:* "I'm just not sure about all this. For my own peace of mind, I would like to get a second opinion."
> *Saying no to medication:* A woman with some discomfort from osteoarthritis reads about the side effects of the medication and decides that sometimes the cure is worse than the symptom. "I think I'll hold off on medication for now and try the aquatic arthritis class at my club first."
>
> From Breitman, P., & Hatch, C. (2000). *How to say no without feeling guilty.* New York, NY: Broadway Books.

opinion. Berent and Evans (1992) offered some phrases that might be helpful:

> *"No!"*
> *"No, thank you, I don't care to. I've never done that and don't want to start."*
> *"I can't do that."*
> *"I make it a habit never to…"*
> *"I make it a habit always to…"*
> *"As a matter of principle, I…"*

Sometimes healthcare consumers believe the recommended treatment regimen is unreasonable. How can they "just say no" (Box 25.1)?

MOMENTS OF CONNECTION…
A Nursing Student Uses the DESC Script to Confront an Unreasonable Request

I babysit regularly and, often at the last minute, the children's mom asks me to stay later than planned. This meant I was late to class. I decided to approach my employer: "I am finding that when I stay later, I arrive late to class, and this is really stressing me out. It would help me if we could stay with the time we planned." She understood and no longer asked me to stay late.

Return to "Active Learning" at the beginning of the chapter and write your responses.

PRACTICING REFUSING UNREASONABLE REQUESTS

Journaling/Skill Building: Exercise 1

If refusing requests is a recurrent issue with you, consider the notion that "you can't improve what you don't measure" (Hedberg, 2010). If this is true, then consider making a brief entry each day in your journal to track your progress on refusing unreasonable requests.

Application: Exercise 2

For each of the following situations, write an assertive refusal. Compare your responses with those of your colleagues and pool your suggestions to come up with the most assertive refusal, or role play one of the situations in class.

1. A colleague with whom you are working the night shift asks you to keep an eye on the clients and an ear out for the telephone and night supervisor while she has a nap. You think this request is unreasonable because you are both being paid to do the job, and, if any trouble occurs, two staff members will be needed.

2. A client is being observed for withdrawal from street drugs. She asks you if she can go down to the cafeteria with her visitor to have a cup of coffee. Your preference is for her to remain on the unit, where you can have frequent contact with her.

3. A client who comes once a week to receive an injection from you asks you if he could come 15 minutes later in the future. Moving back his appointment would inconvenience you, because it would mean you would be late leaving work and would not make your bus connections.

4. A colleague who lives in the same area of the city asks you if he can get a ride to and from work with you. That quiet time in the car by yourself is your only peaceful time in the day. You would find it stressful to have

to make conversation with another person during the commuting time.

REFERENCES

Ayhan, D., & Oz, H. S. (2021). Effect of assertiveness training on the nursing students' assertiveness and self-esteem levels: Application of hybrid education in COVID-19 pandemic. *Nursing Forum, 56*(4), 807–815. doi:10.1111/nuf.12610.

Balzer Riley, J. (2002). *Saying what you mean and meaning what you say.* Scottsdale, AZ: Workshop presented at the Faculty Development Institute.

Berent, I. M., & Evans, R. L. (1992). *The right words: The 350 best things to say to get along with people.* New York, NY: Warner Books.

Buitrago, R. (2013). How to "just say no" to a patient. *Clinical Advisor: For Nurse Practitioners, 16*(9), 92.

Chenevert, M. (1997). *Pro-nurse handbook: Designed for the nurse who wants to thrive professionally.* St. Louis, MO: Mosby.

Ellis, A., & Powers, M. (1998). *A guide to rational living.* Hollywood, CA: Wilshire Book.

Hedberg, A. G. (2010). Strategies and tools for personal growth and health awareness. In A. G. Hedberg (Ed.), *Forms for the therapist.* St. Louis, MO: Elsevier.

Levine, B. (2010). How to say no gracefully. How to Say No Without Feeling Guilty - Tips for Saying No at WomansDay.com.

McDonald, G., Jackson, D., Wilkes, L., & Vickers, L. (2013). Personal resilience in nurses and midwives: Effects of a work-based educational intervention. *Contemporary Nurse, 45*(1), 134.

Meagan. (2021). 7 Self-Care Boundaries (to Finally Start Putting Yourself First) (okaynowbreathe.com).

Oxman, A. D., & Sackett, D. L. (2013). Clinical-trialist rounds: 15. Ways to advance your career by saying "no"— part 3: How to say "no," nicely. *Clinical Trials, 10*, 340.

Paskin, J. (2005). How to handle a crushing deadline. *Money, 34*(11), 44A.

Speed, B. C., Goldstein, B. L., & Goldfried, M. R. (2018). Assertiveness training: A forgotten evidenced-based treatment. *Clinical Psychology: Science and Practice, 25*(1), 1.

Caring Communication with Clients and Colleagues whose Behaviors Are Challenging

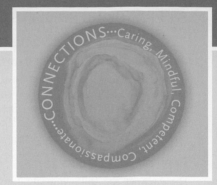

Kathleen Sitzman, PhD, RN, CNE, ANEF, FAAN,
Julia Balzer Riley, RN, MN, AHN-BC, REACE

Healing takes time. We want to rush it. To get back to being normal…But we can't go back. Can't undo. To me, healing is like a garden: the seeds you plant are growing underneath. You can't see anything for a while until enough rain, sun, time, feeding, and weeding—then something new begins to grow.

Nancy Guilmartin (2010)

OBJECTIVES

1. Identify common situations in nursing in which clients or colleagues may demonstrate challenging behaviors.
2. Discuss how to maintain professionalism while engaging in caring communication within the context of distress.
3. Describe caring communication strategies and micro-practices for working with distressed clients and colleagues.
4. Practice caring communication with clients and colleagues whose behaviors are challenging.

? ACTIVE LEARNING

Think about how you will write your answers as you read this chapter.

What?
Write one thing you learned from this chapter.

So What?
How will this affect your nursing practice?

Now What?
How will you implement this new knowledge or skill?

Think About It …

COMMON SITUATIONS IN NURSING IN WHICH CLIENTS OR COLLEAGUES MAY DEMONSTRATE CHALLENGING BEHAVIORS

Mad, sad, glad, and scared…nurses bear witness to all the human emotions. Consider the journey of a person from diagnosis with cancer through treatment and survivorship or end of life and the journey of staff as they travel alongside. Anxiety, anger, sadness, fear, worry, times of hope and joy, and times of sorrow may be shared with everyone whose life is touched. A person may become clinically depressed, feel isolated, or move into spiritual crisis (Dean & Street, 2014).

When the client or the nurse is distressed, clear communication is compromised, which can result in reduced quality of care and increased complaints (Jack et al., 2013). Their behaviors may present challenges to assertive, caring communication. We are called to be present and hold the space for others to express both negative and positive feelings (O'Connor, 2017). When clients and colleagues are distressed, we work to respond in helpful ways, yet we can be stressed by their distress. As we study and reflect on suffering—ours, our colleagues', and our clients'—we look to find meaning in the illness experience (Pollock & Sands, 1997). Nurses witness suffering and distress. Some suffering is inherent in a situation, such as receiving a frightening diagnosis and enduring uncomfortable, even excruciating, side effects of treatment. Other avoidable suffering comes from harm caused by inadequate care or caring connection, or what Dempsey and Wojciechowski (2014) referred to as Compassionate Connected Care: competent, quality, compassionate care that connects clients and staff through a clear mission that values engagement.

Clients convey their anguish verbally and nonverbally. Changes in health status, illness, and hospitalization are just some sources of distress in clients. Their loss of composure is a signal that they are disturbed by what is happening to them.

The changing healthcare climate causes stress for us as nurses and for our colleagues. In addition, nurses may pick up the sadness of clients (called *shadow grief*), which can lead to burnout. We may find that we have less energy, experience no zest for living, and talk about our clients continuously, even on our off hours. How we respond and how our clients respond to distress depends on personal history, culture, and experience. We experience the constraints of time, the emergent nature of a situation, and the unanticipated change (White, Duncan, & Baumle, 2010). We need to develop ways in which to relate to distressed colleagues and clients that soothe their distress without upsetting ourselves. Maintaining our sensitivity to others so that we can respond in a caring way without being overcome and losing our objectivity is one of a nurse's most inviting challenges—the gift of your presence without giving yourself away.

Interpersonal problems experienced by health professionals clearly reveal that our reactions to emotionally laden situations interfere with our ability to act effectively. We need to identify our own triggers, such as unwarranted criticism, and manage our reactions assertively to avoid disturbing our own peace of mind (Robinson-Walker, 2017). Nurses may ignore their responses to being overwhelmed with emotional demands, and this is called *compassion fatigue* (Vaughn, 2001). Untoward reactions can come from within ourselves (feeling unsure or inadequate about how to act), the situation (feeling overcome or impotent), or the distressed person (feeling distress ourselves).

SIMPLIFY AND DEEPEN

Maybe this one moment with this one person is the very reason we're here on Earth, at this time.

"The Caring Moment," Jean Watson

🌹 **MOMENTS OF CONNECTION...**

"We had an 11-year-old boy having a nonmalignant tumor removed from his spine. He was labeled a 'brat' due to his demanding behavior. One day, I had a few extra minutes and went and sat with him. We took out his science book and talked about what was happening with his surgery and about his fears. From that time on, he was much less anxious and became one of our favorites." A few minutes of kindly, authentic presence made a significant difference in this child's level of anxiety and distress (demanding behavior).

Common Events that Cause Stress

Kaufman and Wetmore (1994) suggested four common events that can cause stress: loss of control, change, sense of threat, and unrealized expectations. When nurses work with distressed clients, these are the overarching issues. How a nurse chooses to react when involved in distressing situations will have a direct impact on the level of distress experienced by all involved. The teaching of communication skills and protocols aimed at managing difficult situations implies that if we say the right thing, clients or colleagues will respond with acceptance, gratitude, and understanding, which will result in decreased distress. This is not always the case because distress is a complex event with multiple dimensions. Consider a new view in which distress is an opportunity to offer caring, authentic presence, and equanimity aimed at supporting productive connection, comfort, and problem solving among all involved.

Ascher (1994), in her memoir of grief at the death of her brother from acquired immunodeficiency syndrome, painted a picture that demonstrates the complexity distress can present. She defines grief as a "landscape without gravity." Of her family, she says:

My husband does not know I'm here, afloat... They continue to communicate through normal channels as though we were all here together on the steady plane of everyday life. Grief is outside the scope of language. I can only speak in signs. The furrow of my brow, the tightness of my lips. But when they who love me entreat, "Do you want to talk about it?" I say, "no," and turn away. I could say "ouch," I could say "it hurts." But language seems slight. Grief is physical and it hurts.

Ascher refers to it as a "journey into paralysis." We must remain present, nonjudgmental, and humble at the pain and anguish of suffering clients, families, and colleagues, whose stories we will never fully understand.

WIT AND WISDOM

Asking, "What is this like for you....?" is an open-ended question that demonstrates your presence, your willingness to learn what the experience means to the patient, and your willingness to be in a relationship with someone who is experiencing distress.

Parse (2014)

What Is Caring Communication?

Caring in one form or another is an expected dimension of professional nursing, and there are many theoretical definitions and nuances related to what caring means in different areas or situations. The *caring communication* approaches that we will explore in this chapter are based on Watson's Human Caring Theory, which calls us to establish a firm intent to mindfully and consistently care for self and others through:

- Practicing altruism and kindness with self and others
- Being fully and authentically present in our lives and work
- Accepting and nurturing individual beliefs and practices of self and others
- Cultivating helping-trusting-caring relationships
- Processing positive and negative feelings with awareness that we are not our feelings
- Using all ways of knowing for caring assessment and creative decision making
- Engaging in teaching and learning that honors diverse needs and learning styles
- Creating healing environments that holistically respect human dignity
- Recognizing that assisting with any basic need constitutes a sacred act
- Becoming open to mystery and miracles in everyday life (Adapted from "Watson's 10 Caritas Processes" in Sitzman & Watson, 2018).

These caring tenets apply to the full range of professional behaviors and activities in nursing. Everything we do as nurses *communicates* something to those around us, whether we are interacting with clients, significant others, or colleagues and whether spoken, unspoken, acted-upon, or overlooked. Consciously and continually cultivating a firm intent to care for self and others while enacting the tenets listed previously opens new ways to envision what might be possible and helpful during moments of distress at work and beyond.

CARING COMMUNICATION WHILE MAINTAINING PROFESSIONALISM

Deep caring, as described previously, can sometimes be misunderstood to mean that a nurse should become closer to or more involved with a client than healthy professional boundaries allow. This is not the case because the hallmark of wise and *authentic* caring is when the nurse is consistently grounded on a firm intent to care for self and others while enacting interventions that honor professional context. Sustaining a firm and healthy intent to care is best demonstrated when the caregiver mindfully pays attention to the distressed client or colleague in an effort to determine how best to "care" while appreciating what it means to maintain professional demeanor, privacy, and boundaries. This process will look different depending on the circumstances. A bit of self-disclosure may be helpful and compassionate in one instance but not in another. Warmth and the use of touch might be comfortable to provide for one client and not another. It is

normal and perfectly okay to vary your approach to caring based on the client or colleague you are working with and how you feel in the moment—this is an integral part of self-awareness and self-care. Some clients or colleagues will be more difficult than others, and your feelings and behavior will adjust accordingly. The other aspect to consider is your own temperament. For example, you may not be a person who likes to touch others or you might be a person who is very comfortable touching others, or you might be talkative and outgoing while another person is reserved. It is possible to demonstrate genuine, professional, and appropriate caring regardless of your own temperament. The key is to understand that caring is not a prescribed style of behavior to be displayed to others—it is an internally held stance to care however you are able in whatever circumstance you might find yourself. A lesson I learned many years ago while conducting a research study on caring helps to illustrate this point.

I conducted a small research study about the effective nursing interventions of an occupational health nurse who assessed the workstations of hospital employees to see if workstation improvements could be made to avoid ergonomic injuries. She had an unusually high success rate related to decreasing pain, mitigating injury, and consistent use of ergonomic interventions. I wondered if caring behaviors supported her success. In those days, I believed that caring had to include personal warmth, friendliness, and pleasant conversational banter. This turned out to not necessarily be true. My study showed that, in this case, clients said they felt cared-for and motivated to following the prescribed ergonomic interventions because the nurse that came to assess their workstations paid focused and in-the-moment attention to them through mirroring, eye-contact, and verbal validation of the presenting concern(s). This nurse did not ever touch the client directly, nor did she engage in any conversational banter during any of the observed interventions. She did not display personal warmth or a high level of friendliness. The primary features of every observed exchange were mindfulness, immediacy, and a palpable sense of being wholly attentive and firmly present for each client in that moment (Sitzman, 2001). There was a strong sense that concerns were *fully seen and heard* by the nurse. Results from this study have been validated many times over during my research related to caring science; caring, love, and trust *are best sustained through intention, presence, attentiveness, immediacy, and mindfulness.* Friendliness, warmth, and affection may be components of caring communication, but they are not necessities. This point is particularly helpful to recall when working with people who do not respond well to warmth, affection, or friendliness or when you don't feel inclined to be overtly warm, affectionate, or friendly.

To Sum up…
- Pay full attention.

- Cultivate curiosity rather than thinking you understand what another person is experiencing.
- Suspend judgement and just "be" or "bear witness" in the moment. Sometimes this is all that is needed or wanted by a person experiencing distress.
- Keep in mind that caring, love, and trust are best sustained through *caring intention, presence, attentiveness, immediacy, and mindfulness.* If these dimensions are present within the one doing the caring, then caring communication is the result.

WIT AND WISDOM

Poetry is a way some people share their distress. Ken Saulter (2010), coping with early memory loss, and his wife spoke at Innovations in Dementia Care during which he shared a poem his wife identified as important in their relationship. As you read "Between Us," think about offering writing as an expressive outlet for distress.

Between Us

Losing my memory,
Losing my memory to a terminal disease,
Is getting to be a problem.
Like when I'm in a group
And people talk to me and then,
Suddenly I fall silent,
While my brain skips a beat.
We know it's not a simple senior moment.
Eyes divert to shoe laces or thereabouts,
Anywhere else but the ceiling.
The moment becomes one of deep discomfort.
And here I am, a fraction of a person,
A clown without make-up or costume,
Waiting giant seconds to recover.
I'm told I will not remember
These bricks of separation
In the wall that is, regrettably,
Being built between us.
I worry a lot about forgetting habits, like
My locker combination, after 20 years of use.
And then, someday maybe, remembering where I live;
Or, luckily, maybe not.
But, against our will,
The wall keeps getting higher and higher.
Yet I keep on living, accepting the losses and
Focusing on what I've got, and you.
And trying to lower the wall between us
Or slow it down,
Or build a gate,
Or do something.
(Copyright © Ken Saulter. Used with permission.)

CARING COMMUNICATION PRACTICE EXAMPLES

Before you examine these practice examples, refer to Box 26.1, Examples of What to Say to Convey Caring in a Professional Manner, to begin thinking about how to convey caring in your own words.

Working with a Client in Distress

Mr. James, a 58-year-old avid outdoorsman, has been hunting in the woods near your rural hospital. While climbing steep terrain, he slipped and fell 50 feet down a ragged incline. In addition to suffering multiple bruises and scratches, he broke his glasses and lost his phone. Today he was admitted to your hospital for overnight observation. As you make your first round on the evening shift, you go into his room to introduce yourself:

You: *"Good afternoon, Mr. James. I'm sorry you have to be here under such unfortunate circumstances. How are you feeling right now?"*

Mr. James: *"How long am I going to be here? Can you get me a phone? I need to reach my wife. Somebody's got to bring me my extra glasses. I can't drive…I can't do anything without them. You can have your damn hospital. Just get me a phone so I can make arrangements to get out of here."*

BOX 26.1 Examples of What to Say to Convey Caring in a Professional Manner

- Is everything okay?
- I am here for you.
- I am here to listen and help.
- Please let me know if you want to talk.
- I will never be able to fully understand your pain/experience/anguish, but I am here to support you.
- My thoughts are with you.
- My heart is with you.
- You are important to me.
- I am unsure what would be most useful to you in this moment…
- If I (*do these specific things*), would that be helpful to you, or is there something else I can do?
- Is it okay if I sit here with you for a few minutes?
- Thank you for trusting me with your story/feelings/concerns/anguish.
- Is there anything I can do to help you right now?
- This is a difficult/shocking/horrible/stressful situation, and I am so sorry you are experiencing it.

Adapted from: Sitzman & Watson, 2017.

Mr. James raises his voice as he is talking and turns away from you. He squeezes the bed sheet in his hands and looks exasperated.

You: *"Thank-you for trusting me with your concerns. I'm sure you're eager to talk to your wife and make arrangements to get your glasses and go home. I'll get a phone for you right away. I can imagine that it's frustrating to be without your glasses, so please let us know how we can help you manage until you get the spare ones."*

Working with Upset Colleagues

Joe is the intern on the unit on which you have been a student for the past 6 weeks. Because you are both students working on the unit at the same times, you have become friends. This day Joe looks preoccupied, and you have noticed that he is not his usual good-natured self. He snaps at you for not having your client ready for his physical examination, even though he had not warned you about his plans to do the exam at this time. Later he approaches you with the following:

Joe: *I'm sorry for snapping at you earlier. I'm just not myself. Dayle just found out she's pregnant, and it's all I can think about. I just can't imagine being a father. I can barely cope with being a husband and an intern. It's been the only thing on my mind since I found out 2 days ago. I can't think straight. I can't sleep…I still can't believe it. I don't know what I'm going to do. We want kids, but why now?"*

You: *"Joe, Thank-you for letting me know! It's a challenging situation. It must be overwhelming right now to imagine trying to squeeze in being a father when you are busy enough being a husband and getting your career started. I am here to listen and support."*

Working with Clients Who Are Sad or Depressed

Jim is an 18-year-old client on your unit. He has just had a surgical repair after breaking his leg in a football game. Jim is an all-star athlete who knows he will not be playing any more sports this year. He is worried about getting behind in his schoolwork because of the advanced placement classes he is taking. Every day counts if he is to keep up with the fast pace of the class. This is Jim's senior year in high school, and he is worrying that his grade point average may slip because a football scholarship is now out of the question. He is tearful and seems embarrassed.

You: *"Good morning, Jim. How's it going?"*
Jim: *"It's not…"* (looking away from you and sighing).
You: *"What's wrong?"*

Jim: *"Oh…what's the point? I've got nothing to look forward to. All my plans have gone down the tube."* (Jim's voice is flat, and he makes no eye contact with you.)
You: *"You're really feeling down and that is totally understandable. Breaking your leg was very unexpected and disruptive to your life during this critical time and I am so sorry you are experiencing this. What can I do to help you right now?"*

Working with Colleagues Who Are Sad or Depressed

Petra is a fellow student you have come to know and like. The two of you have been in the same classes in nursing school and have had the same clinical rotations for the past year and a half. Now you are working on an oncology service in which many of the clients are dying of cancer. Petra has been quieter and has kept more to herself this week. She looks pale and lethargic in sharp contrast to her usual witty and energetic self. At coffee break one morning you ask Petra how she is feeling and she responds as follows:

Petra: *"I didn't think it was that noticeable. It's working with cancer patients…I don't think I can take much more of it. My visions of being a nurse are to cure people—to get them well again. It seems all the people we are working with now are dying, and there's no way around it. It's so depressing. How can you stand it? I go home every night, and all I can think is 'Is this all there is to life?' All we do seems so pointless if this is how things end."*
You: *"I have thought about that since being on this unit, too. When this happens, I try to adjust my perspective. I remind myself that the people we see in here are a small sample of the people in our city and there are lots of healthy people out there living active lives. I also try to cultivate the understanding that dying is part of living—life cannot exist without death. I try to focus on helping our clients fully live each day until they die. I think of their time with us as a very special part of their lives. They look to us to be able to listen to them without having to worry about what they say. These insights help me focus on hopefulness and usefulness in a place where it is easy to lose hope and feel there isn't anything I can do to help. Thank-you for trusting me with your feelings. It means a lot to me and I want you to know that I am here for you."*

Working with Clients Who Are Crying

Mrs. Urst is a 35-year-old woman who has just given birth to her second child. Both she and her baby are healthy. Her husband and their 8-year-old son are thrilled with the new addition to their family. You have just entered her room and found her weeping. She has gone through several tissues, and her eyes are red and swollen.

You: *"You have been crying. What's troubling you?"*

Mrs. Urst: *"Ohhhh…"* (sobs and blows nose; laughs and then starts crying again). *"I can't stop. It's just dawned on me that I'm now a mother of two. It's ridiculous…"* (sobs) *"I've known for 9 months, but now I wonder how I'll cope. I've forgotten all the stuff mothers need to know, and if I stay at home, I'll forget all the stuff secretaries are supposed to know. Why did we get ourselves into this predicament? Oh, I'm sorry to burden you. I guess I've just got the 'baby blues'"* (blows nose and bites lip to keep from crying anymore).

You: *"It's likely that your tears are in part due to 'baby blues,' but your whole world has been upset with the arrival of your new daughter; that's bound to take some adjustment. Working out a schedule between two important roles like motherhood and career is complicated. Given time to adjust to your new schedule, I'm certain you can work out something that suits you. I have some time now if you'd like to talk."*

Working with Colleagues Who Are Crying

Don is a nurse on the rehabilitation unit in the long-term care facility in which you are working. When you go into the office to collect your purse, you find him sitting in a chair with his head in his hands. When he sees you coming in, he quickly rubs his eyes and turns in his chair so that you cannot see his face. He gets out a tissue, blows his nose, and says the following:

Don: *"Come on in, Kathy. Guess you caught me crying. It's the news about Mr. Kent that's got to me."* (Looking at you.) *"I really thought he would make it. I can't believe he's dead. He was making so much progress. I never thought I'd say it, but I'll even miss the way he used to act like the king of the unit."*

*Don is referring to Mr. Kent, an elderly resident of your rehabilitation unit who was transferred yesterday to an acute care hospital after a cardiac arrest. Mr. Kent had been on the unit for 8 months, during which time he made himself known by his lively and sometimes overbearing involvement with all the staff. He was a well-liked, integral part of the life of your team. Your colleague Don had often been assigned as Mr. Kent's nurse because of Mr. Kent's request for a male nurse. Don and Mr. Kent had enjoyed friendly arguments about politics.

You: *(You sit down beside Don.) "I can't believe Mr. Kent is dead either, Don. You two had such a close relationship that I can see why you are so sad. You*

gave him a lot of pleasure and companionship during his stay here. It's hard to just keep on working when you lose someone as special as Mr. Kent. Can I help you out with your assignment in any way today, or is there something else I can do to help?"

Working with Clients' Criticism

Mr. Hunter has been a client on your medical burn unit for 6 weeks. He has extensive burns on his arms, upper body, and face as a result of trying to rescue his daughter from a house fire. He has been in isolation for the duration of his hospitalization. Chris, your colleague who has been his primary nurse since his admission, has left for a vacation. As the student having your clinical experience on this unit, you have been assigned to care for Mr. Hunter in Chris' absence. His wounds require extensive debridement and frequent dressing changes.

You are changing a dressing on Mr. Hunter's shoulder when this conversation takes place:

You: *"I'm going to let that soak for 5 minutes, Mr. Hunter. Then I'll remove it and do your other shoulder. Your burns are healing nicely."*

Mr. Hunter: *"That's thanks to Chris. She's a wonderful nurse. You've replaced her on her days off before, and you don't do things like she does. I want you to be careful and do things like they are supposed to be done. You're just a student, and I'm going to watch you carefully; if you do anything out of line, I'm going to report you to your instructor."*

You: *"You're welcome to watch what I do and ask any questions. I'm sure my way of doing things is a little different from Chris's, but I do guarantee that what I'm doing is safe and in keeping with your physician's orders. It is hard when things are done differently by each nurse, and you are likely missing Chris's style because you worked closely together for the 6 weeks you have been here. Do you want to ask me anything about what I've done so far in changing your dressing?"*

Working with Colleagues' Criticism

You are a student nurse who has just spent the past 6 weeks of clinical experience in the obstetric services of the hospital. During that time, your clinical instructor has been meticulously thorough in her supervision and teaching of the skills needed for obstetric nursing. This area of nursing is one you love, and you think you might pursue a career in this field. You believe you are adept at the physical care of both mother and baby, and you have been influential in helping mothers and fathers adjust to caring for their newborns. Your teaching sessions to mothers have been rated as outstanding, and the head nurse in postpartum has indicated that she is pleased with your work.

Despite your certainty that you are doing a good job and the positive feedback from clients and staff, you have never received a word of praise from your clinical instructor. In fact, she takes every opportunity to tell you where you could improve and is petty in her reprimands about your small errors. You are disappointed that your instructor is not more encouraging and enthusiastic about your successes. Today she is meeting with you to give you feedback on the bath class you gave to the fathers. You have had a chance to look over the fathers' evaluation forms, and they clearly state that your manner and content were reassuring in their first experience of bathing their newborns. Your instructor has just listed everything you did wrong and made suggestions about how you could improve such a class in the future.

> Instructor: *"Overall, you need to polish your professionalism. You are much too casual; you always are, for that matter. How do you expect anyone to treat you like a professional if you are lax and don't have a tight rein on things? You need to shape up in that regard so you'll command a lot more respect."*

Here are two assertive responses you might use.

> You: *"I can see you are giving me some advice that you believe is very important, but it's not clear to me. What exactly do you mean by 'professional'? If you explain what you mean, it'll be clearer to me so that I will be more likely to improve."*
>
> You: *"I know that when you give me all those suggestions about improving you are trying to help me be the best obstetric nurse I can be. It's disappointing that you haven't also noted some of the good things I've done and some of the ways in which I've acted professionally. I have received enough super evaluations from the clients and encouraging comments from the staff to support my belief that I am doing some things well. Before I leave this rotation, I would like you to give me some positive feedback in addition to your suggestions for improvement. Will you do that for me?"*

Working with Clients' Hostile Behavior

Debbie is an 18-year-old client on the medical unit where you work. She is a recently diagnosed diabetic and is terrified of receiving her insulin injection. When you try to administer it, she screams and kicks. It requires two staff members to hold her down securely to give her the insulin safely. You know that this situation is unsatisfactory because Debbie will soon be discharged and will have to give herself her own insulin. She will have to overcome her fear and gradually take on more responsibility for her self-care.

You decide to talk with Debbie about your desire for her to be more involved in her diabetes care. You have started the conversation by explaining that you have some ideas about how she can overcome her fear and learn to be more confident in giving herself insulin. Debbie interrupts you with the following:

> Debbie: *"Hold it!"* (Raising her voice.) *"I'm not, repeat, not ever going to give myself insulin. Get out, you bloodsucking vampire! You enjoy torturing me every morning. Well, forget it! Get lost! Go find someone else to bug. Just get off my back about this insulin junk."* (Debbie comes face-to-face with you and looks you right in the eye. She is red in the face and has her fists clenched and raised.)
>
> You: *"I know it's scary to receive a needle every morning, Debbie. It's a big thing to adjust to, especially for someone as active and as healthy as you. I can help you to feel quite confident, and eventually even comfortable, about taking your insulin. What I'd like you to do is to sit down with me right now and listen to my plan. I want you to hear me out, and then you can ask any questions and consider whether you'd like to try it."*

Working with Colleagues' Hostile Behavior

You are a nurse working in an outpatient mental health center. There are small interviewing rooms that can be booked for private interviews with clients and their families. As usual, space is an issue and scheduling of rooms is essential. In the past 3 days your interviews have been 5 minutes longer than the half hour that you had booked. By going over your time, you have delayed the interviews of others. Your colleague Karen has been annoyed but understanding because you are not usually so inconsiderate.

Today you booked the room for 45 minutes so that you could complete your interview without holding up others. However, your client has just revealed some serious information about her marriage and is upset and crying in the interview room. You know you need about 5 minutes over your time to help your client calm down before vacating the interview room. Karen has booked the room after you. She has knocked on the door twice already to remind you that your time is up. When you come out with your client, she blasts you with the following:

> Karen: *"It's about time. This is the fourth time this week that I've had to wait for you to leave the room when I've booked it. This has got to stop. My client's family is here on their lunch hour. You aren't the only one with important things to do, you know."* (Karen's voice is raised and her hands are on her hips.)

You: *"I apologize to all of you (looking at Karen and her clients) for this inconvenience." (Later, at a mutually convenient time when you and Karen are alone, you continue the conversation.) "Karen, I'd like to talk with you about how you handled my overstaying my booking time this morning. Is this a good time or would a little later be better?" (Proceeding after Karen agrees to do so.) "I will really try not to inconvenience you by going over my booked time in the future. I know I put you in a tough spot, and I was very embarrassed that you scolded me in front of our clients in the middle of the hall where everyone could hear. In the future I would appreciate it if you would ask to talk about any complaints you have in private. Then no one will be embarrassed, and we can keep our staff quarrels away from the clients. Could you do this, Karen?"*

Working with Clients' Verbal Abuse

Mrs. Suit is a 60-year-old client who has been admitted to the coronary care unit with chest pain. She has diabetes, which is poorly managed, and arthritis. She has been very demanding, especially on the days when her husband is unable to visit her. Today she has put her call light on repeatedly, and this time she has asked you to bring her fresh water in a glass with a straw. You start out for the kitchen but are waylaid by the distraught son of another client. He is almost in tears and wants to discuss the news of his father's forthcoming surgery with you. You pause to talk with him before you get Mrs. Suit's drink. When you get back to Mrs. Suit's room, she lambastes you as follows:

Mrs. Suit: *"Damnation. You could die here before you get a simple glass of water. You're such a smart-ass; you probably think I'm just a sick old lady, but I've got just as much right to service as anybody in this hospital. What in the hell were you doing, melting some ice? Damn it! Just give me the straw; you're slower than molasses in January. I'll open it myself. If I let you do it, you could take all night. You can go now. You smart-assed nurses think you're so damn important, but you can't even get an old lady a drink of water without messing things up."*

You: *"Mrs. Suit, I'm sorry I was so long in coming with your water. It's not that I don't care about you. I was delayed by an upset family member who needed to talk about his seriously ill father. I'm sure you can understand now why I was delayed. I am free for a few minutes now, though, if there's anything you'd like to talk about."*

Working with Clients' Manipulative Behavior

Mr. Gilmour is a 58-year-old gentleman on your rehabilitative stroke unit. He is a heavy smoker, and, because he burns holes in his clothing, it is the policy to keep his cigarettes at the nursing station, ensure that he wears a non-flammable smoking jacket, and supervise him when he smokes. Because this is a nonsmoking facility, it is necessary for a staff member to take him outside for a cigarette. Mr. Gilmour has a knack of asking for cigarettes at the most inconvenient times. He knows that he is supposed to wait until the report is over before he asks for a smoke, but he invariably bugs the nursing staff at report time. You are the nurse in charge of the day shift, and you want to complete the report to the evening staff so that you can go home. Mr. Gilmour has already interrupted your report three times to ask for a smoke. You gave him a cigarette 30 minutes ago. His fourth manipulative attempt goes like this:

Mr. Gilmour: *"Aw, come on. I'll smoke it right here where you can see me. I promise I won't start a fire. (He moves his wheelchair closer and closer to the small area where you are making the report.) It won't hurt you to give me one little smoke. Come on. No one else cares about these stupid hospital rules. I haven't had one all afternoon. Give a guy a break. I had to go for that stupid x-ray, so I missed my after-lunch smoke. Just one and then I won't bother you again."*

You: *"Mr. Gilmour, please do not interrupt us while we are doing the report. We will finish in 5 minutes if you stop interrupting us. It's only been 30 minutes since your last cigarette, and when our report is finished, one of the evening nurses will take you outside. If you do not leave us alone now, we will delay giving you a cigarette for another hour.*

Working with Colleagues' Manipulative Behavior

You are a nurse in an outpatient clinic that keeps sample medications on hand to give to clients. It is midway through the day. Your colleague Noreen has suffered a splitting headache all night, and she is concerned that it will develop into one of her immobilizing migraine headaches. You are the only one with the keys to the medication cabinet. She approaches you with this request:

Noreen: *"Leslie, I can't take this headache of mine any longer. I feel like my brain has dried up into a hard ball and is knocking against my skull. On the outside it feels as if a vise was locking in on it. I've already tossed up what little supper I could eat. Leslie, could you give me some of that new analgesic for my head? I've used it in the past, and it stops me from vomiting and somehow eases my head, too. My doctor would agree to it, I swear; so won't you please help me out of my misery? It's not like it's a narcotic I'm asking for. What do you* say? I might be of some help to you for the rest of the day if you give me the analgesic."

You: "Noreen, you sound terrible. I think if you're that uncomfortable, you'd better go home. I will not give you any medications, and I don't think you should take anything until you've checked with your doctor. It's been a slow day, and I know I can manage. Who could we call to come and get you?

Self-Care Nudge
Review micro-practices in Box 26.2.

Now, see what you think! Refer to Box 26.3, What Would You Do?

Return to "Active Learning" at the beginning of the chapter and write your responses.

BOX 26.2   Micro-Practices to Use with Self and Others When Distressed*

Centering during hand cleansing/handwashing to use every time you or your client takes a few moments to engage in hand cleansing/handwashing:

Plant both feet firmly in front of the hand cleansing station and begin washing/cleansing your hands while drawing your attention inward.

Breathe in, pause, exhale.
Breathe in, pause, exhale.
Breathe in, pause, exhale.

Now turn your renewed awareness outward and move forward into the remainder of your day.

Three Breaths Visualization requires about 3 minutes to do and can be used during difficult encounters or meetings when calmness or clarity is needed:

Inhale, pause, exhale.
Inhale, pause, exhale.

Some say that the breath is a crossroad between physical and spiritual, that the small pause between inhale and exhale provides a portal for the mind, body, and spirit to enter the elusive mystery of deep awareness.

Breathing is also golden thread that binds us all to the same life force because the air I breathe is also the air you breathe, ebbing, flowing, moving in, around, and through… an almost imperceptible dance of connection in time, place, and circumstance. You can't see the air, but it is most certainly there—invisible to the eye, yet integral to our existence.

Every breath is a miracle—a mostly involuntary, taken-for-granted, yet profoundly miraculous sharing of collective awareness and life force. And it is literally right under your nose!

Taking just a few moments to pause and engaging in three mindful breaths can provide focus and renewal. Let's try it now:

Plant both feet firmly, whether sitting or standing.
Draw your attention inward.
Breathe in, pause, and feel the small pulse of awareness… exhale.
Breathe in, pause, and feel the small pulse of awareness… exhale.
Last time…Breathe in, pause, and feel the small pulse of awareness…exhale.

Now turn your renewed awareness outward and move forward into the remainder of your day.

Blue Sky Visualization takes about 10 minutes and can be used to add perspective, calmness, and clarity when emotions are running high:

Feelings constantly come and go, changing from moment to moment.

It is easy to get attached to emotions as if they are something substantial, unchanging, and enduring. This attachment can cause ongoing pain and discord.

In reality, emotions are as insubstantial as the clouds in the sky.

Please ground yourself by firmly planting your feet or sit bones to the floor.

Breathe in and bring your awareness to your physical body. Squirm and adjust until you feel just right and then settle into calm repose.

Inhale, pause, exhale.
Close your eyes and envision the blue sky.
Your calm, unperturbed core essence is the blue sky.
Breathe in the fresh, cool sparkling air in the clear blue sky that is the true "you."

Now envision a few puffy white clouds drifting by in the sky of your mind.

Reach out to grasp a cloud.
Its cool mist floats between your fingers, and your hand comes up empty.

Inhale, pause, exhale.
Clouds represent the many feelings that pass by your blue core essence.

Clouds look solid and substantial, but if you reach out to hold onto a cloud, it is impossible to grasp it.

It is the same with feelings. They continually go by in the calm blue sky of your mind, impermanent, always moving, changing, dissipating, and reforming.

Feel the cool dampness as they roll by.
Acknowledge the flow of clouds and note that, as they move, reform, and move again, your blue sky core essence remains unperturbed!

Appreciate each cloud for what can be learned from its passing without trying to fruitlessly hang on to any one cloud.

Whether it is negative or positive, none are permanent or graspable.

Just as blue sky is not made of clouds, you are not your feelings.

Inhale, pause, exhale.
Open your eyes with renewed perspective and peace.

BOX 26.3   What Would You Do?

Scenario: You are a new nurse on a cardiac step-down unit while caring for Mr. Whaley, a 70-year-old White man who was admitted yesterday after a cardiac arrest. Upon returning to the bedside later in the morning after providing morning care, Mr. Whaley's wife is present. She turns to you and angrily complains about your care, complaining that her husband has sleep in the corner of his eye, and yells, "Obviously, you don't know what you're doing! I want a new nurse! Someone who has a clue!"

You're caught completely off guard. Consider the following possible responses. Identify the potential value of each of the selections below and describe your rationale.

A. Turn and walk out of the room.

B. "I'm so sorry, I don't know how I missed that. I'll take care of it right away."

C. "Excuse me, but you are over-reacting to this situation."

D. "I can see that you really care about your husband and want him to have the best care possible."

E. "You're angry about your husband's care."

Discussion

This actual situation demonstrates how nurses may receive the brunt of a patient or family member's angst.

A. You may have selected this item because you didn't know how to respond and/or you are setting boundaries because you find it unacceptable to be treated in this angry, accusatory manner. This response is not the best because it does not acknowledge Mrs. Whaley's feelings and has the potential to inflame the situation. In this circumstance, this is not a therapeutic response.

B. Apologizing and rectifying the situation is a satisfactory answer. You are acknowledging Mrs. Whaley's concerns and providing a corrective response. You did not offer an excuse; patient's do not have an interest in excuses, they need to have their concerns acknowledged.

C. Telling Mrs. Whaley that she is over-reacting is a blaming, confrontational response certain to escalate the situation and damage future interactions. This defensive response of blaming the patient is not therapeutic.

D. Looking behind the angry (and superficial) behavior for what is being communicated is an extremely powerful and helpful nursing response that opens the door for further communication. This therapeutic response is reflecting feelings.

E. Acknowledging Mrs. Whaley's angry feelings is also a therapeutic response. She no longer needs to demonstrate her anger because you've 'got it.' You've acknowledged her and her feelings.

...and the Rest of the Story

This actual situation happened to me as a new staff nurse on a cardiac unit after working primarily as a psychiatric nurse. Because of my psychiatric experience, I am more comfortable than most nurses with highly emotional behavior. Consequently, I responded with option D, and this is what unfolded:

The patient's wife (Mrs. W in our scenario) immediately broke down in tears. We sat down and out tumbled her concerns that she had *caused* her husband's cardiac arrest because she neglected to give him his potassium supplement the previous day. Racked with guilt, she was stressed and anxious. Based on this discovery, I called the charge nurse into the conversation, and she was able to allay Mrs. W's concerns using her seasoned professional knowledge and experience.

Mrs. W's initial behavior is a classic example of the defense mechanism of projection. Her personal blame and guilt about not taking adequate care of her husband (neglecting the potassium) was projected onto the nurse. In my experience, projection happens regularly in nursing—and in life. Projections can be conscious, unconscious, or in between (which was probably the circumstance in our scenario).

I want to point out that as a nursing student and new professional nurse, option E is a perfectly acceptable response. Reflecting the feeling of anger will de-escalate angry behavior and potentially allow for further discussion and satisfactory resolution of the problem.

The take-away here is to recognize that all behavior is communication, and looking and responding to what is behind the behavior tends to yield the best patient outcome. The art of nursing is part detective work!

Developed by Susan Hill Crowley, MS/RN (2022) for this text and shared in personal correspondence with text author.

Next-Generation NCLEX® Case Study

Working with Clients' Verbal Abuse

1430: A 55-year-old male experiencing chest and epigastric pain was transported to the emergency department by ambulance. The patient was admitted and prescribed a variety of medical diagnostic testing and cardiac monitoring.

1730: The results of both the diagnostic testing and cardiac monitoring ruled out a myocardial infarction, but he was diagnosed with severe hypertension, hyperlipidemia, hiatus hernia, and obesity. The patient was admitted to a medical unit.

Next Day

1030: The patient was prescribed an antihypertensive medication and an H-blocker as well as being placed on a low-sodium, low-fat diet. The nurse provided mediation education, and the dietitian has provided information regarding his diet and meal planning.

1245: The nurse enters the room in preparation to administer the prescribed medication and observes the patient's uneaten lunch tray at the bedside. Before being able to inquire about the meal, the patient angrily complains about the food, yelling, "No one would eat this stuff. I expect food that I like and tastes good. I don't care whether it's 'good for me' or not. Just take this slop away and leave me alone."

Item Type: Cloze

How should the nurse respond in order to demonstrate an understanding of therapeutic communication in this clinical situation?

The nurse would respond by stating,
_____1_____for the purpose of
_____2_____.

Option 1	Option 2
"You are too upset to talk about this now. I'll be back in an hour and I'll discuss it with you then."	Looking beyond the angry and inappropriate behavior for the basis of the patient's concerns
"I'm sorry you are upset but if you follow your physician's orders you'll be back to normal in no time."	Acknowledging the patient's concerns while offering a short-term solution to the problem
"Only when you stop reacting so rudely can you and your health team work out a solution to your concerns."	Setting boundaries that support a mutually respectful nurse–patient relationship
"When faced with life-altering changes, it usually helps to talk about how you are feeling."	Acknowledging the patient's angry feelings while providing reassurance
"If you want your health to improve, you will need to follow this diet."	Presenting a realistic view of the situation in an assertive manner in order to share the importance of prescribed treatments

Note: The answer keys for the previous NGN case study are given in the back of the book in Appendix III.

PRACTICING CARING COMMUNICATION WITH CLIENTS AND COLLEAGUES WHOSE BEHAVIORS ARE CHALLENGING

Journaling/Skill Building: Exercise 1

Identify a difficult conversation you had in which the client or colleague was sad and one in which he or she was angry. Write a brief journal entry describing what happened and how you responded. Include your assessment of what you said and did and anything you would have done differently. Identify who you can talk with to support you and offer suggestions after these conversations.

Journaling/Skill Building: Exercise 2

Identify a time when you were distressed and someone responded to you in a way that offered you comfort. Write a brief reflective journal entry identifying what brought you comfort. Think of what the other person did or did not do and said or did not say. Consider the person's body language, tone of voice, and the amount of time offered you. Reread what you have written, and identify at least three things you learned from this that could help you be more fully present for a client or colleague who is distressed.

REFERENCES

Ascher, B. L. (1994). *Landscape without gravity: A memoir of grief.* New York, NY: Penguin Books.

Crowley, S. H. (2022). What would you do? Personal correspondence with author.

Dean, M., & Street, R. L., Jr. (2014). A 3-stage model of patient-centered communication for addressing cancer patients' emotional stress. *Patient Education and Counseling, 94,* 143.

Dempsey, C., & Wojciechowski, S. (2014). Reducing suffering through compassionate connected care. *Journal of Nursing Administration, 44*(10), 517.

Guilmartin, N. (2010). *Healing conversations: What to say when you don't know what to say.* San Francisco, CA: Jossey-Bass.

Jack, B. A., O'Brien, M. R., Kirton, J. A., Marley, K., Whelan, A., Baldry, C. R., et al. (2013). Enhancing communication with distressed patients, families and colleagues: The value of the Simple Skills secrets model of communication for the nursing and healthcare workforce. *Nurse Education Today, 33,* 1550.

Kaufman, P., & Wetmore, C. (1994). *The brass tacks manager: Getting down to what really counts in the workplace.* New York, NY: Bantam Doubleday.

O'Connor, M. (2017). Creating caring connections through presence. *Nurse Leader, 15*(5), 347.

Parse, R. R. (2014). *The humanbecoming paradigm: A transformational worldview.* Pittsburgh, PA: A Discovery International Publication.

Pollock, S. E., & Sands, D. (1997). Adaptation to suffering: Meaning and implications for nursing. *Clinical Nursing Research, 6*(1), 171.

Robinson-Walker, C. (2017). Managing our triggers. *Nurse Leader, 15*(6), 372.

Saulter, K. (2010). *Living with dementia: Discovering what matters most today and for our futures. 8th Lillian & James Portman conference, celebrating direct care workers.* Livonia, MI: Innovations in Dementia Care.

Sitzman, K. (2001). Effective ergonomic teaching for positive client outcomes. *American Association of Occupational Health Nurses Journal, 49*(7), 329–335.

Sitzman, K., & Watson, J. (2017). *Watson's caring in the digital world: A guide for caring when interacting, teaching, and learning in cyberspace.* New York, NY: Springer.

Sitzman, K., & Watson, J. (2018). *Caring science, mindful practice: Implementing Watson's human caring theory.* New York, NY: Springer.

Vaughn, S. (2001). Burnout can strike anyone. *Los Angeles Times,* March 25.

White, L., Duncan, G., & Baumle, W. (2010). *Foundations of nursing.* Florence, KY: Cengage Learning.

Confronting Bullying and Incivility with Honesty and Respect

Renee Thompson, DNP, RN, CSP

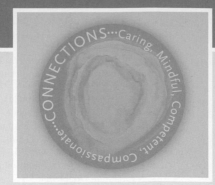

Nurses need to extend the same compassion to each other as we do to our patients.

Dr. Renee Thompson

OBJECTIVES

1. Differentiate characteristics of bullying, incivility, and constructive feedback.
2. Recognize overt and covert behaviors in the workplace through situational observations.
3. Identify strategies to communicate assertively with disruptive colleagues.
4. Execute scripting and naming strategies to confront disruptive behaviors.
5. Practice confronting bullying and incivility with honesty and respect.

A MESSAGE FROM THE AUTHOR

As a clinical nurse and nurse leader for more than 30 years, I had seen my share of bad behavior in healthcare and I finally got to the point where I was no longer willing to sit back and say, "Well, that's just the way it is in nursing." I had to do something about it. What I've learned over the years is that talking about bullying and incivility is, well, uncomfortable. The topic is unpleasant for many reasons, mainly

because nobody would expect to witness or experience bad behavior in an industry dedicated to active learning.

INTRODUCTION

New nurses are typically afraid of two things when they start their first job: making a mistake and being eaten alive by the other nurses. When new nurses are about to start their first job as professional nurses, many ask the same questions: "What if the nurses are mean? Does my preceptor want to be a preceptor? Do the nurses on the unit like new nurses?" Unfortunately, they have every right to be concerned about how they will be treated when they start their new job.

Consider this scenario. Tarah, a new nurse, was treated with cruelty on her first day of work. Tarah arrived on the unit at 6:45 am and approached the unit clerk sitting at the desk in the nurses' station. After waiting uncomfortably for a few minutes, the unit clerk finally looked up and asked Tarah what she wanted. Tarah told the unit clerk she was new and that today was her first day on the unit. Tarah asked the unit clerk if her preceptor, Rosita, was available. The unit clerk, who didn't smile and barely acknowledged Tarah's presence, turned to a group of nurses sitting in the nurses' station and said, "Hey, Rosita. Your 'baby' nurse

ACTIVE LEARNING

Think about how you will write your answers as you read this chapter.

What?
Write one thing you learned from this chapter.

So What?
How will this affect your nursing practice?

Now What?
How will you implement this new knowledge or skill?

Think About It …

is here." Rosita looked up and said, "Great," sarcastically, walked over to Tarah and said, "Look. I hate being a preceptor. Just don't get in my way and try not to kill anyone. Okay?" The look on Tarah's face was shock and horror.

Nurse-to-nurse bullying is a problem. Bullying is pervasive, destructive, and an embarrassment to the nursing profession. Unfortunately, bullying and incivility have been around for a long time. Many theories exist regarding why nurses are so unkind to each other and what bullying looks like, but little has been done to stop the behavior. Bullying, therefore, continues to plague the nursing profession.

A study conducted at a Canadian University (MacDonald et al., 2022) found that incivility toward nursing students was endured and not reported, with 70% of the students noting experiencing incivility in clinical practice. Not only do these behaviors jeopardize patient safety, they also jeopardize the nursing workforce. A cross-sectional study (n = 450) by Al Muharraq, Baker, and Alallah (2022) found a significant positive correlation between workplace bullying and nursing turnover. One-third of the respondents stated they intended to leave their current jobs.

You may find it interesting that, first, you are not alone if you have experienced this. This is an age-old problem in the nursing profession. Many nursing professionals and leaders have researched this phenomenon. Consider some of these poignant research studies, indicating strong evidence of what a pervasive problem this is and how to deal with it!

One of the reasons this issue has continued for so long is because we, nurses, tolerate it. We turn the other cheek; make comments such as, "That's just the way he is." "Don't let him bother you." "It's just their way." Some managers keep bullies on staff because they are either great clinicians or work a lot of overtime. Therefore, they're more likely to justify and tolerate their behavior. It's not right. However, it is the truth. Until we can come together as a profession, take ownership of our behavior, hold others accountable, and stop accepting bullying behavior as "normal," it will continue.

You can do something about it if faced with cruelty from your nurse colleagues.

When developing a nurse residency program for an extensive health system, I conducted many focus groups with student nurses, new nurses, and nurses who precepted. They needed to transition into professional practice successfully. However, they wanted to talk about how badly the other nurses treated them.

As I listened to their stories of intimidation, sabotage, condescension, and unnecessary criticism, they reminded me of my own experiences with bullying and incivility. In those moments, I decided enough was enough; that I had to do something about bullying and incivility in nursing.

Nursing is a wonderful profession—both challenging and rewarding. You've worked hard through nursing school. You deserve to work in an environment that's supportive and nurturing. Instead of worrying that the nurses will be mean and demonstrate intolerance to you being new, you should be focusing on learning how to deliver high-quality, safe, and effective care. As a senior nursing student or recently graduated new nurse, now is the time to learn the strategies to protect yourself against any bully that may be waiting for you in your first job as a professional nurse.

The content in this chapter will equip you with strategies to help you address any incidents of bullying or incivility from your colleagues. Isn't it time nurses stop treating each other with cruelty and start supporting each other?

GETTING CLEAR ON DEFINITIONS

Bullying, incivility, lateral or *horizontal violence,* and *disruptive* or *toxic behaviors* are terms used to describe similar behaviors; however, they are not the same. Many nurses refer to their colleagues as bullies or say that they are being bullied when, in reality, they are working with someone who is being uncivil or disruptive at the moment.

Some questions come to mind here. What about conflict? When does conflict cross the line into bullying? Does it? Working in healthcare is stressful. When under stress, we can all misbehave. How do you know if your peer is bullying you or if they are just having a bad day?

Not everything is bullying, and when we call everything bullying, we lessen our chances of addressing actual bullying. Therefore, understanding what bullying is and what it's not is important to employ the appropriate tactics when addressing it.

So, let's get clear on what bullying is and what it is not.

Disruptive Behavior

When we think of disruption in healthcare, we tend to think of someone or something stopping the flow of care. This disruption can be a person (patient or coworker) or a situation (unexpected admission or additional assignment). However, in the context of disruptive behaviors, we can quickly see how frequent disruptions (and disrupters) can impact work relationships and, ultimately, patient care. *Disruptive behaviors* are commonly used as an umbrella term when discussing behaviors before going deeper into specifics.

According to The Joint Commission, the following represent disruptive behaviors:

- Reluctance or refusal to answer questions, return phone calls, or respond to pages
- Physical threats
- Verbal outbursts
- Impatience with questions
- Refusing assigned tasks
- Uncooperative attitudes during routine activities

Condescending language and all unprofessional and disrespectful behaviors can be first termed *disruptive* when you think about it.

In June of 2021, The Joint Commission found these disrespectful behaviors and more like these to be so prevalent that they updated the original 2016 Sentinel Event Alert 40: Behaviors that undermine a culture of safety to include new workplace standards, which provide a framework to guide hospitals in defining workplace violence and developing prevention systems and structures.

Incivility

Incivility is considered low-level, rude, inconsiderate, and unprofessional conduct. A teenager occupying a seat on the bus who doesn't give up a seat for an oncoming elderly person, a peer who interrupts you mid-sentence to interject her opinion, or a friend who is consistently late for dinner or other events, etc. is considered disrespectful and rude.

Common behaviors in the workplace that may be categorized as incivility include:

- Engaging in condescending body language
- Texting or talking during someone else's presentation
- Mocking a coworker
- Using gossip as a way to retaliate
- Excluding certain people from social events

Bullying

Bullying is different from incivility. Bullying is the repeated pattern of disruptive behavior with the intentional or unintentional attempt to do harm. Although there is a legal definition for harassment and discrimination, there is no legal definition for bullying in the United States.

For a behavior to be considered bullying, the following needs to be present:

- *Target:* Bullies tend to focus on either one person or a small group of people. For example, you start your first nursing job alongside four new nurses. Carl is welcoming to everyone else. However, he is rude, dismissive, and condescending to you (one person). Carl is harsh, dismissive, and condescending to you all (small group).
- *Harm:* The behavior has to be harmful in some way. For example, during a clinical rotation, you inform a nurse that you have been assigned as her student nurse today, and she rolls her eyes at you. Is this harmful to you? Technically, eye-rolling is not harmful and therefore not considered bullying. However, if Meleka deliberately fails to inform you that the physician just wrote an order for the patient to be NPO and you give the patient crackers and peanut butter, which then causes a delay in care, who is this harmful to? Now we can see harm to the patient.

- *Repetition:* For a behavior to be considered bullying, it must be repeated over time. What we're doing now is establishing a pattern of behavior.

When you look at the list of disruptive and uncivil behaviors, they can all be considered bullying if repeated, if there is intent to harm (intentional or unintentional), and if there is an intended target. Many nurses are often surprised to hear this—that it is deliberate or unintentional! When we understand that intent does not matter, it helps pave the way for us to be less of a diagnostician trying to figure out "why" and assume a more proactive role in doing something about this.

What Is Not Considered Bullying?

"My instructor is a bully!," Shawn screamed when he exploded into the Dean's office. "She wrote me up for calling off and I'm sick of her bullying me! YOU need to do something about her!"

Is Shawn's instructor a bully?

Maybe.

Not everything is bullying or incivility. When we label everything as bullying, we do a disservice to actual bullying. Let's get clear about what bullying is not.

Bullying is not:

- *Being held accountable for performance or behavior:* Many student nurses reach out to me, complaining that their instructor is bullying them because they were given a bad grade or given an "unsafe" during clinical. Again, this is not bullying. Perhaps the instructor is just holding students accountable to a higher standard of care.
- *Constructive feedback:* Especially during the orientation period, new nurses should expect to receive ongoing and relentless positive and constructive feedback. However, new nurses commonly claim that their preceptors are bullying them when they are just giving constructive feedback. Constructive feedback can be hard to take because it needs to be honest and direct. This can hurt, but we must improve our skills.
- *Conflict and expressing a different opinion:* Just because you have conflict or disagree with a coworker or your boss doesn't mean they are bullies. Conflict is different. Conflict is not bullying.
- *Having a bad day and getting "testy" with your coworkers:* Let's face it, nurses work in stressful environments filled with unpredictability and complexity. We are not always on our best behavior. I challenge you to claim that you've never done or said anything unprofessional at work when under stress. It's a human thing. However, we are not all bullies! And we are not perfect!

See Box 27.1, Is It Bullying or Something Else?, to help make these distinctions.

The next time you think someone is bullying you, stop and ask yourself these questions:
1. Is this person just holding me accountable for my performance or behavior?
2. Is this conflict or a difference of opinion?
3. Am I the only person being treated this way?
4. Is the behavior harmful to me?
5. Have I seen this behavior before?

Bottom Line

Whether bullying, incivility, or someone just having a bad day—these behaviors need to be addressed because they impact relationships and the work environment.

Recognize Disruptive Behaviors in the Workplace

Now that you know what bullying is and what it is not, it's time to explore the different ways disruptive behaviors present themselves in the workplace.

OVERT VERSUS COVERT BEHAVIOR

Two basic categories of disruptive behaviors exist: overt and covert. Overt behaviors are easier to observe, whereas covert behaviors are subtler.

Overt Behaviors

Any behavior that can be observed is considered overt. Smiling, laughing, running, and cursing are overt behaviors; we can observe and describe these behaviors in similar ways. During shift report, your coworker, Tammy, loudly criticizes you for not completing the pre-op checklist before the end of your night shift. She points her finger at you, yells, "How could you be so stupid?", and then refuses to take report on the remaining patients. She storms down the hallway, huffing and puffing.

Whoever was standing nearby would be able to describe Tammy's behavior in the same way.

Characteristics of overt behaviors include:
- Yelling
- Criticizing
- Cursing
- Blaming
- Silent treatment
- Threatening
- Name calling
- Physical violence

Covert Behaviors

Most of us would rather deal with overt behaviors than covert. Covert behaviors aren't always initially apparent; they are more complex. They're sneaky and highly passive-aggressive in which someone gets their anger out in "crooked" ways. In contrast to overt behavior in which others can observe the action, only the person themselves can witness the behavior in covert behavior.

Characteristics of covert behaviors include:
- Excluding others
- Withholding information
- Using sarcasm
- Favoritism
- Retaliation
- Sabotaging others
- Unfair work assignment
- Taking credit for someone else's work
- Being nice to someone's face but mocking them behind their back

What about eye-rolling? What category does eye-rolling fall under?

It depends. If you are discussing an idea with a colleague and they immediately roll their eyes at you, it's overt. However, it's covert if they act genuinely interested but then roll their eyes when you turn around.

Keep in mind that any of these behaviors could be considered bullying if they meet the criteria of being targeted, harmful, and repeated. See Box 27.2, Disruptive Behavior Assessment, to look at your own experience.

Moving from Witnessing to Action

The next section reviews how to handle these behaviors—whether overt or covert. It's not always easy. However, it is possible!

Having a trusted colleague or friend to share in confidence the behaviors you are experiencing is a great first step. As a special note, it will be most effective for you if you share your perspectives in a "non-gossipy" kind of way. For example, rather than saying, "Can you believe how the charge nurse treated me today? They're always giving me the worst assignments," it's more effective to say, "I've been having difficulty in communicating with the charge nurse, who seems to give assignments unfairly. I may be over-reacting and I'd like to bounce this off you." See the difference? In the first scenario, you want empathy. In the second assignment, you want help.

CONFRONTING DISRUPTIVE BEHAVIORS BY COMMUNICATING ASSERTIVELY

In nursing school, you learn anatomy and physiology, body systems, disease processes, treatments, evidence-based

BOX 27.2   Disruptive Behavior Assessment

To determine the frequency that you've experienced disruptive behaviors, please review the following list of behaviors, and answer based on the rating scale:

Workplace Behavior — Use the following ratings:

1 – Never	2 – Rarely	3 – Occasionally	4 – Frequently	5 – Very frequently

Regarding individuals in your department, how often have you *experienced* these behaviors?

Being yelled at, criticized, or cursed at in front of others

Having a coworker roll their eyes at you

Receiving an uneven workload assignment, seemingly based on favoritism

Having a coworker break confidence by sharing private or embarrassing information

Having a coworker withhold information that leads to a negative impact on performance

1. Being excluded by certain individuals from routine lunches or celebratory or social events
2. Having accomplishments downplayed, such as awards or advanced degrees
3. Being ignored or given the silent treatment by certain individuals
4. Being treated nicely to your face but mocked or insulted behind your back
5. Hearing individuals name-calling or making ethnic slurs, jokes, or inappropriate sexual comments
6. Being micromanaged and repeatedly reminded of your mistakes
7. Being the target of gossip or false rumors
8. Receiving threats of physical violence
9. Being retaliated against for speaking up
10. Being made to feel stupid or incompetent

If you scored between 15 and 30, you have had mild exposure to disruptive behaviors.

If you scored between 31 and 59, you have had moderate exposure to disruptive behaviors.

If you scored between 60 and 75, you have had severe exposure to disruptive behaviors.

practice, and even the art and science of caring. However, not as much focus has been placed on learning how to communicate effectively, especially in difficult situations. Yet, as nurses, we work in high-stress, demanding, and complex environments involving life and death situations that depend on skillful communication among healthcare professionals. Add a few bullies into the mix and even the most skilled person can get quickly caught off guard and unsure how best to respond. And newest nurses are the most vulnerable as they often want to show their best sides, understandably so, and not upset the apple cart when dealing with disruptive situations.

The good news is that by understanding that learning how to communicate effectively is just as important as the cardiovascular system and then engaging in deliberate skill development, you can learn how best to communicate in most situations. The following section will get you started.

Understanding Communication Styles

Human beings utilize one of four primary communication styles: aggressive, passive, passive-aggressive, or assertive. Each style can be further described as how honest and respectful they are.

For example, aggressive communicators are honest, but not very respectful. They often do not consider the impact of their behaviors on others.

Passive communicators are not direct, because they either don't want to hurt your feelings or are afraid of how you will react if they do.

Then there are the passive-aggressive communicators— you know, the people who are so nice to your face, but as soon as you turn around, they are setting up booby traps behind your back. They are neither honest nor respectful. They get their anger out in "crooked" ways.

Finally, there are assertive communicators. Assertive communicators are honest, direct, and respectful at the same time. This style enables professionals to express themselves with confidence, allows them to deflect negative conversations, and minimizes the negative impact when faced with disruptive behaviors. Assertiveness is not a personality trait. It's a communication style that allows healthcare team members to work together to achieve common goals.

Although we each have our natural communication style, the only style healthcare professionals should be using in healthcare is the assertive style.

The following content will help you develop assertive communication skills regardless of your natural style.

Assertive Communication Characteristics

Assertive communicators use cooperative language such as "we," "together," and "us."

They offer specific information and avoid generalizations.

- Nonspecific: "Lois, you always give me an unfair workload!"
- Specific: "Lois, you've assigned me four patients in isolation for the last four days while the other nurses on

the unit were assigned only one. Is there a reason for this?"

They use open and honest statements.

- "George, I've never cared for a patient with a 3-way catheter before, and I'm not comfortable managing Mr. Lester's catheter independently. Will you come with me?"
- "I need your help with…."

They display an even and confident tone of voice and avoid yelling.

They actively listen without interruption.

- Looks person in the eye
- Allows time for listening without interruption

Assertive communicators focus on the issue or problem, not the person.

- "The problem is…"
- "Is this what's best for our patients?"

They use nonjudgmental verbal and nonverbal language.

- "Help me to understand why…."
- "Is there a reason for…."
- Displays open posture

They actively initiate actions that need to be done.

- "I am willing to do…."
- "Let's figure out a way to…."

They negotiate, bargain, and compromise.

- "What are our options for solving this problem?"
- "How can we compromise?"
- "What alternatives do we have?"

Most importantly, assertive communicators are honest and respectful in all conversations.

Confronting Disruptive Behaviors

Now that you understand the characteristics of assertive communication, you are ready to address bullying and incivility. Two of the most powerful strategies we'll explore are "Name it" and "Script it."

Name It

The single most powerful action you can take to address disruptive behavior in the moment is to name someone's behavior. Confronting someone's behavior as it happens can stop them immediately and prevent an escalation of that behavior. People who feel a sense of power during their tirades gain momentum as they disrupt. Interrupting someone midstream and naming their behavior can act as a defibrillator, short-circuiting the verbal assault.

Likewise, when you work with a colleague who uses covert tactics and is secretly trying to sabotage you, rolling their eyes behind your back or undermining your credibility, acknowledging that you are aware of their behavior by naming it exposes their unprofessional conduct honestly and respectfully. They may think their efforts are going unnoticed until you name them.

> **WIT AND WISDOM**
> *Before we can change things, we must call them by their real name.*
> **Confucius**

Naming It Examples

"You are *raising your voice* at me so loudly in front of patients and their families."

"I saw you *roll your eyes* at me when I asked you for help with a patient."

"During our staff meeting, when our manager introduced Sarah and me as new graduate nurses, I *heard you say something under your breath* and *saw you roll your eyes.*"

"I am willing to talk about my mistake when you are willing to speak privately and *without raising your voice.*"

"You told me to go home even though I hadn't finished my work—that you would pick up the slack. However, I found out you were complaining about me during the night. I would appreciate it if you would give me direct feedback instead of *talking about me behind my back.*"

Action Step: Observe your coworkers' behaviors for the next few weeks. Identify the behaviors as overt or covert. Write down how you would "name" that behavior.

ASSERTIVE SCRIPTING

If you're like many people, when someone says something to you that embarrasses you, you don't know what to say in the moment. You may freeze and not say anything or say something you'll regret later. This is understandable. But the next day, in the shower, you can think of all sorts of things to say. By then, it's too late. That is why scripting ahead of time is a powerful tool to confront disruptive behavior.

The reason is that when we are caught off guard and treated in a very negative way, that is, yelled at, openly criticized, treated with condescension, or threatened, we may immediately go into fight or flight mode. To protect ourselves, our amygdala responds first and immediately wants to either "clobber the jerk" or freeze. Then, after the experience travels through our amygdala, it reaches our prefrontal cortex that responds by thinking, "maybe clobbering the jerk isn't such a good idea." Hence, the next day in the shower, you can think of a better response.

Scripting enables you to identify a behavior that you've experienced, identify an appropriate response beforehand, practice that response, and then, even when your emotions are high and the amygdala is on full attack, respond appropriately by utilizing that script.

The following represent assertive scripts to address everyday situations in healthcare.

Public Criticism

- I'm not comfortable discussing this here. Let's go somewhere private where patients and family members cannot hear us.
- Excuse me. In my opinion, this needs to be addressed in private.
- I see you are getting angry. Let's discuss this elsewhere (or some other time).
- Excuse me, could we talk in private about this?
- I'm not comfortable talking to you right now.
- Help me understand why you are criticizing me in front of everyone.
- I think we need to discuss this later.
- I am willing to receive feedback as long as you are willing to deliver it privately and respectfully.
- I'm so uncomfortable with your language that I cannot hear what you are saying.

Ethnic or Sexual Jokes

- It makes me uncomfortable when you say things like that.
- How would you feel if this was said about you?
- I'm offended when you share jokes about _____.
- If you were in their shoes, how would you feel if this was said about you?

Exclusion

- In the future, would you please include me in the meeting/event?
- Help me understand why I was not included in _____.
- I'm not sure you realize, but I never received an invite for the _____.
- Is there a reason why I wasn't invited?

Gossip

- I don't feel right that you are talking about _____ when they are not in the room.
- Have you considered talking to them?
- I don't think it is fair to talk about someone who is not in the room.
- Maybe we don't have all of the details.
- I know I wouldn't appreciate it if someone talked about me.
- Do we know this is a fact?
- Should we be talking about this here or anywhere for that matter?
- Why are we talking about this? This sounds like gossip to me.
- I think this conversation is not for me to hear or know.

Angry or Frustrated Coworker

- How can we resolve this?

- I see you are upset.
- Is something bothering you? You seem upset/angry/stressed.
- (Name), Do you have a minute? I can see you're frustrated. Do you want to talk about it?
- I can see you're upset. Do you want to go back into the breakroom to speak?
- You seem overwhelmed. How can I help?

Unfair Assignments

- I'm not comfortable with this assignment because…
- I don't have the skills required for this assignment.
- I'm not sure you realize that I already have a heavy patient load.
- In my opinion, this assignment is unsafe.
- Would you be willing to review my assignment? I have concerns about the workload.

Unsafe Practice

- Are you OK going over what just happened?
- I want to show you what I've learned about that.
- I know you're busy; maybe you don't realize you skipped a step.
- So that I understand…
- Can we review this together? I want to make sure we are both practicing correctly.
- Before we continue, can we discuss_____?

🌹 MOMENTS OF CONNECTION…
Scripting Works!

My daughter, Kaitlin, worked as a schoolteacher. One of her peers would say rude things to her but only in front of the other teachers, never when they were alone. My daughter felt embarrassed and didn't know how to respond. She didn't want to reply in a way that would be considered rude, yet at the same time she didn't want to look passive either. Because of my expertise in addressing disruptive behaviors, my daughter called me for help. I told her to use this script the next time her peer said something rude to her: "I'm offended by that comment." I told her to practice saying that script repeatedly until it was automatic. My daughter was ready! Sure enough, her peer repeated something rude in front of others. This time, my daughter looked her in the eye and said, "I'm offended by that comment." Her peer was caught off guard and tried to defend herself. "Oh, you know I'm only joking." My daughter again replied, "I'm offended by that comment." She then walked away. Kaitlin worked with that person for another year. Her peer never said anything rude to her again. Scripting works—not 100% of the time, but it works!

Bonus Strategies to Become More Assertive

In addition to assertive communication, naming the behavior, and utilizing powerful scripts, there are a few additional strategies for you to consider as you navigate the complexities of human behavior in the workplace.

Engage in Positive Self-Talk

Your internal dialogue can have a profound effect on your external dialogue. There is a connection between what you think and what you say and do. If you are concerned that you will become a target of bullying, the more time you spend thinking about successfully addressing bullying behavior, the more likely you will succeed. Tell yourself, "I can do this." Visualize yourself walking tall, looking at others using direct eye contact, and communicating assertively.

Rehearse Your Response

Once you understand the assertive communication style, script a few responses to negative situations you commonly encounter and practice saying your lines. Like an actor, the more you practice your lines, the more comfortable you will be during the performance. If it helps, practice this on someone you trust and have them respond. Doing this in "real time" can help.

Practice assertive communication in relatively benign and more manageable situations before using it on someone you're nervous around. Engage in positive thoughts; envision your success. Rehearse your response until you can say it clearly and firmly.

Self-Care Nudge

Step away. *Almost everything will work again if you unplug it for a few minutes, including you.*

Anne Lamott

Walk Away

Some aggressive communicators love an audience. Like a theatrical performance, they need to have an audience for the performance to continue. Walking away takes away their audience and their power. Seldom will you see someone continue screaming, yelling, or criticizing somebody without an audience.

It takes moral courage to walk away from a bully yelling or openly criticizing you. Walking away is a crucial step to stopping their behavior without getting into a confrontation. One tip: When you walk away, sometimes it helps to say something like, "I want you to know that this is uncomfortable for me, so I am walking away. Please let me know when you XYZ [e.g., want to talk about this in a quiet tone]."

Exercise: Write your signature on a piece of paper. Now, switch hands and write your signature with your nondominant hand. Difficult, right? Although uncomfortable, awkward, and challenging, you can do it. With practice and time, your signature might look similar to your dominant hand.

Combating bullying and incivility isn't easy, but you can do it. Just like practicing your signature with your nondominant hand, it may feel awkward and uncomfortable. Still, with practice over time and a dose of moral courage, you can decrease your attractiveness as a target.

As you start your first job as a nurse, please remember that bullying undermines a culture of respect and safety. If you find yourself being bullied despite your efforts to avoid becoming a target, speak up. Remember, you deserve to work in a nurturing and supportive environment that is free from bullying behaviors that rob you of productive and joyous work!

WHAT IF YOU'RE THE BULLY?

Numerous studies show that anywhere from 70% to 90% of all nurses have experienced or witnessed bullying in the workplace (Daly, Flynn-Magee & Rodney, 2020; King et al., 2021). Who are these "bullies"? We are. But unfortunately, some of us don't realize it.

I read this example a few years ago about a guy who was curious about who the "mean guy" was in the neighborhood. People were always talking about how mean this guy was who lived on our block. But I decided to see for myself. I went to his door, but he said he wasn't the mean guy; the mean guy lived in the house over there. "No, you stupid idiot," I said, "that's my house."

What I know about humans is that we are all myopic. We only see the world through our own eyes and often fail to consider that we might also be part of the problem. When we can actually turn the mirror back on ourselves and objectively see how others perceive us, only then are we able to transform.

How Do You Know If You're the Bully?

The first step is to be honest enough to consider your behaviors and ask if they might be regarded as unprofessional. Take an introspective look at your behaviors to see if they contribute to bullying and incivility in the workplace. It's a difficult thing to open yourself for scrutiny and awareness of your behaviors, but such openness is a quality of both maturity and professionalism. Refer to Box 27.3, Am I a Bully? Take a self-assessment to take a look at your own behavior.

SIMPLIFY AND DEEPEN

If you want others to be happy, practice compassion. If you want to be happy, practice compassion.

The Dalai Lama

BOX 27.3 Am I a Bully? Take a Self-Assessment

Please use the following ratings:

1 – Never	2 – Rarely	3 – Occasionally	4 – Frequently	5 – Very frequently

In my work environment…

1. I roll my eyes or make mean faces behind other people's backs.
2. I enjoy confrontations with people I know I can dominate.
3. I talk about other people in negative ways when they are not around.
4. I have purposely not invited somebody to a work party or event.
5. I have made fun of others because they are different.
6. I go out of my way to help some of my coworkers but not others.
7. If I'm in charge, I deliberately give the more straightforward assignments to nurses I like.
8. I justify behaviors that help new nurses "toughen up."
9. I sometimes ridicule a new or inexperienced coworker.
10. Sometimes, I make people cry at work.
11. Other people seem unreasonably upset by the things I say or do.
12. I think most of my coworkers are incompetent.
13. Other people seem scared to give me their opinions.
14. New or inexperienced nurses rarely ask me for help more than once or twice.
15. I've been told that I intimidate other people.

There's no shame in finally realizing you've been treating others in an unprofessional and inappropriate way if you do everything you can to change. Sometimes the ability to change requires professional help. All healthcare organizations offer employee assistance programs, typically at no or low-cost. Why not get some help?

If you have recognized bully behavior in yourself, avoid spending excess energy on guilt and self-deprecation. Nurses who bully don't always make a conscious decision to treat their coworkers poorly. Sometimes they adopt bullying behaviors to cope with the demands of the job, to protect themselves from others (the best defense is a good offense), or because they have personal issues that infect their work environment. There is no shame in realizing you've been behaving like a bully. The shame lies when you know it but do nothing to change it.

You can't fix something if you don't even know it's broken.

WIT AND WISDOM

What makes the dawn come up like thunder? Courage!

The Cowardly Lion in *The Wizard of Oz*

In Closing

Thank you for choosing to become a nurse. Although you will have days that will challenge you beyond your imagination, you will have more days when you know you've made a difference in someone's life. You deserve to start your career in a nurturing and supportive environment that is free from bullies! Remember that addressing bullying behavior takes courage, practice, and support from others. Many nurses are passionate about eliminating bullying behavior in the workplace.

We all have to do our part to stop the cycle of bullying, disruptive, and uncivil behaviors in healthcare. Like the Cowardly Lion in *The Wizard of Oz*, tackling bullying and incivility in nursing takes courage. Courage is similar to your bicep muscle. The more you use it, the bigger and stronger it gets. I hope this chapter helps put this often-confusing topic into new perspectives. You deserve the best.

When we all understand how to make this happen, patient and work relationships will thrive—and so will you!

Return to "Active Learning" at the beginning of the chapter and write your responses.

Next-Generation NCLEX® Case Study

Identifying the Difference between Bullying, Incivility, and Honesty

A newly licensed registered nurse, RT, was hired by a local community hospital. RT has completed the classroom portion of the institution's orientation program and is currently being oriented to a medical unit where they will be permanently assigned. After 3 weeks on the unit the nurse manager has arranged for a meeting with RT to discuss whether the orientation program and process has met RT's needs as a newly licensed nurse. While reporting being generally satisfied with the orientation, RT shares that another nurse named TY has exhibited concerning behaviors. The nurse manager assures RT that inappropriate behavior, including bullying and incivility, will not be tolerated and asks for examples of TY's behaviors that are concerning to RT.

Item Type: Matrix

Use an X to indicate whether each statement about TY, made by RT, is an example of incivility, bullying, or constructive feedback. Each statement will have only one answer.

Statement	Incivility	Bullying	Constructive Feedback
"Tells assistive personnel that I'm difficult to work with because I am new"			
"Imitates my lisp when talking to me"			
"Identifies me continuously as the unit's new nurse who is being oriented"			

Statement	Incivility	Bullying	Constructive Feedback
"States I'll be reprimanded if I don't arrive to shift report on time"			
"Says I'm rude when I don't laugh at jokes about people of various ethnicities"			
"Tells me how to improve my time management skills"			
"Disagrees on how much time I spend on basic client care"			

Note: The answer keys for the above NGN case study are given in the back of the book in Appendix III.

 PRACTICING CONFRONTING BULLYING AND INCIVILITY WITH HONESTY AND RESPECT

Skill Building: Exercise 1

Spend some time over the next few weeks observing people's behaviors in your life. Then identify them as either overt or covert. Pay attention to the cashier at your local grocery store and how they interact with customers. Observe the behaviors of your friends, family, and colleagues. Can you identify and categorize their behaviors? The more you can easily recognize behaviors, the quicker you will be able to address them.

Skill Building: Exercise 2

Identify the behavior category in the following examples by circling overt or covert.

Situation: You are a student nurse assigned to Mr. Rossi who is a patient admitted yesterday with new-onset atrial fibrillation. Zane is the nurse assigned to Mr. Rossi. While assessing Mr. Rossi's breath sounds, you notice crackles bibasilar. The report you received from Zane indicated that his lungs were clear. You approach Zane and tell them you heard crackles bibasilar during Mr. Rossi's assessment and that you think this is a new finding.

Behavior 1: Zane interrupts you and says, "I'm sure his lungs are clear. I just listened 10 minutes ago." Zane walks away and takes a lunch break.

Overt   Covert

Behavior 2: Zane listens attentively, thanks you for sharing the information, and tells you he will assess Mr. Rossi "right away." As soon as you turn around, Zane rolls his eyes and tells another nurse, "These baby nurses think they know everything." Zane doesn't reassess Mr. Rossi.

Overt   Covert

Behavior 3: Zane doesn't make eye contact with you and says, "Go tell your instructor about Mr. Rossi's breath sounds. Isn't that his job?"

Overt   Covert

Behavior 4: Zane listens to you, immediately assesses Mr. Rossi, calls the physician and says, "I just assessed Mr. Rossi and discovered he now has crackles bibasilar." Zane ignores you for the rest of the day.

Overt   Covert

Behavior 5: Zane smiles and says, "Oh yeah. I didn't tell you about it this morning during report. I wanted to see if you could figure it out on your own."

Overt   Covert

Answers to overt and covert situations:

Behavior 1: The Answer Is Overt

Rationale: Interrupting is considered an overt behavior. Interrupting devalues the speaker, making them feel their opinion doesn't matter.

Zane openly downplays your assessment of Mr. Rossi and leaves the unit! Zane's overt behavior sends a message to you that Zane doesn't believe you and your assessment doesn't matter to him.

If answered incorrectly: Incorrect.

Behavior 2: The Answer Is Covert

Rationale: You think Zane is receptive to your input regarding Mr. Rossi. Outwardly, Zane appears interested and seems to value your input. You may think Zane is supportive and nurturing because of what you observed. However, as soon as you turned your back, Zane behaved differently. The problem with this behavior is that it is unseen by you. Zane's behavior is covert.

Behavior 3: The Answer Is Overt

Rationale: Not making eye contact with someone speaking to you can be considered rude. It's as if the person is saying, "You're not worthy of my attention." Zane doesn't accept responsibility for Mr. Rossi and "punts" the issue to your instructor.

Behavior 4: The Answer Is Covert

Rationale: Zane does demonstrate concern for Mr. Rossi by validating your assessment. Initially, it appears that Zane values your input. However, Zane takes full credit for "discovering" Mr. Rossi's change in breath sounds. Zane offers you no acknowledgment by ignoring you.

Behavior 5: The Answer Is Covert

Rationale: Zane is testing you in this situation, but, initially, you're not aware. He is sabotaging you by withholding critical information regarding Mr. Rossi. You're not aware you're "taking a test" until Zane tells you whether you've passed or failed.

REFERENCES

Al Muharraq, E. H., Baker, O. G., & Alallah, S. M. (2022). The prevalence and the relationship of workplace bullying and nurses turnover intentions: A cross sectional study. *SAGE Open Nursing, 8.* https://doi.org/10.1177/23779608221074655.

Daly, Z., Flynn-Magee, K., & Rodney, P. (2020). A call to revisit and address the history of bullying in nursing education. *Quality Advancement in Nursing Education - Avancées en formation infirmière, 6*(3), 9. https://doi.org/10.17483/2368-6669.1249.

King, C., Rossetti, J., Smith, T. J., Smyth, S., Moscatel, S., Raison, M., et al. (2021). Workplace incivility and nursing staff: An analysis through the lens of Jean Watson's Theory of Human Caring. *International Journal for Human Caring, 25*(4), 283–291.

MacDonald, C. M., Hancock, P. D., Kennedy, D. M., MacDonald, S. A., Watkins, K. E., & Baldwin, D. D. (2022). Incivility in practice-incidence and experiences of nursing students in eastern Canada: A descriptive quantitative study. *Nurse Education Today*, 105263.

Resources for Exploration

The Institute for Safe Medical Practices (2014). Disrespectful Behaviors: Their Impact, Why They Arise and Persist, and How to Address Them (Part II). https://www.ismp.org/resources/disrespectful-behaviors-their-impact-why-they-arise-and-persist-and-how-address-them-part?id=78.

The Joint Commission. (Updated 2021). Sentinel event alert 40: Behaviors that undermine a culture of safety. https://www.jointcommission.org/resources/patient-safety-topics/sentinel-event/sentinel-event-alert-newsletters/sentinel-event-alert-issue-40-behaviors-that-undermine-a-culture-of-safety/#.YmHI8OjMKUk.

The Healthy Workforce Institute. For more resources, tools, and tips regarding how to cultivate a professional and respectful work culture. https://healthyworkforceinstitute.com/.

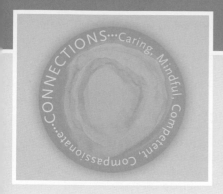

28

Managing Team Conflict Assertively and Responsibly

For good ideas and true innovation, you need human interaction, conflict, argument, debate.

Margaret Heffernam

OBJECTIVES

1. Define conflict.
2. Identify four categories of conflict.
3. Identify the steps of win–win conflict resolution.
4. Contrast win–win, lose–win, and win–lose methods of handling team conflict.

5. Identify the characteristics of five multigenerational team members and their effect on the team.
6. Participate in selected exercises to build assertive conflict-resolution skills.

? ACTIVE LEARNING

Think about how you will write your answers as you read this chapter.

What?
Write one thing you learned from this chapter.

So What?
How will this affect your nursing practice?

Now What?
How will you implement this new knowledge or skill?

Think About It ...

DEFINITION OF CONFLICT

From your work in Chapter 3, you have learned more about your own communication strengths, styles of approaching conflict, and information about the application of emotional intelligence, all of which can contribute to better communication and a positive team climate in interprofessional teams (Agreli, Peduzzi, & Baily, 2017; Azizan, Darus, & Othman, 2017; Codier & Codier, 2017). Research demonstrated that workplace conflict is one of the main sources of nurses'

stress and has been for many years (Stecker & Stecker, 2014). Conflict, often referred to as a bad thing, is a natural part of interactions and can improve relationships and promote organizational growth. Donnelly (2018), editor of the journal *Holistic Nursing Practice*, suggested we embrace disagreement and negativity as a strategy for problem solving. She advised that next time a colleague expresses a negative view, you should listen carefully, ask questions to clarify, and separate the emotions from the possibilities.

Smooth functioning of interprofessional teams is essential for safe, quality care in a complex, high-risk industry (Stucky, Wymer, & House, 2021), and unprecedented stressors from the COVID-19 pandemic make working together challenging (Tannenbaum, Traylor, Thomas, & Salas, 2021). Dealing effectively with conflict is a core competency. Conflict may be viewed as a feeling, a disagreement, a real or perceived incompatibility of interests, inconsistent worldviews, or a set of behaviors (Mayer, 2012). Conflict arises when interdependency exists, and conflict resolution is necessary to build positive relationships with others and to meet our own needs. Whenever two people come together, there is the potential for conflict. Although conflict is inevitable, it can have advantageous outcomes when it is handled in assertive and responsible ways. Conflict resolution can build interdependence and professional collaboration and can help team members better address the big-picture issues. Building positive coworker relationships, teamwork, and collaboration supports clear communication, which has a direct effect on patient safety. New staff who enter an established healthcare team need support to be integrated into the team to encourage mutual respect and positive relationships (McKibben, 2017). In Chapter 4 you read about the importance of interprofessional education and team communication skills in prevention of medical errors. The Joint Commission Center for Transforming Healthcare (Zhani, 2010) reported that an "estimated 80% of serious medical errors involve miscommunication between caregivers when responsibility for patients is transferred or handed off." In their Hand-Off Communication Project, participating hospitals found that more than 37% of hand-offs were defective, preventing the receiver of the information from safely caring for the patient. After implementing targeted solutions to the hand-off communication, the result was a 52% reduction in defective hand-offs.

SIMPLIFY AND DEEPEN

You need your own love to save your heart.

Rithvik Singh

Cushnie (1988) identified four categories of conflict intensifying in degree of difficulty from first to last: facts, methods, goals, and values.

Facts

Conflicts about facts are differences about data. These disagreements can be resolved by terminating the debate and seeking information from reliable sources.

Methods

Conflicts about methods are differences about how something is done. A conflict about methods occurs when there is no absolute standard shared by all parties affected by the issue. Resolving conflicts of this kind includes acknowledging that there is more than one way to accomplish the same goal or task. A way to minimize this type of conflict is to establish criteria for method selection.

Goals

Goal conflicts are differences about desired outcomes. Discussion often reveals that parties share a common concern. If they are able to identify a common goal, this redefinition opens up new opportunities for problem solving.

Values

Differences in belief systems are the most complex type of conflict, and a high level of motivation is required from involved parties to understand each other's beliefs. If the parties can avoid the divisiveness of allocating others' viewpoints to rigid categories of "right" or "wrong" and find compatible goals, then they are on their way to conflict management (Cushnie, 1988).

TYPES OF CONFLICT

Several forms of conflict are seen (Kinder, 1981):

- Intrapersonal conflict occurs within an individual.
- Interpersonal conflict occurs between two individuals or among members of a group.
- Intragroup conflict occurs within an established group.
- Intergroup conflict is the struggle between groups.

This chapter focuses on interpersonal conflict in a workplace or school setting.

Healthcare teams are composed of people with many different backgrounds. A variety of professional outlooks are found in a team of nurses, physicians, clergy, nutritionists, occupational and physical therapists, social workers, and others. In addition to the differences in socialization of these professionals, they carry personal views based on sex, age, cultural origin, socioeconomic situation, and life experience. This potpourri is a potential source of conflict in any healthcare team.

This variety results in different perceptions about an issue and the role and obligations each should fulfill. When team members do not agree about a situation or their respective roles, then the potential for conflict is great.

Team members often have different (or opposing) ideological views about a given situation. Their views may come from having different objectives or from endorsing different priorities among the objectives. Conflict results when team members do not agree on what to do, how to do it, and when to do it. Review Chapter 22 for the stages of group behavior. Remember that group conflict is healthy and expected in the storming stage.

Occasionally, conflict resurfaces between team members who have had a long history of disagreement. The level of trust and collaboration has been worn down between these people, and their competitiveness is sharpened. Such a situation fuels conflict.

CONFLICT-RESOLUTION APPROACHES

You know you cannot avoid conflict. What you can avoid is feeling impotent or uncomfortable when you encounter situations involving conflict. By now you are familiar with assertive and responsible communication. These approaches can help you resolve conflicts in constructive ways.

Resolving a conflict means acting in such a way that an agreement is reached that is acceptable, and even pleasing, to both parties. If both parties cannot agree on a resolution, the conflict will continue. When conflict drags out and team members do not see a hopeful resolution, then helplessness prevails. Any healthcare team that is stuck in this hopeless situation is not working at its full capacity. Harrington-Mackin (1994) advised dealing with conflicts in a timely way and suggested that most people find it difficult to openly discuss and work through conflicts. Instead, they accumulate grudges and use techniques such as procrastination and sniping to "get even." Client care and morale suffer when conflicts remain unresolved.

You can approach conflict resolution in three ways: win–win, lose–win, or win–lose. Although win–win is preferable, there may be times when a workable compromise is the best solution to avoid having both parties lose. Throughout this book, the point has been made that assertiveness is a matter of choice. There may be times when you feel obligated to insist on your solution to a problem, such as in parenting a small child. There may be times when you choose to allow the other person to win, such as when you recognize that a colleague has been pushed to the limit and your position seems less important than their peace of mind.

The win–win approach to conflict resolution requires you to be assertive and responsible. This approach results in a solution with which you and your colleagues are happy. Not only is the outcome satisfactory, but adopting a win–win approach uses your full creativity and often results in a unique and innovative resolution.

The lose–win approach is one in which you allow your colleagues to resolve the conflict at your expense. Either you are not happy with the outcome or you permit your colleagues to walk all over you. This approach is nonassertive and irresponsible.

The win–lose approach is the opposite of the lose–win approach. You may resolve the conflict in a way that is satisfying to you, but, in the process, you bulldoze over the rights of your colleagues. This approach is aggressive and irresponsible.

Any win–lose/lose–win approach creates forces that aggravate the struggle and do little to discover constructive solutions acceptable to all involved. A conflict is more constructive when the outcome is satisfying to all the participants than when it is satisfying to only some. Conflict at some point is inevitable, so it helps to know how to use it as an opportunity to be constructive, because the alternatives have unpleasant consequences.

A win–win conflict management strategy covers each of the following steps (Flanagan, 1995):

1. View the problem in terms of needs (what is required) instead of solutions (what should be done) to facilitate a mutual problem-solving approach; detach yourself from biases and stay focused on the actual data.
2. Consider the problem as a mutual one to be solved, requiring the active involvement of all affected persons.
3. Describe the conflict as specifically as possible, using undistorted data.
4. Identify the differences between concerned parties before attempting to resolve the conflict.
5. See the conflict from another point of view.
6. Use brainstorming to arrive at possible solutions instead of adopting the first or most convenient idea.
7. Select the solution that best meets both parties' needs and considers all possible consequences.
8. Reach an agreement about how the conflict is to end and not recur.
9. Plan who will do what and where, as well as when it will be done.
10. After the plan has been implemented, evaluate the problem-solving process, and review how well the solution turned out.

Table 28.1 summarizes three approaches to conflict. The assertive, responsible attitude toward conflict and approach

TABLE 28.1	Assertive/Responsible versus Nonassertive/Irresponsible Ways of Handling Team Conflict			
Characteristic Win	**Win–Win**	**Lose–Win**	**Win–Lose**	
Attitude toward conflict	Assumes conflict is inevitable and occurs whenever people work together	Assumes conflicts are sent to try us	Sees conflict as a challenge to be won	
	Assumes that conflict can be managed so that creative solutions are achieved	Assumes that, in a conflict, the other person always wins	Considers that manipulation is needed to win conflicts and that it is never ceasing and thinks fighting is required to get what you want	

Continued

TABLE 28.1 **Assertive/Responsible versus Nonassertive/Irresponsible Ways of Handling Team Conflict—cont'd**

Characteristic Win	Win–Win	Lose–Win	Win–Lose
	Assumes that controversy involves everything in the issue and increases members' commitment	Assumes that it is a foregone conclusion that the plan to resolve the conflict will satisfy only others	Believes the other person is trying hard to win
	Assumes that conflict can be resolved in ways that are satisfying to all team members	Wonders why there must be conflict in the workplace	—
Approach to conflict resolution	Uses a systematic problem-solving approach	Decides in advance that the other person will win and gives up	Keeps fighting with biased information that supports his or her own viewpoint
Data collection	Examines his or her own thoughts and feelings objectively	Prematurely closes data collection	Seeks, examines, and submits only data that support his or her own desired resolution
	Listens emphatically to colleagues' points of view	Assumes it is hopeless to collect data because of an irrational belief that others will win regardless	—
	Seeks relevant information from appropriate resources (literature, consultants)	Dwells on how bad things will be if the conflict is not resolved	—
	Shares knowledge of the conflict with all others involved	Passively participates in information sharing	—
	Remains objective	—	—
Assessment	Formulates an accurate definition of the conflict	Defines the conflict in terms of how it affects colleagues	Does not seek out colleagues' assessments of the conflict
	Shares assessment with colleagues	Defines conflict from his or her own point of view	Overwhelmingly argues for his or her own assessment of the conflict
	Acknowledges colleagues' perceptions of the conflict	—	—
Resolution generation	Considers resolutions that satisfy all involved	Contributes little to this planning because of the assumption that the winner will tell the loser what to do	Only considers or supports plans that agree with his or her own interpretation of the conflict
	Chooses resolutions that maximize the benefits and minimize the drawbacks	—	Sabotages plans that oppose his or her own view
Evaluation	Maintains vigilance to ensure that resolution continues to satisfy self and colleagues on the team	Complains that resolution could never be successful; disgruntled	Ignores the fact that others are not satisfied with the resolution

to conflict resolution (win-win) is contrasted with the non-assertive, irresponsible approaches (lose-win and win-lose).

ASSERTIVE AND RESPONSIBLE WAYS TO OVERCOME CONFLICT

On healthcare teams, conflict can involve all members or only a few. How to manage conflict using a win–win approach in both these instances is explored.

> **WIT AND WISDOM**
> One-liners to start a tough conversation:
> *I'm puzzled by…*
> *I'm curious about what your thoughts were on…*
> *Could you help me understand…?*
> *I need your help (name of person you are addressing)…*

Conflict Situation Involving the Entire Healthcare Team

1. Before you can do anything to resolve a conflict, you need to fully understand the conflict, including your own thoughts and feelings about the situation, as well as the thoughts of your colleagues. If you try to resolve a conflict without completing an assessment, you will probably overlook an important factor that could result in an unsatisfactory resolution.

Example: You believe clients have the right to be informed about any untoward side effects they might experience when taking a prescribed medication. On your unit, few clients are told in advance of the potential side effects. This omission is incompatible with your beliefs about good nursing care and client rights. You discover that many of your colleagues, including the other nurses and physicians on your team, prefer to keep knowledge of side effects from clients so that they will be more likely to take the medication. Here the conflict is incompatible activities (informing versus not informing) and incompatible beliefs about clients' rights (autonomy versus dependency).

2. To fully understand your side of the conflict, you need to examine your own thoughts and feelings. You cannot complete this step in a hurry. You need to sit down (with paper and pencil if necessary) and discover your answers to the questions that follow.

What Is It About This Conflict that Bothers Me?

In considering the conflict, you might have some of the following thoughts:

- "It bothers me that clients are not warned about side effects that might result from the medications."

- "It's not right that they don't have full knowledge of the treatment and that they are taking the pills without fully understanding the implications."

- "I believe that it is dishonest to withhold information about side effects from clients."

- "I believe that people have the responsibility to decide what they should do about their health. By withholding information, we are keeping the control of clients' health in our hands."

Answering this question makes it clearer what the conflict means to you. You have a strong belief that clients should be given the information they need to make the best decision about what health behavior to adopt.

Our initial reaction to a conflict situation is often influenced more by emotion than by intellect. The tension or anxiety creates a fight-or-flight stress response, and the intensity of the stress response varies in relation to the degree of threat perceived (Cushnie, 1988). Taking time to sort out your emotional reactions as you just did helps you control your emotions and increases your effectiveness in conflict management.

What Resolution to This Conflict Would Be Satisfactory for Me?

It is important to answer this question. Often, we know there is a conflict but are uncertain about how we want it resolved. The clearer you can be in answering these questions, the more articulate you will be to others about your stand on the issue.

In thinking about how you would like to have the conflict resolved, you come up with the following idea:

- "The most satisfactory resolution for me would be to institute a policy that all clients will be informed in advance about any possible side effects of any medication prescribed for them."

3. Discover what your colleagues' responses are to the same two questions you just answered yourself. This step requires you to invest time and energy, but you need this information to have a complete understanding of the conflict. The best approach is to arrange a time to sit down with your colleagues and obtain this information.

What Is It About This Conflict that Bothers Them?

Your colleagues may come up with some of the following ideas:

- "If we told every client about possible side effects, it would take too much time."

- "If clients knew all the possible side effects, they might not take the medications and then they would never benefit from them."

- "I believe that we should not scare clients by telling them everything that can go wrong. After all, they're already sick. Why add to their worries?"

You are learning that your colleagues have their clients' interests at heart when your colleagues avoid telling their clients about the side effects. They have raised a significant point about the time factor as well. Discovering alternative viewpoints expands your awareness of conflict you encounter.

What Resolution to the Conflict Would Be Satisfactory for Your Colleagues?

These are some examples of what your colleagues might tell you:

- "The only solution I can see is to tell only those clients who ask about the side effects."
- "I think we should give out information only about the most common and significant side effects so that clients will be inclined to take their medications."
- "I think we should continue as usual. I've never known any client who was upset about not knowing the side effects of the medications. They need the medications to get well."

These suggestions from your colleagues tell you that they value something more than client autonomy; they value compliance and recovery from illness. You have learned that some of your colleagues are agreeable to informing clients about side effects under certain circumstances.

Finding the answers to these questions will require your best interpersonal communication skills. When you are invested in an issue, it becomes harder to see other points of view. In a conflict situation it is important to listen actively to what your colleagues have to say and check that you have understood their side of the issue.

4. In addition to information obtained from the thoughts and feelings of the people involved in the conflict, you may need information from other sources. In this example, you could seek the counsel of the hospital's legal advisor about the rights of your clients. There may be a clients' rights committee that could advise you.

For example, your legal counsel may advise you that "clients have the right by law to be informed of any likely untoward effects of any treatment regimen, unless such information would be considered by the caregivers to be threatening to the client's well-being." A guideline such as this is sufficiently nonspecific so that your healthcare team would have to make its own interpretation of its application.

5. Once you have fully explored how you and your colleagues feel about the conflict and have acquired any other relevant information, the next step is to search for a resolution that will be satisfactory to all of you. This is no easy feat; the win–win approach takes time and effort.

One creative approach at this stage is to brainstorm. Out of brainstorming is likely to come a creative and original resolution to your conflict. It is important that everyone involved in the conflict has an opportunity to contribute ideas about how to resolve it. In this example, there should be representation from nurses, physicians, and clients.

In the brainstorming process, it is important that every idea be considered and that no ideas be ridiculed or eliminated. Using this rule means that team members must acknowledge and respect each other's ideas. This action of listening to one another helps to diffuse any hostility that may have arisen as the conflict grew. In a conflict, competition often reigns, with individuals wanting to get their own way; brainstorming ensures that team members communicate in a cooperative way.

In this situation, the following suggestions for resolution of the conflict were put forward:

- Give information about side effects only to clients who ask for it.
- Before clients start on a medication, require that they be able to recite its benefits and side effects.
- Leave a copy of a drug description manual in the clients' common room so that any clients who wish to check on the side effects of a medication can do so.
- Give clients copies of the telephone numbers of the pharmaceutical companies so that they can call a representative and obtain any information about drugs that are prescribed for them.
- Have the pharmacist prepare information sheets about the side effects of clients' drugs that would be available for them to keep and review.
- Give a card to every client admitted to the unit that defines the right-to-know policy concerning side effects of treatments and medications and indicates that clients need only ask the staff to receive this information.
- Wait until clients experience side effects and then clearly explain them.
- Initiate a policy of inviting questions from clients about the side effects of a medication.

You can see that the suggestions represent a variety of points of view.

6. The next step is to choose an acceptable resolution from the many suggestions put forth. The most expedient action to take on this unit is to form a committee composed of staff members representing both sides of the conflict, as well as clients and administrators of the unit.

You are selected as a member who favors informed consent. Another nurse with the point of view that informing clients can cause unnecessary problems is also selected. The head nurse, one physician, and a representative from the clients' rights committee complete the membership.

This committee has the responsibility to develop a policy about what information to give clients concerning side effects of their medications. The decision it makes must meet certain criteria in a win–win approach to conflict resolution. It must satisfy both points of view, be feasible to carry out on the unit (in terms of cost and staffing abilities), and be legally sound.

7. The next step is to systematically review the pros and cons of the eligible resolutions remaining. At this stage, team members must remain open to others' points of view and give all members a chance to defend or refute points. When a group is trying to reach the best decision, it must create a climate that allows members to speak freely.

Consider the effect that the possibility of territoriality or competition among members might have on communication. Members sabotage each other by providing misleading or biased information that results in mistrust. When the communication breaks down this way, it is unlikely that the best decision will be chosen because the database will be incomplete and inaccurate. It takes a concerted effort by the members and the leader to ensure that all points of view are encouraged and respected.

8. After considerable discussion, the group narrows down the choices for resolution to the following:

   - Give a card to clients when they are admitted to the unit that advises them that they have the right to know the side effects of any medications and that they need only ask the staff to receive this information.
   - Initiate a policy in which nurses and physicians invite questions from clients about the side effects of their medications at the time clients are started on a new medication.
   - Require that before clients start taking a medication, they be able to recite its benefits and side effects.

After much deliberation, the committee decides that distributing cards for clients would be too expensive. The members come up with the idea of adding a paragraph to address these issues to the "Permission for Treatment" sheet that all clients must sign on admission.

This action appeals to all members of the committee. They believe that it would inform clients of their rights at the beginning of their hospital stay and instill the idea that their questions would be welcomed and answered in a clear way.

The second decision made by the committee is to endorse the following suggestion as unit policy:

Each time clients start on a new medication they will be informed of the benefits, untoward side effects, and any special instructions for taking the medication in a simple, clear way. At this time, they will be invited and encouraged to ask any questions.

The committee takes a lot of time to arrive at this decision. None of the committee members has difficulty with the suggestion of telling clients about the benefits of medications, but they are reluctant to explain the potential hazards. After looking at the issue from many angles, all members agree that it is unfair to give clients only half of the picture. A compromise is drawn in which all concur that only the most likely side effects will be explained to clients and the probability of their occurrence will be specified. Any known corrective action will also be made known to clients (e.g., taking a laxative for constipation, drinking extra fluids and chewing gum for dryness in the mouth, and avoiding abrupt movements for vertigo).

Committee members agree that the workload for launching this new policy will be shared between physicians and nurses. A physician prescribing a new medication will be responsible for explaining the rationale, benefits, and risks to clients and will invite questions. This delegation will mean that nurses alone will not incur the extra time that implementing this policy will demand.

In addition, it has been decided that the medication nurse will follow up the physician's explanation when the first dose of the medication is administered. At that time the nurse will find out what the clients understand about the benefits and risks, confirm the facts, correct the errors, and invite any further questions. Sharing the responsibility between physicians and nurses makes the time commitment feasible for both parties.

The committee stresses that no health professional should be expected to remember the side effects of a multitude of medications. Referring to pharmaceutical references and consulting with the hospital pharmacist are encouraged.

The committee's chosen resolutions are satisfactory to all team members and are feasible from an administrative point of view.

9. The process does not stop at the point of agreeing on a resolution. Once the plan is implemented, a follow-up evaluation must be performed to determine whether the healthcare team remains satisfied with the implementation of the resolution. Questions to consider in completing this evaluation might include the following:

   - Do those who felt strongly that clients have a right to know about side effects believe that clients are being correctly informed?
   - Do those who objected because it could be time consuming and frightening for clients believe that the new plan avoids these negative consequences?
   - Are clients of the opinion that their rights are being respected?
   - Is the resolution being carried out without undue drawbacks in terms of cost effectiveness and staffing patterns?

Each time clients start on a new medication they will be informed of the benefits and untoward effects in a simple, clear way. At this time, they will be invited and encouraged to ask any questions.

In this example, the committee decides to meet 6 weeks after the resolution has been adopted to evaluate its effectiveness.

This healthcare team handled its conflict using a win–win conflict-resolution strategy. All sides were asked to contribute their opinions to resolve the conflict. This action was assertive because it prevented any one side from coloring the picture or totally biasing the issue. It was responsible because it considered all the data available in the conflict situation: thoughts and feelings of both parties and objective data from a legal perspective.

Self-Care Nudge

Try alternate nostril breathing for stress relief for yourself, and teach it to patients. Close one nostril with your finger, breathe through the other nostril. Then close that nostril and exhale through the opposite nostril. Repeat slowly several times (Jahan et al., 2020). Find a video online.

Conflict Situation Involving Two Team Members

In contrast to the previous situation, conflict situations can be isolated to a small segment of the healthcare team. An example in which two team members are in conflict is examined next.

Example: You and David are two nursing students on the same medical unit in a general hospital. You are a student in an early stage of your clinical experience, and David is in his graduating year. You are studying the concept of loss and its effects on body image. You wish to have Mr. Partain as your client because he has recently had a severe myocardial infarction, and it is unlikely that he will be able to resume his former job. Because he has suffered a loss in physical function that affects other areas of his life, he would make an excellent candidate for your assignment.

David has been assigned as Mr. Partain's nurse and has been caring for him for the past 3 days. When you ask David if he would switch and let you take on Mr. Partain's care, David refuses on the grounds that he needs to learn about postcardiac care for an assignment he is doing.

At the moment, Mr. Partain is the most suitable candidate for both these students. There is a conflict over limited resources in this situation.

1. The first step is to uncover all the information about the conflict. Accomplishing this task involves being open and listening actively. One technique for ensuring that you really understand the conflict from the other's point

of view is to reflect with empathy each statement your colleague makes. Here is an example:

David: *"I think we have a problem here because I need to continue my care of Mr. Partain to understand how postcardiac clients adjust to the limited activity and cope with the fear of resuming normal functioning. I can't change with you."*

At this point, it would be tempting for you to argue that you, too, need to study Mr. Partain's recovery to understand his loss. Such a defensive approach would escalate your conflict. Instead, to understand the conflict from David's point of view, all you are allowed to do at this point is to reflect his thoughts and feelings with empathy. You will soon get your turn to state things from your point of view.

You: *"You want to continue nursing Mr. Partain for a longer period of time so that you really understand the reaction of postcardiac patients to changes in their activity levels."*

This response allows your colleague to feel understood and encourages him to reveal more of his point of view.

David: *"This is one of my last assignments before I graduate, and I'm afraid if I give up Mr. Partain now, I will not find another postcardiac client with whom to do my assignment."*

You: *"I can see why you do not wish to switch with me. You're concerned that he may turn out to be the last such client before graduation and you need the experience."*

In addition to allowing David to feel understood, reflecting with empathy obliges you to fully understand the conflict from his point of view. Without this information, you could not come up with the most effective resolution.

You are entitled to describe the conflict from your point of view, and you therefore explain to David the importance of Mr. Partain to your own client assignment. You have no control over whether David will listen with empathy to your side of the conflict, but your previous active listening will increase the chances.

2. Once you understand the conflict, the next step is to work out a satisfactory resolution. The resolution most acceptable to both you and David (to be Mr. Partain's primary nurse) is mutually incompatible. You need to generate another suitable resolution. Unlike the situation in the first example, there is limited time in which to do so. You propose the following suggestions to David:

- When David is off duty, you will take over as the nurse in charge of Mr. Partain's care.
- You will share with David any information you have on loss as it applies to the postcardiac client in return for being able to ask him questions about Mr. Partain's adjustment.

David accepts your suggestions and offers the following ones that might be helpful to you:

- You can be present when he is talking to Mr. Partain (if the client agrees) so that you can apply some of what he gleans to your study of the concepts of loss and body image.
- You can consider the case of Mrs. Tenn, a diabetic client on the unit, who is upset that her diabetes prevents her from becoming pregnant again. Mrs. Tenn might make a suitable client for your study of loss.
- He will give you a copy of his paper when it is completed because your topics overlap and you might find it helpful.

This brainstorming has generated several possible resolutions that have benefits for both of you. If you and David adopt all the suggestions, both of you will gain more than you could have if you each went your separate ways. In addition to achieving your learning goals, you both will have the opportunity to learn from each other and possibly develop a closer friendship.

3. After adopting any resolution to a conflict, it is important to check to see if the plan continues to meet your expectations. The bottom line in this situation is that both you and David complete your assignments. Any additional happenings will be bonuses.

You can see that two of the important processes in effective conflict resolution are empathy and problem-solving. Making these two strategies influential in your conflict-resolution approach ensures that you will be assertive and responsible.

 MOMENT OF CONNECTION...

A Nursing Student Tackles Team Conflict

We were working on our group mental health project, and one of my classmates always has an attitude that is nonproductive and makes the assignment even harder. Instead of getting angry and bottling up my emotions, I decided to address the issue right away. After a couple of minutes of attitude, I interrupted her to tell her that her attitude was a problem. Either she could change her tone or dismiss herself. I said it in an assertive, not aggressive tone. I said what everybody else in the group wanted to say but did not from lack of courage or a desire to keep peace. That night I was upset, thinking I

had been aggressive and maybe we should have just put up with her. The next day we met again and for the first time, no attitude! It was very exciting for all of us, and we actually finished the project that day. I love practicing assertiveness and have been doing it when I need to. It is making a real difference in my life.

THE MULTIGENERATIONAL TEAM

Nursing involves unique challenges and opportunities in the blend of team members from different generations. Misperceptions about the motivation of nurses older or younger can cause conflict when we expect everyone to have our point of view. Moss (2018) suggested different generations have different definitions of what is thought of as common language and recommended discourse between generations about respect, accountability, loyalty, and coaching.

Our workforce has five generations: traditionalists, veterans, or the silent generation, born from 1937 to 1945; Baby Boomers, born from 1945 to 1964; Generation X (or latch-key), born from 1965 to 1976; Generation Y (Millennials or Net Generation), born from 1977 to 1991; and Generation Z (or iGeneration), born 1992 to 2012 (Anthony, 2006; Bell, 2013; Kupperschmidt, 2006; Sherman, 2006; Weston, 2006).

Although depending on generalizations about different generations can be problematic, it is helpful to begin to look at some commonalities among these five groups.

Traditionalists were raised to value a strong work ethic, seeing nursing as a "calling." They pride themselves on doing a good job, believing in discipline and respect. They are team players and realists. Of the nursing workforce in the United States, 10% is older than 65 years, which is more than ever before with increased life expectancies and economic changes.

Baby Boomers, 55% of Western society's workforce, were raised more permissively and were encouraged to be independent, seeing nursing as a "profession." They are idealists, are inner directed, and tend to be workaholics.

Generation X was raised in two-career families; may have been latch-key children; may have lived in a single-parent home; and, having seen no evidence of job security in nursing, see themselves as free agents with a responsibility to build skills for their own marketability. They have seen their parents' commitment to work not paying off in their professional or personal lives. They are cynical and want balance and respect for their personal priorities.

Generation Y, or the Millennial Generation, has been raised in a time of violence with digital technology and multiculturalism, with their childhood protected and family supported with preschool and after-school programs.

They multitask and expect instant feedback and customization. They are used to 24/7 global Internet access. Nursing is seen as an occupation or job in which there should be cutting-edge technology and a quick response to problems.

Generation Z, the iGeneration or digital natives, have always known handheld computers and cell phones. This generation is now in nursing school or are new graduates and expect to be able to work or study while texting, surfing the "Net," or participating in a social network. They have watched international disasters on television, were in high school during the 2008 global recession, are close to family, and are confident and open to change (Bell, 2013; Kupperschmidt, 2006; Weston, 2006).

Conflict arises when nurses from one generation blame the other for having "an attitude" rather than a different worldview based on different life experiences. The framework of clarify, articulate, request, encourage (CARE) confrontations, discussed in Chapter 24, is a helpful approach to beginning a dialogue about differences, perceptions, and expectations. Traditionalists bring attention to details and best use of resources. Boomers can assist with consensus building and mentoring. Nurses from Generation X bring the entrepreneurial spirit and skill with technology. Generation Y is sensitive to different cultures and is comfortable with new technology (Kupperschmidt, 2006). Generation Z nurses can work with Generation Y to help earlier generations with shortcuts to using informational technology. Earlier generations can help younger generations with face-to-face communication skills (Bell, 2013). Nurses who begin to see these differences as gifts to round out the skills of the team will be able to broaden their perspective and work better as a team with the goal of quality patient care and high team spirit.

CONFLICT RESOLUTION AND THE NURSING PROFESSION

Conflict can be a positive force for nursing if it is used to foster growth-producing change in the profession and in the organizations in which nurses work. In addition to being knowledgeable about managing conflicts, nurses must develop a positive attitude toward conflict by recognizing the potential gains to be realized from it. We need to become more astute at predicting potential conflicts. A study of the complex needs of healthcare teams indicated that team members expect nurses to communicate clearly to ensure quality decisions and to promote team synergy (Propp et al., 2010). Misunderstandings, lack of clarity, and discomfort with differences can fuel conflict. "Virtual" teams, people in different geographic locations communicating electronically, are now in place. Ferrazzi (2014) reported that with the right team, the right leadership, the right touch points, and the right technology, team productivity can be maximized.

Evidence-Based Strategies for Teamwork during a Crisis

Building upon 30 years study and advising teams, Tannenbaum et al. (2021) offer seven recommendations for effective teamwork in a pandemic or other crisis situation:

1. Acknowledge big and small successes to build "collective efficacy," a belief in the team's ability to be successful.
2. Ensure shared mindsets (i.e., updated priorities, clarified responsibilities, and updated information) for interventions.
3. Remember the people who are behind the scenes. Offer recognition for those in supportive roles, those making sure that there are adequate supplies and that families are kept up to date.
4. Watch out for each other and monitor each other for safe practices. In high-stress situations, people can lose team focus. Offer a prebrief at the shift beginning. Watch for team members who are tired, and make asking for and offering help common behaviors.
5. Promote psychological safety of team members. Support assertive behavior of speaking up and disagreeing without fear of punishment. This helps a team be more effective through open problem solving.
6. Support team members' concerns about their "home" team, their family. During the pandemic, team members helped identify resources for financial, emotional, or material support for children and families of staff.
7. Boost resilience. When conflicts have arisen, staff members take the time to "mend" the situation. Keeping updated and preparing for anticipated stressors help support the team's effectiveness.

We are all in this together.

🌸 MOMENTS OF CONNECTION…
When "Just Listen to the Doctor" Won't Work

"As a pain management nurse, I was concerned about a very sick client who needed a refill for his morphine pump. Our physician said the client had to come into the clinic. Other staff said that, since I work full time, the doctor would not get reimbursement if the client did not make a clinic visit, so I should 'just listen to the doctor.' I told the doctor that I could do a home visit and do the refill there. He gave his permission, and I received an orientation from the home health agency staff. I visited the home four times to refill the pump as the dosage was increased. The client and his wife were so happy. He died last month. Yes, it would have been easier to comply without question, but even though everyone anticipated that there would be a problem, there really was no conflict, just a difference of opinion."

Return to "Active Learning" at the beginning of the chapter and write your responses.

PRACTICING MANAGING TEAM CONFLICT ASSERTIVELY AND RESPONSIBLY

Application: Exercise 1

Reflecting on what you learned about yourself in Chapter 3, discuss how your personal strengths, emotional intelligence, and approach to conflict might positively affect your positive contribution to the interprofessional healthcare team. Identify personal challenges or areas for growth in working with teams from what you learned.

Skill Building/Critical Thinking: Exercise 2

In your journal, make a list of people in your professional and personal life who represent each of the five generations discussed. Reflect on where you fit in the generations, and write an entry about differences you have seen in behavior or attitude, assumptions you have made, and what you have learned from beginning to understand the other four generations.

Quality and Safety Education for Nurses Learning Strategy: Exercise 3 QSEN

Observe interactions among the multiple team members involved in caring for your client. Describe the interactions concerning how differences of opinion or conflict are handled. Select one example to describe how it was handled.

- How would you describe the interactions and relationships among the group?
- How would you describe the chain of command or hierarchy?
- What could be improved?
- What lessons can you learn about your own team interactions?
- How did these interactions affect safety?
- What effect will this interaction have on future interactions among this group?

REFERENCES

Agreli, H. F., Peduzzi, M., & Baily, C. (2017). Contributions of team climate in the study of interprofessional collaboration: A conceptual analysis. *Journal of Interprofessional Care, 31*(6), 679.

Anthony, M. (2006). Overview and summary: The multigenerational workforce: boomers and Xers and Nets, oh my! *Online Journal of Issues in Nursing, 11*(2), 11.

Azizan, F. L., Darus, A., & Othman, N. (2017). Team coordination influencing team effectiveness: A study of nursing team. *International Journal of Management Research and Review, 7*(9), 893.

Bell, J. A. (2013). Five generations in the nursing workforce. *Journal for Nurses in Professional Development, 29*(4), 205.

Codier, E., & Codier, D. D. (2017). Could emotional intelligence make patients safer? *American Journal of Nursing, 117*(7), 58.

Cushnie, P. (1988). Conflict: developing resolution skills. *Association of Perioperative Registered Nurses Journal, 47*(3), 732.

Donnelly, G. F. (2018). Embracing negativity to improve work environments. *Holistic Nursing Practice, 32*(3), 21.

Ferrazzi, K. (2014). Managing yourself: Getting virtual teams right. *Harvard Business Review,* 120–123.

Flanagan, L. (1995). *What you need to know about today's workplace: A survival guide for nurses.* Washington, DC: American Nurses Association.

Harrington-Mackin, D. (1994). *The team building tool kit: Tips, tactics, and rules for effective workplace teams.* New York, NY: American Management Association.

Jahan, I., Begum, M., Akhter, S., Islam, Z., Jahan, N., & Haque, M. (2020). Effects of alternate nostril breathing exercise on respiratory functions in healthy young adults leading stressful lifestyle. *Journal of Population Therapeutics and Clinical Pharmacology, 27*(1), e104–e114, Mar 19, 2020. doi:10.15586/jptcp.v27i1.668.

Kinder, J. S. (1981). *Conflict and diploma nursing education, management of conflict.* New York, NY: National League for Nursing.

Kupperschmidt, B. R. (2006). Address multigenerational conflict: Mutual respect and confronting as strategy. *Online Journal of Issues in Nursing, 11*(2), 14.

Mayer, B. S. (2012). *The dynamics of conflict resolution: A guide to engagement and intervention.* San Francisco, CA: Jossey-Bass.

McKibben, L. (2017). Conflict management: Importance and implications. *British Journal of Nursing, 26*(2), 100.

Moss, K. D. (2018). Decoding: Generational discourse—cracking the code to improve communication across generations. *Nurse Leader, 16*(1), 34.

Propp, K. M., Apker, J., Zabava Ford, W. S., Wallace, N., Serbenski, M., & Hofmeister, N. (2010). Meeting the complex needs of the health care team: Identification of nurse–team communication practices perceived to enhance patient outcomes. *Quality Health Research, 20*(1), 15.

Sherman, R. O. (2006). Leading a multigenerational nursing workforce: Issues, challenges, and strategies. *Online Journal of Nursing Issues, 11*(2), 13.

Stecker, M., & Stecker, M. M. (2014). Disruptive staff interactions: A serious source of interprovider conflict and stress in health care settings. *Issues of Mental Health Nursing, 35*(7), 533.

Stucky, C. H., Wymer, J. A., & House, S. (2021). Nurse leaders: Transforming interprofessional relationships to bridge healthcare quality and safety. *Nurse Leader, 2022.* https://doi.org/10.1016/j.mnl.2021.12.003.

Tannenbaum, S. I., Traylor, A. M., Thomas., E. J., & Salas, E. (2021). Managing teamwork in the face of pandemic: Evidence-based tips. *British Medical Journal of Quality and Safety, 30*, 59–63. doi:10.1136/bmjqs-2020-011447.

Weston, M. J. (2006). Integrating generational perspectives in nursing. *Online Journal of Nursing Issues, 11*(2), 12.

Zhani, E. E. (2010). Joint Commission Center for Transforming Healthcare tackles miscommunication among caregivers: Top U.S. hospitals identify causes, develop targeted solutions to save lives, News Release (globenewswire.com).

29

Communicating at the End of Life

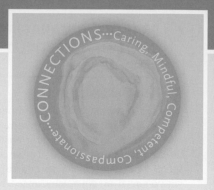

Laughter, tears, and silence came like healing waves into the hospital room. I think one of the keys to dying well is creating space and giving permission for these three healing friends to do their work.

Jarem Sawatsky in Dancing with elephants: Mindfulness training for those living with dementia, chronic illness, or an aging brain (2017)

OBJECTIVES

1. Identify fears about communicating with clients near the end of life.
2. Discuss strategies for caring communication near the end of life.
3. Identify strategies for creative expression for clients at the end of life and their families.
4. Identify strategies for the nurse to deal with grief.
5. Discuss the role of self-care for the nurse when working with clients at the end of life and their families.
6. Participate in exercises to build strategies for caring communication with clients near the end of life and their families.

❓ ACTIVE LEARNING

Think about how you will write your answers as you read this chapter.

What?
Write one thing you learned from this chapter.

So What?
How will this affect your nursing practice?

Now What?
How will you implement this new knowledge or skill?

Think About It ...

THE IMPORTANCE OF COMMUNICATION IN END-OF-LIFE CARE

The COVID-19 pandemic challenged nurses and families to cope with separation and isolation in ways we could not imagine. Nurses used their phones to initiate video contact between families and their loved ones. Nurses rolled wheelchairs to a window for the family and patient to see each other. Nurses were often caught in the middle, having to reinforce strict visitation rules in the face of a disease no one really understood. When touch and presence has been so important and families could not always be there, nurses sat and held the hand of the dying patient. We know the importance of mindfulness, being fully present without judgment. We continually reflect on how to support students of nursing and nurses who are growing their communication skills and have made great strides.

Jeffers et al. (2022) conducted a qualitative study of students' participation in high-fidelity simulation with a focus on difficult end-of-life communication. Jeffers reviews educational initiative: the End-of-Life Nursing Education Consortium (ELNEC), which continually updates its education for palliative care. Goldsmith & Wittenberg (2020) discuss the COMFORT curriculum acronym that stands for communication, orientation and options, family, openings, relating, and team and provides seven modules. Kopp and Mayberry (2022) study the reliability of an end-of-life communication rubric.

Review Chapter 25 for the application of Watson's caring theory with specific suggestions for communication with distressed patients and family. These principles apply to all caring communication. They can support you throughout your career as you gain more clinical experience and become more comfortable with the value of caring mindfulness.

CONSIDERATIONS FOR THE NURSE IN END-OF-LIFE CARE

"A willingness to go there," is an invitation from a study of rural and urban palliative care nurses' communication strategies for spiritual care of patients and families. The themes that emerged include "the capacity to act, a willingness to enter into the unknown and the ability to have deep meaningful conversations with patients regardless of the path it might yield" (Minton, Isaacson, Varilek, Stadick, & O'Connell-Persuad, 2018, p. 173). In caring for people at the end of life, there are two terms you need to understand: *hospice care* and *palliative care*. Hospice care is the model for quality, compassionate care for people facing a life-limiting illness or injury…a team-oriented approach to expert medical care, pain management, and emotional and spiritual support expressly tailored to the patient's needs and wishes. Support is provided to the patient's loved ones as well…the belief that each of us has the right to die pain-free and with dignity and that our families will receive the necessary support to allow us to do so (National Hospice and Palliative Care Association, 2015).

Hospice care is provided in the home, residential settings, and designated hospice houses, based on the understanding that dying is a normal part of the life cycle. Hospice promotes the idea of "living until you die." This movement is credited to Dame Cicely Saunders and is the foundation of the emerging field of palliative care. Medicare and Medicaid may provide support for hospice care, which is usually offered in what are believed to be the last 6 months of life. Palliative care is "the active total care of patients whose disease is not responsive to curative treatment. Control of pain, of other symptoms, and of psychological, social, and spiritual problems is paramount. The goal of palliative care is achievement of the best possible quality of life for patients and their families" (World Health Organization, 1990). Palliative care can be given at the same time as treatments to cure or treat the disease (MedlinePlus, 2018).

Why might you, as a nurse, be uncomfortable or unsure about how to communicate with clients who are approaching the end of their lives? Stop a moment to consider this, then see Box 29.1 and reflect on the following ideas:

BOX 29.1   When It Is Hard to Open the Patient's Door…

- We are afraid of facing our own mortality.
- We are afraid that we won't know the "right" thing to say.
- We are afraid that we will say the wrong thing.
- We may have little personal experience with someone who is dying.
- We may have unresolved grief over losses and deaths in our own lives.
- We may be afraid that our emotions will overwhelm us and that we might cry.
- We may be afraid that we will be blamed for the person's death.
- We may be afraid that we will dishonor the family or client because we do not understand the client's culture.
- We may be uncomfortable with just "being" with the client rather than "doing" things.
- We may simply not know what to do, and it is the not knowing that frightens us.

From American Association of Colleges of Nursing and City of Hope National Medical Center. (2017). *Training program facility guide*, Duarte, CA: End-of-Life Nursing Education Consortium (ELNEC); Matzo, M. L., Sherman, D. W., Sheehan, D. C., Ferrell, B. R., & Penn, B. (2003). Communication skills for end-of-life nursing care. *Nursing Education Perspectives, 24*(4), 176.

Yes, when we work with the dying, we can no longer deny our own mortality. Yet, from becoming clearer about the finite nature of life, we can make better choices about how to live our own lives with more beauty, connection, and meaning. When we accept our own mortality, we can be more fully present for our clients. We can listen without fear of being inadequate at this sacred time in life…and the listening is enough. We are not called to give answers but to give of ourselves as a companion for the journey (Nouwen, 2005).

Why is it hard to watch someone we love or have come to love die? People we love become a part of us. When they die, it is as though a part of us has died, too. The separation is the source of the grief. On holidays, birthdays, or the anniversary of the death of a loved one, we are more clearly aware of the loved one's absence. By "remembering" them, we make them a part of ourselves again. "Remembering them means letting their spirits inspire our daily lives" (Nouwen, 2005). Some people experience an even greater closeness after death. Grief counselors may encourage the bereaved to talk to the person who has died and to listen to what they think would be the response, and they may suggest reflecting on how knowing the person changed his or her life (Loomis, 2009).

 MOMENTS OF CONNECTION...

I Felt Broken and Helpless...a Student Nurse Faces Death

On the oncology unit, I cared for a young mother in her 30s whose cancer had metastasized to her bones. She was such a sweet wife and mother. All the prayers I could pray just kept coming to my mind because I did not want her to die. Up until that point, she had been a very strong person and accepted what was going on as God's will. When I came into her room, she burst into tears. I felt so broken and helpless. I sat at the end of her bed, held her hand, and rubbed her leg for comfort. She cried and cried as I remained silent for about 20 minutes. She talked about her fears of dying and leaving her three little girls and her husband. We cried together, and I had the opportunity to educate her about hospice. She was discharged to hospice the next day. We hugged each other as we said goodbye, and I felt as if I had been a part of something so special. I will never forget her.

Self-Care Nudge

Leave work at work. Develop a routine to detach from work, perhaps starting with washing your hands before you leave. The ability to rest and relax helps you to have a more positive outlook in life. Worrying, ruminating over the day, does work no good and harms you. Some nurses report having a special memento hanging from their rear-view mirror in the car as a cue. A ritual of changing your clothes immediately when you get home can help. Set the intention, make a plan, let it become a habit.

CARING COMMUNICATION NEAR THE END OF LIFE

The Process

Communication at the end of life is a process of interactions through which a relationship is created. These interactions are an exchange of thoughts, ideas, and feelings communicated verbally and nonverbally. "Dying is more than a medical event; it is a spiritual event" (Young & Koopsen, 2005). Staff and family can help create an environment in which personal transformation, reconciliation, and the expression of love can occur. Essential qualities of being with the dying are acceptance, being calm and open-minded, listening deeply, and proactive intervention and

advocacy on behalf of clients and their families (Norlander, 2008; Seno, 2010). Consider the following:
1. Be present for the person, relating to the person and not the illness.
2. Pay attention by listening without judgment to the needs, wishes, and personal wisdom of the dying person. Compassionate listening means setting aside your own discomfort and those automatic, reassuring responses that help the listener more than the person who is dying. Compassionate listening is letting the person talk in whatever way he or she needs to talk (Davis, Paleg, & Fanning, 2004). It is OK to laugh with your client or by just sit silently.
3. Show compassion by gentle touch, using lotion on your hands, or by giving a back rub. Offer a cool cloth when your client is perspiring.

Create a peaceful environment, perhaps lowering the lights or opening the blinds to let in the light if desired. These considerations create a climate in which thoughts and feelings can be shared openly (Corr, Nabe, & Corr, 2003; Young & Koopsen, 2005) (Box 29.2).

It is interesting and perhaps comforting to know that research confirms the existence of deathbed visions and deathbed coincidences involving the appearance or apparition of a dying person to someone close to them at the

BOX 29.2   My Commitment to You and Your Family When I Care for You at the End of Life

- I will be truthful.
- I will not abandon you.
- I will ask you what is important to you.
- I will do my best to help you meet your goals.
- I will respond to your questions in a timely manner.
- I will ask you what you need and what I can do for you.
- I will be an active part of your healthcare team.
- I will seek help when I don't know what to do.
- I will reflect on how I would want a beloved family member to be treated.
- I will listen to you with compassion.
- I will work on my own issues with grief to better serve you.
- I will pay attention to my own self-care so I can pay full attention to you.
- I will bring my best self to you, including my tears and my laughter.

Modified from American Association of Colleges of Nursing and City of Hope National Medical Center (2017). *Training program facility guide.* Duarte, CA: End-of-Life Nursing Education Consortium (ELNEC).

time of death or a strong feeling that the person has died and is "all right." This supports what appears to be a need for "spiritual connection and meaning, requiring compassionate understanding and respect from those who provide end-of-life care" (Fenwick & Brayne, 2011).

> **WIT AND WISDOM**
>
> *Ira Byock, in his book Dying Well, offers five tasks that facilitate peacefulness at the end of life.*
> *These are saying, "Forgive me," "I forgive you," "I love you," "Thank you," and "Good-bye."*
>
> **Ira Byock (1998)**

Wisdom from a Hospice Nurse

As a nurse author, I have had the added privilege of the experience of working part-time as an expressive arts facilitator with hospice clients, their family, and staff. As are other nurses, I am in awe of the ability to do this work as our mission in nursing. After 5 years of experience of contact with one nurse whose comfort with dying and touching support of patients is remarkable, I asked her to share her observations, experience, and beliefs with you. This is the demonstration of how one hospice nurse sees her work and makes sense of it. Elizabeth Labbate shares her experiences throughout this chapter where noted (Boxes 29.3 and 29.4). When you understand more about the dying process, you can better reassure the client and inform the family, who values sensitive, specific presentation of what to expect at the end of life (Boucher et al., 2010; Zomorodi & Lynn, 2010).

> **WIT AND WISDOM**
>
> *And When You Are Ready…to explore the spiritual transformation of the dying process, consider these stages of surrender and transformation: qualities of grace; letting go; radiance; focusing inward; silence; a sense of the sacred; wisdom; intensity; and, in the end, a merging with Spirit.*
> *Singh, K. D. (2000). The grace in dying: A message of hope, comfort, and spiritual transformation.*
>
> **New York, NY: HarperOne**

STRATEGIES FOR CREATIVE EXPRESSION

The expressive arts offer creative ways for clients and families to access emotion. The National Organization for Arts in Health (NOAH) has developed the *Core Curriculum for Arts in Health Professionals* (Albright & Carytsas, 2021) to support this work. In end-of-life care, offering materials for collage from magazines can evoke personal stories and create legacy pieces for the family. Bring a few magazines

---

BOX 29.3 When Death Is Near: A Hospice Nurse's Observations for the Nurse, Client, and Family

Some know for months that the end is coming but do not talk about it. Some believe that to speak of it is to hasten it. They may see death negatively, not be ready for it, or not have spiritual beliefs and may be afraid. Some people may withdraw as they become aware of their impending death. They may be quieter as they process and evaluate their life and have less interest in worldly things such as television and then family and friends. They may nap more and then may sleep most of the day. Family may not recognize this process. Now touch and facial expression become important. Nutrition is less important as the body shuts down. At this time feeding a person more than they desire causes more pain and suffering. Teach the family that this is a natural process. Offer liquids and soft food.

Early on, the person cannot hold his or her eyes open, but can still be awakened. Some professionals believe seeing departed family members is a hallucination. I believe the person is more easily confused as he or she wanders from this world to the next. The person often speaks to deceased loved ones, reaches with hands, picks items in the air, and talks about unfamiliar places and events. Blood pressure may lower, and the pulse and respirations may increase or decrease dramatically. Perspiration increases, skin may be cool and moist, and its color may change from normal to flushed, or cool and blue, or yellow. Nail beds may be blue. Breathing may stop only to restart with abdominal breaths and pursed lips. With congestion comes the "death rattle," or fluid that the person may be unable to clear, sounding more upsetting than it is to the client.

There may be restlessness from less oxygen and a sense that the end is near. Just before the active dying process, a brief energy surge may occur, giving family false hope. Some believe this is spiritual energy expressed as physical energy. Now eyes may be open but unseeing. Consciousness may decrease until the person is unresponsive. The sense of hearing may be acute, and the person may feel your touch. Continue to communicate with the person until death. Treat a person with respect and dignity up until and even past the very last breath.

Elizabeth Labbate, MS, RN, LMT, CHPN. Used with permission.

---

that might be of interest to your client and scissors, glue, and colored paper or mat board. Have the client select words or images that are appealing and glue them to the

BOX 29.4   This I Believe about Death and Dying: A Gift from One Hospice Nurse's Experience of the Mystery of Death

As patients enter the final hours, some need direction to leave this world. They talk about "wanting to go," believe that they have accomplished all that they need to in this lifetime, and are ready for "God" to take them; they feel frustrated that they do not die just then. When their bodies are shutting down, if the person believes in a life after death, tell them to look for their deceased loved ones and to take their hands. I remember a patient telling me that his sister was visiting. He told her to lose weight. She had been dead a year. He was so intent on telling her what to do that he missed seeing the hand she extended. We were able to redirect him to take her hand. He passed quickly and peacefully. Many patients live until all issues are resolved and then pass peacefully. Others, after a life review, make remarkable transitions in resolving conflict. Some stop years of fighting and decide that "all is forgiven." Often, the patient is given an understanding of why situations happened that they were not privy to during their lifetime. Some fight until the last moment, saying, "I'm not going," as if talking with someone. Patients who have not decided that it is their time to leave may have a difficult time leaving. This is especially true of younger people. The person may fight until the body cannot sustain life, lapse into a coma, or collapse and die.

Personal choices become evident. Some die with their family present. Others die alone. Having the personal choice of time determines who is present at our death. Some tell me it is too painful for family to be present. Family members might sit vigil for 72 hours nonstop, leave the room for a few minutes, and the loved one dies. Or the patient will hold on longer than expected, until family finally arrives and greets them, and then may die within a few minutes.

Elizabeth Labbate, MS, RN, LMT, CHPN. Used with permission.

background, helping whenever needed. Then ask the client if a story comes to mind from the art. Families can be offered a time to create a memory box about their loved one. Cigar boxes serve as a surface for collage and a keepsake box for mementos.

You were introduced to mandalas in the introduction of this text and on the front cover. Coloring mandala designs can be relaxing. Mandala coloring books are available. Find mandalas online to print at https://www.free-mandalas.net/ or by searching "free mandalas to color."

Offer colored pencils, markers, or watercolors and watercolor paper. Having your client or family member simply paint lines of blue and green and purple can be self-soothing. Suggest that even imagining this process can help when you have difficulty sleeping (Hayes, 2006).

Before the client is actively dying, favorite music may assist with reminiscence and storytelling. When you do not know the client well, you can try using the client's age to calculate in what year the patient was 20 years old and introduce music of that era. Closer to the time of death, music that has been found to be helpful comes from the field of music thanatology, which is a subspecialty of palliative care, such as *Rosa Mystica*, a CD from the Chalice of Repose Project (Schroeder-Sheker, 2011).

Encourage clients and families to keep a journal or write poetry if that appeals to them. If you decide to give a journal to a patient or family member, have the person write something on the first page to take away the fear of getting started or "messing it up." Poetry magnets can help. Have the person just choose words that appeal to him or her and arrange them into a poem, assuring the person that there is no right way to make a poem and that rhyme is unnecessary (see Box 29.5 A Poem…No More).

BOX 29.5   A Poem…No More

This poem is generously shared by a colleague in Sage-ing® International. Elizabeth Bell is a Certified Sage-ing Leader, supporting people in the second half of life through a conscious aging process of life review and life repair of the past, and facing one's mortality and fears of death to live more fully in the present (see https://www.sage-ing.org/).

No More
He lay there
breathed by a machine,
his body nourished
by liquid nutrition through a tube
hanging from a pole
with a dozen other dripping promises in bags
to keep him alive
His spirit fighting for life.
his alert eyes seeking and finding his wife,
speaking his I love you.
Daily the wife sits vigil by his side
watching, loving and returning
the I love you.
The doctors making their rounds
serve up yet another cup of hope…
"once we can get the infection
in his lungs cleared up…"

BOX 29.5   A Poem...No More—cont'd

this leading to the seemingly
unstoppable momentum of
medical treatment.
And Hope accompanied by her sister Expectation,
waits to hear the daily recitation of test results,
better–same–worse.
The wife riding
the tortuous waves of
hope and despair,
of knowing and not knowing
how to proceed,
if to proceed.
Until the day
when his body spoke clearly,
it's over—there is no more to give.
His spirit asking to be released
and the wife then knowing
with certainty amidst the deep pain—
"stop," she says, "no more."

Elizabeth Bell (2018). Used with permission.

In her career, Deborah Grassman (2012), a hospice nurse in the Veterans Administration, personally took care of 10,000 dying veterans. Her book, *The Hero Within: Redeeming the Destiny You Were Born to Fulfill*, offers in-depth processes to help dying people find peace with such tools as life review, letter writing, and other healing rituals.

 MOMENTS OF CONNECTION...

A psychiatrist working with clients for more than 30 years talks about helping them deal with their fears about dying, saying this was not taught in his medical training. When asked, "Where will I go when I die?" a response he gives is that when we die, we return to the place we were before we were born (Yalom, 2009).

 MOMENTS OF CONNECTION...

Sarah, a 77-year-old woman with lung cancer, was a patient in a hospice house. I offered her art materials for card making, and as she painted, she began to talk about her life. She seemed sad, and we talked about to whom she might send the card. I asked her if there was anyone in her life with whom there were things left unsaid. She teared up and said she wished she could just tell her daughter that she loved her and that she knew her daughter always felt criticized by her. We talked about how she might be able to do that. Later she arranged for her daughter to visit and afterward talked about how much better she felt.

 MOMENTS OF CONNECTION...
Using Music

Suzanne, a 71-year-old hospice patient, had just been admitted to an assisted living facility and spoke little. She answered questions vaguely because of memory loss. Her affect was bland, and she seldom made eye contact. The expressive arts facilitator from hospice talked with her about what music she liked from the 1950s and brought the music. Suzanne brightened and was able to sing all the lyrics to her favorite song, "Chantilly Lace" by the Big Bopper. She began to talk about how much she loved the opera *Carmen* and that living near New York City she had been taught about opera in junior high school and had taken field trips to the opera in the city. The facilitator was able to find a CD with selections from the opera. Suzanne became animated and related the story of the opera.

SIMPLIFY AND DEEPEN

God grant me the serenity to accept the things I cannot change, the courage to change the things I can, and the wisdom to know the difference.

Strategies for Nurses to Deal with Grief

Nurses often develop close relationships with patients and their families. When patients die, often nurses grieve this loss, which may be overwhelming. Knowing loss and grief is a part of nursing; we must recognize this and build in strategies to deal with this.

Kubler-Ross's classic work *On Death and Dying* (1969), proposed five stages of grief: denial; anger, bargaining, depression, and acceptance. The presentation of these stages as linear has been criticized as experiences teaches that these may come and go in a different order, some never experienced (Nathoo & Ellis, 2019). Other theories have been proposed, but understanding these phases can help us observe our own reactions and those of patients, family, and colleagues.

Houck (2014) reports an educational intervention to help nurses cope with grief and compassion fatigue. Cumulative unresolved grief can lead to emotional exhaustion, physical complaints, and emotional detachment from patients. Her work suggests nurses have the personal responsibility to:

1. Recognize and acknowledge loss and grief and allow time to grieve
2. Engage in self-care for body-mind-emotional-spiritual wellness
3. Seek professional assistance when grief continues to interfere with personal and professional life

Her work suggests organizations can support staff through areas for meditation, ceremonies for remembrance, and educational programs about grief and loss.

SELF-CARE FOR NURSES WORKING WITH CLIENTS AT THE END OF LIFE

Holistic self-care is the foundation of holistic nursing. As you care for yourself, so you care for your clients. As you care for yourself, so you care for your colleagues. When we work with clients and their families at the end of life, the experience touches us at a very deep level and calls on us to give of ourselves in new ways. We stretch to grow. We ponder and reflect on our own life and its meaning. We sigh a breath of relief that it is not our time or the time of our loved ones. We go home and tuck our children into bed more tightly. We look at our family and friends with softened eyes. We experience gratitude. All this takes energy, and, like all of nursing, although this is noble work, we are not the only nurse who can be present. When we are off duty physically, we need to find ways to maintain healthy boundaries from our work. We do work hard, and now we need to play hard. We need time for respite and activities with no social value—time that is just *fun*.

Creative expression strategies are valuable tools for self-care for nurses, too. Nurses at international meetings of Sigma Theta Tau, the nursing honor society, were given an opportunity to submit examples of their own art-making, including submissions such as visual arts, fabric art, prose, and poetry (Wendler, 2005). Reading for pleasure, listening to music, playing an instrument, writing music or poetry, visual arts, dance, sculpture, quilting, cooking, gardening, and walking in nature are valuable strategies. Praying, reading inspirational materials, playing with pets, and gardening are supportive. What do you do? Mak, Fluharty & Fancourt (2021) studied the use of the arts as coping tools during the COVID-19 pandemic and highlighted the value of the arts for coping during stressful situations. See Chapter 30 for more information on resilience to stay present in the challenges of nursing.

Dame Cicely Saunders wrote, "How people die remains in the memories of those who live on." Let this theme guide you as you work with clients near the end of life. Ask yourself how you can contribute to a positive experience for the family, creating memories that can be carried into the bereavement period and beyond (Kueblerr, Berry, & Heidrich, 2002).

Return to "Active Learning" at the beginning of the chapter and write your responses.

PRACTICING CARING COMMUNICATION IN END-OF-LIFE CARE

Self-Assessment: Exercise 1

Consider the following quote from Mark Twain: "The fear of death follows from the fear of life. A man who lives fully is prepared to die at any moment." Jarem Sawatsky, living with a neurodegenerative disease, poses this question in his book, *Dancing with Elephants: Mindfulness Training for Those Living with Dementia, Chronic Illness, or an Aging Brain* (Sawatsky, 2017): What things in your life create joy and love? He suggested that if we want to offer these things to others, we need to make time for them in our lives. In your journal, begin your list as you work to live fully.

Creative Expression/Discussion: Exercise 2

Reflect on this quote by Harriett Beecher Stowe: "The bitterest tears shed over graves are for words left unsaid and deeds left undone." Depending on your life experience, you may or may not be able to relate to this quote, but all of us have words of gratitude that have not been shared. Try this gratitude practice:
A. Sit quietly, eyes closed, and bring to mind the people in your life for whom you are grateful.
B. Identify one person to whom you would like to express your gratitude. Compose a handwritten letter and send it or give it to the person.

Creative Expression/Discussion: Exercise 3

Online, search YouTube to watch the movie *Tuesdays with Morrie,* which is the story of a man who wants to relate his experience at the end of life as a legacy. Watch the movie with several other students or colleagues, and then discuss its implications for your work with clients at the end of life.

Creative Expression/Reflection: Exercise 4

Online, search *Listen to the Fall of Freddie* on YouTube. Listen to the book *The Fall of Freddie the Leaf* by Leo Buscaglia, which is an allegory about life and death through the format of a children's book on the life of a leaf throughout the seasons. Write a reflective journal entry on what you learned in this comparison of the life of a person through the story of a leaf.

Creative Expression/Reflection: Exercise 5

As a class, watch the full-length movie *Wit* (rent online). Caution: this is a very powerful, emotional film. Note especially the role of Susie Monahan, Vivian's nurse. This is used as a teaching film in medical and nursing schools. Reflect topics for discussion in the following as you view the video.

Discussion Guide for the Movie *Wit*, Starring Emma Thompson. Summary: The movie was adapted from the 1999 Pulitzer Prize winning play by Margaret Edson. It chronicles the journey of Vivian Bearing, an English professor with a biting wit, who educates but also alienates her students. With her teaching and life both rigidly under control, Vivian would never let her defenses down until the day comes when they are taken down for her. Diagnosed with a devastating illness, Vivian agrees to undergo a series of procedures that are brutal, extensive, and experimental. For 8 months, her life must take an uncharted course. No longer a teacher but a subject for others to study, Vivian Bearing is about to discover a fine line between life and death.

1. Identify your own response to the video. Discussing your own feelings about Vivian, the patient, and about the care being given is a place to begin.
2. How does the communication by healthcare staff reflect what you have been learning in this text? Consider the different healthcare professionals whose behavior and conversation you observe.
3. Watch for scenes in which Vivian's nurse connects with her and advocates for her as an individual, rather than a research subject, and comment on what behaviors/conversation strike you.

Adapted from http://services.medicine.uab.edu/public-documents/palliativecare/film/wit_study_guide.pdf. (No longer available online.)

REFERENCES

Albright, A., & Carytsas, F. P. (Eds.). (2021). *Core curriculum for arts in health professionals*. San Diego: National Organization of Arts in Healthcare (NOAII).

Bell, E. (2018). A poem…No more. Personal correspondence with author.

Boucher, J., Bova, C., Sullivan-Bolyai, S., Theroux, R., Klar, R., Terrien, J., et al. (2010). Next-of-kin's perspectives of end-of-life care. *Journal of Hospice and Palliative Nursing, 12*(1), 41.

Byock, I. (1998). *Dying well*. New York, NY: Riverhead Books.

Corr, C. A., Nabe, C. M., & Corr, D. M. (2003). *Death and dying, life and living* (4th ed.). Belmont, CA: Thomson/Wadsworth.

Davis, M., Paleg, K., & Fanning, P. (2004). *How to communicate workbook: Powerful strategies for effective communication at work and home*. New York, NY: MJF Books.

Fenwick, P., & Brayne, S. (2011). End-of-life experiences: Reaching out for compassion, communication, and connection—meaning of deathbed visions and coincidences. *American Journal of Hospice and Palliative Care, 28*(1), 7.

Goldsmith, J. V., Wittenberg, E., & Parnell, T. A. (2020). The COMFORT communication model: A nursing resource to advance health literacy in organizations. *Journal of Hospice & Palliative Nursing, 22*(3). doi:10.1097/NJH.0000000000000647.

Grassman, D. L. (2012). *The hero within: Redeeming the destiny you were born to fulfill*. St. Petersburg, FL: Vandamere Press.

Hayes, P. M. (2006). *Art therapy and anxiety: Healing through imagery*. Tampa, FL: Cross Country Education Seminar.

Jeffers, S., Lippe, M. P., Justice, A., Ferry, D., Borowik, K., & Connelly, C. (2022). Nursing student perceptions of end-of-life communication competence: A qualitative descriptive study. *Journal of Hospice & Palliative Nursing*. doi:10.1097/NJH.0000000000000849. Published ahead of print 2/17/22.

Kopp, M. L., & Mayberry, A. L. M. (2022). An end-of-life communication performance rubric: Reliability Assessment. *Journal of Hospice and Palliative Nursing, 23*(5), 429–434. doi:10.1097/NJH.0000000000000772.

Kubler-Ross, E. (1969). *On death and dying*. New York: Macmillan.

Kuebler, K. K., Berry, P. H., & Heidrich, D. E. (2002). *End-of-life care: Clinical practice guidelines*. Philadelphia, PA: WB Saunders.

Loomis, B. (2009). End-of-life issues: Difficult decisions and dealing with grief. *Nursing Clinics of North America, 44*(2), 223.

Mak, H. W., Fluharty M., & Fancourt, D. (2021). Predictors and impact of arts engagement during the COVID-19 pandemic: Analyses of data from 19,384 adults in the COVID-19 social study. *Front Psychol, 12*, 626263. doi:10.3389/fpsyg.2021.626263.

Matzo, M. L., Sherman, D. W., Sheehan, D. C., Ferrell, B. R., & Penn, B. (2003). Communication skills for the end-of life nursing care. *Nursing Education Perspectives, 24*(4), 176.

MedlinePlus. (2018). What is palliative? https://medlineplus.gov/ency/patientinstructions/000536.htm.

Minton, M. E., Isaacson, M. J., Varilek, M., Stadick, J. L., & O'Connell-Persaud, S. (2018). A willingness to go there: Nurses and spiritual care. *Journal of Clinical Nursing, 27*, 173.

Nathoo, D., & Ellis, J. (2019). Theories of loss and grief experienced by the patient, family, and healthcare professional: A personal account of a critical event. *Journal of Cancer Education, 34*, 831–835. https://doi.org/10.1007/s13187-018-1462-1.

National Hospice and Palliative Care Association. (2015). Hospice care. http://www.nhpco.org/about/hospice-care.

Norlander, L. (2008). *To comfort always: A nurse's guide to end-of-life care*. Indianapolis, IN: Sigma Theta Tau International.

Nouwen, H. J. M. (2005). *The dance of life: Weaving sorrows and blessings into one joyful step*. Notre Dame, IN: Ave Maria Press.

Sawatsky, J. (2017). *Dancing with elephants: Mindfulness training for those living with dementia, chronic illness, or an aging brain*. Rosemary Beach, FL: Red Canoe Press.

Schroeder-Sheker, T. (2011). The chalice of repose project. http://www.chaliceofrepose.org/history.htm.

Seno, V. L. (2010). Being with dying: Authenticity in end-of-life encounters. *American Journal of Hospice and Palliative Care, 27*, 377. (Original work published online May 3, 2010.).

Wendler, C. (Ed.). (2005). *The heART of nursing: Expressions of creative art in nursing*. Indianapolis, IN: Sigma Theta Tau International.

World Health Organization. (1990). *Cancer pain relief and palliative care. Report of a WHO expert committee*, 804 (p. 1). World Health Organization Technical Report Series.

Yalom, I. D. (2009). *Staring at the sun: Overcoming the terror of death*. San Francisco, CA: Jossey-Bass.

Young, C., & Koopsen, C. (2005). *Spirituality, health, and healing*. Thorofare, NJ: SLACK Incorporated.

Zomorodi, M., & Lynn, M. R. (2010). Critical care nurses' behaviors with end-of-life-care. *Journal of Hospice and Palliative Care Nursing, 12*(2), 89.

30

Continuing the Commitment to the Journey

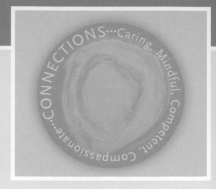

As human beings, our greatness lies not so much in being able to remake the world…as in being able to remake ourselves.

Mahatma Gandhi

OBJECTIVES

1. Identify practices of the resilient nurse.
2. Examine proactive approaches to reality shock, the transition from student to graduate.
3. Identify three competencies for achieving life balance.
4. Identify commonalities among "living legacy" responses from nurses with 50 or more years of experience.
5. Identify strategies for renewal.
6. Discuss the importance of commitment to nursing to continue to build communication skills.

❓ ACTIVE LEARNING

Think about how you will write your answers as you read this chapter.

What?
Write one thing you learned from this chapter.

So What?
How will this affect your nursing practice?

Now What?
How will you implement this new knowledge or skill?

Think About It …

PUTTING IT ALL TOGETHER

As I revise this last chapter, I reflect on lessons learned, research, and personal experience of the healthcaring experience of the last several years, facing a global pandemic. How do nurses cope? How does anyone cope? We are mindful, being present in this moment without judgment. We are compassionate, being empathetic without such attachment to the outcome that we can no longer be of use to those

we serve, those we love, and ourselves. We focus on that for which we are grateful. We extend kindness to ourselves and to others. Yes, we have been challenged, but that does not change who we are as nurses and as people and what we need to do to continue our commitment to caring and to service. Dr. Betty Ferrell (2021), in an editorial, reminds us of Remen's definition of service. "Service honors life as sacred, a holy mystery with an unknown purpose. In service, we belong to life and to that purpose: we are all connected; all suffering is like my suffering, all joy is like my joy."

Take a deep breath and imagine yourself in the nursing role of which you dream. What will you be doing? How will you look? What will you feel? Where will you be? This chapter invites you to be proud of your accomplishments and to be confident about the contribution you are and will continue to be making. It encourages you to respect the challenge of making your way in the work world; to pay attention to specific, successful strategies that have helped those who have gone before you; and to continue your commitment to learning and growing through your day-to-day experiences. It challenges you to assume responsibility for your own self-care. The American Nurses Association's (ANA's) *Code of Ethics* Provision 5 (2021, p. 14) (ANA, 2021) tells us we owe ourselves the care we provide for patients.

So, you are not being selfish to make time for yourself to eat healthy foods, to get enough sleep, for a spiritual/religious practice, to play, and to be with friends and family—in fact, you are ethically responsible to do so.

As you become more comfortable with your ability to communicate, you will soon become increasingly aware of how complex a venture it is. Beyond the technique comes the art, the intuitive application of what you know. This concluding chapter asks you to consider the commitments necessary to move on in your chosen profession: to remain open and sensitive to the human condition, to renew your energy, and to embrace change. To do these, you must find balance in life as you explore the challenges of moving from the role of student to graduate: from transitioning from the clear expectations of school to the ambiguity of nursing practice; from a low nurse-to-client ratio to the conflicting needs of many patients; and from perhaps a focused role as student to stressors from additional life changes such as marriage, having children, moving, and adjusting to a new, perhaps first, job (Tingle, 2001).

WHAT IS A RESILIENT NURSE?

As you read this final chapter and focus on creating success in your chosen profession, the research on resilience in nursing and other helping professions offers information to guide you. Resilience is the process of adapting to adversity, trauma, and stress in your professional and personal life.

It is "bouncing back" from challenging experiences in the everyday life of a nurse (American Psychological Association [APA], 2018).

Read Box 30.1 and reflect on your work with this text to see what you already know about resilience. This information is a distillation of many articles on resilience and well-being in students and nurses and on my own experience.

REALITY SHOCK: THE TRANSITION TO NURSING PRACTICE

Marlene Kramer (1974) conducted a classic study of the problem of "reality shock," which is when young graduates find themselves in a work situation, thinking they were going to be prepared, and finding that they were not. Understanding these findings provides you with an opportunity to be more proactive in your approach to the work world, although it may not make it easier to deal with the emotions encountered in this transition toward personal and professional development. Although this may not be the exact situation in which you will find yourself, it is useful to examine her findings and the research that has followed.

As a student, you learn how to be successful in the role of student, moving from novice to expert in that role by the time you graduate. In a new work setting, you again become the novice. Kramer described the development of the professional–bureaucratic conflict in which the nurse faces the challenge of not being able to give the desired

---

BOX 30.1   What Does It Mean to Be a Resilient Nurse?

Mindfulness practices, to be present in the moment without judging the situation, and knowing who you are, which support critical thinking

Authenticity, to learn more about yourself, and to show up as yourself using your strengths and honoring the need for being, in a "beginner's mind," open to learning

Reframing, looking for the lesson in the problem, cognitive restructuring to combat the belief that you can be perfect, and understanding you are human as are others

Using humor to help you keep your perspective and not taking yourself so seriously

Building and using your support systems so you have a "safe harbor"

Collaborating with your interprofessional team...you are not alone in wanting and working for safe, competent, and compassionate healthcare

Practicing self-care, including integrative/complementary therapies such as relaxation, imagery, yoga, breath

work, a sleep ritual to get enough sleep, simple exercise, and managing your own chronic illness

Finding meaning in your work through learning new skills and connecting with clients, family, and colleagues with compassion, caring, and gratitude/appreciation

Reflective practice to learn from your experience

Assertive communication to set boundaries for yourself and establish your professional identity

Toughening up to bear witness to human suffering, knowing that your presence, your listening, and your "being," even when you cannot "do," holds the space for healing

Look for the positive in a situation and in your own role in it

Practice forgiveness and nonjudgment of yourself and others

Learn to take a breath and just "let it go"...go home, get some sleep, eat a good meal, take a walk, start over with an attitude of curiosity about tomorrow; wonder, don't worry.

Adapted from Ashcraft & Gatto, 2018; Devney, 2018; Gallison, 2018; Grant & Kinman, 2014; Hart, Brann, & De Chesnay, 2014; Kelly & Adams, 2018; Kemper & Hill, 2017; Prince-Paul & Kelley, 2017; Raso, 2018; Reyes, Andrusyszyn Iwasiw, Forchuck, & Babenko-Mould, 2015; Stephens, 2013; Zuzelo, 2018.

BOX 30.2   Phases of Reality Shock

1. *Honeymoon phase:* Enthusiasm, excitement, high energy.
2. *Shock phase:* The realization that nursing is not what you expected; anger, frustration, disappointment, fatigue, being critical, having a negative life view.
3. *Recovery phase:* A realization that there is more than one perspective in the work situation, returning sense of humor.
4. *Resolution phase:* Choosing a way to resolve the conflicts between the subcultures of school and work, with different values and emphasis. (Behaviors in this phase may include frequent job changes; fleeing work by returning to school; quitting nursing; burnout, the result of unresolved work conflict with chronic complaining; or bicultural adaptation, which is a constructive form of resolution that integrates both value systems.)

---

amount of time to an individual client. Kramer identified four phases of this culture shock (Box 30.2).

Emotions you may experience during this transition include "exhilaration, anger, grief, excitement, resentment, nervousness, euphoria, self-doubt, or satisfaction" (Tingle, 2001). Understand that a range of feelings is normal. To deal with stress at this time, self-care is important. For example, take a break during your shift and eat your meal off the unit if possible, making sure that your clients' immediate needs are met before you leave them in someone else's care. Your confidence will grow over time. Be patient with yourself. Tingle (2001) summarized transition strategies through the mnemonic NURSES:

Never fail to ask for help!
Use available facility resources!
Reenergize with professional associations!
Stay in contact with friends!
Evaluate your own growth realistically!
Stay focused on your goals!

A study of 612 newly licensed registered nurses in New York identified several themes in these nurses' experience: colliding expectations between nurses' personal view of nursing and their lived experience; the need for speed and not enough time to get everything done and get to know the patients; high expectations and too much work and responsibility; mistreatment by physicians, rudeness, and criticism; and yet a theme of hope that, after the first 6 months of difficult transition, things were better and the nurses were more resilient (Pellico, Brewer, & Kovner, 2009). A study in Norway of job satisfaction and job values among new nurses found that the transition from school to work was less dramatic than initially assumed (Daehlen, 2008).

PROACTIVE APPROACHES TO REALITY SHOCK: THE TRANSITION FROM STUDENT TO NURSE

Communication is important at this time of transition. When you have questions, be clear about what you are asking and take time to decide who is the most appropriate person to ask. More experienced staff may assume you know steps you do not, so do not hesitate to keep asking until you get the information you need. If a situation is urgent, then communicate this. Listen carefully to answers you receive and repeat the answer to make sure your anxiety has not prevented you from listening.

Kramer (1974) offered the following suggestions to achieve bicultural adaptation: Evaluate situations in the workplace by looking at all sides of the issue, consider how your behavior will affect other colleagues, and identify appropriate and attainable goals.

Other proactive strategies, when interviewing for a job, include the following: Dress up to show respect for the organization or people interviewing you, and demonstrate enthusiasm for *this* job even if it is not your dream job; keep answers short and concise—do not ramble; do not volunteer personal information; inquire about the length of the orientation and internships or preceptor programs for new graduates; do your homework about the organization's philosophy and mission statement (usually available online); and ask about the next steps after the interview (Tuckerton, 2013). When you accept a position, ask questions about the history of the organization, focus on gaining a reputation for competence in skills and interpersonal relationships, and identify someone who will understand what you are experiencing and let you express your feelings. This should not be someone with whom you work but someone you trust to keep a confidence. Additionally, expect to be tested as the "new kid on the block" and avoid being defensive; understand that other staff members also feel pressure and experience stress; and keep a journal to record the thoughts, feelings, reflections, and ideas you have about how things could be changed. These are ideas you might share when you have earned the respect of your colleagues (Dyess & Sherman, 2009).

ACHIEVING GENERATIVE BALANCE

Guterman (1994) proposed a model he calls *generative balancing*, which focuses on three competencies: "creating success, finding meaning, and renewal…All three competencies are necessary for balancing, and the real thrill, the excitement of the ride—just as in life—comes from the movement, not from finding a steady-point," but from balance.

In a classic column, Ann Landers related an essay that compares life to a journey on a train. The essay advises that the focus of life should not be the station or the destination, but rather the journey itself.

SIMPLIFY AND DEEPEN

Simple pleasures are the last healthy refuge in a complex world.

Oscar Wilde

Creating Success

To create success, set goals to see the station or the destination. Guzzetta (1998) compared her journey of holistic nursing practice to weaving a tapestry: "master weavers of a tapestry have described the weaving of a tapestry as a calling, as transformation, as healing, or as a sacred work." What would your tapestry of success as a nurse contain? How would you embellish and color it to reflect your unique contribution?

Achievement of success, however, is often not enough in itself. "Balance comes from a life view that provides joy along the way," says Rabbi Harold Kushner (2002). Consider his quotation, "Nobody on his deathbed ever said, 'I wish I had spent more time on my business.'" Nursing provides many opportunities for success, such as clinical practice, administration, teaching, research, advanced practice, and many emerging roles for the nurse entrepreneur. Balance comes from attention to all three components of the model and setting the intention to care for yourself, knowing that the foundation of holistic nursing is self-care for the nurse.

Self-Care Nudge

What would be one thing you can do for fun? Put it on your calendar this week.

Finding Meaning
Meaning for the Nurse

To find meaning is essential for the nurse. Arnold (1989) saw this process as crucial for the nurse to prevent burnout, which she proposes is an existential crisis, and for the patient, who needs the nurse in the role of "meaning maker." Arnold's work confirms what many career nurses have come to view as the essence of nursing.

Arnold (1989) suggested that many nursing students grow up with a set of values and beliefs that translate into rules and regulations. Faith may be seen as a gift that is tied to good behavior. Do the right things and all will be well. When nurses are faced with seemingly meaningless tragedies or have stressors that accumulate, the following occurs: "The nurse's spiritual perspective is thrown off balance. Beliefs previously used no longer provide an internal guide on which to base decisions." It may become hard to pray or attend religious services. Traditional passive beliefs in a higher power may "not necessarily lend any understandable meaning to life experience. If one thinks of spirituality in such narrow terms, the essence of spirituality as a relationship with a higher power is lost." Through the resolution of this existential crisis comes the following: "a total acceptance and commitment to stewardship, anchored by a reasoned loyalty and trust in a higher purpose. What is needed is a broader perspective, a transcendent level of meaning that reorders the incomprehensible circumstances of pain and suffering that a nurse experiences on a daily basis." An examination of nurses' stories from their work with disenfranchised people, clients who frighten us or who are afraid, revealed four dimensions of meaning: the reward of meaning as overcoming challenges through facing our own fears and prejudices; the reward of meaning from a sense of having been called to the work; the reward of meaning as a legacy of caring connected with family experience or tragedy; and the reward of meaning from the experience of common humanity, which is the belief that each person has a right to care and respect (Zerwekh, 2000).

Kushner (2001) faced just such an existential crisis when his own child died of progeria, a disease of premature aging. He questioned his own beliefs: How could he, a rabbi, a good person, have such a senseless tragedy occur in his life? In his book *When Bad Things Happen to Good People*, he concluded that you cannot control the events in your life, only the attitude that you take toward life. Kushner discussed three ways that he found to give meaning to life: belong to people, accept pain as a part of life, and know that you have made a difference. These are all a part of your life as a nurse if you remain open and sensitive to the human condition (Kushner, 2002).

To belong to people is to have a few people who are a permanent part of your life, people with whom you share yourself. Nurses sometimes lament their poor relationships with family members. Until you can work through these relationships, claim close friends as new relatives.

To accept pain as a part of life is also to be able to experience the contrasting joy. To be fully present with a client or family member is to be open to sharing suffering, but also to be open to rejoicing in the triumph of coping and changing in the face of crisis.

To know you have made a difference can be a comfort when you are unable to control the course of life's events.

Savor the thank-yous you get. Save the notes and cards you receive and place them in a book. Later, these notes will bring you renewed joy and pride.

The Nurse as Meaning Maker

The ability to develop a belief system, an inner process, as a way of understanding or explaining events that seem beyond human understanding is reflected in interpersonal communication with clients and family. A nurse who is not exactly sure what she believes reports that when a client's family was distressed, she spontaneously said, "There are some things that are beyond our understanding, but I believe that life has a purpose." Listen to colleagues as they comfort family and clients, and you will experience a demonstration of their belief systems.

 MOMENTS OF CONNECTION...

Nursing...Days of Wonder

"I worked in the intensive care unit and took care of an elderly man who was dying. He was a brilliant philosopher and teacher. We spent many evenings talking, and he touched me in ways I did not think were possible. He died one evening when I was not working. I was sad for days. One morning I saw his surgeon who asked me if I would like to see the autopsy results. When I went with him, I was shocked to see we were in the actual autopsy. When I saw the body, I realized for the first time what death was all about. This body was just a shell, and his eyes were vacant. I knew all his experiences and stories and brilliant knowledge were with me and everyone else with whom he had come into contact. The experience allowed me to accept my father's death a few years later and [helped] me in my work with the dying."

Creating a Living Legacy

Consider that your work throughout your career in nursing creates a living legacy. Nursing students at Lakeview College of Nursing, Danville, Illinois, complete a research legacy project each year that might be adopted by the class that follows. One project was a fundraising event to contribute money for healthcare expenses for a child with chronic illness. As longtime nurses reflect on their work, they can see their living legacy (see Box 30.3).

Remember that our work in nursing is always about the patient, not about us. We are called to take care of ourselves, center ourselves, set our worries aside, show up, and be present for those we serve. Arnold (1989) advocated involvement as a part of life but recognized that detachment and renewal of energy are necessary to maintain personal wellness and the continued ability to nurture our own interpersonal relationships. Loss of meaning can cause spiritual distress, but setting impossible standards of perfection in your professional and personal life can be overwhelming and exhausting. The level of intimacy in communication in nursing can take its toll on energy reserves; thus, attention to renewal is essential.

Renewing Energy

Now that the inevitable stressors facing nurses today have been discussed, it is time to actively consider how you can add energy, fun, and laughter to your life. Consider a body–mind–spirit approach.

The Body

Find a physical activity you like and do it on a regular basis but not obsessively. Dance, play tennis, walk, or run; the list is endless. Start with 10 minutes twice a day—just move. Begin a yoga practice for stress relief. Gentle stretching and

---

BOX 30.3   **Living Legacy**

Nurses with 50 or more years of experience share their wisdom in response to these three questions:

1. When you think of communication in nursing, what message would you like to give to students of nursing and new graduates?
2. What is one thing you learned the hard way that you would like to share to grow our profession?
3. What words of wisdom would you like to share from your experience?

The respondents' education varies: diploma, baccalaureate, master's, and doctoral graduates. Their experience ranges from staff nurse in a variety of specialties and settings to other roles such as quality improvement,

education, entrepreneur, managers, night supervisor, administrator, Medicare appeals, and a federal position. One has practiced in Canada for most of her career. Some are still in practice, and others have retired. *As you review their responses, look for commonalities.*

Ann Rinaldi: Listen, listen, listen with kindness, compassion, and caring. Patients are not interested in who you are nor in your personal life. They want to know how you will care for them. From a personal experience as a patient having a difficult experience, prepare your patient with what is going to happen, as many patients are scared to death and information may allay their fears. It is a God-given privilege to care for the sick. Act like it!

BOX 30.3   Living Legacy—cont'd

Roberta Rauer: What I want to emphasize is your patients already see you as an authority figure and rely on you to give them good information and to listen. One caveat is don't share personal information; talk about shared interests, sports, movies. A little humor goes a long way in nursing, just as in everyday life does a smile and a pleasant word.

Denise Geolot Sherer: Communication skills are life skills—never underestimate their importance. They are a key to success: interpersonal skills, affect, attitude, demeanor, and body language. How and what you communicate to patients and colleagues can impact the plan of care and patient outcomes. Nursing is an integral part of healthcare but is not always appreciated. Research documents nursing's role in increasing access to cost effective quality care. Nurses need to expand their sphere of influence and be a part of the larger discussion of healthcare providers, insurers, policy makers, regulators, and professional associations, trying to identify and solve today's complex healthcare problems of cost, quality, and access. Nursing is a wonderful profession, and, in the course of my career, it took unexpected turns. Each provided opportunities that resulted in a career that was interesting, exciting, and fulfilling. My advice to new graduates is to be open to opportunities and to take risks. The rewards are wonderful.

Kaarlyn Shilliday: Communicate with patients and colleagues as you would want for yourself: words, tone of voice, sincere appreciation, and a thank you. When problems arise at work—and they always do—take a breath, don't react immediately, go away to reflect on your part in the problem, swallow your pride, and share your part of the problem. Learn to say you are sorry. It has been a grand 50 years. I've been so privileged to work in a field surrounded by so many hard-working, dedicated, interesting, and kind people.

Betty Laing: Treat patients as you would like to be treated if you were in their role. It works! Patients are responsive to a good listener, a touch, or a reassuring word. It all communicates caring. Technology and knowledge are necessary, but caring is the core of a committed nurse. When I was 10, I was in a hospital after a car accident. It was the nurse's caring and skill that led me into nursing. Caring and respect applies to colleagues,

too. There is no perfect working environment. Try not to focus on the negatives. Nurses have the ability to enrich "the young" nurses and their environment as they grow and blossom in their career. Opportunity abounds!

Carol Washburn: You don't have to have all of the answers or even the "right" words. In times of crisis and hardship, simple communication is most effective. Long explanations are often not heard. A touch, a warm smile, and eye contact that come from a place of honesty can be the most meaningful. Remember, building relationships between the caregivers provides strength and support to caregivers and enhances the support for the patient exponentially. As a young nurse, I felt I had to be strong, decisive, and an independent thinker and did not see the opportunity the love and support of the team offered, especially from those who were more experienced. Meaningful relationships amongst the team offers patients and loved ones a safe place to ask questions and express feelings. Remember in our task-oriented world to take a moment to be present with yourself and with another human being. Small moments have been the most meaningful to me when I allow them. When I was a night supervisor, I would take early morning phone calls from nurses who were sick and wouldn't be coming to work. One middle of the night call came from a nurse whose parent had died. She was sobbing with sorrow over the phone. I just listened. That brief moment on the phone created a bond between us that lasted throughout the time we worked together. Our communication was enhanced, enabling us to provide better care to the patients. Just a brief moment in time over a telephone. Be present and cherish them.

Kathy West: Realize that your patients do not always understand their disease status. They may not understand the difference between a positive TB test and active TB status or that TB is a treatable disease. Remember there are workplace politics in healthcare. One needs to know how to identify when these are in place and how to best deal with them. I made the choice not to play the games—that made moving up the ladder very difficult. Remember, know who you are and what you want to achieve. Hopefully, you have entered healthcare as a calling. That is important in the delivery of quality patient care.

deep breathing are relaxing and promote sleep (Fontaine, 2014). Look in the mirror. Do you like what you see? Are you a role model for health and wellness? Do you see your body as sacred?

The Mind

Consider working to develop a mindfulness practice, "purposefully paying attention in the present moment with a sense of acceptance and nonjudgment" (Bazarko, 2014).

This is achieved through mindfulness meditation, yoga, walking meditation, engaging in a creative process, and spending time in nature (Bazarko, 2014). This is a self-care practice to help you be more present with your patients and yourself. The ANA's publication *Mindfulness and You: Being Present in Nursing Practice* (Bazarko, 2014) is a good introduction available for purchase as a download or in hard copy. The University of Virginia has a Contemplative Sciences Center to integrate such practices as mindfulness in nursing, medicine, and throughout the university and the community.

Choose music or movies or reading material that renew your energy. Add play, laughter, and humor to your life (see Chapter 14). Embellish your world with beauty in your home. In a workshop for healthcare givers and volunteers in hospice and palliative care, three creative self-care strategies were introduced. Here are the strategies and a participant's comment regarding each: journal writing, "What I can do with words! I just needed to know where to start"; expressive art, "Being able to express myself in art puts me in touch with feelings I wasn't aware of"; and music therapy, "Music gave me a sense of freedom I had forgotten I ever had" (Murant, 2000). Journal, play with art, and listen to music to suit or shift your mood.

 MOMENTS OF CONNECTION...

A Nursing Student Is "Putting It All Together"

Today my best friend's mother had a hysterectomy. This gave me an opportunity to practice therapeutic communication. My friend was so anxious and upset. She cried and visited her mom before and after work. She kept talking about it even when her mom was out of surgery and stable. I practiced what I remembered from the book on demonstrating warmth, being empathetic, being caring and genuine, being present, allowing for silence and tears, providing caring touch, and showing compassion and understanding. I taught her some strategies to reduce anxiety and offered reassurance by telling her I know the care is excellent in this hospital. She got visibly calmer. I was so glad to be able to offer these things, and, although I won't have a deep personal relationship with my patients, I am confident that I will be able to communicate in ways that are supportive.

The Spirit

Nourish your spirit by taking time to read inspirational material or stories. Take time to be silent and to just be and not do. Set aside a regular time to contemplate life. Review the chapters on imagery and relaxation. Write your own mission statement for your personal and professional life

(Kenney, 1998). Mine is to "re-spirit, re-inspire, and re-vitalize nurses to provide sensitive care and find humor and joy and meaning along the journey." See Jones' (1998) *The Path: Creating Your Mission Statement for Work and for Life* for specific directions to help you write your mission statement.

> **WIT AND WISDOM**
>
> *I like to think of men and women as artists of their own lives, working with what comes to hand through accident or talent to compose and recompose a pattern in time that expresses who they are and what they believe in—making meaning even as they are studying and working and raising children, creating and recreating themselves.*
>
> **Bateson (2010)**

CONTINUING CONNECTIONS

Read and think about Box 30.4, providing reflections from each of the 30 chapters in this book.

A few final points demonstrate continuing the commitment and the risks and joy it entails.

One nurse concluded that, although nurses may wear many hats, they all maintain the "commitment to the art of nursing" (Schettle, 1998). Nurses are taking on many expanded clinical and administrative roles to make an impact on healthcare delivery in complex integrated delivery systems, and yet they maintain the commitment to quality care for clients and families and to the promotion of wellness for individuals and communities; through electronic communication, they move on to global concerns for healthcare. Nurses are asked to develop education for house-wide hospital education. Nurses are moving into industry to design corporate wellness programs. Nurses are advocating for healthcare through political roles. They are bringing information technology to healthcare through informatics. These new roles demand new skills and a commitment to the goal of being a lifelong learner.

The examples in this text deal with one issue at a time. Clinical situations present the complex lives of real people struggling with many of life's challenges at once. To face this complexity and what may seem like impossible situations, nurses must grow with their clients and families. Honest, clear communication takes a commitment to continue to grow, to deal with change, and to stay connected with people. The rewards are substantial. Work can bring joy, but the cost is too great if you lose the joy that comes from having a rich personal life, interests to pursue, and people to whom you are connected. Consider these final exercises to help you along the journey.

BOX 30.4 Putting It All Together...On Reflection

Chapter 1: Practice assertive communication, which does not guarantee that you will get what you want but increases the probability that you will.

Chapter 2: Take a breath and listen, letting go of having to have answers and being willing to not know.

Chapter 3: Offer your support and information when appropriate, and remember that people make their own decisions.

Chapter 4: Learn more about yourself to be more understanding of others.

Chapter 5: Focus on things we have in common rather than on differences.

Chapter 6: Smile from your eyes and your heart, a valuable demonstration of warmth.

Chapter 7: Shared respect is a good foundation for health caring.

Chapter 8: Share your authentic self. Authenticity is the absence of self-deception.

Chapter 9: Be clear that we can try to put ourselves in another's place, but true empathy is expressed with humility, knowing we can never succeed.

Chapter 10: Use self-disclosure in the service of the client, family, or colleague.

Chapter 11: Pay attention. Details do matter, and being specific can save lives.

Chapter 12: Ask questions for what you need to know. Be aware that clients are vulnerable and trust you not to ask for more information than you need.

Chapter 13: Remember that expressing an opinion and giving advice are not the same.

Chapter 14: Learn to laugh at yourself, to not take yourself so seriously.

Chapter 15: Work on meeting your own spiritual needs to be able to offer support for another to express theirs.

Chapter 16: Remember that if you refuse to ask for support and help from others when you need it, you deny them the good feeling you get when you are able to help another.

Chapter 17: Understand that a small amount of anxiety helps you focus, learn, and grow.

Chapter 18: Remember Ashleigh Brilliant's adage: "I may not be totally perfect, but parts of me are excellent."

Chapter 19: When you must stop at a traffic light or wait in a store, reframe this as a time to practice deep breathing and relaxation.

Chapter 20: Consider that your neurophysiology does not know the difference between your being in Hawaii and imagining you are there. Take an instant vacation.

Chapter 21: Remember *The Little Engine that Could:* I think I can, I think I can, I think I can.

Chapter 22: When working in a group, claim your value by sharing your knowledge and ideas.

Chapter 23: Remember that digital communication is a convenience, but a handwritten note is a legacy.

Chapter 24: Consider that sometimes when you confront a person, you grow the relationship and become closer.

Chapter 25: You get to choose when to turn down an unreasonable request and when to choose to fulfill it. It is a matter of choice as long as you know you can say no. Sometimes yes is the right answer.

Chapter 26: Remember that today someone else may be distressed; tomorrow it might be you.

Chapter 27: Remember that you deserve to be treated with respect. Sometimes you must teach others that.

Chapter 28: Consider that conflict and differing opinions can generate better solutions.

Chapter 29: Reflect on this quote: "He not busy being born is busy dying" (Bob Dylan). We are all in this together.

Chapter 30: Consider this thought: As I care for myself, so I care for others.

Good-bye and blessings for your journey.

Return to "Active Learning" at the beginning of the chapter and write your responses.

 ## PRACTICING CONTINUING THE COMMITMENT TO THE JOURNEY

Create a Care Plan for Yourself: Exercise 1

You spend a lot of time creating care plans for your patients. Create a holistic care plan for yourself. Here is a format and some examples.

For my body today I will: Eat a healthy breakfast/drink 8 cups of water.

For my mind today I will: Practice mindfulness by pausing, paying attention to my breath, walking mindfully between patient rooms/read one chapter in a book of my choice.

For my spirit today I will: Walk outside for a few minutes and appreciate nature as a sign of something greater than myself/start and end my day listing three things or people for whom I am grateful.

(Inspired by the work of Elena Aguilar on resilience for educators [Aguilar, 2018a, b])

Self-Assessment/Skill Building: Exercise 2

List all the roles you play in your life such as nurse or student, daughter or son, spouse, parent, and community volunteer. Then draw two circles 4 inches in diameter. Divide the first circle into portions like a pie with as many pieces as you have roles, with each portion sized in proportion to the amount of time you spend in each role. When you are finished, consider if your use of time reflects your values. After this reflection, divide the second circle into portions according to how you would prefer to spend your time. If there are discrepancies between the two distributions of your time, consider alterations you might choose to make.

Reflective Practice: Exercise 3

Begin a journal of your own moments of connection to clients, colleagues, loved ones, and yourself. What went well today? What surprised me? What did I accomplish today? How did I make a difference today? What am I grateful for today? What can I do differently next time? What brought me a sense of wonder, awe, or joy today?

Creative Expression: Exercise 4

Begin a "joy box," an "antidepression kit," to collect mementos, motivational clippings, thank-you notes, small toys, and things that lift your spirits. Encourage a child in your life to do the same thing; call it a treasure box. Consider collaging the box with images that bring joy.

Creative Expression: Exercise 5

Create a collage of your own healing journey. Glue pictures cut from magazines, greeting cards, copies of special photographs, and bits of memorabilia to a heavy piece of cardboard or mat board. Take time to reflect on the meanings of your selections. Write about what you learned. If you are in a class, share your thoughts briefly with others doing the collage. This activity can be used with clients and family members for a variety of purposes. To tap the power of your inner wisdom, using your dominant hand (your writing hand), write three questions about the collage for yourself, such as, "What lessons do I need to learn?" Using your nondominant hand, answer the questions. Reflect on your responses.

Professional and Personal Development: Exercise 6

Define a goal you have for yourself. Write it in positive terms, such as "to pass my examination for licensure." Envision yourself having successfully completed the goal. Write a journal entry about your future self. How do you look? How do you sound? Do you carry yourself in a different way? Hold this vision of yourself (Bolton, Field, & Thompson, 2006).

Creative Expression: Exercise 7

As a self-care practice, go outside and sit in a beautiful spot in nature such as park, a garden, or the woods. Pay attention to what you experience. Write a haiku poem about what you experience. This short 17-syllable poem is a traditional Japanese poetry form from the eighth century. "The philosophy behind haiku says that, in losing oneself in involvement in the natural world, the writer becomes open to learning everything of importance, thereby open to gaining peace and acceptance of life's vicissitudes" (Bolton et al., 2006). The first line of a haiku has five syllables, the second line has seven syllables, and the third line has five syllables. Example: Breeze blowing through trees. In and out and up and down. Some leaves cling, some fall.

Quality and Safety Education for Nurses Learning Strategy: Exercise 8 QSEN

All nurses are on a journey toward professional excellence and maturity. Developing capacity as a leader in patient safety and to be able to contribute to and lead cultures of safety progresses as one gains experience. Using the image of transportation, draw a picture of how you hope to continue your journey of developing as a leader in safety culture over the next 5 years.

- Where do you hope to be in 5 years as a mode of transportation to reach your desired destination?
- What do you need to change to be successful to reach your goal, and what speed limits may apply?
- What are stops along the way?
- What are possible detours and roadblocks?
- How will you manage your forward progress?
- Who are possible mentors to help guide your progress?

REFERENCES

Aguilar, E. (2018). *Onward: Cultivating emotional resilience in educators.* San Francisco, CA: Jossey-Bass.

Aguilar, E. (2018). *The onward workbook: Daily activities to cultivate your emotional resilience and thrive.* San Francisco, CA: Jossey-Bass.

American Nurses Association (ANA). (2021). *Nursing scope and standards of practice* (4th ed.). Silver Springs, MD: ANA.

American Psychological Association (APA). (2018). The road to resilience. *Building your resilience* (apa.org).

Arnold, E. (1989). Burnout as a spiritual issue: Rediscovering meaning in nursing practice. In V. B. Carson (Ed.), *Spiritual dimensions of nursing practice.* Philadelphia, PA: WB Saunders.

Ashcraft, P., & Gatto, S. (2018). Curricular interventions to promote self-care in prelicensure nursing students. *Nurse Educator, 43*(3), 140.

Bateson, M. C. (2010). *Composing a further life: The age of active wisdom.* New York, NY: Knopf.

Bazarko, D. (2014). *Mindfulness and you: Being present in nursing practice.* Silver Spring, MD: American Nurses Association (nursingworld.org).

Bolton, G., Field, V., & Thompson, K. (2006). *Writing works: A resource book for therapeutic writing workshops and activities.* London, UK: Jessica Kingsley Publishers.

Daehlen, M. (2008). Job satisfaction and job values among beginning nurses: A questionnaire survey. *International Journal of Nursing Studies, 45*(12), 1789.

Devney, A. M. Rapid anxiety reduction tools for nursing staff, faculty and students. *COJ Nurse Healthcare, 2*(5). COJNH.000546.2018. doi:10.31031/COJNH.2018.02.000546.

Dyess, S. M., & Sherman, R. O. (2009). The first year of practice: New graduate nurses' transition and learning needs. *Journal of Continuing Education in Nursing, 40*(9), 403.

Ferrell, B. R. (2021). From the editor: 2021 - A reflection on service. *Journal of Hospice & Palliative Care, 23*(6). doi:10.1097/NJH.0000000000000809.

Fontaine, K. L. (2014). *Complementary & alternative therapies for nursing practice.* Upper Saddle River, NJ: Prentice Hall.

Gallison, B. (2018). Connecting holistic nursing practice with relationship-based care: A community hospital's journey. *Nurse Leader, 16*(3), 181–185.

Grant, L., & Kinman, G. (2014). Emotional resilience in the helping professions and how it can be enhanced. *Health and Social Care Education, 3*(1), 23.

Guterman, M. S. (1994). *Common sense for uncommon times: The power of balance in work, family, and personal life.* Palo Alto, CA: CPP Books.

Guzzetta, C. E. (1998). Weaving a tapestry of holism. *Journal of Cardiovascular Nursing, 12*(2), 18.

Hart, P. L., Brann, J. D., & De Chesnay, M. (2014). Resilience in nurses: An integrative review. *Journal of Nursing Management, 22*, 720.

Jones, L. B. (1998). *The path: Creating your mission statement for work and for life.* New York, NY: Hyperion.

Kelly, L. A., & Adams, J. M. (2018). Nurse leader burnout: How to find your joy. *Nurse Leader, 16*(1), 24.

Kemper, K. J., & Hill, E. (2017). Training in integrative therapies increases self-efficacy in providing nondrug therapies and self-confidence in offering compassionate care. *Journal of Evidenced-Based Complementary & Alternative Medicine, 22*(4), 618.

Kenney, E. G. (1998). Creating fulfillment in today's workplace: A guide for nurses. *American Journal of Nursing, 98*(5), 44.

Kramer, M. L. (1974). *Reality shock: Why nurses leave nursing.* St. Louis, MO: CV Mosby.

Kushner, H. (2001). *When bad things happen to good people.* New York, NY: Schocken Books.

Kushner, H. (2002). *When all you've ever wanted isn't enough: A search for a life that matters.* New York, NY: Fireside.

Murant, G. M. (2000). Creativity and self-care for caregivers. *Journal of Palliative Care, 16*(2), 44.

Pellico, L. H., Brewer, C. S., & Kovner, C. T. (2009). What newly licensed registered nurses have to say about their new experiences. *Nursing Outlook, 57*(4), 194.

Prince-Paul, M., & Kelley, C. (2017). Mindful communication: Being present. *Seminars in Oncology Nursing, 33*(5), 475.

Raso, R. (2018). Wellness, stress, balance…and resilience. *Nursing Management, 42*(29), 6.

Reyes, A. T., Andrusyszyn, M., Iwasiw, C., Forchuk, C., & Babenko-Mould, Y. (2015). Resilience in nursing education: An integrative review. *Journal of Nursing Education, 54*(8), 438.

Schettle, S. (1998). A nurse's reflection: Nursing in the '90s—old hats, new ways. *American Journal of Nursing, 98*(5), 16J.

Stephens, T. M. (2013). Nursing student resilience: A concept clarification. *Nursing Forum, 48*(2), 125.

Tingle, C. A. (2001). Workplace advocacy as a transition tool. *Student Nurse Advisor, 1*(16).

Tuckerton, R. (2013). *15 minutes to a better interview: What I wish every job candidate knew.* Createspace Independent Publishing Platform.

Zerwekh, J. V. (2000). Caring on the ragged edge: Nursing persons who are disenfranchised. *Advances in Nursing Science, 22*(4), 47.

Zuzelo, P. R. (2018). Nurses' sleepiness and sleeplessness: The epidemic of insufficient sleep. *Holistic Nursing Practice, 32*(3), 172.

Chapter Objectives in This Book Mapped to the American Association of Colleges of Nursing (AACN) 2021 Essentials Domains

Kathleen Sitzman, PhD, RN, CNE, ANEF, FAAN

Download a PDF copy of the AACN Essentials here: https://www.aacnnursing.org/AACN-Essentials.

Educators who incorporate this book into a course may use this quick overview of chapter objectives with related

AACN Essentials Domains to streamline content development and tracking.

Chapters with Objectives	Applicable AACN Essentials *Domains and Competencies*
Chapter 1: Responsible, Assertive, Caring Communication in Nursing 1. Complete a Holistic Self-Care Assessment. 2. Identify the functions of interpersonal communication in nursing. 3. Distinguish between assertive, nonassertive, and aggressive communication. 4. Identify a three-step process to build assertiveness skills. 5. Identify assertive rights. 6. Identify irrational beliefs that impede assertive communication. 7. Explain the describe, express, specify, consequences (DESC) script for developing an assertive response. 8. Identify three types of assertions. 9. Identify three essential criteria for presenting an assertive response. 10. Describe the behavior of an assertive nurse. 11. List the advantages of assertive communication. 12. Describe responsible communication in nursing. 13. Discuss the role of caring in nursing. 14. Participate in exercises to build skills in responsible, assertive, caring communication.	D1[a](1.1,[b] 1.2); D2(2.1, 2.2, 2.3, 2.5, 2.6); D6(6.1 6.4); D9(9.1, 9.2, 9.3, 9.5); D10(10.1, 10.3)

Chapters with Objectives	Applicable AACN Essentials Domains and Competencies
Chapter 2: The Client–Nurse Relationship: A Helping Relationship 1. Identify the purpose of the client–nurse relationship. 2. Complete a self-assessment of your communication skills. 3. Identify Peplau's three phases of the nurse–patient relationship. 4. Describe the cognitive, affective, and psychomotor abilities that nurses and clients bring to the therapeutic encounter. 5. Discuss clients' rights as consumers of healthcare service. 6. Identify characteristics of a successful client–nurse relationship. 7. Identify therapeutic communication techniques. 8. Identify nontherapeutic communication techniques. 9. List dos and don'ts in the client–nurse relationship. 10. Identify behavioral dimensions indicative of bonding in the client–nurse relationship. 11. Discuss the FOCUSED model for being present. 12. Identify qualities of a story catcher. 13. Discuss listening skills. 14. Participate in exercises to build skills in the client–nurse relationship.	D1(1.1); D2(2.1, 2.2); D9(9.1, 9.2, 9.5)
Chapter 3: Starting with YOU: Understanding Yourself to Build a Foundation for Learning about Communication 1. Recognize the need for self-assessment as a starting point for building communication skills. 2. Learn to identify your own personal strengths. 3. Describe how each person's unique combination of personal strengths can be applied to concepts of communication. 4. Identify four key domains of emotional intelligence, and use tools to identify competency levels. 5. Describe interventions for improving low emotional intelligence scores. 6. List five major modes of conflict management and identify your preferred mode. 7. Identify personal strengths that could be used to learn to use all modes of conflict management as appropriate to the situation. 8. Begin to apply concepts of self-understanding to building responsible, assertive, caring communication skills.	D9(9.1); D10(10.1, 10.2)
Chapter 4: Solving Problems Together 1. Define mutuality in nurse–client relationships. 2. Compare the steps of the nursing process (assessment, diagnosis, planning, implementation, and evaluation [ADPIE]) with the National Council of State Boards of Nursing (NCSBN). Clinical Judgment Measurement Model (NCJMM). 3. Identify the core competencies of interprofessional collaborative practice. 4. Discuss mutual problem solving to involve the client in the implementation of the nursing process. 5. Complete exercises to practice a mutual problem-solving approach to the nursing process. 6. Participate in exercises to build skills in solving problems with clients.	D1(1.1, 1.3); D2(2.1, 2.2, 2.3, 2.5, 2.6, 2.8, 2.9); D5(5.3); D6(6.1, 6.2, 6.4); D9(9.1, 9.2. 9.3, 9.5); D10(10.3)

Continued

Chapters with Objectives	Applicable AACN Essentials *Domains and Competencies*
Chapter 5: Understanding Each Other: Communication and Culture 1. Define culture, ethnicity, and ethnocentrism. 2. Define cultural humility. 3. Discuss reasons why nurses need to become informed about the healthcare beliefs and behaviors of diverse cultures. 4. Discuss two common personally held beliefs and values that may interfere with nurses' recognition and appreciation of the healthcare beliefs and behaviors of diverse cultures. 5. Describe your own cultural background and its influence on your healthcare beliefs and behaviors. 6. Identify the components of communication suggested for assessment in Purnell's model for cultural competence. 7. Discuss techniques that enhance communication with clients from diverse cultures. 8. Apply communication techniques to improve the care of clients from diverse cultures. 9. Discuss how the variables of age and gender relate to culture and communication. 10. Participate in exercises to build skills in understanding each other.	D1(1.2, 1.2, 1.3); D2(2.1, 2.2); D5(5.3); D6(6.1, 6.4); D9(9.1, 9.2, 9.3, 9.5, 9.6); D10(10.2)
Chapter 6: Demonstrating Warmth 1. Discuss the benefits of warmth in communication with clients and colleagues. 2. Identify behaviors that demonstrate warmth. 3. Review a tool to analyze warmth in interpersonal communications. 4. Describe a variety of ways in which warmth is displayed and articulate the importance of warmth in human interactions. 5. Become aware of opportunities to embellish your life with warmth in day-to-day encounters with clients and colleagues. 6. Participate in exercises to build skills in demonstrating warmth.	D2(2.1, 2.2)
Chapter 7: Showing Respect 1. Discuss the benefits of respect in the relationships in healthcare. 2. Identify behaviors that demonstrate respect in relationships. 3. Define workplace bullying. 4. Participate in exercises to build skills in demonstrating respect.	D1(1.3); D2(2.2, 2.9); D5(5.3); D9(9.1, 9.2, 9.5); D10(10.1, 10.2, 10.3)
Chapter 8: Being Genuine 1. Differentiate between genuine and nongenuine behavior. 2. Discuss the importance of being genuine with clients and colleagues. 3. Participate in exercises to build skills in demonstrating genuineness.	D1(1.3); D2(2.1, 2.9); D10(10.1, 10.2)
Chapter 9: Being Empathetic 1. Define empathy. 2. Identify the preverbal, verbal, and nonverbal aspects of empathy. 3. Discuss the benefits of empathy with clients and colleagues. 4. Identify six steps to empathic communication. 5. Examine steps in breaking bad news. 6. Practice a centering exercise. 7. Participate in exercises to build skills in demonstrating empathy.	D1(1.1); D2(2.1, 2.2); D9(9.1, 9.2, 9.5, 9.6); D10(10.1, 10.2)

Chapters with Objectives	Applicable AACN Essentials *Domains and Competencies*
Chapter 10: Honoring Professional Boundaries 1. Discuss professional boundaries in nursing. 2. Define self-disclosure in the helping relationship. 3. Define immediacy in the helping relationship. 4. Identify guidelines for appropriate self-disclosure by the nurse. 5. Discuss helpful self-disclosures. 6. Participate in exercises to build and deepen an understanding of professional boundaries.	D1(1.1, 1.3); D2(2.1, 2.2); D6(6.1, 6.3); D9(9.1, 9.2, 9.3, 9.4, 9.5)
Chapter 11: Being Specific 1. Define specificity. 2. Identify the usefulness of specificity and its effect on communication behavior. 3. Explore an online resource for the use of the SBAR tool. 4. Identify strategies to communicate with specificity. 5. Discuss tips for handoff in nursing change of shift report. 6. Contrast the placebo effect and the nocebo effect. 7. Participate in exercises to build skills in specificity.	D1(1.1); D2(2.1, 2.2, 2.3, 2.4, 2.5, 2.9); D9(9.1, 9.3, 9.5)
Chapter 12: Asking Questions 1. Discuss the importance of the skill of asking effective questions. 2. Discuss the importance of patients feeling safe to ask questions. 3. Define closed, open, and indirect questions. 4. Identify six points to keep in mind when asking questions. 5. Identify common errors in asking questions and strategies to avoid them. 6. Identify behaviors that support patients asking questions. 7. Participate in exercises to assess and build skills in asking questions.	D1(1.1, 1.2, 1.3); D2(2.1, 2.2, 2.3, 2.7, 2.9); D9(9.5, 9.6); D10(10.3)
Chapter 13: Expressing Opinions 1. Distinguish between giving advice and expressing opinions. 2. Identify strategies to express opinions in an assertive way. 3. Discuss examples of sharing positive regard for others. 4. Identify the effects on empowerment of expressing opinions. 5. Participate in exercises to build skills in expressing opinions.	D1(1.1, 1.3); D2(2.1, 2.2, 2.7, 2.9); D5(5.3); D6(6.1, 6.2, 6.3, 6.4); D9(9.1, 9.2, 9.5); D10(10.2)
Chapter 14: Using Humor 1. Define therapeutic humor. 2. Distinguish between positive and negative humor. 3. Identify three criteria for the appropriate use of humor in healthcare. 4. Discuss the functions of humor in healthcare. 5. Identify strategies to implement humor in healthcare. 6. Identify three ways humor can be used to promote positive communication in healthcare. 7. Discuss creative ways to add humor and play to relieve stress, build relationships, and promote creativity. 8. Identify possible health benefits of laughter. 9. Participate in exercises to build skills in the appropriate uses of humor.	D1(1.1, 1.2, 1.3); D2(2.1, 2.2); D9(9.2); D10(10.1, 10.2)

Continued

Chapters with Objectives	Applicable AACN Essentials *Domains and Competencies*
Chapter 15: Embracing the Spiritual Journey of Healthcaring: Meaning Making 1. Define spiritual care. 2. Review the personal Spiritual Assessment Tool, and begin to complete it. 3. Examine the Faith and Belief: Importance, Community, and Address in Care (FICA) tool for taking a spiritual history. 4. Discuss themes of spirituality. 5. Discuss strategies to nurture the spirit. 6. Identify nursing interventions to meet the spiritual needs of the client and family. 7. Describe behaviors that the nurse can use to adopt a hopeful perspective and offer hope. 8. Discuss the role of the nurse in helping the client find meaning in illness. 9. Participate in exercises to build skills in meeting spiritual needs in health.	D1(1.1, 1.2, 1.3); D2(2.1, 2.2, 2.9); D10(1.1)
Chapter 16: Requesting Support 1. Discuss the relationship between social support and health. 2. Complete a support system assessment. 3. Distinguish between assertive, nonassertive, and aggressive requests for support. 4. Practice making requests for support in selected exercises.	D1(1.1); D2(2.5, 2.6, 2.9); D5(5.2, 5.3); D6(6.1, 6.2, 6.3, 6.4); D9(9.1. 9.2, 9.3, 9.6); D10(10.1, 10.2, 10.3)
Chapter 17: Overcoming Evaluation Anxiety 1. Define evaluation anxiety. 2. Describe characteristics of evaluation anxiety. 3. Identify strategies to handle job performance appraisals assertively. 4. Discuss techniques to decrease test anxiety. 5. Identify benefits of criticism. 6. Identify assertive strategies to handle difficult situations in student performance evaluations. 7. Participate in exercises to overcome evaluation anxiety.	D10(10.1)
Chapter 18: Working with Feedback 1. Discuss the importance of feedback in communication. 2. Identify strategies for giving feedback. 3. Discuss steps for receiving feedback to promote self-growth. 4. Practice seeking, giving, and receiving feedback in selected exercises.	D2(2.1, 2.2, 2.6, 2.7, 2.9); D5(5.3); D6(6.1, 6.2, 6.4); D9(9.1, 9.2, 9.3); D10(10.1)
Chapter 19: Using Relaxation Techniques to Become More Mindful 1. Define mindfulness. 2. Discuss the hungry, angry, lonely, and tired (HALT) approach for resiliency and stress management. 3. Discuss the importance of relaxation skills for the nurse. 4. Identify stressors in nursing. 5. Describe guidelines for beginning to practice meditation to elicit the relaxation response. 6. Identify the steps of progressive relaxation for deep relaxation. 7. Identify brief, practical strategies for immediate relaxation. 8. Identify brief stretching exercises to promote relaxation. 9. Practice relaxation techniques to become more mindful.	D10(10.1, 10.2)

Chapters with Objectives	Applicable AACN Essentials *Domains and Competencies*
Chapter 20: Incorporating Imagery into Professional Practice and Self-Care 1. Define imagery or visualization. 2. Practice imagery using the tart lemon exercise. 3. Discuss the history of the use of imagery. 4. Identify uses of imagery in clinical practice. 5. Identify brief imagery exercises to cope with stressful situations. 6. Discuss the use of imagery techniques to improve communication skills. 7. Participate in selected exercises to build skills in using imagery in professional practice and self-care.	D1(1.1, 1.2); D2(2.1, 2.2, 2.8); D9(9.2); D10(10.1)
Chapter 21: Incorporating Positivity into Life and Work 1. Define positivity. 2. Define self-talk and its influence on behavior. 3. Discuss the relationship between self-talk and interpersonal communication. 4. Discuss the use of affirmations as a strategy to create positive self-talk. 5. Practice positive self-talk to develop confidence in communication skills and nursing practice.	D1(1.1, 1.2); D2(2.1, 2.2); D10(10.1, 10.2)
Chapter 22: Learning to Work Together in Groups 1. Identify three essential conditions for group effectiveness. 2. Identify four stages of group development. 3. Examine how different mental processes affect behavior in groups. 4. Identify maintenance roles of group members. 5. Identify task roles of group members. 6. Identify individual roles of group members that impede group progress. 7. Apply the concept of emotional intelligence to groups. 8. Discuss why meetings are important. 9. Identify examples of virtual meetings. 10. Identify tools to promote effectiveness in meetings. 11. Discuss characteristics of effective groups. 12. Describe strategies to organize a committee. 13. Participate in exercises to build skills in working together in groups.	D1(1.1); D2(2.9); D6(6.1, 6.2, 6.3, 6.4); D9(9.2, 9.3, 9.5); D10(10.1, 10.2, 10.3)
Chapter 23: Navigating the Complex World of Digital Communication 1. Discuss practical strategies to convey and sustain caring in digital settings. 2. Discuss three ways that social media impacts nursing. 3. Describe organizational policies to support the safe use of smartphones in healthcare. 4. Name three clinical applications that are beneficial to professional nursing practice. 5. Name several ways to appropriately use nonclinical applications in the clinical setting. 6. Describe three types of digital learning used in nursing. 7. Name one reputable search engine for digital research of nursing topics. 8. Discuss the benefits of clinical documentation utilizing an electronic health record. 9. Describe the dangers of digital communication and how to avoid them. 10. Discuss the nursing implications of increased healthcare consumer use of the Internet.	D1(1.1, 1.2); D2(2.1, 2.2); D5(5.2, 5.3); D8(8.1, 8.2, 8.3, 8.4), 8.5; D9(9.1, 9.2, 9.3, 9.4, 9.5); D10(10.2)

Continued

Chapters with Objectives	Applicable AACN Essentials *Domains and Competencies*
Chapter 24 Learning Confrontation Skills 1. Identify the benefits of confrontation skills. 2. Discuss the steps of the Clarify, Articulate, Request, Encourage (CARE) model of confrontation. 3. Identify the relationship between confrontation skills and empowerment. 4. Practice confrontation in selected exercises to build confidence in the skills.	D1(1.1, 1.2); D2(2.1, 2.2, 2.9); D5(5.2, 5.3); D6(6.1, 6.2, 6.4)
Chapter 25: Refusing Unreasonable Requests 1. Discuss the importance of the right to refuse unreasonable requests from clients and colleagues. 2. Distinguish between assertive, nonassertive, and aggressive refusals. 3. Participate in exercises to build skills to refuse unreasonable requests.	D9(9.5); D10(10.1, 10.2)
Chapter 26: Caring Communication with Clients and Colleagues whose Behaviors Are Challenging 1. Identify common situations in nursing in which clients or colleagues may demonstrate challenging behaviors. 2. Discuss how to maintain professionalism while engaging in caring communication within the context of distress. 3. Describe caring communication strategies and micro-practices for working with distressed clients and colleagues. 4. Practice caring communication with clients and colleagues whose behaviors are challenging.	D1(1.1, 1.2); D2(2.1, 2.2); D5(5.2, 5.3); D6(6.1, 6.2, 6.4); D9(9.1, 9.2, 9.5)
Chapter 27: Confronting Bullying and Incivility with Honesty and Respect 1. Differentiate characteristics of bullying, incivility, and constructive feedback. 2. Recognize overt and covert behaviors in the workplace through situational observations. 3. Identify strategies to communicate assertively with disruptive colleagues. 4. Execute scripting and naming strategies to confront disruptive behaviors. 5. Practice confronting bullying and incivility with honesty and respect.	D1(1.1, 1.2, 1.3); D6(6.1, 6.2, 6.4); D9(9.1, 9.5); D10(10.1, 10.2)
Chapter 28: Managing Team Conflict Assertively and Responsibly 1. Define conflict. 2. Identify four categories of conflict. 3. Identify the steps of win–win conflict resolution. 4. Contrast win–win, lose–win, and win–lose methods of handling team conflict. 5. Identify the characteristics of five multigenerational team members and their effect on the team. 6. Participate in selected exercises to build assertive conflict-resolution skills.	D6(6.1, 6.2, 6.4)
Chapter 29: Communicating at the End of Life 1. Identify fears about communicating with clients near the end of life. 2. Discuss strategies for caring communication near the end of life. 3. Identify strategies for creative expression for clients at the end of life and their families. 4. Identify strategies for the nurse to deal with grief. 5. Discuss the role of self-care for the nurse when working with clients at the end of life and their families. 6. Participate in exercises to build strategies for caring communication with clients near the end of life and their families.	D1(1.1, 1.2, 1.3); D2(2.1, 2.2, 2.3, 2.5, 2.6, 2.7, 2.8, 2.9); D9(9.2)

Chapters with Objectives	Applicable AACN Essentials *Domains and Competencies*
Chapter 30: Continuing the Commitment to the Journey 1. Identify practices of the resilient nurse. 2. Examine proactive approaches to reality shock, the transition from student to graduate. 3. Identify three competencies for achieving life balance. 4. Identify commonalities among "living legacy" responses from nurses with 50 or more years of experience. 5. Identify strategies for renewal. 6. Discuss the importance of commitment to nursing to continue to build communication skills.	D10(10.1, 10.2, 10.3)

[a]D with an accompanying number = AACN Essential Domain. Here is an example: D1 = Domain 1: Knowledge for Nursing Practice.

[b]Numbers in parenthesis that follow the Domain number represent applicable competencies within each Domain. Here is an example: D1(1.1, 1.2) means that Competencies 1.1 and 1.2 within the D1 Domain are applicable to chapter objectives.

Holistic Self-Care Assessment

Add your scores to receive a score for "Where I am now" and a score for "How I want it to be" for each of the components of the assessment.

Physical

Where I am Now	Almost Always	Sometimes	Almost Never	How I Want It to Be
Exercise 3–5 times a week for 20 minutes	2	1	0	
Eat nutritious foods daily	2	1	0	
Play without guilt	2	1	0	
Practice relaxation daily	2	1	0	
Energy level is effective for daily activities	2	1	0	
Do not smoke	2	1	0	
Drink in moderation	2	1	0	
Have regular physical and dental checkups	2	1	0	
Sleep 8 hours most nights	2	1	0	
Practice safe sex	2	1	0	
PHYSICAL SCORE	——			——

Mental

Where I Am Now	Almost Always	Sometimes	Almost Never	How I Want It to Be
Am open and receptive to new ideas and life patterns	2	1	0	
Read a broad range of subjects	2	1	0	
Am interested in and knowledgeable about many topics	2	1	0	
Use my imagination in considering new choices or possibilities	2	1	0	
Prioritize my work and set realistic goals	2	1	0	
Enjoy developing new skills and talents	2	1	0	
Ask for suggestions and help when I need it	2	1	0	
MENTAL SCORE	——			——

Emotions

Where I Am Now	Almost Always	Sometimes	Almost Never	How I Want It to Be
Assess and recognize my own feelings	2	1	0	
Have a nonjudgmental attitude	2	1	0	
Express my feelings in appropriate ways	2	1	0	
Include my feelings when making decisions	2	1	0	
Can remember and acknowledge most events of my childhood including painful as well as happy ones	2	1	0	
Listen to and respect the feelings of others	2	1	0	
Recognize my intuition	2	1	0	
Listen to inner self-talk	2	1	0	
EMOTIONS SCORE	——			——

Relationships

Where I Am Now	Almost Always	Sometimes	Almost Never	How I Want It to Be
Share my opinions and feelings without seeking the approval of others or fearing outcomes	2	1	0	
Create and participate in satisfying relationships	2	1	0	
Sexuality is part of my relationship	2	1	0	
Have a balance between my work and family life	2	1	0	
Am clear in expressing my needs and desires	2	1	0	
Am open and honest with people without fearing the consequences	2	1	0	
Do my part in establishing and maintaining relationships	2	1	0	
Focus on positive topics in relationships	2	1	0	
RELATIONSHIPS SCORE	——			——

Choices

Where I Am Now	Almost Always	Sometimes	Almost Never	How I Want It to Be
Manage my time to meet my personal goals	2	1	0	
Am committed and disciplined whenever I take on new projects	2	1	0	
Follow through and work on decisions with clarity and action steps	2	1	0	
Am usually clear on decisions	2	1	0	
Take risks	2	1	0	
Can accept circumstances that are beyond my control	2	1	0	
Take on no more new tasks than I can successfully handle	2	1	0	
Recognize shortcomings of people and events for what they are	2	1	0	
CHOICES SCORE	——			——

Spirit

Where I Am Now	Almost Always	Sometimes	Almost Never	How I Want It to Be
Operate from the perspective that life has value, meaning, and direction	2	1	0	
Know at some level a connection with the universe	2	1	0	
Know some power greater than myself	2	1	0	
Feel a part of life and living frequently	2	1	0	
Recognize that the different roles of my life are expressions of my true self	2	1	0	
Know how to create balance and feel a sense of connectedness	2	1	0	
Know that life is important and that I make a difference	2	1	0	
SPIRIT SCORE		——		——

Modified from: L. Keegan and B. Dossey, Self-Care: A Program to Improve Your Life © 2004, Holistic Nursing Consultants. Used with permission.

NGN Case Study Answers

CHAPTER 1: RESPONSIBLE, ASSERTIVE, CARING COMMUNICATION IN NURSING

Assertive Communication

Answer(s):

Option 1	Option 2
Lack of assertiveness	**Ineffective pain control**
Depression	**Improper nutrition**
Immobility	Diminished sense of self worth
Aging	Impaired skin integrity

Rationales: Assertiveness, a key to successful relationships between the client, the family, the nurse, and other members of the interprofessional healthcare team, reduces interpersonal stress, builds team relationships, improves nursing care, and promotes client safety. Assertiveness is the ability to express one's own thoughts, ideas, and feelings without undue anxiety and without any expense to others. It involves being clear and respectful in language and behavior regarding what is needed. Assertive behavior, which is an active behavior, is contrasted with nonassertive (or passive) behavior in which individuals disregard their own needs and rights. The immediate priority is for the client to feel comfortable and confident in effectively expressing her needs in an assertive manner. This will help the nursing staff to address her pain control and nutrition needs effectively, which can benefit the client's recovery process.

While the client is challenged by immobility issues, this is not the priority need. The client may be experiencing some degree of depression; however, that is a mood disorder diagnosis and is not evident in this case. The normal aging process does not result in ineffective communication about needs.

Without further assessment, it cannot be assumed that the client has a diminished sense of self-worth. Although skin integrity is important, this issue can be addressed by implementing appropriate pain control to minimize discomfort when care is provided. Nutrition interventions to enhance the client's nutrition status, which contributes to wound healing, can also be implemented.

Cognitive Skill: Prioritizing Hypotheses

CHAPTER 26: CARING COMMUNICATION WITH CLIENTS AND COLLEAGUES WHOSE BEHAVIORS ARE CHALLENGING

Working with Clients' Verbal Abuse

Answer(s):

Option 1	Option 2
"You are too upset to discuss this now. I'll be back in an hour and we will talk then."	**Looking beyond the angry and inappropriate behavior for the basis of the patient's concerns**
"I'm sorry you are upset, but if you follow your physician's orders you'll be back to normal in no time."	Acknowledging the patient's concerns while offering a short-term solution to the problem
"Only when you stop reacting so rudely can we work out a solution to your concerns."	Setting boundaries that support a mutually respectful nurse–patient relationship
"When faced with life-altering changes, it usually helps to talk about how you are feeling."	Acknowledging the patient's angry feelings while proving reassurance.
"If you want your health to improve, you will need to follow this diet."	Presenting a realistic view of the situation in an assertive manner in order to share the importance of prescribed treatments.

Rationales: Clients and those who love them convey their anguish and fear verbally and nonverbally. Changes in health status, illness, and hospitalization are just some sources of distress they are likely to experience. Their loss of composure is a signal that they are disturbed by what is happening over which they have little or no control. As nurses we need to develop ways in which to relate to distressed clients and their loved ones that soothe their distress without upsetting ourselves. Maintaining sensitivity to others so that we can respond in a caring way without being overcome and losing our objectivity is one of a nurse's most inviting challenges—the gift of your presence without giving yourself away. The correct option looks behind the angry (and superficial) behavior for what is being communicated. This is an extremely powerful and helpful nursing response that opens the door for further communication. The option to come back later while offering future communication is not the best response because it does not acknowledge the patient's feelings and has the potential to inflame the situation and so is not therapeutic. Offering reassurances that the situation will improve is not therapeutic since it is beyond the nurse's control. Telling the patient that he or she is overreacting is a blaming, confrontational response that is certain to escalate the situation and damage future interactions. This response also infers conditions for quality care, which is not therapeutic. Placing full responsibility for the patient's health on their shoulders is not realistic, and this option fails to acknowledge the patient's concerns.

Cognitive Skill: Take Action

CHAPTER 27: CONFRONTING BULLYING & INCIVILITY WITH HONESTY AND RESPECT

Identifying the Difference Between Bullying, Incivility, and Honesty

Answer(s):

Statement	Incivility	Bullying	Honest Feedback
Tells the Unlicensed Assistive Personnel (UAPs) that I'm difficult to work with		X	
Regularly imitates my lisp when talking to me	X		
Continuously identifies me as the unit's nurse-in-training		X	

Statement	Incivility	Bullying	Honest Feedback
Insists I'll be reprimanded if I don't get to shift report on time			X
Tells me I'm rude when I don't laugh at demeaning ethnic jokes	X		
Is always telling me how to improve my time management skills			X
Strongly disagrees on how much time I should spend on basic client care			X

Rationales: The patterns of behavior associated with bullying are different from those associated with incivility and constructive feedback. Incivility is low-level, rude, inconsiderate, immature, disrespectful, and unprofessional conduct. A person displaying incivility in the workplace often directs belittling, dismissive, and/or mocking comments or behaviors toward another staff member. Incivility is also displayed when an individual intentionally ignores, socially excludes, and/or gossips about others in the workplace. Bullying takes place when inappropriate comments or behavior is focused on a single person or a small group of people who usually share a common trait. The action must also be repeated over a period of time to be identified as a pattern of behavior. Finally, bullying behavior has to be harmful in some manner, either to a staff member or to a client. The bully may not intend to cause harm, but if harm occurs, the behavior is considered bullying. Constructive or honest feedback is an important learning tool, especially when given to nurses during orientation periods. During the orientation period, new nurses should expect to receive ongoing, objective, and constructive feedback. This type of feedback, although delivered in a direct, matter-of-fact manner, is different than bullying. Constructive or honest feedback is not meant to be hurtful, as it is provided as a means to improve the skills of the person who is receiving the feedback.

Cognitive Skill: Analyze Cues

INDEX

Page numbers followed by "*f*" indicate figures, "*b*" indicate boxes, and "*t*" indicate tables.